a LANGE medical book

Vaughan & Asbury's

GENERAL OPHTHALMOLOGY

. . . Now do you not see that the eye embraces the beauty of the whole world? It is the lord of astronomy and the maker of cosmography; it counsels and corrects all the arts of mankind; it leads men to the different parts of the world; it is the prince of mathematics, and the sciences founded on it are absolutely certain. It has measured the distances and sizes of the stars; it has found the elements and their locations; it . . . has given birth to architecture, and to perspective, and to the divine art of painting. Oh excellent thing, superior to all others created by God! . . . What peoples, what tongues will fully describe your true function? The eye is the window of the human body through which it feels its way and enjoys the beauty of the world. Owing to the eye the soul is content to stay in its bodily prison, for without it such bodily prison is torture.

Leonardo da Vinci (1452–1519)

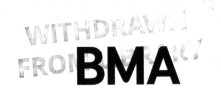

Vaughan & Asbury's
GENERAL OPHTHALMOLOGY

NINETEENTH EDITION

Edited by

Paul Riordan-Eva, FRCOphth
Consultant Ophthalmologist
King's College Hospital, London, United Kingdom

James J. Augsburger, MD
Professor of Ophthalmology
Dr. E. Vernon and Eloise C. Smith Chair of Ophthalmology
Department of Ophthalmology
University of Cincinnati College of Medicine,
Cincinnati, Ohio

Mc
Graw
Hill
Education

New York   Chicago   San Francisco   Athens   London   Madrid   Mexico City
Milan   New Delhi   Singapore   Sydney   Toronto

Notice

Medicine is an ever-changing science. As new research and clinical experience broaden our knowledge, changes in treatment and drug therapy are required. The authors and the publisher of this work have checked with sources believed to be reliable in their efforts to provide information that is complete and generally in accord with the standards accepted at the time of publication. However, in view of the possibility of human error or changes in medical sciences, neither the authors nor the publisher nor any other party who has been involved in the preparation or publication of this work warrants that the information contained herein is in every respect accurate or complete, and they disclaim all responsibility for any errors or omissions or for the results obtained from use of the information contained in this work. Readers are encouraged to confirm the information contained herein with other sources. For example and in particular, readers are advised to check the product information sheet included in the package of each drug they plan to administer to be certain that the information contained in this work is accurate and that changes have not been made in the recommended dose or in the contraindications for administration. This recommendation is of particular importance in connection with new or infrequently used drugs.

This book was set in Minion Pro by Cenveo® Publisher Services.
The editors were Brian Belval and Christie Naglieri.
The production supervisor was Richard Ruzycka.
Project management was provided by Kritika Kaushik, Cenveo Publisher Services.
The cover designer was RANDOMATRIX.
LSC Communications was printer and binder.

This book is printed on acid-free paper.

This edition of
General Ophthalmology
is dedicated with gratitude and in memory of

Roderick ("Rick") Biswell, MD,
(1937-2015)
who was a chapter author for many previous editions.

Contents

Authors

Ahmed Al-Maskari, FRCOphth
Anterior Segment Fellow, Moorfields Eye Hospital,
    London, United Kingdom

James J. Augsburger, MD
Professor of Ophthalmology, Dr E Vernon and Eloise C
    Smith, Chair of Ophthalmology, Department of
    Ophthalmology, College of Medicine, University of
    Cincinnati, Cincinnati, Ohio

David F. Chang, MD
Clinical Professor, University of California,
    San Francisco

Steve Charles, MD
Clinical Professor of Ophthalmology, Department of
    Ophthalmology, University of Tennessee, Memphis,
    Tennessee

August Colenbrander, MD
Affiliate Senior Scientist, Rehabilitation Engineering Center,
    Smith-Kettlewell Eye Research Institute, San Francisco,
    California

Zélia M. Corrêa, MD, PhD
Professor of Ophthalmology, Mary Knight Asbury Chair of
    Ophthalmic Pathology and Ocular Oncology,
    Department of Ophthalmology, College of Medicine,
    University of Cincinnati, Cincinnati, Ohio

Emmett T. Cunningham, Jr., MD, PhD, MPH
Director, The Uveitis Service, Department of
    Ophthalmology, California Pacific Medical Center,
    San Francisco, California

Dustin Curts, MD
Department of Ophthalmology, Owen Sound Hospital,
    Owen Sound, Ontario, Canada

Frederick W. Fraunfelder, MD, MBA
Chairman and Roy E Mason and Elizabeth Patee Mason
    Distinguished Professor of Ophthalmology, Mason Eye
    Institute, University of Missouri School of Medicine,
    Columbia, Missouri

Francisco J. Garcia-Ferrer, MD
Division Chief, Ophthalmology, Mercy Hospital, St Louis,
    Missouri

Richard A. Harper, MD
Professor, Department of Ophthalmology,
    University of Arkansas for Medical Sciences,
    Little Rock, Arkansas

William G. Hodge, MD, MPH, PhD, FRCSC
Professor, Ophthalmologist-in-Chief, Department of
    Ophthalmology, Ivey Eye Institute, Schulich School of
    Medicine, University of Western Ontario, London,
    Ontario, Canada

Munir M. Iqbal, MD
Ophthalmology Resident, Department of Ophthalmology,
    Ivey Eye Institute, Schulich School of Medicine,
    Western University, London, Ontario, Canada

Daniel F. P. Larkin, MD, FRCOphth
Consultant Ophthalmologist, Moorfields Eye Hospital,
    London, United Kingdom

Raeba Mathew, FRCS
Specialist Ophthalmologist, Department of Ophthalmology,
    Canadian Specialist Hospital, Dubai,
    United Arab Emirates

Lindsey M. McDaniel, MD
Department of Ophthalmology, Mason Eye Institute,
    University of Missouri School of Medicine,
    Columbia, Missouri

James McHugh, FRCOphth
Ophthalmology Trainee, Department of Ophthalmology,
    King's College Hospital, London, United Kingdom

W. Walker Motley, MS, MD
Clinical Assistant Professor of Ophthalmology,
    Department of Ophthalmology, University of Cincinnati,
    Cincinnati, Ohio

Jonathan Pargament, MD
Fellow, American Society of Ophthalmic Plastic and
    Reconstructive Surgery, Center for Facial Appearances,
    Salt Lake City, Utah

Carlos Pavesio, MD, FRCOphth
Consultant Ophthalmologist, Medical Retina, Moorfields
    Eye Hospital, London, United Kingdom

Edward Pringle, MRCP, FRCOphth
Consultant Ophthalmologist, Department of Ophthalmology, King's College Hospital, London, United Kingdom

Paul Riordan-Eva, FRCOphth
Consultant Ophthalmologist, Department of Ophthalmology, King's College Hospital, London, United Kingdom

John F. Salmon, MD, FRCS
Consultant Ophthalmologist, Department of Ophthalmology, University of Oxford, Oxford, United Kingdom

Sobha Sivaprasad, FRCOphth
Professor of Ophthalmology, Moorfields Eye Hospital, London, United Kingdom

Gwen K. Sterns, MD
Clinical Professor of Ophthalmology, Department of Ophthalmology, University of Rochester School of Medicine and Dentistry, Rochester, New York

Alastair Stuart, BMBS FRCOphth
Corneal Fellow, Moorfields Eye Hospital and Moorfields Eye Centre at St George's Hospital, London, United Kingdom

M. Reza Vagefi, MD
Assistant Professor of Ophthalmology, Department of Ophthalmology, UCSF School of Medicine, San Francisco, California

Preface

For almost six decades, General Ophthalmology has served as a concise, current, and authoritative review of the subject for medical students, ophthalmology residents, practicing ophthalmologists, nurses, optometrists, and colleagues in other fields of medicine and surgery, as well as health-related professionals. The nineteenth edition has been revised and updated in keeping with that goal. It contains the following changes from the eighteenth edition:

- All relevant illustrations in color
- Major revision of Chapters 6 (Cornea), 10 (Retina), 13 (Orbit), 14 (Neuro-Ophthalmology), 16 (Immunologic Diseases of the Eye), 20 (Causes and Prevention of Vision Loss) and 23 (Lasers in Ophthalmology).

We are grateful to Toby Chan, Victor Chong, Eleanor Faye, Allan Flach, Emily Fletcher, Douglas Fredrick, Elizabeth Graham, William Hoyt, Lisa Nijm, Adnan Pirbhai, Shefalee Shukla Kent, John Shock, Ivan Schwab and John Sullivan for their contributions to previous editions. We warmly welcome our new authors, Ahmed Al-Maskari, Dustin Curts, Munir Iqbal, Frank Larkin, Raeba Mathew, Lindsey McDaniel, James McHugh, Jonathan Pargament, Sobha Sivaprasad and Alastair Stuart.

Paul Riordan-Eva, FRCOphth
James J. Augsburger, MD
December 2016

Acknowledgments

Margot Riordan-Eva

Elliott Riordan-Eva

Natasha Riordan-Eva

Anastasia Riordan-Eva

Patricia Cunnane

Patricia Pascoe

Geraldine Hruby

Anatomy & Embryology of the Eye

Paul Riordan-Eva, FRCOphth

A thorough understanding of the anatomy of the eye, orbit, visual pathways, upper cranial nerves, and central pathways for the control of eye movements is a prerequisite for proper interpretation of diseases having ocular manifestations. Furthermore, such anatomic knowledge is essential to the proper planning and safe execution of ocular and orbital surgery. Whereas most knowledge of these matters is based on anatomic dissections, either postmortem or during surgery, noninvasive techniques—particularly magnetic resonance imaging (MRI), ultrasonography, and optical coherence tomography (OCT)—are increasingly providing additional information. Investigating the embryology of the eye is more difficult because of the relative scarcity of suitable human material, and thus there is still great reliance on animal studies with the inherent difficulties in inferring parallels in human development. Nevertheless, a great deal is known about the embryology of the human eye, and—together with the recent expansion in molecular genetic—this has led to a much deeper understanding of developmental anomalies of the eye.

I. NORMAL ANATOMY

THE ORBIT (FIGURES 1–1 AND 1–2)

The orbital cavity is schematically represented as a pyramid of four walls that converge posteriorly. The medial walls of the right and left orbit are parallel and are separated by the nose. In each orbit, the lateral and medial walls form an angle of 45°, which results in a right angle between the two lateral walls. Anteriorly, parts of the **frontal bone, zygomatic (malar) bone**, and **maxilla** form a sturdy approximately circular bony aperture that is slightly smaller in cross-sectional dimension than the base of the pyramid, thus providing protection to the globe.

The volume of the adult orbit is approximately 30 mL, and the eyeball occupies only about one-fifth of the space. Fat and muscle account for the bulk of the remainder.

The anterior limit of the orbital cavity is the **orbital septum**, which acts as a barrier between the lids and orbit (see Lids later in this chapter).

The orbits are related to the paranasal sinuses. The thin orbital floor and paper-thin medial wall (lamina papyracea) are easily damaged by direct trauma to the globe, resulting in a "blowout" fracture with herniation of orbital contents inferiorly into the maxillary antrum or medially into the ethmoid sinus. Infection within the ethmoid and sphenoid sinuses can spread into the orbit or affect the optic nerve respectively. Defects in the roof (eg, neurofibromatosis) may result in visible pulsations of the globe transmitted from the brain.

▶ Orbital Walls

The roof of the orbit is composed principally of the orbital plate of the frontal bone. The lacrimal gland is located in the lacrimal fossa in the anterior lateral aspect of the roof. Posteriorly, the lesser wing of the sphenoid bone containing the optic canal completes the roof.

The lateral wall is separated from the roof by the superior orbital fissure, which divides the lesser from the greater wing of the sphenoid bone. The anterior portion of the lateral wall is formed by the orbital surface of the zygomatic bone. This is the strongest part of the bony orbit. Suspensory ligaments, the lateral palpebral tendon, and check ligaments have connective tissue attachments to the lateral orbital tubercle.

The orbital floor is separated from the lateral wall by the inferior orbital fissure. The orbital plate of the maxilla forms the large central area of the floor and is the region where blowout fractures most frequently occur. The frontal process of the maxilla medially and the zygomatic bone laterally complete the inferior orbital rim. The orbital process of the **palatine bone** forms a small triangular area in the posterior floor.

The boundaries of the medial wall are less distinct. The **ethmoid bone** is paper-thin but thickens anteriorly as it meets the **lacrimal bone**. The body of the sphenoid forms the most posterior aspect of the medial wall, and the angular

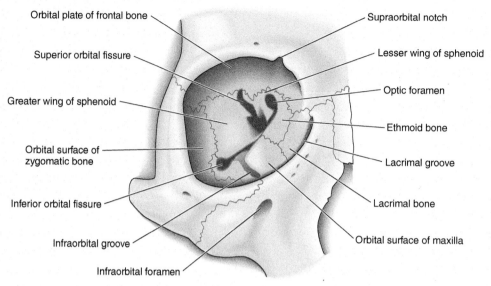

Orbital plate of frontal bone

Superior orbital fissure

Greater wing of sphenoid

Orbital surface of
zygomatic bone

Inferior orbital fissure

Infraorbital groove

Infraorbital foramen

Supraorbital notch

Lesser wing of sphenoid

Optic foramen

Ethmoid bone

Lacrimal groove

Lacrimal bone

Orbital surface of maxilla

▲ **Figure 1–1.** Anterior view of bones of right orbit.

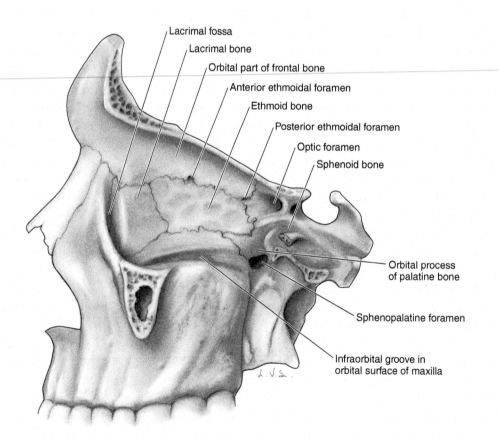

Lacrimal fossa

Lacrimal bone

Orbital part of frontal bone

Anterior ethmoidal foramen

Ethmoid bone

Posterior ethmoidal foramen

Optic foramen

Sphenoid bone

Orbital process
of palatine bone

Sphenopalatine foramen

Infraorbital groove in
orbital surface of maxilla

▲ **Figure 1–2.** Medial view of bony wall of left orbit.

process of the frontal bone forms the upper part of the posterior lacrimal crest. The lower portion of the posterior lacrimal crest is made up of the lacrimal bone. The anterior lacrimal crest is easily palpated through the lid and is composed of the frontal process of the maxilla. The lacrimal groove lies between the two crests and contains the lacrimal sac.

▶ Orbital Apex (Figure 1–3)

The apex of the orbit is the main portal for all nerves and vessels to the eye and the site of origin of all extraocular muscles except the inferior oblique. The **superior orbital fissure** lies between the body and the greater and lesser wings of the sphenoid bone. The superior ophthalmic vein and the lacrimal, frontal, and trochlear nerves pass through the lateral portion of the fissure that lies outside the annulus of Zinn. The superior and inferior divisions of the oculomotor nerve and the abducens and nasociliary nerves pass through the medial portion of the fissure within the annulus of Zinn. The optic nerve and ophthalmic artery pass through the optic canal, which also lies within the annulus of Zinn. The inferior ophthalmic vein frequently joins the superior ophthalmic vein before exiting the orbit. Otherwise, it may pass through any part of the superior orbital fissure, including the portion adjacent to the body of the sphenoid that lies inferomedial to the annulus of Zinn, or through the inferior orbital fissure.

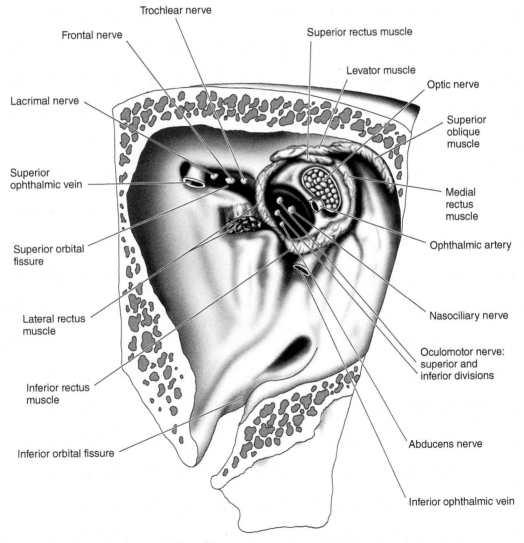

▲ **Figure 1–3.** Anterior view of apex of right orbit.

Blood Supply (Figures 1–4, 1–5, and 1–6)

The principal arterial supply of the orbit derives from the ophthalmic artery, the first major branch of the intracranial portion of the internal carotid artery. This branch passes beneath the optic nerve and accompanies it through the optic canal into the orbit. The first intraorbital branch is the central retinal artery, which enters the optic nerve about 8–15 mm behind the globe. Other branches of the ophthalmic artery include the lacrimal artery, supplying the lacrimal gland and upper lid; muscular branches to the various muscles of the orbit; long and short posterior ciliary arteries; medial palpebral arteries to both lids; and the supraorbital and supratrochlear arteries. The short posterior ciliary arteries supply the choroid and parts of the optic nerve. The two long posterior ciliary arteries supply the ciliary body and anastomose with each other and with the anterior ciliary arteries to form the major arterial circle of the iris. The anterior ciliary arteries are derived from the muscular branches to the rectus muscles. They supply

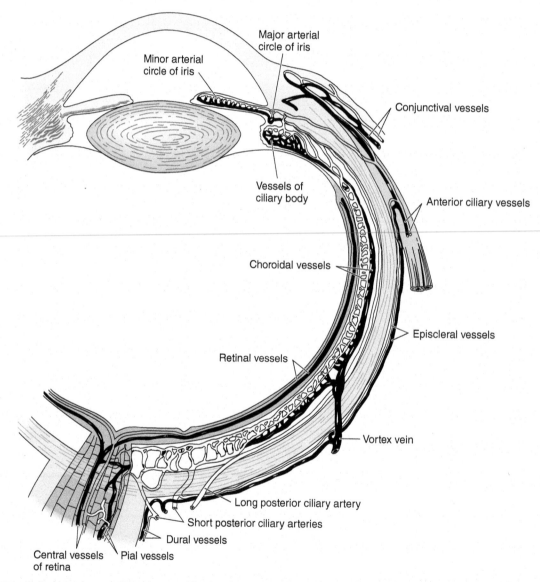

▲ **Figure 1–4.** Vascular supply to the eye. All arterial branches originate with the ophthalmic artery. Venous drainage is through the cavernous sinus and the pterygoid plexus.

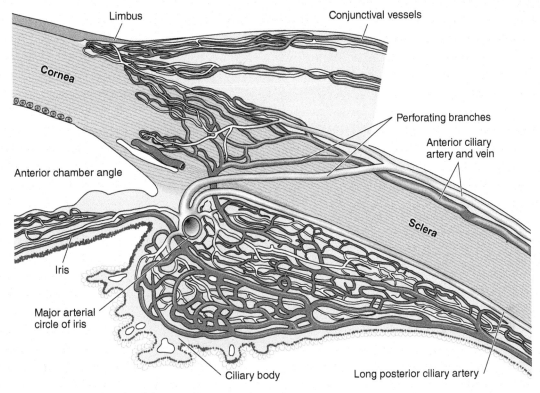

Limbus

Conjunctival vessels

Cornea

Perforating branches

Anterior ciliary
artery and vein

Anterior chamber angle

Sclera

Iris

Major arterial
circle of iris

Ciliary body

Long posterior ciliary artery

▲ Figure 1–5. Vascular supply of the anterior segment.

the anterior sclera, episclera, limbus, and conjunctiva and contribute to the major arterial circle of the iris. The most anterior branches of the ophthalmic artery contribute to the formation of the arterial arcades of the lids, which make an anastomosis with the external carotid circulation via the facial artery.

The venous drainage of the orbit is primarily through the superior and inferior ophthalmic veins, into which drain the vortex veins, the anterior ciliary veins, and the central retinal vein. The ophthalmic veins communicate with the cavernous sinus via the superior orbital fissure and the pterygoid venous plexus via the inferior orbital fissure. The superior ophthalmic vein is initially formed from the supraorbital and supratrochlear veins and from a branch of the angular vein, all of which drain the skin of the periorbital region. This provides a direct communication between the skin of the face and the cavernous sinus, thus forming the basis of the potentially lethal cavernous sinus thrombosis, secondary to superficial infection of the periorbital skin.

THE EYEBALL

The normal adult globe is approximately spherical, with an anteroposterior diameter averaging 24 mm.

THE CONJUNCTIVA

The conjunctiva is the thin, transparent mucous membrane that covers the posterior surface of the lids (the palpebral conjunctiva) and the anterior surface of the sclera (the bulbar conjunctiva). It is continuous with the skin at the lid margin (a mucocutaneous junction) and with the corneal epithelium at the limbus.

The **palpebral conjunctiva** lines the posterior surface of the lids and is firmly adherent to the tarsus. At the superior or inferior margin of the tarsus, the conjunctiva is reflected posteriorly (at the superior and inferior fornices) and covers the episcleral tissue to become the bulbar conjunctiva.

The **bulbar conjunctiva** is loosely attached to the orbital septum in the fornices and is folded many times. This allows the eye to move and enlarges the secretory conjunctival surface. (The ducts of the lacrimal gland open into the superior temporal fornix.) Except at the limbus (where Tenon's capsule and the conjunctiva are fused for about 3 mm), the bulbar conjunctiva is loosely attached to Tenon's capsule and the underlying sclera.

A soft, movable, thickened fold of bulbar conjunctiva (the **semilunar fold**) is located at the inner canthus and corresponds to the nictitating membrane of some lower animals.

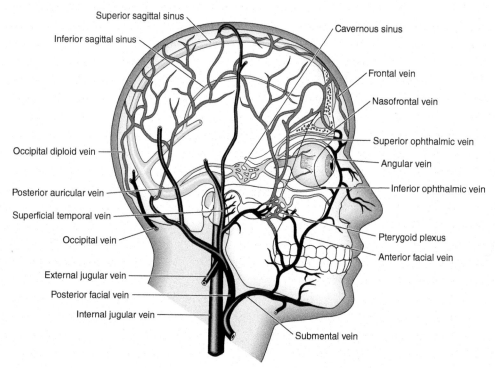

▲ Figure 1–6. Venous drainage system of the eye.

A small, fleshy, epidermoid structure (the **caruncle**) is attached superficially to the inner portion of the semilunar fold and is a transition zone containing both cutaneous and mucous membrane elements.

▶ Histology

The **conjunctival epithelium** consists of two to five layers of stratified columnar epithelial cell—superficial and basal. Conjunctival epithelium near the limbus, over the caruncle, and near the mucocutaneous junctions at the lid margins consists of stratified squamous epithelial cells. The **superficial epithelial cells** contain round or oval mucus-secreting goblet cells. The mucus, as it forms, pushes aside the goblet cell nucleus and is necessary for proper dispersion of the precorneal tear film. The **basal epithelial cells** stain more deeply than the superficial cells and may contain pigment near the limbus.

The **conjunctival stroma** is divided into an adenoid (superficial) layer and a fibrous (deep) layer. The **adenoid layer** contains lymphoid tissue and, in some areas, may contain "follicle-like" structures without germinal centers. The adenoid layer does not develop until after the first 2 or 3 months of life. This explains why in the newborn inclusion conjunctivitis is papillary, whereas thereafter it is follicular. The **fibrous layer** is composed of connective tissue that attaches to the tarsal plate. This explains the appearance of the papillary reaction in inflammations of the conjunctiva. The fibrous layer is loosely arranged over the globe.

The **accessory lacrimal glands** (glands of Krause and Wolfring), which resemble the lacrimal gland in structure and function, are located in the stroma. Most of the glands of Krause are in the upper fornix, and the remainder are in the lower fornix. The glands of Wolfring lie at the superior margin of the upper tarsus.

▶ Blood Supply, Lymphatics, & Nerve Supply

The conjunctival arteries are derived from the anterior ciliary and palpebral arteries. The two arteries anastomose freely and—along with the numerous conjunctival veins that generally follow the arterial pattern—form a considerable conjunctival vascular network. The conjunctival lymphatics are arranged in superficial and deep layers and join with the lymphatics of the lids to form a rich lymphatic plexus. The conjunctiva receives its nerve supply from the first (ophthalmic) division of the fifth nerve. It possesses a relatively small number of pain fibers.

TENON'S CAPSULE (FASCIA BULBI)

Tenon's capsule is a fibrous membrane that envelops the globe from the limbus to the optic nerve (see Figure 1–19). Adjacent to the limbus, the conjunctiva, Tenon's capsule, and episclera are fused together. More posteriorly, the inner surface of Tenon's capsule lies against the sclera, and its outer aspect is in contact with orbital fat and other structures within the extraocular muscle cone. At the point where Tenon's capsule is pierced by tendons of the extraocular muscles in their passage to their attachments to the globe, it sends a tubular reflection around each of these muscles. These fascial reflections become continuous with the fascia of the muscles, the fused fasciae sending expansions to the surrounding structures and to the orbital bones. The fascial expansions are quite tough and limit the action of the extraocular muscles, and are therefore known as **check ligaments** (see Figure 1–20). They regulate the direction of action of the extraocular muscles and may act as their functional mechanical origins, possibly with active neuronal control (active pulley hypothesis). The

lower segment of Tenon's capsule is thick and fuses with the fascia of the inferior rectus and the inferior oblique muscles to form the suspensory ligament of the eyeball (Lockwood's ligament), upon which the globe rests.

THE SCLERA & EPISCLERA

The **sclera** is the fibrous outer protective coating of the eye, consisting almost entirely of collagen (Figure 1–7). It is dense and white, and continuous with the cornea anteriorly and the dural sheath of the optic nerve posteriorly. Across the posterior scleral foramen are bands of collagen and elastic tissue, forming the **lamina cribrosa**, between which pass the axon bundles of the optic nerve. The outer surface of the anterior sclera is covered by a thin layer of fine elastic tissue, the

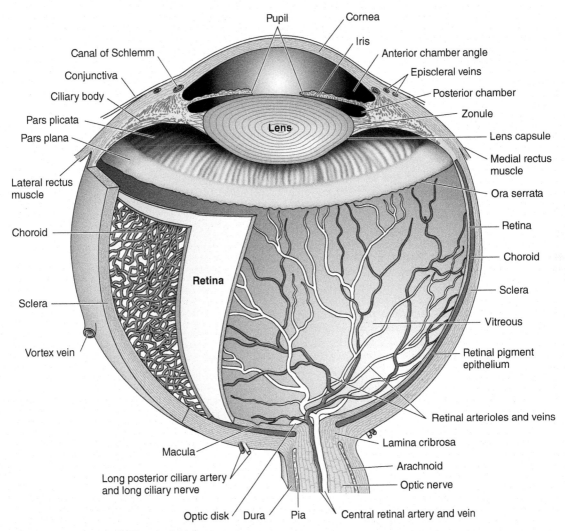

▲ **Figure 1–7.** Internal structures of the human eye.

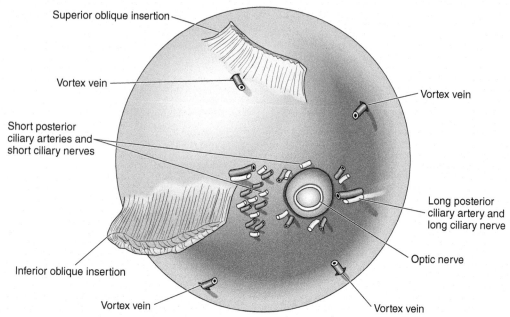

▲ **Figure 1–8.** Posterior view of left eye.

episclera, which contains numerous blood vessels that nourish the sclera. The brown pigment layer on the inner surface of the sclera is the lamina fusca, which forms the outer layer of the suprachoroidal space.

At the insertion of the rectus muscles, the sclera is about 0.3 mm thick; elsewhere it is about 0.6 mm thick. Around the optic nerve, the sclera is penetrated by the long and short posterior ciliary arteries and the long and short ciliary nerves (Figure 1–8). The long posterior ciliary arteries and long ciliary nerves pass from the optic nerve to the ciliary body in a shallow groove on the inner surface of the sclera at the 3 and 9 o'clock meridians. Slightly posterior to the equator, the four vortex veins draining the choroid exit through the sclera, usually one in each quadrant. About 4 mm posterior to the limbus, slightly anterior to the insertion of the respective rectus muscle, the four anterior ciliary arteries and veins penetrate the sclera. The nerve supply to the sclera is from the ciliary nerves.

Histologically, the sclera consists of many dense bands of parallel and interlacing collagen bundles, each of which is 10–16 µm thick and 100–140 µm wide. The histologic structure of the sclera is remarkably similar to that of the corneal stroma (see the next section), but it is opaque rather than transparent mainly because of irregularity of the collagen lamellae and higher water content.

THE CORNEA

The cornea is a transparent tissue comparable in size and structure to the crystal of a small wristwatch (Figure 1–9). It is inserted into the sclera at the limbus, the circumferential depression at this junction being known as the scleral sulcus. The average adult cornea is 550 µm thick in the center, although there are racial variations, and about 11.7 mm in diameter horizontally and 10.6 mm vertically. From anterior to posterior, it has five distinct layers (Figure 1–10): the epithelium (which is continuous with the epithelium of the bulbar conjunctiva), Bowman's layer, the stroma, Descemet's membrane, and the endothelium. The epithelium has five or six layers of cells. Bowman's layer is a clear acellular modified portion of the stroma. The corneal stroma accounts for about 90% of the corneal thickness. It is composed of intertwining lamellae of collagen fibrils 10–250 µm in width and 1–2 µm in height that run almost the full diameter of the cornea. They run parallel to the surface of the cornea and, by virtue of their regularity, are optically clear. The lamellae lie within a ground substance of hydrated proteoglycans in association with the keratocytes that produce the collagen and ground substance. Descemet's membrane, constituting the basal lamina of the corneal endothelium, has a homogeneous appearance on light microscopy but a laminated appearance on electron microscopy due to structural differences between its prenasal and postnatal portions. It is about 3 µm thick at birth but increases in thickness throughout life, reaching 10–12 µm in adulthood. The endothelium has only one layer of cells, but this is responsible for maintaining the essential deturgescence of the corneal stroma. The endothelium is quite susceptible to injury as well as undergoing loss of cells with age: the normal density reducing from 23,000 cells/mm² at birth to 2000 cells/mm² in old age. Endothelial repair is limited to enlargement and sliding of existing cells, with little

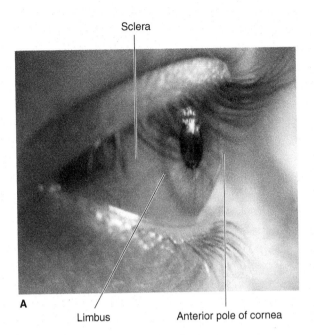

Sclera

Limbus   Anterior pole of cornea

A

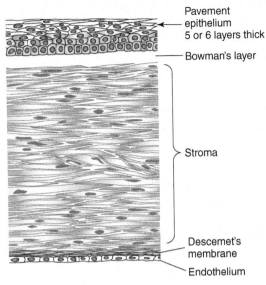

Pavement epithelium 5 or 6 layers thick

Bowman's layer

Stroma

Descemet's membrane

Endothelium

▲ **Figure 1–10.** Transverse section of cornea.

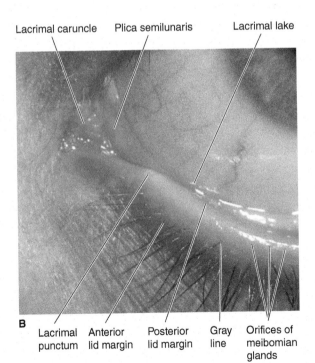

Lacrimal caruncle   Plica semilunaris   Lacrimal lake

B

Lacrimal punctum | Anterior lid margin | Posterior lid margin | Gray line | Orifices of meibomian glands

▲ **Figure 1–9. (A, B)** External landmarks of the eye. The sclera is covered by transparent conjunctiva.

capacity for cell division. Failure of endothelial function leads to corneal edema.

Sources of nutrition for the cornea are the vessels of the limbus, the aqueous, and the tears. The superficial cornea also gets most of its oxygen from the atmosphere. The sensory nerves of the cornea are supplied by the first (ophthalmic) division of the fifth (trigeminal) cranial nerve.

The transparency of the cornea is due to its uniform structure, avascularity, and deturgescence.

THE UVEAL TRACT

The uveal tract is composed from anterior to posterior of the iris, the ciliary body, and the choroid (Figure 1–7). It is the middle vascular layer of the eye and is protected by the cornea and sclera. It contributes blood supply to the retina.

▷ Iris

The **iris** is a shallow cone pointing anteriorly with a centrally situated round aperture, the **pupil**. It is positioned in front of the lens, dividing the **anterior chamber** from the **posterior chamber**, each of which contains aqueous humor that passes through the pupil. There are no epithelial cells covering the anterior stroma. The sphincter and dilator muscles develop from the anterior epithelium, which covers the posterior surface of the stroma and represents an anterior extension of the retinal pigment epithelium. The heavily pigmented posterior epithelium represents an anterior extension of the neuroretina.

The arterial blood supply to the iris is from the major circle of the iris (Figure 1–4). Iris capillaries have a non-fenestrated endothelium, and hence do not normally leak intravenously injected fluorescein. Sensory nerve supply to the iris is via fibers in the ciliary nerves.

The iris controls the amount of light entering the eye. Pupillary size is principally determined by a balance between constriction due to parasympathetic activity transmitted via the third cranial nerve and dilation due to sympathetic activity (see Chapter 14).

The Ciliary Body

The **ciliary body**, roughly triangular in cross section, extends forward from the anterior end of the choroid to the root of the iris (about 6 mm). It consists of a corrugated anterior zone, the pars plicata (2 mm), and a flattened posterior zone, the pars plana (4 mm). The ciliary processes arise from the pars plicata (Figure 1–11). They are composed mainly of capillaries and veins that drain through the vortex veins. The capillaries are large and fenestrated, and hence leak intravenously injected fluorescein. There are two layers of ciliary epithelium: an internal nonpigmented layer, representing the anterior extension of the neuroretina, and an external pigmented layer, representing an extension of the retinal pigment epithelium. The ciliary processes and their covering ciliary epithelium are responsible for the formation of aqueous.

The **ciliary muscle** is composed of a combination of longitudinal, radial, and circular fibers. The function of the circular fibers is to contract and relax the zonular fibers, which originate in the valleys between the ciliary processes (Figure 1–12). This alters the tension on the capsule of the lens, giving the lens a variable focus for both near and distant objects in the visual field. The longitudinal fibers of the ciliary muscle insert into the trabecular meshwork to influence its pore size.

The arterial blood supply to the ciliary body is derived from the major circle of the iris. The nerve supply is via the short ciliary nerves.

The Choroid

The choroid is the posterior segment of the uveal tract, between the retina and the sclera. It is composed of three layers of choroidal blood vessels: large, medium, and small. The deeper the vessels are placed in the choroid, the wider their lumens (Figure 1–13). The internal portion of the choroid vessels is known as the choriocapillaris. Blood from the choroidal vessels drains via the four vortex veins, one in each of the four posterior quadrants. The choroid is bounded internally by Bruch's membrane and externally by the sclera. The suprachoroidal space lies between the choroid and the sclera. The choroid is firmly attached posteriorly to the margins of the optic nerve. Anteriorly, the choroid joins with the ciliary body.

The aggregate of choroidal blood vessels serves to nourish the outer portion of the retina (Figure 1–4). The nerve supply to the choroid is via the ciliary nerves.

THE LENS

The lens is a biconvex, avascular, colorless, and almost completely transparent structure, about 4 mm thick and 9 mm in diameter. It is suspended behind the iris by the zonule, which connects it with the ciliary body. Anterior to the lens is the aqueous; posterior to it, the vitreous.

The lens capsule is a semipermeable membrane (slightly more permeable than a capillary wall) that will admit water and electrolytes. A subcapsular epithelium is present anteriorly (Figure 1–14). With age, subepithelial lamellar fibers are continuously produced, so that the lens gradually becomes larger and less elastic throughout life. The nucleus and cortex are made up of long concentric lamellae, the lens nucleus being harder than the cortex. The suture lines formed by the end-to-end joining of these lamellar fibers are Y-shaped when viewed with the slitlamp (Figure 1–15). The Y is upright anteriorly and inverted posteriorly.

Each lamellar fiber contains a flattened nucleus. These nuclei are evident microscopically in the peripheral portion of the lens near the equator and are continuous with the subcapsular epithelium.

The lens is held in place by a suspensory ligament known as the zonule (zonule of Zinn), which is composed of numerous fibrils that arise from the surface of the ciliary body and insert into the lens equator.

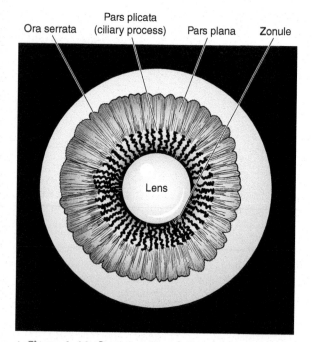

Ora serrata   Pars plicata (ciliary process)   Pars plana   Zonule

Lens

▲ **Figure 1–11.** Posterior view of ciliary body, zonule, lens, and ora serrata.

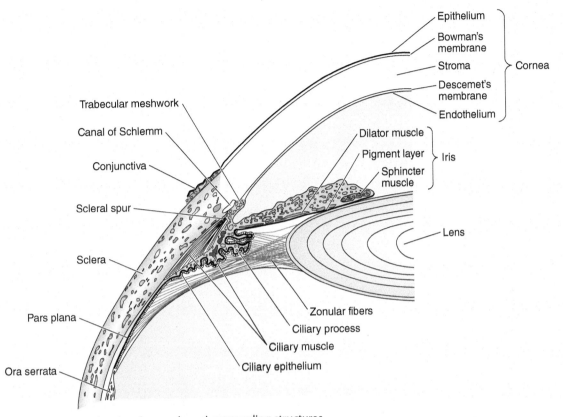

▲ **Figure 1–12.** Anterior chamber angle and surrounding structures.

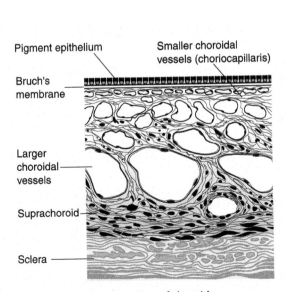

▲ **Figure 1–13.** Cross section of choroid.

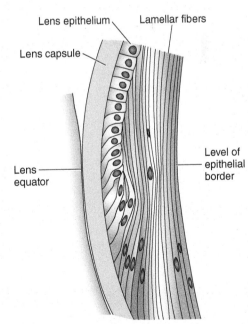

▲ **Figure 1–14.** Magnified view of lens showing termination of subcapsular epithelium (vertical section).

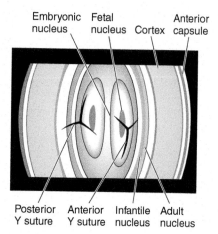

Figure 1–15. Zones of lens showing Y sutures.

The lens consists of about 65% water, about 35% protein (the highest protein content of any tissue of the body), and a trace of minerals common to other body tissues. Potassium is more concentrated in the lens than in most tissues. Ascorbic acid and glutathione are present in both oxidized and reduced forms.

There are no pain fibers, blood vessels, or nerves in the lens.

THE AQUEOUS

Aqueous humor is produced by the ciliary body. Entering the posterior chamber, it passes through the pupil into the anterior chamber (Figure 1–7) and then peripherally toward the anterior chamber angle. The physiology of the aqueous is discussed in Chapter 11.

THE ANTERIOR CHAMBER ANGLE

The anterior chamber (iridocorneal) angle lies at the junction of the peripheral cornea and the root of the iris (Figures 1–12 and 1–16). Its main anatomic features are Schwalbe's line, the trabecular meshwork (which overlies Schlemm's canal), and the scleral spur.

Schwalbe's line marks the termination of the corneal endothelium. The trabecular meshwork is triangular in cross section, with its base directed toward the ciliary body. It is composed of perforated sheets of collagen and elastic tissue, forming a filter with decreasing pore size as the canal of Schlemm is approached. The internal portion of the meshwork, facing the anterior chamber, is known as the uveal meshwork; the external portion, adjacent to the canal of Schlemm, is called the corneoscleral meshwork. The longitudinal fibers of the ciliary muscle insert into the trabecular meshwork. The scleral spur is an inward extension of the sclera between the ciliary body and Schlemm's canal, to

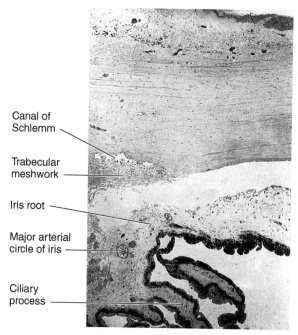

Figure 1–16. Photomicrograph of anterior chamber angle and related structures. (Used with permission from I. Wood and L. Garron.)

which the iris and ciliary body are attached. Efferent channels from Schlemm's canal (about 30 collector channels and up to 12 aqueous veins) communicate with the episcleral venous system.

THE RETINA

The retina is a thin, semitransparent, multilayered sheet of neural tissue that lines the inner aspect of the posterior two-thirds of the wall of the globe. It extends almost as far anteriorly as the ciliary body, ending at that point in a ragged edge, the ora serrata (Figure 1–12). In adults the ora serrata is about 6.5 mm behind Schwalbe's line on the temporal side and 5.7 mm behind it nasally. The outer surface of the sensory retina is apposed to the retinal pigment epithelium, and thus related to Bruch's membrane, the choroid, and the sclera. In most areas, the retina and retinal pigment epithelium are easily separated to form the subretinal space, such as occurs in retinal detachment. But at the optic disk and the ora serrata, the retina and retinal pigment epithelium are firmly bound together, thus limiting the spread of subretinal fluid in retinal detachment. This contrasts with the potential suprachoroidal space between the choroid and sclera, which extends to the scleral spur. Choroidal detachments thus extend beyond the ora serrata, under the pars plana and pars plicata. The epithelial layers of the inner surface of the ciliary body and the posterior surface of the iris represent anterior extensions of the retina and retinal pigment epithelium. The inner surface of the retina is apposed to the vitreous.

The layers of the retina, starting from its inner aspect, are: (1) internal limiting membrane; (2) nerve fiber layer, containing the ganglion cell axons passing to the optic nerve; (3) ganglion cell layer; (4) inner plexiform layer, containing the connections of the ganglion cells with the amacrine and bipolar cells; (5) inner nuclear layer of bipolar, amacrine, and horizontal cell bodies; (6) outer plexiform layer, containing the connections of the bipolar and horizontal cells with the photoreceptors; (7) outer nuclear layer of photoreceptor cell nuclei; (8) external limiting membrane; (9) photoreceptor layer of rod and cone inner and outer segments; and (10) retinal pigment epithelium (Figure 1–17). The inner layer of Bruch's membrane is actually the basement membrane of the retinal pigment epithelium.

The retina is 0.1 mm thick at the ora serrata and 0.56 mm thick in parts of the posterior pole. In the center of the posterior retina is the 5.5- to 6.0-mm-diameter macula, defined clinically as the area bounded by the temporal retinal vascular arcades. It is known to anatomists as the area centralis, being defined histologically as that part of the retina in which the ganglion cell layer is more than one cell thick. The macula lutea is defined anatomically as the 3-mm-diameter area containing the yellow luteal pigment xanthophyll. The 1.5-mm-diameter fovea is characterized histologically by thinning of the outer nuclear layer and absence of the other parenchymal layers as a result of the oblique course of the photoreceptor cell axons (Henle fiber layer) and the centrifugal displacement of the retinal layers that are closer to the inner retinal surface. In the center of the macula, 4 mm lateral to the optic disk, is the 0.3-mm-diameter foveola, clinically apparent as a depression that creates a particular reflection when viewed ophthalmoscopically. It is the thinnest part of area of the retina (0.25 mm), containing only cone photoreceptors, and corresponds to the retinal avascular zone on fluorescein angiography. The histologic features of the fovea and foveola provide for fine visual discrimination, with the foveola providing optimal visual acuity. The normally empty extracellular space of the retina is potentially greatest at the macula. Diseases that lead to accumulation of extracellular material particularly cause thickening of this area (macular edema).

The retina receives its blood supply from two sources: the choriocapillaris immediately outside Bruch's membrane, which supplies the outer third of the retina, including the outer plexiform and outer nuclear layers, the photoreceptors, and the retinal pigment epithelium; and branches of the central retinal artery, which supply the inner two-thirds (Figure 1–4). The foveola is supplied entirely by the choriocapillaris and is susceptible to irreparable damage when the retina is detached. The retinal blood vessels have a nonfenestrated endothelium, which forms the inner blood-retinal barrier, whereas the endothelium of choroidal vessels is fenestrated. The outer blood-retinal barrier lies at the level of the retinal pigment epithelium.

THE VITREOUS

The vitreous is a clear, avascular, gelatinous body that comprises two-thirds of the volume and weight of the eye. It fills the space bounded by the lens, retina, and optic disk (Figure 1–7). The outer surface of the vitreous—the hyaloid membrane—is normally in contact with the following structures: the posterior lens capsule, the zonular fibers, the pars plana epithelium, the retina, and the optic nerve head. The base of the vitreous maintains a firm attachment throughout life to the pars plana epithelium and the retina immediately behind the ora serrata. The attachment to the lens capsule and the optic nerve head loosens in adulthood.

The vitreous is about 99% water. The remaining 1% includes two components, collagen and hyaluronan, which give the vitreous a gel-like form and consistency because of their ability to bind large volumes of water.

THE EXTERNAL ANATOMIC LANDMARKS

Accurate localization of the position of internal structures with reference to the external surface of the globe is important in many surgical procedures. The distance of structures

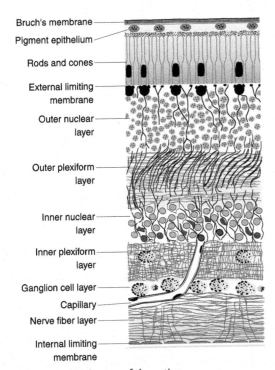

Bruch's membrane
Pigment epithelium
Rods and cones
External limiting membrane
Outer nuclear layer
Outer plexiform layer
Inner nuclear layer
Inner plexiform layer
Ganglion cell layer
Capillary
Nerve fiber layer
Internal limiting membrane

▲ **Figure 1–17.** Layers of the retina.

from the limbus as measured externally is less than their actual length. Externally, the ora serrata is situated approximately 5.5 mm from the limbus on the medial side and 7 mm on the temporal side of the globe. This corresponds to the level of insertion of the rectus muscles. Injections into the vitreous cavity through the pars plana should be given 3.5–4.0 mm from the limbus in the phakic eye and 3–3.5 mm from the limbus in the pseudophakic or aphakic eye. The pars plicata, which is the target for cyclodestructive procedures in the treatment of intractable glaucoma, occupies the 2–3 mm directly posterior to the limbus.

THE EXTRAOCULAR MUSCLES

Six extraocular muscles control the movement of each eye: four rectus and two oblique muscles.

Rectus Muscles

The four rectus muscles originate at a common ring tendon (annulus of Zinn) surrounding the optic nerve at the posterior apex of the orbit (Figure 1–3). They are named according to their insertion into the sclera on the medial, lateral, inferior, and superior surfaces of the eye. The principal action of the respective muscles is thus to adduct, abduct, depress, and elevate the globe (see Chapter 12). The muscles are about 40-mm long, becoming tendinous 4–8 mm from the point of insertion, where they are about 10 mm wide. The approximate distances of the points of insertion from the corneal limbus are: medial rectus, 5.5 mm; inferior rectus, 6.5 mm; lateral rectus, 7 mm; superior rectus, 7.5 mm (Figure 1–18). With the eye in the primary position, the vertical rectus muscles make an angle of about 23° with the optic axis.

Oblique Muscles

The two oblique muscles primarily control torsional movement and, to a lesser extent, upward and downward movements of the globe (see Chapter 12).

The **superior oblique** is the longest and thinnest of the ocular muscles. It originates above and medial to the optic foramen and partially overlaps the origin of the levator palpebrae superioris muscle. The superior oblique has a thin, fusiform belly (30-mm long) and passes anteriorly in the form of a tendon (10-mm long) to its trochlea, or pulley. It is then reflected backward and downward as a further length of tendon to attach in a fan shape to the sclera beneath the superior rectus. The trochlea is a cartilaginous structure attached to the frontal bone 3 mm behind the orbital rim. The superior oblique tendon is enclosed in a synovial sheath as it passes through the trochlea.

The **inferior oblique** muscle originates from the nasal side of the orbital wall just behind the inferior orbital rim and lateral to the nasolacrimal duct. It passes outside the

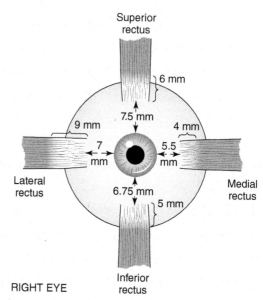

▲ **Figure 1–18.** Approximate distances of the rectus muscles from the limbus, and the approximate lengths of tendons.

inferior rectus and inside the lateral rectus muscle to insert with a short tendon into the posterolateral sclera just over the macular area. The muscle is about 35-mm long.

In the primary position, the muscle plane of the superior and inferior oblique muscles forms an angle of 51–54° with the optic axis.

Fascia

All the extraocular muscles are ensheathed by fascia. Near the points of insertion of these muscles, the fascia is continuous with Tenon's capsule, and fascial condensations to adjacent orbital structures (check ligaments) act as the functional origins of the extraocular muscles (Figures 1–19 and 1–20).

Nerve Supply

The oculomotor nerve (III) innervates the medial, inferior, and superior rectus muscles and the inferior oblique muscle. The abducens nerve (VI) innervates the lateral rectus muscle; the trochlear nerve (IV) innervates the superior oblique muscle.

Blood Supply

The blood supply to the extraocular muscles is derived from the muscular branches of the ophthalmic artery. The lateral rectus and inferior oblique muscles are also supplied by branches from the lacrimal artery and the infraorbital artery, respectively.

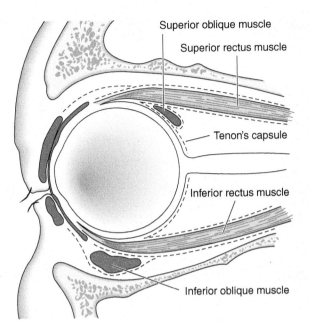

▲ **Figure 1–19.** Fascia about muscles and eyeball (Tenon's capsule).

THE OCULAR ADNEXA

1. BROWS

The brows are folds of thickened skin covered with hair. The skin fold is supported by underlying muscle fibers. The glabella is the hairless prominence between the brows.

2. LIDS

The upper and lower lids (palpebrae) are modified folds of skin that can close to protect the anterior eyeball (Figure 1–21). Blinking helps spread the tear film, which protects the cornea and conjunctiva from dehydration. The upper lid ends at the eyebrows; the lower lid merges into the cheek.

The lids consist of five layers: skin, striated muscle (orbicularis oculi), areolar tissue, fibrous tissue (tarsal plates), and mucous membrane (palpebral conjunctiva) (Figure 1–22).

▶ Structures of the Lids

A. Skin

The skin of the lids differs from skin on most other areas of the body in that it is thin, loose, and elastic and possesses few hair follicles and no subcutaneous fat.

B. Orbicularis Oculi Muscle

The function of the orbicularis oculi muscle is to close the lids. Its muscle fibers surround the palpebral fissure in

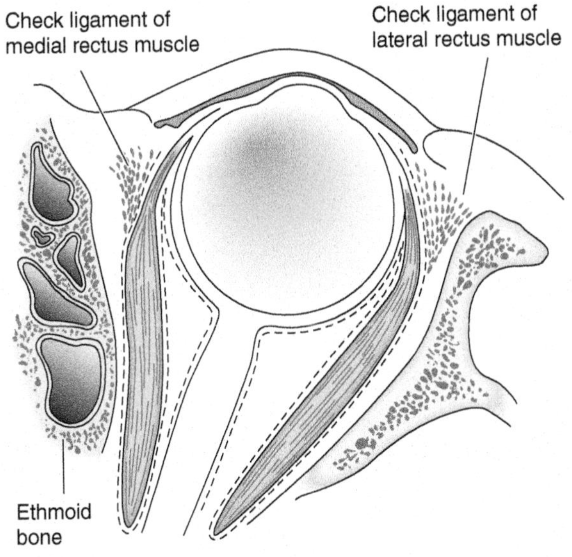

▲ **Figure 1–20.** Check ligaments of medial and lateral rectus muscles, right eye (diagrammatic).

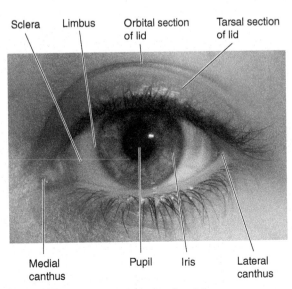

▲ **Figure 1–21.** External landmarks of the eye.

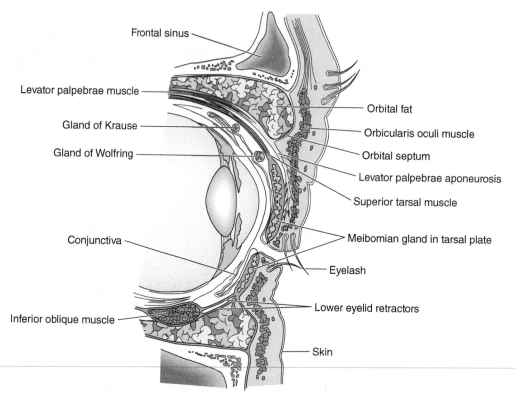

Figure 1–22. Cross section of the lids. (Used with permission from C Beard.)

concentric fashion and spread for a short distance around the orbital margin. Some fibers run onto the cheek and the forehead. The portion of the muscle that is in the lids is known as its pretarsal portion; the portion over the orbital septum is the preseptal portion. The segment outside the lid is called the orbital portion. The orbicularis oculi is supplied by the facial nerve.

C. Areolar Tissue

The submuscular loose areolar tissue that lies deep to the orbicularis oculi muscle communicates with the subaponeu-rotic layer of the scalp.

D. Tarsal Plates

The main supporting structure of the lids is a dense fibrous tissue layer that—along with a small amount of elastic tissue—is called the tarsal plate. The lateral and medial angles and extensions of the tarsal plates are attached to the orbital margin by the lateral and medial palpebral ligaments. The upper and lower tarsal plates are also attached by a condensed, thin fascia to the upper and lower orbital margins. This thin fascia forms the orbital septum.

E. Palpebral Conjunctiva

The lids are lined posteriorly by a layer of mucous membrane, the palpebral conjunctiva, which adheres firmly to the tarsal plates. A surgical incision through the gray line of the lid margin (see the next section) splits the lid into an anterior lamella (margin) of the skin and the orbicularis muscle and a posterior lamella (margin) of the tarsal plate and the palpebral conjunctiva.

▶ Lid Margins

The free lid margin is 25- to 30-mm long and about 2 mm wide. It is divided by the gray line (mucocutaneous junction) into anterior and posterior margins.

A. Anterior Margin

1. **Lashes**—The lashes project from the margins of the lids and are arranged irregularly. The upper lashes are longer and more numerous than the lower lashes and turn upward; the lower lashes turn downward.
2. **Glands of Zeis**—These are small, modified sebaceous glands that open into the hair follicles at the base of the lashes.
3. **Glands of Moll**—These are modified sweat glands that open in a row near the base of the lashes.

B. Posterior Margin

The posterior lid margin is in close contact with the globe, and along this margin are the small orifices of modified sebaceous glands (meibomian, or tarsal, glands).

C. Lacrimal Punctum

At the medial end of the posterior margin of each of the upper and lower lids is a small elevation with a central small opening (punctum) through which tears pass to the corresponding canaliculus and thence to the lacrimal sac.

▶ Palpebral Fissure

The palpebral fissure is the elliptic space between the two open lids. The fissure terminates at the medial and lateral canthi. The lateral canthus is about 0.5 cm from the lateral orbital rim and forms an acute angle. The medial canthus is more elliptic than the lateral canthus and surrounds the lacrimal lake (Figure 1–21), in which lies the lacrimal caruncle, a yellowish elevation of modified skin containing large modified sweat glands and sebaceous glands that open into follicles that contain fine hair (Figure 1–9), and the **plica semilunaris**, a vestigial remnant of the third lid of lower animal species.

In the Asian population, a skin fold known as the **epicanthus** passes from the medial termination of the upper lid to the medial termination of the lower lid, hiding the caruncle. Epicanthus may be present normally in young infants of all races and disappears with the development of the nasal bridge but persists throughout life in Asians.

▶ Orbital Septum

The orbital septum is the fascia behind that portion of the orbicularis muscle that lies between the orbital rim and the tarsus and serves as a barrier between the lid and the orbit.

The orbital septum is pierced by the lacrimal vessels and nerves, the supratrochlear artery and nerve, the supraorbital vessels and nerves, the infratrochlear nerve (Figure 1–23), the anastomosis between the angular and ophthalmic veins, and the levator palpebrae superioris muscle.

The superior orbital septum blends with the tendon of the levator palpebrae superioris and the superior tarsus; the inferior orbital septum blends with the inferior tarsus.

▶ Lid Retractors

The lid retractors are responsible for opening the lids. They are formed by a musculofascial complex, with both striated and smooth muscle components, known as the levator complex in the upper lid and the capsulopalpebral fascia in the lower lid.

In the upper lid, the striated muscle portion is the **levator palpebrae superioris**, which arises from the apex of the orbit and passes forward to divide into an aponeurosis and a deeper portion that contains the smooth muscle fibers of **Müller's (superior tarsal) muscle** (Figure 1–22). The aponeurosis elevates the anterior lamella of the lid, inserting into the posterior surface of the orbicularis oculi and through this into the overlying skin to form the upper lid skin crease. Müller's muscle inserts into the upper border of the tarsal plate and the superior fornix of the conjunctiva, thus elevating the posterior lamella.

In the lower lid, the main retractor is the inferior rectus muscle, from which fibrous tissue extends to enclose the inferior oblique muscle and insert into the lower border of the tarsal plate and the orbicularis oculi. Associated with this aponeurosis are the smooth muscle fibers of the inferior tarsal muscle.

The smooth muscle components of the lid retractors are innervated by sympathetic nerves. The levator and inferior rectus muscles are supplied by the third cranial

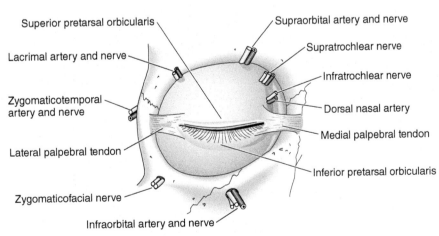

▲ **Figure 1–23.** Vessels and nerves to extraocular structures.

(oculomotor) nerve. Ptosis is thus a feature of both Horner's syndrome and third nerve palsy.

Levator Palpebrae Superioris Muscle

The levator palpebrae muscle arises with a short tendon from the undersurface of the lesser wing of the sphenoid. The tendon blends with the underlying origin of the superior rectus muscle. The levator belly passes forward, forms an aponeurosis, and spreads like a fan. The muscle, including its smooth muscle component (Müller's muscle), and its aponeurosis form an important part of the upper lid retractor (see previous section). The palpebral segment of the orbicularis oculi muscle acts as its antagonist.

The two extremities of the levator aponeurosis are called its medial and lateral horns. The medial horn is thin and is attached below the frontolacrimal suture and into the medial palpebral ligament. The lateral horn passes between the orbital and palpebral portions of the lacrimal gland and inserts into the orbital tubercle and the lateral palpebral ligament.

The sheath of the levator palpebrae superioris is attached to the superior rectus muscle inferiorly. The superior surface, at the junction of the muscle belly and the aponeurosis, forms a thickened band (Whitnall's ligament) that is attached medially to the trochlea and laterally to the lateral orbital wall, the band forming the check ligaments of the muscle.

The levator is supplied by the superior branch of the oculomotor nerve (III). Blood supply to the levator palpebrae superioris is derived from the lateral muscular branch of the ophthalmic artery.

Sensory Nerve Supply

The sensory nerve supply to the lids is derived from the first and second divisions of the trigeminal nerve (V). The lacrimal, supraorbital, supratrochlear, infratrochlear, and external nasal nerves are branches of the ophthalmic division of the fifth nerve. The infraorbital, zygomaticofacial, and zygomaticotemporal nerves are branches of the maxillary (second) division of the trigeminal nerve.

Blood Supply & Lymphatics

The blood supply to the lids is derived from the lacrimal and ophthalmic arteries by their lateral and medial palpebral branches. Anastomoses between the lateral and medial palpebral arteries form the tarsal arcades that lie in the submuscular areolar tissue.

Venous drainage from the lids empties into the ophthalmic vein and the veins that drain the forehead and temple (Figure 1–6). The veins are arranged in pretarsal and posttarsal plexuses.

Lymphatics from the lateral segment of the lids run into the preauricular and parotid nodes. Lymphatics draining the medial side of the lids empty into the submandibular lymph nodes.

3. THE LACRIMAL APPARATUS

The lacrimal complex consists of the lacrimal gland, accessory lacrimal glands, lacrimal puncta, lacrimal canaliculi, lacrimal sac, and nasolacrimal duct (Figure 1–24).

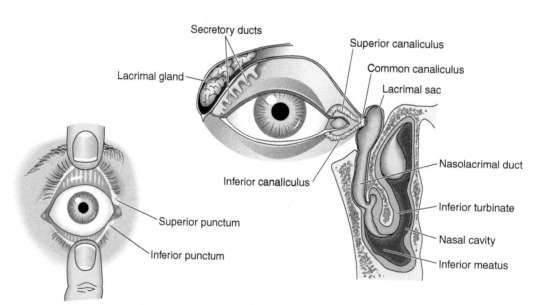

▲ **Figure 1–24.** The lacrimal drainage system.

The lacrimal gland consists of the following structures:

1. The almond-shaped **orbital portion**, located in the lacrimal fossa in the anterior upper temporal segment of the orbit, is separated from the palpebral portion by the lateral horn of the levator palpebrae muscle. To reach this portion of the gland surgically, one must incise the skin, the orbicularis oculi muscle, and the orbital septum.

2. The smaller **palpebral portion** is located just above the temporal segment of the superior conjunctival fornix. Lacrimal secretory ducts, which open by approximately 10 fine orifices, connect the orbital and palpebral portions of the lacrimal gland to the superior conjunctival fornix. Removal of the palpebral portion of the gland cuts off all of the connecting ducts, and thus prevents secretion by the entire gland.

The accessory lacrimal glands (glands of Krause and Wolfring) are located in the substantia propria of the palpebral conjunctiva.

Tears drain from the lacrimal lake via the upper and lower puncta and canaliculi to the lacrimal sac, which lies in the lacrimal fossa. The nasolacrimal duct continues downward from the sac and opens into the inferior meatus of the nasal cavity, lateral to the inferior turbinate. Tears are directed into the puncta by capillary attraction and gravity and by the blinking action of the lids. The combined forces of capillary attraction in the canaliculi, gravity, and the pumping action of Horner's muscle, which is an extension of the orbicularis oculi muscle to a point behind the lacrimal sac, all tend to continue the flow of tears down the nasolacrimal duct into the nose.

Blood Supply & Lymphatics

The blood supply of the lacrimal gland is derived from the lacrimal artery. The vein that drains the gland joins the ophthalmic vein. The lymphatic drainage joins with the conjunctival lymphatics to drain into the preauricular lymph nodes.

Nerve Supply

The nerve supply to the lacrimal gland is by (1) the lacrimal nerve (sensory), a branch of the trigeminal first division; (2) the great petrosal nerve (parasympathetic secretory), which comes from the superior salivary nucleus and is a branch of the facial nerve; and (3) sympathetic nerves in the deep petrosal nerve and accompanying the lacrimal artery and the lacrimal nerve. The greater and deep petrosal nerves form the nerve of the pterygoid canal (Vidian nerve).

Related Structures

The **medial palpebral ligament** connects the upper and lower tarsal plates to the frontal process at the inner canthus anterior to the lacrimal sac. The portion of the lacrimal sac below the ligament is covered by a few fibers of the orbicularis oculi muscle. These fibers offer little resistance to swelling and distention of the lacrimal sac. The area below the medial palpebral ligament becomes swollen in acute dacryocystitis, and fistulas commonly open in the area.

The angular vein and artery lie just deep to the skin, 8 mm to the nasal side of the inner canthus. Skin incisions made in surgical procedures on the lacrimal sac should always be placed 2–3 mm to the nasal side of the inner canthus to avoid these vessels.

THE OPTIC NERVE

The trunk of the optic nerve consists of about 1 million axons that arise from the ganglion cells of the retina and form the nerve fiber layer. The optic nerve emerges from the posterior surface of the globe through the posterior scleral foramen, a short, circular opening in the sclera about 1 mm below and 3 mm nasal to the posterior pole of the eye (Figure 1–8). The nerve fibers become myelinated on leaving the eye, increasing the diameter from 1.5 mm (within the sclera) to 3 mm (within the orbit). The orbital segment of the nerve is 25- to 30-mm long; it travels within the optic muscle cone, via the bony optic canal, and thus gains access to the cranial cavity. The intracanalicular portion measures 4–9 mm. After a 10-mm intracranial course, the nerve joins the opposite optic nerve to form the optic chiasm.

Eighty percent of the optic nerve consists of visual fibers that synapse in the lateral geniculate body on neurons whose axons terminate in the primary visual cortex of the occipital lobes. Twenty percent of the fibers are pupillary and bypass the geniculate body en route to the pretectal area. Since the ganglion cells of the retina and their axons are part of the central nervous system, they will not regenerate if severed.

Sheaths of the Optic Nerve (Figure 1–25)

The fibrous wrappings that ensheathe the optic nerve are continuous with the meninges. The pia mater is loosely attached to the nerve near the chiasm and only for a short distance within the cranium, but it is closely attached around most of the intracanalicular and all of the intraorbital portions. The pia consists of some fibrous tissue with numerous small blood vessels (Figure 1–26). It divides the nerve fibers into bundles by sending numerous septa into the nerve substance. The pia continues to the sclera, with a few fibers running into the choroid and lamina cribrosa.

The arachnoid comes in contact with the optic nerve at the intracranial end of the optic canal and accompanies the nerve to the globe, where it ends in the sclera and overlying dura. This sheath is a diaphanous connective tissue membrane with many septate connections with the pia mater, which it closely resembles. It is more intimately associated with pia than with dura.

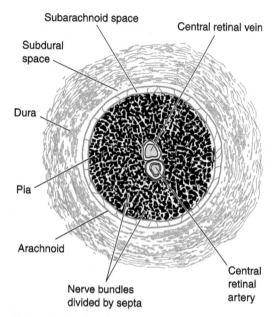

Figure 1–25. Cross section of the optic nerve.

The dura mater lining the inner surface of the cranial vault comes in contact with the optic nerve as it leaves the optic canal. As the nerve enters the orbit from the optic canal, the dura splits, with one layer (the periorbita) lining the orbital cavity and the other forming the outer dural covering of the optic nerve. The dura becomes continuous with the outer two-thirds of the sclera. The dura consists of tough, fibrous, relatively avascular tissue lined by endothelium on the inner surface.

The subdural space is between the dura and the arachnoid; the subarachnoid space is between the pia and the arachnoid. Both are more potential than actual spaces under normal conditions but are direct continuations of their corresponding intracranial spaces. Increased cerebrospinal fluid pressure results in dilatation of the subarachnoid component of the optic nerve sheaths. The meningeal layers are adherent to each other and to the optic nerve and the surrounding bone within the optic foramen, making the optic nerve resistant to traction from either end.

▶ Blood Supply (Figure 1–26)

The surface layer of the optic disk receives blood from branches of the retinal arterioles. In the region of the lamina cribrosa, comprising the prelaminar, laminar, and retrolaminar segments of the optic nerve, the arterial supply is from the short posterior ciliary arteries. The anterior intraorbital optic nerve receives some blood from branches of the central retinal artery. The remainder of the intraorbital nerve, as well as the intracanalicular and intracranial portions, are supplied by a pial network of vessels derived from the various branches of the ophthalmic artery and other branches of the internal carotid.

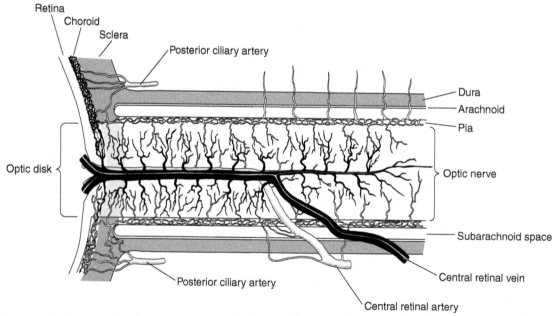

Figure 1–26. Blood supply of the optic nerve. (Redrawn from: Hayreh SS: *Trans Am Acad Ophthalmol Otolaryngol.* 1974;78:240.)

THE OPTIC CHIASM

The optic chiasm is located at the junction of the floor and anterior wall (lamina terminalis) of the third ventricle. It is variably situated near the top of the diaphragm of the sella turcica, most often posteriorly, lying 1 cm above it and continuing the 45° upward angulation of the optic nerves after their emergence from the optic canals (Figure 1–27). The internal carotid arteries lie just laterally, adjacent to the cavernous sinuses. The chiasm is made up of the junction of the two optic nerves and provides for crossing of the nasal fibers to the opposite optic tract and passage of temporal fibers to the ipsilateral optic tract. The macular fibers are arranged similarly to the rest of the fibers except that their decussation is farther posteriorly and superiorly. The chiasm receives many small blood vessels from the neighboring circle of Willis.

THE RETROCHIASMATIC VISUAL PATHWAYS

Each optic tract begins at the posterolateral angle of the chiasm and sweeps around the upper part of the cerebral peduncle to end in the lateral geniculate nucleus. Afferent pupillary fibers leave the tract just anterior to the nucleus and pass via the brachium of the superior colliculus to the midbrain. (The pupillary pathway is diagrammed in Figure 14–2.) Afferent visual fibers terminate on cells in the lateral geniculate nucleus that give rise to the geniculocalcarine tract. This tract traverses the posterior limb of the internal capsule and then fans out into a broad bundle called the optic radiation. The fibers in this bundle curve backward around the anterior aspect of the temporal horn of the lateral ventricle and then medially to reach the calcarine cortex of the occipital lobe, where they terminate. The most inferior fibers, which carry projections from the superior aspect of the contralateral half of the visual field, course anteriorly into the temporal lobe in a configuration known as Meyer's loop. Lesions of the temporal lobe that extend 5 cm back from the anterior tip involve these fibers and can produce superior quadrantanopic field defects.

The primary visual cortex (area V1) occupies the upper and lower lips and the depths of the calcarine fissure on the medial aspect of the occipital lobe. Each lobe receives input from the two ipsilateral half-retinas, representing the contralateral half of the binocular visual field. Projection of the visual field onto the visual cortex occurs in a precise retinotopic pattern. The macula is represented at the medial posterior pole, and the peripheral parts of the retina project

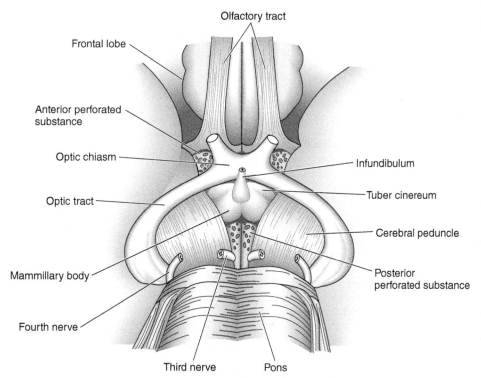

▲ **Figure 1–27.** Relationship of optic chiasm from inferior aspect. (Redrawn from: Duke-Elder WS: *System of Ophthalmology*, vol 2. Mosby, 1961.)

to the most anterior part of the calcarine cortex. On either side of area V1 lies area V2, and then area V3. V2 appears to function in a manner very similar to V1. Area V4, situated on the medial surface of the cerebral hemisphere but more anterior and inferior than V1 in the region of the fusiform gyrus, is primarily concerned with color processing. Motion detection localizes to area V5 at the junction of the occipital and temporal lobes, lateral to area V1.

THE OCULOMOTOR NERVE (III)

The oculomotor nerve leaves the brainstem between the cerebral peduncles and passes near the posterior communicating artery of the circle of Willis. Lateral to the pituitary gland, it is closely approximated to the optic tract, and here it pierces the dura to course in the lateral wall of the cavernous sinus. As the nerve leaves the cavernous sinus, it divides into superior and inferior divisions. The superior division enters the orbit within the annulus of Zinn at its highest point and adjacent to the trochlear nerve (Figure 1–3). The inferior division enters the annulus of Zinn low and passes below the optic nerve to supply the medial and inferior rectus muscles. A large branch from the inferior division extends forward to supply the inferior oblique. A small twig from the proximal end of the nerve to the inferior oblique carries parasympathetic fibers to the ciliary ganglion.

THE TROCHLEAR NERVE (IV)

The thinnest of the cranial nerves, the trochlear nerve (Figure 1–3) is the only nerve to originate on the dorsal surface of the brainstem. The fibers decussate before they emerge from the brainstem just below the inferior colliculi, where they are subject to injury from the tentorium. The nerve pierces the dura behind the sella turcica and travels within the lateral walls of the cavernous sinus to enter the superior orbital fissure medial to the frontal nerve. From this point it travels within the periorbita of the roof over the levator muscle to the upper surface of the superior oblique muscle.

THE TRIGEMINAL NERVE (V) (FIGURE 1–3)

The trigeminal nerve originates from the pons, and its sensory roots form the trigeminal ganglion. The first (ophthalmic) of the three divisions passes through the lateral wall of the cavernous sinus and divides into the lacrimal, frontal, and nasociliary nerves. The **lacrimal nerve** passes through the upper lateral aspect of the superior orbital fissure, outside the annulus of Zinn, and continues its lateral course in the orbit to terminate in the lacrimal gland, providing its sensory innervation. Slightly medial to the lacrimal nerve within the superior orbital fissure is the frontal nerve, which is the largest of the first division of branches of the trigeminal nerve. It also crosses over the annulus of Zinn and follows a course over the levator to the medial aspect of the orbit, where it divides into

the supraorbital and supratrochlear nerves. These provide sensation to the brow and forehead. The nasociliary nerve is the sensory nerve of the eye. After entering through the medial portion of the annulus of Zinn, it lies between the superior rectus and the optic nerve. Branches to the ciliary ganglion and those forming the ciliary nerves provide sensory supply to the cornea, iris, and ciliary body. The terminal branches are the infratrochlear nerve, which supplies the medial portion of the conjunctiva and lids, and the anterior ethmoidal nerve, which provides sensation to the tip of the nose. Thus, the skin on the tip of the nose may be affected with vesicular lesions prior to the onset of herpes zoster ophthalmicus.

The second (maxillary) division of the trigeminal nerve passes through the foramen rotundum and enters the orbit through the inferior orbital fissure. It passes through the infraorbital canal, becoming the **infraorbital nerve**, and exits via the infraorbital foramen, supplying sensation to the lower lid and adjacent cheek. It is frequently damaged in fractures of the orbital floor.

THE ABDUCENS NERVE (VI)

The abducens nerve (Figure 1–3) originates between the pons and medulla and pursues an extended course, having the longest intracranial course of any cranial nerve, up the clivus to the posterior clinoid, penetrates the dura, and passes within the cavernous sinus. (All other nerves course through the lateral wall of the cavernous sinus.) After passing through the superior orbital fissure within the annulus of Zinn, the nerve continues laterally to innervate the lateral rectus muscle.

THE FACIAL NERVE (VII)

The facial nerve exits the brainstem at the lower border of the pons, the greater petrosal nerve forming part of the separate portion known as the nervus intermedius, and passes through the internal acoustic meatus with the vestibulocochlear (VII) nerve into the facial canal. At the geniculate ganglion, the greater petrosal nerve, which contains parasympathetic secretomotor fibers, joins the lesser petrosal nerve to form the nerve of the pterygoid canal (Vidian nerve) and pass through the pterygopalatine ganglion, where the parasympathetic fibers synapse, to reach the lacrimal gland. The facial nerve exits the facial canal at the stylomastoid foramen, passes through the parotid gland, and then branches out across the face to supply the muscles of facial expression, including orbicularis oculi.

II. EMBRYOLOGY OF THE EYE

The eye is derived from three of the primitive embryonic layers: surface ectoderm, including its derivative—the neural crest; neural ectoderm; and mesoderm. Endoderm does not enter into the formation of the eye. Mesenchyme, derived from mesoderm or the neural crest, is the term for embryonic connective tissue. Most of the mesenchyme of the head and neck is derived from the neural crest.

The **surface ectoderm** gives rise to the lens, the lacrimal gland, the epithelium of the cornea, conjunctiva and adnexal glands, and the epidermis of the lids.

The **neural crest**, which arises from the surface ectoderm in the region immediately adjacent to the neural folds of neural ectoderm, is responsible for the formation of the corneal keratocytes, the endothelium of the cornea and the trabecular meshwork, the stroma of the sclera, the vitreous, and the optic nerve meninges. It is also involved in the formation of the orbital cartilage and bone, the orbital connective tissues and nerves, the extraocular muscles, and the subepidermal layers of the lids.

The **neural ectoderm** gives rise to the optic vesicle and optic cup and is thus responsible for the formation of the retina and retinal pigment epithelium, the pigmented and nonpigmented layers of ciliary epithelium, the posterior epithelium, the dilator and sphincter muscles of the iris, and the optic nerve fibers and glia.

The **mesoderm** contributes to the vitreous, extraocular and lid muscles, and the orbital and ocular vascular endothelium.

Optic Vesicle Stage

The embryonic plate is the earliest stage in fetal development during which ocular structures can be differentiated. At 2 weeks, the edges of the neural groove thicken to form the neural folds. The folds then fuse to form the neural tube, which sinks into the underlying mesoderm and detaches itself from the surface epithelium. The site of the optic groove or optic sulcus is in the cephalic neural folds on either side of and parallel to the neural groove, which forms when the neural folds begin to close at 3 weeks (Figure 1–28).

At 4 weeks, just before the anterior portion of the neural tube closes completely, neural ectoderm grows outward and toward the surface ectoderm on either side to form the spherical optic vesicles. The optic vesicles are connected to the forebrain by the optic stalks. At this stage also, a thickening of the surface ectoderm (lens plate) begins to form opposite the ends of the optic vesicles.

Optic Cup Stage

As the optic vesicle invaginates to produce the optic cup, the original outer wall of the vesicle approaches its inner wall. The invagination of the ventral surface of the optic stalk and of the optic vesicle occurs simultaneously and creates a groove, the optic (embryonic) fissure. The margins of the optic cup then grow around the optic fissure. At the same time, the lens plate invaginates to form first a cup and then a hollow sphere known as the lens vesicle. By 6 weeks, the lens vesicle separates from the surface ectoderm and lies free in the rim of the optic cup.

The optic fissure allows mesodermal mesenchyme to enter the optic stalk and eventually to form the hyaloid system of the vitreous cavity. As invagination is completed, the optic fissure narrows and closes, leaving one small permanent opening at the anterior end of the optic stalk through which the hyaloid artery passes. At 4 months, the retinal artery and vein pass through this opening.

Once the optic fissure has closed, the ultimate general structure of the eye has been determined. Further development consists in differentiation of the individual optic structures. In general, differentiation of the optic structures occurs more rapidly in the posterior than in the anterior segment of the eye during the early stages and more rapidly in the anterior segment during the later stages of gestation.

EMBRYOLOGY OF SPECIFIC STRUCTURES

Lids & Lacrimal Apparatus

The lids develop from mesenchyme except for the epidermis of the skin and the epithelium of the conjunctiva, which are derivatives of surface ectoderm. The lid buds are first seen at 6 weeks growing in front of the eye, where they meet and fuse by 8 weeks. They separate during the fifth month. The lashes and meibomian and other lid glands develop as downgrowths from the epidermis.

The lacrimal and accessory lacrimal glands develop from the conjunctival epithelium. The structures of the lacrimal drainage system (canaliculi, lacrimal sac, and nasolacrimal duct) are also surface ectodermal derivatives, which develop from a solid epithelial cord that becomes buried between the maxillary and nasal processes of the developing facial structures. This cord canalizes just before birth.

Sclera & Extraocular Muscles

The sclera and extraocular muscles are formed from condensations of mesenchyme encircling the optic cup and are identifiable by 7 weeks. Development of these structures is well advanced by the fourth month. Tenon's capsule appears about the insertions of the rectus muscles at 12 weeks and is complete at 5 months.

Anterior Segment

The anterior segment of the globe is formed by the invasion of the neural crest mesenchymal cells into the space between the surface ectoderm, which develops into the corneal epithelium, and the lens vesicle, which has become separated from it. The invasion occurs in three stages: the first is responsible for formation of the corneal endothelium, the second for formation of the iris stroma, and the third for formation of the corneal stroma. The anterior chamber angle

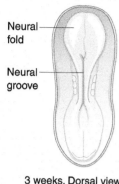

Neural fold

Neural groove

3 weeks. Dorsal view. Neural folds beginning to close.

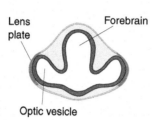

Lens plate

Forebrain

Optic vesicle

4 weeks. Transverse section. Formation of optic vesicles and lens plates.

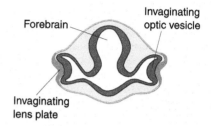

Forebrain

Invaginating optic vesicle

Invaginating lens plate

4½ weeks. Transverse section. Invagination of optic vesicles and lens plates.

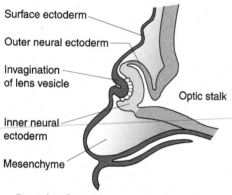

Surface ectoderm

Outer neural ectoderm

Invagination of lens vesicle

Optic stalk

Inner neural ectoderm

Mesenchyme

5 weeks. Cross section. Development of optic cup and lens vesicle.

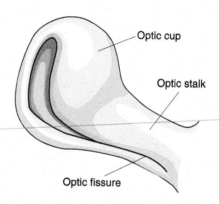

Optic cup

Optic stalk

Optic fissure

6 weeks. External view. Closure of optic fissure through which hyaloid vessels enter the optic cup.

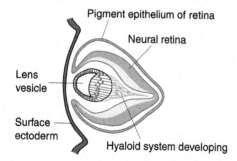

Pigment epithelium of retina

Neural retina

Lens vesicle

Surface ectoderm

Hyaloid system developing

7 weeks. Cross section. Differentiation of layers of neural ectoderm into pigment epithelium and neural retina and expansion of lens vesicle.

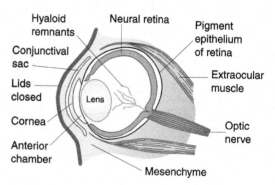

Hyaloid remnants

Neural retina

Pigment epithelium of retina

Conjunctival sac

Lids closed

Lens

Extraocular muscle

Cornea

Optic nerve

Anterior chamber

Mesenchyme

8 weeks. Cross section. Fusion of lids and development of extraocular muscles from mesenchyme.

▲ **Figure 1–28.** Embryologic development of ocular structures.

is formed from a residual condensation of mesenchyme at the anterior rim of the optic cup. The mechanism of formation of the anterior chamber itself—and hence the angle structure—is still debated but seems to involve patterns of migration of neural crest cells and subsequent changes in their structure rather than cleavage of mesodermal tissue, as previously thought.

The corneal epithelium and endothelium are first apparent at 6 weeks, when the lens vesicle has separated from the surface ectoderm. Descemet's membrane is secreted by the flattened endothelial cells by 11 weeks. The stroma slowly thickens and forms an anterior condensation just under the epithelium that is recognizable at 4 months as Bowman's layer. A definite corneoscleral junction is present at 4 months.

The double row of iris epithelium is a forward extension of the anterior rim of the optic cup. This grows forward during the third month to lie posterior to the neural crest cells that form the iris stroma. These two epithelial layers become pigmented in the iris, whereas only the outer layer is pigmented in the ciliary body. By the fifth month, the sphincter muscle of the pupil is developing from the anterior epithelial layer of the iris near the pupillary margin. Soon after the sixth month, the dilator muscle appears in the anterior epithelial layer near the ciliary body.

The anterior chamber of the eye first appears at 7 weeks and remains very shallow until birth. At 10 weeks, Schlemm's canal appears as a vascular channel at the level of the recess of the angle and gradually assumes a relatively more anterior location as the angle recess develops. The iris, which in the early stages of development is quite anterior, gradually lies relatively more posteriorly as the chamber angle recess develops, most likely because of the difference in the rate of growth of the anterior segment structures. The trabecular meshwork develops from the loose mesenchymal tissue lying originally at the margin of the optic cup. The aqueous drainage system is ready to function before birth.

Lens

Soon after the lens vesicle lies free in the rim of the optic cup (6 weeks), the cells of its posterior wall elongate, encroach on the empty cavity, and finally fill it (7 weeks). At about 6 weeks, a hyaline capsule is secreted by the lens cells. Secondary lens fibers elongate from the equatorial region and grow forward under the subcapsular epithelium, which remains as a single layer of cuboidal epithelial cells, and backward under the lens capsule. These fibers meet to form the lens sutures (upright Y anteriorly and inverted Y posteriorly), which are complete by the seventh month. (This growth and proliferation of secondary lens fibers continues at a decreasing rate throughout life; the lens therefore continues to enlarge slowly, causing compression of the lens fibers.)

Ciliary Body & Choroid

The ciliary epithelium is formed from the same anterior extension of the optic cup that is responsible for the iris epithelium. Only the outer layer becomes pigmented. The ciliary muscle and blood vessels are derived from mesenchyme.

At 3½ weeks, a network of capillaries encircles the optic cup and develops into the choroid. By the third month, the intermediate and large venous channels of the choroid are developed and drain into the vortex veins to exit from the eye.

Retina

The outer layer of the optic cup remains as a single layer and becomes the pigment epithelium of the retina. Pigmentation begins at 5 weeks. Secretion of the inner layer of Bruch's membrane occurs by 6 weeks. The inner layer of the optic cup undergoes a complicated differentiation into the other nine layers of the retina. This occurs slowly throughout gestation. By the seventh month, the outermost cell layer (consisting of the nuclei of the rods and cones) is present as well as the bipolar, amacrine, and ganglion cells and nerve fibers. The macular region is thicker than the rest of the retina until the eighth month, when the macular depression begins to develop. Macular development is not complete anatomically until 6 months after birth.

Vitreous

A. First Stage

(Primary vitreous, 3–6 weeks.) At about 3 weeks, cells and fibroblasts derived from mesenchyme at the rim of the optic cup or associated with the hyaloid vascular system, together with minor contributions from the embryonic lens and the inner layer of the optic vesicle, form the vitreous fibrils of the primary vitreous. Ultimately, the primary vitreous comes to lie just behind the posterior pole of the lens in association with remnants of the hyaloid vessels (Cloquet's canal).

B. Second Stage

(Secondary vitreous, 6–10 weeks.) The fibrils and cells (hyalocytes) of the secondary vitreous are thought to originate from the vascular primary vitreous. Anteriorly, the firm attachment of the secondary vitreous to the internal limiting membrane of the retina constitutes the early stages of formation of the vitreous base. The hyaloid system develops a set of vitreous vessels as well as vessels on the lens capsule surface (tunica vasculosa lentis). The hyaloid system is at its height at 2 months and then atrophies from posterior to anterior.

C. Third Stage

(Tertiary vitreous, 10 weeks on.) During the third month, the marginal bundle of Drualt is forming. This consists of vitreous fibrillar condensations extending from the future ciliary epithelium of the optic cup to the equator of the lens. Condensations then form the suspensory ligament of the lens, which is well developed by 4 months. The hyaloid system atrophies completely during this stage.

Optic Nerve

The axons of the ganglion cells of the retina form the nerve fiber layer. The fibers slowly form the optic stalk (7 weeks) and then the optic nerve. Mesenchymal elements enter the surrounding tissue to form the vascular septa of the nerve. Myelination extends from the brain peripherally down the optic nerve and at birth has reached the lamina cribrosa. Myelination is completed by age 3 months.

Blood Vessels

Long ciliary arteries bud off from the hyaloid system at 6 weeks and anastomose around the optic cup margin with the major circle of the iris by 7 weeks. The hyaloid artery gives rise to the central retinal artery and its branches (4 months). Buds arise in the region of the optic disk and gradually extend to the peripheral retina, reaching the ora serrata at 8 months. The branches of the central retinal vein develop simultaneously. The hyaloid system has atrophied completely by the eighth month.

III. GROWTH & DEVELOPMENT OF THE EYE

Eyeball

At birth, the eye is larger in relation to the rest of the body than is the case in children and adults, but in relation to its ultimate size (reached at 7–8 years), it is comparatively short,

averaging 16.6 mm in anteroposterior diameter. This would make the eye markedly myopic rather than the usual mild hyperopia if it were not for the greater refractive power due to steeper corneal curvature and more spherical lens.

Cornea

The newborn infant has a relatively large cornea that reaches adult size by the age of 2 years. It is steeper than the adult cornea, and its curvature is greater at the periphery than in the center. (The reverse is true in adults.)

Lens

At birth, the lens is more nearly spherical in shape than later in life, producing a greater refractive power that helps to compensate for the short anteroposterior diameter of the eye. The lens grows throughout life as new fibers are added to the periphery from lens epithelial cells, making it flatter.

The consistency of the lens material changes throughout life. At birth, it may be compared with soft plastic; in old age, the lens is of a glass-like consistency. This accounts for the greater resistance to change of shape for accommodation with age.

Iris

At birth, there is little or no pigment in the stroma of the anterior iris, but the epithelium, particularly the posterior layer, is heavily pigmented. Nevertheless, reflection of light by the stroma gives the eyes of most infants a bluish color. Iris color is subsequently determined by pigmentation and thickness of the stroma, the latter influencing visibility of the epithelial pigment.

Ophthalmologic Examination

2

David F. Chang, MD

Of all the organs of the body, the eye is most accessible to direct examination. Visual function can be quantified by simple subjective testing. The external anatomy of the eye is visible to inspection with the unaided eye and with fairly simple instruments. With more complicated instruments, the interior of the eye is visible through the clear cornea. The eye is the only part of the body where blood vessels and central nervous system tissue (retina and optic nerve) can be viewed directly. Important systemic effects of infectious, autoimmune, neoplastic, and vascular diseases may be identified from ocular examination.

The purpose of sections I and II of this chapter is to provide an overview of the ocular history and basic complete eye examination as performed by an ophthalmologist. In section III, more specialized examination techniques will be presented.

I. OCULAR HISTORY

The **chief complaint** is characterized according to its duration, frequency, intermittency, and rapidity of onset. The location, severity, and circumstances surrounding its onset are important, as is identifying any other ocular and nonocular symptoms that may require specific enquiry. Current eye medications and current and past ocular disorders are determined.

The **past medical history** must include enquiry about vascular disorder—such as diabetes and hypertension—and systemic medications, particularly corticosteroids because of their adverse ocular effects. Finally, any drug allergies should be recorded.

The **family history** is pertinent for ocular disorders, such as strabismus, amblyopia, glaucoma, or cataracts, and retinal problems, such as retinal detachment or macular degeneration. Medical diseases such as diabetes may be relevant as well.

COMMON OCULAR SYMPTOMS

A basic understanding of ocular symptomatology is necessary for performing a proper ophthalmologic examination. Ocular symptoms can be divided into three basic categories: abnormalities of vision, abnormalities of ocular appearance, and abnormalities of ocular sensation—pain and discomfort.

Symptoms and complaints should always be fully characterized. Was the **onset** gradual, rapid, or asymptomatic? (For example, was blurred vision in one eye not discovered until the opposite eye was inadvertently covered?) Was the **duration** brief, or has the symptom continued until the present visit? If the symptom was intermittent, what was the frequency? Is the **location** focal or diffuse, and is involvement unilateral or bilateral? Finally, does the patient characterize the **degree** as mild, moderate, or severe?

One should also determine what therapeutic measures have been tried and to what extent they have helped. Has the patient identified circumstances that trigger or worsen the symptom? Have similar instances occurred before, and are there any other associated symptoms?

The following is a brief overview of ocular complaints. Representative examples of some causes are given here and discussed more fully elsewhere in this book.

ABNORMALITIES OF VISION

▶ Visual Loss

Loss of visual acuity may be due to abnormalities anywhere along the optical and neurologic visual pathway. One must therefore consider refractive (focusing) error, lid ptosis, clouding or interference from the ocular media (eg, corneal edema, cataract, or hemorrhage in the vitreous or aqueous space), and malfunction of the retina (macula), optic nerve, or intracranial visual pathway.

A distinction should be made between decreased central acuity and peripheral vision. The latter may be focal, such as a scotoma, or more expansive, as with hemianopia. Abnormalities of the intracranial visual pathway usually disturb the visual field more than central visual acuity.

Transient loss of central or peripheral vision is frequently due to circulatory changes anywhere along the neurologic visual pathway from the retina to the occipital cortex, for example amaurosis fugax and migrainous scotoma.

The degree of visual impairment may vary under different circumstances. For example, uncorrected nearsighted refractive error may seem worse in dark environments. This is because pupillary dilation allows more misfocused rays to reach the retina, increasing the blur. A central focal cataract may seem worse in sunlight. In this case, pupillary constriction prevents more rays from entering and passing around the lens opacity. Blurred vision from corneal edema may improve as the day progresses owing to corneal dehydration from surface evaporation.

▶ Visual Aberrations

Glare or **halos** may result from uncorrected refractive error, scratches on spectacle lenses, excessive pupillary dilation, and hazy ocular media, such as corneal edema or cataract. **Visual distortion** (apart from blurring) may be manifested as an irregular pattern of dimness, wavy or jagged lines, and image magnification or minification. Causes may include the aura of migraine, optical distortion from strong corrective lenses, or lesions involving the macula and optic nerve. **Flashing** or **flickering** lights may indicate retinal traction (if instantaneous) or migrainous scintillations that last for several seconds or minutes. **Floating spots** may represent normal vitreous strands due to vitreous "syneresis" or separation (see Chapter 9) or the pathologic presence of pigment, blood, or inflammatory cells. **Oscillopsia** is a shaking field of vision due to ocular instability.

It must be determined whether **diplopia (double vision)** is monocular or binocular (ie, disappears if one eye is covered). **Monocular diplopia** is often a split shadow or ghost image. Causes include uncorrected refractive error, such as astigmatism, or focal media abnormalities, such as cataracts or corneal irregularities (eg, scars, keratoconus). **Binocular diplopia** (see Chapters 12 and 14) can be vertical, horizontal, diagonal, or torsional. If the deviation occurs or increases in one gaze direction as opposed to others, it is called "incomitant." Neuromuscular dysfunction or mechanical restriction of globe rotation is suspected. "Comitant" deviation is one that remains constant regardless of the direction of gaze. It is usually due to childhood or long-standing strabismus.

ABNORMALITIES OF APPEARANCE

Complaints of "red eye" call for differentiation between redness of the lids and periocular area versus redness of the globe. The latter can be caused by subconjunctival hemorrhage or by vascular congestion of the conjunctiva, sclera, or episclera (connective tissue between the sclera and conjunctiva). Causes of such congestion may be either external surface inflammation, such as conjunctivitis and keratitis, or intraocular inflammation, such as iritis and acute glaucoma (see Inside Front Cover). Color abnormalities other than redness may include jaundice and hyperpigmented spots on the iris or outer ocular surface.

Other changes in appearance of the **globe** that may be noticeable to the patient include focal lesions of the ocular surface, such as a pterygium, and asymmetry of pupil size (anisocoria). The **lids** and **periocular tissues** may be the source of visible signs, such as edema, redness, focal growths, and lesions, and abnormal position or contour, such as ptosis. Finally, the patient may notice bulging or displacement of the globe, such as with exophthalmos.

PAIN & DISCOMFORT

"Eye pain" may be periocular, ocular, retrobulbar (behind the globe), or poorly localized. Examples of **periocular** pain are tenderness of the lid, tear sac, sinuses, or temporal artery. **Retrobulbar** pain can be due to orbital inflammation of any kind. Certain locations of inflammation, such as optic neuritis or orbital myositis, may produce pain on eye movement. Many **nonspecific** complaints, such as "eyestrain," "pulling," "pressure," "fullness," and certain kinds of "headaches," are poorly localized. Causes may include fatigue from ocular accommodation or binocular fusion or referred discomfort from nonocular muscle tension or fatigue.

Ocular pain itself may seem to emanate from the surface or from deeper within the globe. Corneal epithelial damage typically produces a superficial sharp pain or foreign body sensation exacerbated by blinking. Topical anesthesia will immediately relieve this pain. Deeper internal aching pain occurs with acute glaucoma, iritis, endophthalmitis, and scleritis. The globe is often tender to palpation in these situations. Reflex spasm of the ciliary muscle and iris sphincter can occur with iritis or keratitis, producing brow ache and painful "photophobia" (light sensitivity). This discomfort is markedly improved by instillation of cycloplegic/mydriatic agents (see Chapter 22).

▶ Eye Irritation

Superficial ocular discomfort usually results from surface abnormalities. Itching, as a primary symptom, is often a sign of allergic sensitivity. Symptoms of **dryness**, burning, grittiness, and mild foreign body sensation can occur with dry eyes or other types of mild corneal irritation. **Tearing** may be of two general types. Sudden reflex tearing is usually due to irritation of the ocular surface. In contrast, chronic watering and "epiphora" (tears rolling down the cheek) may indicate abnormal lacrimal drainage (see Chapter 4).

Ocular **secretions** are often diagnostically nonspecific. Severe amounts of discharge that cause the lids to be glued shut upon awakening usually indicate viral or bacterial conjunctivitis. More scant amounts of mucoid discharge can also be seen with allergic and noninfectious irritations. Dried matter and crusts on the lashes may occur acutely with conjunctivitis or chronically with blepharitis (lid margin inflammation).

II. BASIC OPHTHALMOLOGIC EXAMINATION

The purpose of the ophthalmologic physical examination is to evaluate both the function and the anatomy of the two eyes. Function includes vision and nonvisual functions, such as eye movements and alignment. Anatomically, ocular problems can be subdivided into three areas: those of the adnexa (lids and periocular tissue), the globe, and the orbit.

VISION

Just as assessment of vital signs is a part of every physical examination, any ocular examination must include assessment of vision, regardless of whether vision is mentioned as part of the chief complaint. Good vision results from a combination of an intact neurologic visual pathway, a structurally healthy eye, and proper focus of the eye. An analogy might be made to a video camera, requiring a functioning cable connection to the monitor, a mechanically intact camera body, and a proper focus setting. Vision can be divided broadly into central and peripheral, quantified by visual acuity and visual field testing, respectively. Clinical assessment of visual acuity and visual field is subjective rather than objective, since it requires responses on the part of the patient.

▶ Visual Acuity Testing

Visual acuity can be tested either for distance or near, conventionally at 20 ft (6 m) and 14 in (33 cm) away, respectively, but distance acuity is the general standard for comparison. For diagnostic purposes, visual acuity is always tested separately for each eye, whereas binocular visual acuity is useful for assessing functional vision (see Chapter 25), such as for assessing the eligibility to drive.

Visual acuity is measured with a display of different-sized optotypes shown at the appropriate distance from the eye. The familiar "Snellen chart" is composed of rows of progressively smaller letters, each row designated by a number corresponding to the distance in feet (or meters) from which a normal eye can read the letters of the row. For example, the letters in the "40" row are large enough for the normal eye to see from 40 ft away. Although wall-mounted illuminated charts or projection systems are commonly used, wall-mounted LCD screens provide better standardization and calibration (Figure 2–1).

Visual acuity is scored as a fraction (eg, "20/40"). The first number represents the testing distance between the chart and

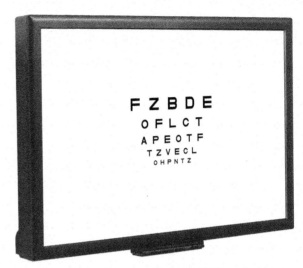

▲ **Figure 2–1.** LCD screen displaying Snellen visual acuity chart with 20/40 letters at the top. (Used with permission from M&S Technologies.)

the patient, and the second number represents the smallest row of letters that the patient's eye can read. Hence, normal vision is 20/20, and 20/60 acuity indicates that the patient's eye can only read from 20 ft letters large enough for a normal eye to read from 60 ft.

Charts containing numerals can be used for patients not familiar with the English alphabet. The "illiterate E" chart is used to test small children or if there is a language barrier. "E" figures are randomly rotated in each of four different orientations throughout the chart. For each target, the patient is asked to point in the same direction as the three "bars" of the E (Figure 2–2). Most children can be tested in this manner beginning at about age 3½ years.

Uncorrected visual acuity is measured without glasses or contact lenses. **Corrected** acuity means that these aids were worn. Since poor uncorrected distance acuity may simply be due to refractive error, corrected visual acuity is a more relevant assessment of ocular health.

▶ Pinhole Test

If the patient needs glasses or if his or her glasses are unavailable, the corrected acuity can be estimated by testing vision through a "pinhole." Refractive blur (eg, myopia, hyperopia, astigmatism) is caused by multiple misfocused rays entering through the pupil and reaching the retina. This prevents formation of a sharply focused image.

Viewing the Snellen chart through a placard of multiple tiny pinhole-sized openings prevents most of the misfocused rays from entering the eye. Only a few centrally aligned focused rays will reach the retina, resulting in a sharper image. In this manner, the patient may be able to read within

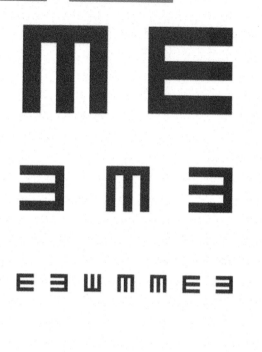

▲ **Figure 2–2.** "Illiterate E" chart.

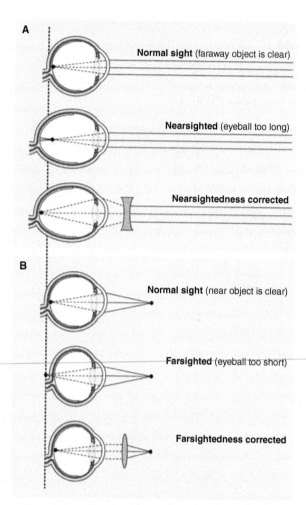

one or two lines of what would be possible if proper corrective glasses were being used.

Refraction

The unaided distant focal point of the eye varies among normal individuals depending on the shape of the globe and the cornea (Figure 2–3). An **emmetropic** eye is naturally in optimal focus for distance vision. An **ametropic** eye (ie, one with myopia, hyperopia, or astigmatism) needs corrective lenses to be in proper focus for distance. This optical abnormality is called **refractive error**.

Refraction is the procedure by which any refractive error is characterized and quantified (see Chapter 21), allowing the best measure of corrected visual acuity. In addition, it is the most reliable means to distinguish between blurred vision caused by refractive error or by other abnormalities of the visual system. Thus, in addition to being the basis for prescription of corrective glasses or contact lenses, refraction serves a crucial diagnostic function.

Testing Poor Vision

The patient unable to read the largest ("20/200") letter on a Snellen chart should be moved closer to the chart until that letter can be read. The distance from the chart is then recorded as the first number. Visual acuity of "5/200" means

▲ **Figure 2–3.** Common imperfections of the optical system of the eye **(refractive errors)**. Ideally, light rays from a distant target should automatically arrive in focus on the retina if the retina is situated precisely at the eye's natural focal point. Such an eye is called **emmetropic**. In **hyperopia** ("farsightedness"), the light rays from a distant target instead come to a focus behind the retina, causing the retinal image to be blurred. A biconvex (+) lens corrects this by increasing the refractive power of the eye and shifting the focal point forward. In **myopia** ("nearsightedness"), the light rays come to a focus in front of the retina, as though the eyeball is too long. Placing a biconcave (–) lens in front of the eye diverges the incoming light rays; this effectively weakens the optical power of the eye enough so that the focus is shifted backward and onto the retina. (Redrawn and adapted from Ganong WF: *Review of Medical Physiology*, 15th ed. McGraw-Hill, 1991.)

that the patient can identify correctly the largest letter from a distance of 5 ft but not further away. An eye unable to read any letters is tested by the ability to count fingers. "CF at 2 ft" indicates that the eye was able to count fingers held 2 ft away but not farther away. If counting fingers is not possible, the eye may be able to detect a hand moving vertically or horizontally ("HM," or "hand motions" vision). The next lower level of vision would be the ability to perceive light ("LP," or "light perception"). An eye that is totally blind is recorded as having no light perception ("NLP").

Visual Field Testing

Visual field testing should be included in every complete ophthalmologic examination because even dense visual field abnormalities may not be apparent to the patient. Since the visual fields of the two eyes overlap, for diagnostic purposes, each eye must be tested separately. Binocular visual field testing is useful in assessment of functional vision (see Chapter 25).

Assessment of visual fields can be quickly achieved using **confrontation testing**. The patient is seated facing the examiner with one eye covered while the examiner closes the opposite eye (eg, the patient's left eye is covered and the examiner's right eye is closed so that the patient's right eye looks into the examiner's left eye). Presentation of targets at a distance halfway between the patient and the examiner allows direct comparison of the field of vision of each eye of the patient and the examiner. Since the patient and examiner are staring eye to eye, any loss of fixation by the patient will be noticed.

For gross assessment, the examiner briefly shows a number of fingers of one hand (usually one, two, or four fingers) peripherally in each of the four quadrants. The patient must identify the number of fingers flashed while maintaining straight-ahead fixation. The upper and lower temporal and the upper and lower nasal quadrants are all tested in this fashion for each eye.

A 5-mm-diameter red sphere or disk attached to a handle as the target allows detection and quantification of more subtle visual field defects, particularly if areas of abnormal reduction in color (desaturation) are sought.

In disease of the right cerebral hemisphere, particularly involving the parietal lobe, there may be **visual neglect** (visual inattention) in which there is no comparable visual field loss on testing of each eye separately, but objects are not identified in the left hemifield of either eye if objects are simultaneously presented in the right hemifield. The patient functions as if there is a left homonymous hemianopia. Visual neglect is detected by **simultaneous confrontation testing**. The examiner holds both hands out peripherally, one on each side. The patient, with both eyes open, is asked to signify on which side (right, left, or both) the examiner is intermittently wiggling his or her fingers. The patient will still be able to detect the fingers in the left hemifield when wiggled alone but not when the fingers in the right hemifield are wiggled simultaneously.

More sophisticated means of visual field testing, important for detection of subtle visual field loss, such as in the diagnosis of early glaucoma and for quantification of any visual field defect, are discussed later in this chapter.

PUPILS

Basic Examination

The pupils should be symmetric, and each one should be examined for size, shape (circular or irregular), and reactivity to both light and accommodation. Pupillary abnormalities may be due to (1) neurologic disease, (2) intraocular inflammation causing either spasm of the pupillary sphincter or adhesions of the iris to the lens (posterior synechiae), (3) markedly raised intraocular pressure causing atony of the pupillary sphincter, (4) prior surgical alteration, (5) the effect of systemic or eye medications, and (6) benign variations of normal.

To avoid accommodation, the patient is asked to fixate on a distant target as a penlight is directed toward each eye. Dim lighting conditions help to accentuate the pupillary response and may best demonstrate an abnormally small pupil. Likewise, an abnormally large pupil may be more apparent in brighter background illumination. The **direct response** to light refers to constriction of the illuminated pupil. The reaction may be graded as either brisk or sluggish. The **consensual response** is the normal simultaneous constriction of the opposite nonilluminated pupil. The neuroanatomy of the pupillary pathway is discussed in Chapter 14.

Swinging Penlight Test for Relative Afferent Pupillary Defect

As a light is swung back and forth in front of the two pupils, one can compare the reactions to stimulation of each eye, which should be equal. If the neural response to stimulation of the left eye is impaired, the pupil response in *both eyes* will be reduced on stimulation of the left eye compared to stimulation of the right eye. As the light is swung from the right to the left eye, both pupils will begin to dilate normally as the light is moved away from the right eye and then not constrict or paradoxically *widen* as the light is shone into the left eye (since the direct response in the left eye and the consensual response in the right eye are reduced compared to the consensual response in the left eye and direct response in the right eye from stimulation of the right eye). When the light is swung back to the right eye, both pupils will begin to dilate as the light is moved away from the left eye and then constrict normally as the light is shone into the right eye. This phenomenon is called a relative afferent pupillary defect. It is usually a sign of optic nerve disease but may occur in retinal disease. Importantly, it does not occur in media opacities such as corneal disease, cataract, and vitreous hemorrhage. Because the pupils are normal in size and may appear to react normally when each is stimulated alone, the swinging flashlight test is the only means of demonstrating a relative afferent pupillary defect. Also, because the pupils react equally, detection of a relative afferent pupillary defect requires inspection of only one pupil and can still be achieved when one pupil is structurally damaged or cannot be visualized, as in dense corneal opacity. Relative afferent pupillary defect is further discussed and illustrated in Chapter 14.

OCULAR MOTILITY

The objective of ocular motility testing is to evaluate the alignment of the eyes and their movements, both individually ("ductions") and in tandem ("versions"). A more complete discussion of ocular motility testing and eye movement abnormalities is presented in Chapters 12 and 14.

▶ Testing Alignment

Normal patients have binocular vision. Since each eye generates a visual image separate from and independent of that of the other eye, the brain must be able to fuse the two images in order to avoid "double vision." This is achieved by having each eye positioned so that both foveas are simultaneously fixating on the object of regard.

A simple test of binocular alignment is performed by having the patient look toward a penlight held several feet away. A pinpoint light reflection, or "reflex," should appear on each cornea and should be centered over each pupil if the two eyes are straight in their alignment. If the eye positions are convergent, such that one eye points inward ("esotropia"), the light reflex will appear temporal to the pupil in that eye. If the eyes are divergent, such that one eye points outward ("exotropia"), the light reflex will be located more nasally in that eye. This test can be used with infants.

The **cover test** (see Chapter 12) is a more accurate method of verifying normal ocular alignment. The test requires good vision in both eyes. The patient is asked to gaze at a distant target with both eyes open. If both eyes are fixating together on the target, covering one eye should not affect the position or continued fixation of the other eye.

To perform the test, the examiner suddenly covers one eye and carefully watches to see that the second eye does not move (indicating that it was fixating on the same target already). If the second eye was not identically aligned but was instead turned abnormally inward or outward, it could not have been simultaneously fixating on the target. Thus, it will have to quickly move to find the target once the previously fixating eye is covered. Fixation of each eye is tested in turn.

An abnormal cover test is expected in patients with diplopia. However, diplopia is not always present in many patients with long-standing ocular misalignment. When the test is abnormal, prism lenses of different power can be used to neutralize the refixation movement of the misaligned eye (prism cover test). In this way, the amount of eye deviation can be quantified based on the amount of prism power needed.

▶ Testing Extraocular Movements

The patient is asked to follow a target with both eyes as it is moved in each of the four cardinal directions of gaze. The examiner notes the speed, smoothness, range, and symmetry of movements and observes for unsteadiness of fixation (eg, nystagmus).

Impairment of eye movements can be due to neurologic problems (eg, cranial nerve palsy), primary extraocular muscular weakness (eg, myasthenia gravis), or mechanical constraints within the orbit limiting rotation of the globe (eg, orbital floor fracture with entrapment of the inferior rectus muscle). Deviation of ocular alignment that is the same amount in all directions of gaze is called "comitant." It is "incomitant" if the amount of deviation varies with the direction of gaze.

EXTERNAL EXAMINATION

Before studying the eye under magnification, a general external examination of the ocular adnexa (eyelids and periocular area) is performed. Skin lesions, growths, and inflammatory signs such as swelling, erythema, warmth, and tenderness are evaluated by gross inspection and palpation.

The positions of the eyelids are checked for abnormalities, such as ptosis or lid retraction. Asymmetry can be quantified by measuring the central width (in millimeters) of the "palpebral fissure"—the space between the upper and lower lid margins. Abnormal motor function of the lids, such as impairment of upper lid elevation or forceful lid closure, may be due to either neurologic or primary muscular abnormalities.

Malposition of the globe, such as proptosis, may occur in orbital disease. Palpation of the bony orbital rim and periocular soft tissue should always be done in instances of suspected orbital trauma, infection, or neoplasm. The general facial examination may contribute other pertinent information as well. Depending on the circumstances, checking for enlarged preauricular lymph nodes, sinus tenderness, temporal artery prominence, or skin or mucous membrane abnormalities may be diagnostically relevant.

SLITLAMP EXAMINATION

▶ Basic Slitlamp Biomicroscopy

The slitlamp (Figure 2–4) is a table-mounted binocular microscope with a special adjustable illumination source attached. A linear slit beam of incandescent light is projected onto the globe, illuminating an optical cross section of the eye (Figure 2–5). The angle of illumination can be varied along with the width, length, and intensity of the light beam. The magnification can be adjusted as well (normally 10× to 16× power). Since the slitlamp is a binocular microscope, the view is "stereoscopic," or three-dimensional.

The patient is seated while being examined, and the head is stabilized by an adjustable chin rest and forehead strap. Using the slitlamp alone, the anterior half of the globe—the "anterior segment"—can be visualized. Details of the lid margins and lashes, the palpebral and bulbar conjunctival surfaces, the tear film and cornea, the iris, and the aqueous can be studied. Through a dilated pupil, the crystalline lens and the anterior vitreous can be examined as well.

Because the slit beam of light provides an optical cross section of the eye, the precise anteroposterior location of abnormalities can be determined within each of the clear ocular structures (eg, cornea, lens, vitreous body). The highest magnification setting is sufficient to show the abnormal presence of cells within the aqueous, such as red or white blood cells or pigment granules. Aqueous turbidity, called "flare," resulting from increased protein concentration can be detected in the presence of intraocular inflammation. Normal aqueous is optically clear, without cells or flare.

▶ Adjunctive Slitlamp Techniques

The eye examination with the slitlamp is supplemented by the use of various techniques. Tonometry is discussed separately in a subsequent section.

A. Lid Eversion

Lid eversion, to examine the undersurface of the upper lid, can be performed either at the slitlamp or without the aid of that instrument. It should always be done if the presence of a superficial foreign body is suspected but not already identified (see Chapter 19). A semirigid plate of cartilage called the tarsus gives each lid its contour and shape. In the upper lid, the superior edge of the tarsus lies centrally about 8–9 mm above the lashes. On the undersurface of the lid, it is covered by the tarsal palpebral conjunctiva.

The patient is positioned and instructed to look down. The examiner gently grasps the upper lashes with the thumb and index finger of one hand while using the other hand to position an applicator handle just above the superior edge of the tarsus (Figure 2–6). The lid is everted by applying slight downward pressure with the applicator as the lash margin is simultaneously lifted. The patient continues to look down, and the lashes are held pinned to the skin overlying the superior orbital rim as the applicator is withdrawn. The tarsal conjunctiva is then examined under magnification. To undo eversion, the lid margin is gently stroked downward as the patient looks up.

B. Fluorescein Staining

Fluorescein is a specialized dye that stains the cornea and highlights any irregularities of its epithelial surface. Sterile paper strips containing fluorescein are wetted with sterile saline or local anesthetic and touched against the inner surface of the lower lid, instilling the yellowish dye into the tear film.

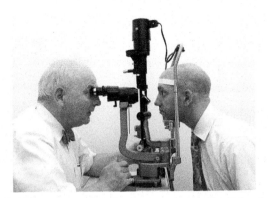

▲ **Figure 2–4. Slitlamp examination.** (Photo by Richard Leung and Matthew Richardson. Used with permission from King's College Hospital, London.)

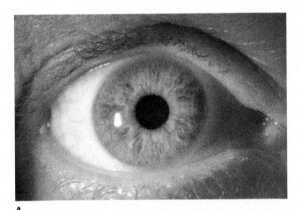

A

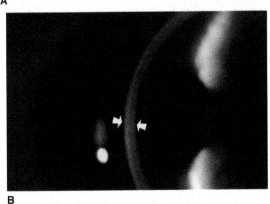

B

▲ **Figure 2–5. Slitlamp photographs of a normal right eye. A:** Diffuse illumination provides a detailed view of the lids, ocular surface, and iris. **B:** Slit beam illumination provides a cross-sectional view of the cornea (between the arrowheads) (also see Figure 6–10). (Photos by Richard Leung and Matthew Richardson. Used with permission from King's College Hospital, London.)

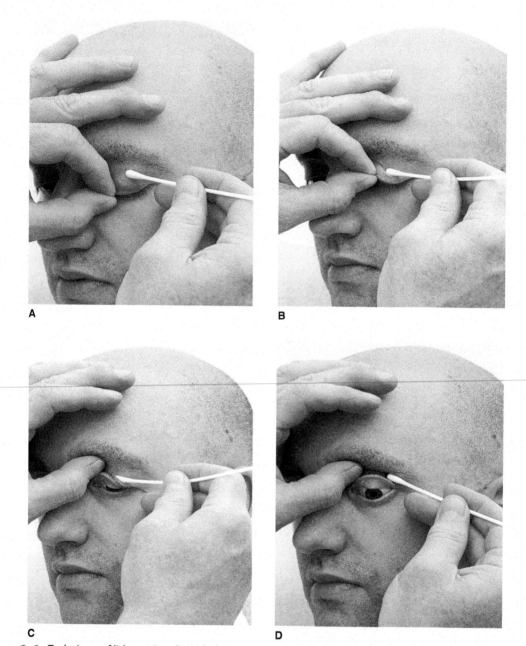

Figure 2–6. Technique of lid eversion. **A:** With the patient looking down, the upper lashes are grasped with one hand as an applicator stick is positioned at the superior edge of the upper tarsus (at the upper lid crease). **B** and **C:** As the lashes are lifted, slight downward pressure is simultaneously applied with the applicator stick. **D:** The thumb pins the lashes against the superior orbital rim, allowing examination of the undersurface of the tarsus. (Photos by Richard Leung and Matthew Richardson. Used with permission from King's College Hospital, London.)

The illuminating light of the slitlamp is made blue with a filter, causing the dye to fluoresce.

A uniform film of dye should cover the normal cornea. If the corneal surface is abnormal, excessive amounts of dye will absorb into or collect within the affected area. Abnormalities can range from tiny punctate dots, such as those resulting from excessive dryness or ultraviolet light damage, to large geographic defects in the epithelium, such as those seen in corneal abrasions or infectious ulcers.

C. Special Lenses

Special lenses enhance and further magnify slitlamp examination of the eye's interior.

Gonioscopy is examination of the anterior chamber angle that requires a goniolens (Figure 2-7). The Goldmann and Posner–Zeiss goniolenses have angled mirrors to provide a line of view parallel with the iris surface and peripherally into the junction between the iris and cornea, which cannot be viewed directly (see Chapter 21). Magnified details of the anterior chamber angle are viewed stereoscopically. By rotating the mirror, the entire 360° circumference of the angle can be examined. The same lens can be used to direct laser treatment toward the angle as therapy for glaucoma. The optics of the Koeppe lens allows a direct view of the anterior chamber angle.

The **Goldmann three-mirror lens** has two other mirrors besides the gonioscopy mirror. When the pupil is dilated, they allow examination and laser treatment of the mid-peripheral and far peripheral retina through 360°. The central portion of the lens allows examination of the vitreous and examination and laser treatment of the central retina.

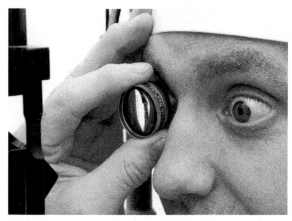

▲ **Figure 2–8.** Examination of the posterior segment with the slitlamp and Volk-style (indirect biomicroscopy) lens. (Photo by Richard Leung and Matthew Richardson. Used with permission from King's College Hospital, London.)

The stereoscopic and magnified view provides the optimal view of the macula and disk.

The patient's side of each of these contact lenses has a concavity designed to fit directly over the topically anesthetized cornea. If necessary, a clear, viscous solution of methylcellulose is placed in the concavity of the lens prior to insertion onto the patient's eye. This eliminates interference from optical interfaces, such as bubbles, and provides mild adhesion of the lens to the eye for stabilization.

The Volk-style (indirect biomicroscopy) range of lenses (Figure 2–8), with its wide variety of magnifications and fields of view, allows stereoscopic examination of the posterior segment of the eye without the need for contact with the globe.

TONOMETRY

The globe can be thought of as an enclosed compartment through which there is a constant circulation of aqueous humor. This fluid maintains the shape and a relatively uniform pressure within the globe. Tonometry is the method of measuring intraocular pressure using calibrated instruments. The normal range is 10–21 mm Hg. With any method of tonometry, care must be taken to avoid pressing on the globe, which artificially increases intraocular pressure.

▶ Applanation Tonometry

In **applanation tonometry**, intraocular pressure is determined by the force required to flatten the cornea. The higher the intraocular pressure, the greater is the force required.

The **Goldmann tonometer** (Figure 2-9) attaches to the slitlamp. Following topical anesthesia and instillation of fluorescein, the patient is positioned at the slitlamp and the

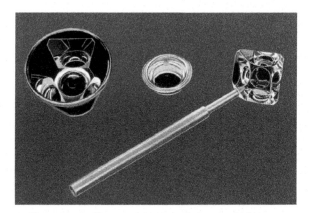

▲ **Figure 2–7.** Three types of goniolenses. **Left:** Goldmann three-mirror lens. Besides the goniomirror, there are also two peripheral retinal mirrors and a central fourth mirror for examining the central retina. **Center:** Koeppe lens. **Right:** Posner–Zeiss-type lens. (Photo used with permission from M. Narahara.)

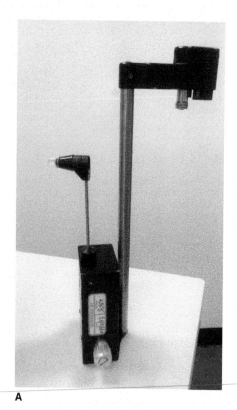

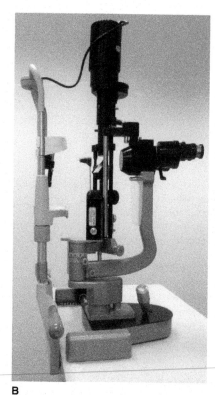

A

B

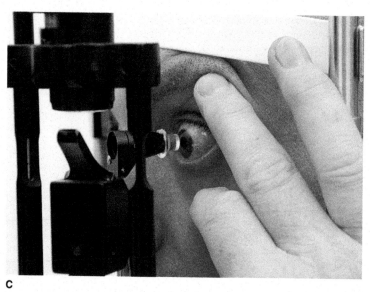

C

▲ **Figure 2–9.** Applanation tonometry. **A:** Goldmann tonometer. **B:** Tonometer attached to slitlamp. **C:** Applanating the cornea. (Photos by Richard Leung and Matthew Richardson. Used with permission from King's College Hospital, London.)

Dial reading greater than pressure of globe

Dial reading less than pressure of globe

Dial reading equals pressure of globe

▲ **Figure 2–10.** Appearance of fluorescein semicircles, or "mires," through the slitlamp ocular, showing the end point for applanation tonometry.

tonometer is swung into place. To visualize the fluorescein, the cobalt blue filter is used with the brightest illumination setting. After grossly aligning the tonometer in front of the cornea, the examiner looks through the slitlamp ocular just as the tip contacts the cornea. A manually controlled counterbalanced spring varies the force applied by the tonometer tip. Upon contact, the tonometer tip flattens the central cornea and produces a thin circular outline of fluorescein. A prism in the tip visually splits this circle into two semicircles that appear green while viewed through the slitlamp oculars. The tonometer force is adjusted manually until the two semicircles just overlap (Figure 2–10). This visual end point indicates that the cornea has been flattened by the set standard amount. The amount of force required to do this is translated by the scale into a pressure reading in millimeters of mercury.

Accuracy of intraocular pressure measurement is affected by central corneal thickness. The thinner the cornea, the more easily it is indented, but the calibration of tonometers generally assumes a cornea of standard thickness. If the cornea is relatively thin, the actual intraocular pressure is higher than the measured value, and if the cornea is relatively thick, the actual intraocular pressure is lower than the measured value. Thus ultrasonic measurement of corneal thickness (pachymetry) may be helpful in assessment of intraocular pressure. The **Pascal dynamic contour tonometer**, a contact but nonapplanating technique, measures intraocular pressure independent of corneal thickness.

Other applanation tonometers are the **Perkins tonometer**, a portable mechanical device with a mechanism similar to the Goldmann tonometer; the **Tono-Pen**, a portable electronic applanation tonometer that is reasonably accurate but requires daily recalibration; and the **pneumatotonometer**, which is particularly useful when the cornea has an irregular surface. The Perkins tonometer and Tono-Pen are commonly used when examination at the slitlamp is not feasible, for example, in emergency rooms in cases of orbital trauma with retrobulbar hemorrhage and in operating rooms during examinations under anesthesia. The **Schiotz tonometer** is a simple, relatively inexpensive, easily portable, hand-held instrument. It can be used in any clinic or emergency room setting, at the hospital bedside, or in the operating room,

but it requires greater expertise and uses preset weights that provide a discontinuous scale of measurement such that it is now rarely used.

All contact tonometers require topical anesthetic and disinfection of the instrument tip prior to use. (Tonometer disinfection techniques are discussed in Chapter 21.)

▶ **Noncontact Tonometry**

The **noncontact ("air-puff") tonometer** is not as accurate as applanation tonometers. A small puff of air is blown against the cornea. The air rebounding from the corneal surface hits a pressure-sensing membrane in the instrument. This method does not require anesthetic drops, since no instrument touches the eye. Thus, it can be more easily used by optometrists or technicians and is useful in screening programs.

DIAGNOSTIC MEDICATIONS

▶ **Topical Anesthetics**

Eye drops such as proparacaine, tetracaine, and benoxinate provide rapid-onset, short-acting topical anesthesia of the cornea and conjunctiva. They are used prior to ocular contact with diagnostic lenses and instruments such as the tonometer. Other diagnostic manipulations using topical anesthetics will be discussed later. These include corneal and conjunctival scrapings, lacrimal canalicular and punctal probing, and scleral depression.

▶ **Mydriatic (Dilating) Drops**

The pupil can be pharmacologically dilated by either stimulating the iris dilator muscle with a sympathomimetic agent (eg, 2.5% phenylephrine) or by inhibiting the sphincter muscle with an anticholinergic eye drop (eg, 0.5% or 1% tropicamide) (see Chapter 22). Anticholinergic medications also inhibit accommodation (cycloplegic). This may aid the process of refraction but causes further inconvenience for the patient. Therefore, drops with the shortest duration of action (usually several hours) are used for diagnostic applications. Combining drops from both pharmacologic classes produces the fastest onset (15–20 minutes) and widest dilation.

Because dilation can cause a small rise in intraocular pressure, tonometry should always be performed before these drops are instilled. There is also a small risk of precipitating an attack of acute angle-closure glaucoma if the patient has preexisting narrow anterior chamber angles (between the iris and cornea). Such an eye can be identified by oblique illumination with a penlight (see Chapter 11). Finally, excessive instillation of these drops should be avoided because of the systemic absorption that can occur through the nasopharyngeal mucous membranes following lacrimal drainage.

A more complete discussion of diagnostic drops is found in Chapter 22.

DIRECT OPHTHALMOSCOPY

▶ Instrumentation

The hand-held direct ophthalmoscope provides a monocular image, including a 15× magnified view of the fundus. Because of its portability and the detailed view of the disk and retinal vasculature it provides, direct ophthalmoscopy is a standard part of the general medical examination. The intensity, color, and spot size of the illuminating light can be adjusted, as well as the ophthalmoscope's point of focus. The latter is changed using a wheel of progressively higher-power lenses that the examiner dials into place. These lenses are sequentially arranged and numbered according to their power in diopters. Usually the (+) converging lenses are designated by black numbers and the (–) divergent lenses are designated by red numbers.

▶ Anterior Segment Examination

Using the high plus lenses, the direct ophthalmoscope can be focused to provide a magnified view of the conjunctiva, cornea, and iris. The slitlamp allows a far superior and more magnified examination of these areas, but it is not portable and may be unavailable.

▶ Red Reflex Examination

If the illuminating light is aligned directly along the visual axis, more obviously when the pupil is dilated, the pupillary aperture normally is filled by a homogeneous bright reddish-orange color. This **red reflex**, equivalent to the "red eye" effect of flash photography, is formed by reflection of the illuminating light by the fundus through the clear ocular media—the vitreous, lens, aqueous, and cornea. It is best observed by holding the ophthalmoscope at arm's length from the patient as he looks toward the illuminating light and dialing the lens wheel to focus the ophthalmoscope in the plane of the pupil.

Any opacity located along the central optical pathway will block all or part of the red reflex and appear as a dark spot or shadow. If a focal opacity is seen, have the patient look momentarily away and then back toward the light. If the opacity is still moving or floating, it is located within the vitreous (eg, small hemorrhage). If it is stationary, it is probably in the lens (eg, focal cataract) or on the cornea (eg, scar).

▶ Fundus Examination

The primary value of the direct ophthalmoscope is in examination of the fundus (Figure 2–11). The view may be impaired by cloudy ocular media, such as a cataract, or by a small pupil. Darkening the room usually causes enough

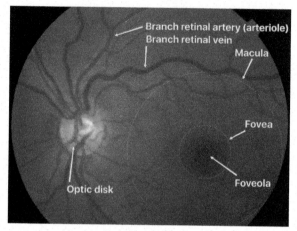

▲ **Figure 2–11.** Normal fundus. Note that the retinal vessels all stop short of and do not cross the fovea.

natural pupillary dilation to allow evaluation of the central fundus, including the disk, the macula, and the proximal retinal vasculature. Pharmacologically dilating the pupil greatly enhances the view and permits a more extensive examination of the peripheral retina.

Examination of the fundus is also optimized by holding the ophthalmoscope as close to the patient's pupil as possible (approximately 1–2 in), just as one can see more through a keyhole by getting as close to it as possible. This requires using the examiner's right eye and hand to examine the patient's right eye and the left eye and hand to examine the patient's left eye (Figure 2–12).

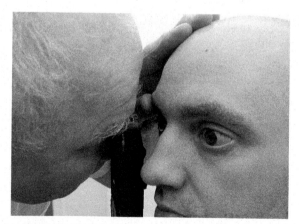

▲ **Figure 2–12.** Direct ophthalmoscopy. The examiner uses the right eye to evaluate the patient's right eye. (Photo by Richard Leung and Matthew Richardson. Used with permission from King's College Hospital, London.)

The spot size and color of the illuminating light can be varied. If the pupil is well dilated, the large spot size of light affords the widest area of illumination. With an undilated pupil, however, much of this light would be reflected back toward the examiner's eye by the patient's iris, interfering with the view, and the pupil will constrict. For this reason, the smaller spot size of light is usually better for undilated pupils.

The refractive error of the patient's and the examiner's eyes will determine the lens power needed to bring the fundus into optimal focus. If the examiner wears spectacles, they can be left either on or off. The patient's spectacles are usually left off, but it may be helpful to leave them on if there is high refractive error.

As the patient fixates on a distant target with the opposite eye, the examiner first brings retinal details into sharp focus. Since the retinal vessels all arise from the disk, the latter is located by following any major vascular branch back to this common origin. At this point, the ophthalmoscope beam will be aimed slightly nasal to the patient's line of vision, or "visual axis." One should study the shape, size, and color of the disk, the distinctness of its margins, and the size of the pale central "physiologic cup." The ratio of cup size to disk size is of diagnostic importance in glaucoma (Figures 2–13 and 2–14). Sizes and distances within the fundus are often measured in "disk diameters" (DD). (The typical optic disk is generally 1.5–2 mm in diameter.) Thus, one might describe a "1 DD area of hemorrhage located 2.5 DD inferotemporal to the fovea."

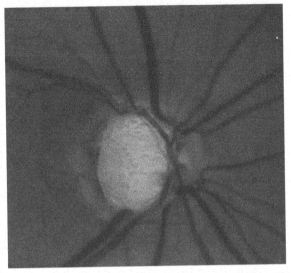

▲ **Figure 2–14.** Cup-to-disk ratio greater than 0.9 in end-stage glaucoma. The normal disk tissue is compressed into a peripheral thin rim surrounding a huge pale cup.

The fovea (Figure 2–11) is located approximately two DD temporal to the edge of the disk. A small pinpoint white reflection or "reflex" marks the central fovea. This is surrounded by a more darkly pigmented and poorly circumscribed area called the foveola. The retinal vascular branches

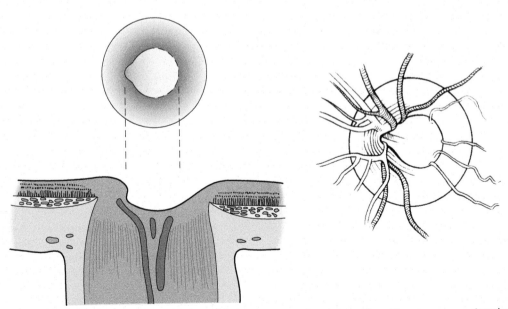

▲ **Figure 2–13.** Diagram of a moderately cupped disk viewed on end and in profile, with an accompanying sketch for the patient's record. The width of the central cup divided by the width of the disk is the "cup-to-disk ratio." The cup-to-disk ratio of this disk is approximately 0.5.

approach from all sides but stop short of the foveola. Thus, its location can be confirmed by the focal absence of retinal vessels or by asking the patient to stare directly into the light.

The major branch retinal vessels define the boundaries of the macula. They are examined and followed as far distally as possible in each of the four quadrants (superior, inferior, temporal, and nasal). The veins are darker and wider than their paired arteries (anatomically arterioles). The vessels are examined for color, tortuosity, and caliber, as well as for associated abnormalities, such as aneurysms, hemorrhages, or exudates. The green "red-free" filter assists in the examination of the retinal vasculature and the subtle striations of the nerve fiber layer as they course toward the disk (see Chapter 14).

To examine the retinal periphery, which is greatly enhanced by dilating the pupil, the patient is asked to look in the direction of the quadrant to be examined. Thus, the temporal retina of the right eye is seen when the patient looks to the right, while the superior retina is seen when the patient looks up. When the globe rotates, the retina and the cornea move in opposite directions. As the patient looks up, the superior retina rotates downward into the examiner's line of vision.

INDIRECT OPHTHALMOSCOPY

Instrumentation

The binocular indirect ophthalmoscope (Figure 2–15) complements and supplements the direct ophthalmoscopic examination. Since it requires wide pupillary dilation and is difficult to learn, this technique is used primarily by ophthalmologists. The patient can be examined while seated, but the supine position is preferable.

The indirect ophthalmoscope is worn on the examiner's head and allows binocular viewing through a set of lenses of fixed power. A bright adjustable light source attached to the headband is directed toward the patient's eye. As with direct ophthalmoscopy, the patient is told to look in the direction of the quadrant being examined. A convex lens is hand-held several inches from the patient's eye in precise orientation so as to simultaneously focus light onto the retina and an image of the retina in midair between the patient and the examiner. Using the preset head-mounted ophthalmoscope lenses, the examiner can then "focus on" and visualize this midair image of the retina.

Comparison of Indirect & Direct Ophthalmoscopy

Indirect ophthalmoscopy is so called because one is viewing an "image" of the retina formed by a hand-held "condensing lens." In contrast, direct ophthalmoscopy allows one to focus on the retina itself. Compared with the direct ophthalmoscope (15× magnification), indirect ophthalmoscopy provides a much wider field of view (Figure 2–16) with less

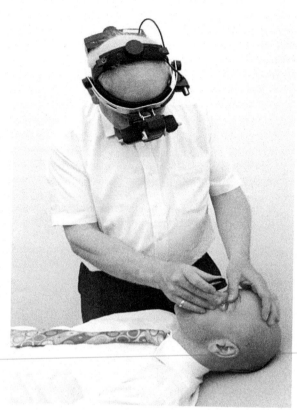

▲ **Figure 2–15.** Examination with head-mounted binocular indirect ophthalmoscope. A 20-diopter hand-held condensing lens is used. (Photo by Richard Leung and Matthew Richardson. Used with permission from King's College Hospital, London.)

overall magnification (approximately 3.5× using a standard 20-diopter hand-held condensing lens). Thus, it presents a wide panoramic fundus view from which specific areas can be selectively studied under higher magnification using either the direct ophthalmoscope or the slitlamp with special auxiliary lenses.

Indirect ophthalmoscopy has three distinct advantages over direct ophthalmoscopy. One is the brighter light source that permits much better visualization through cloudy media. A second advantage is that by using both eyes, the examiner enjoys a stereoscopic view, allowing visualization of elevated masses or retinal detachment in three dimensions. Finally, indirect ophthalmoscopy can be used to examine the entire retina, even out to its extreme periphery, the ora serrata. This is possible for two reasons. Optical distortions caused by looking through the peripheral lens and cornea interfere very little with the indirect ophthalmoscopic examination compared with the direct ophthalmoscope. In addition, the

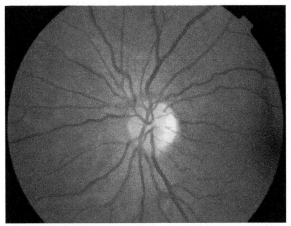

A

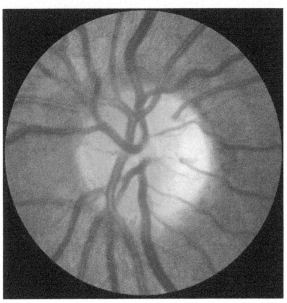

B

▲ **Figure 2–16.** Comparison of view within the same fundus using the indirect ophthalmoscope **(A)** and the direct ophthalmoscope **(B)**. The field of view with the latter is approximately 10°, compared with approximately 37° using the indirect ophthalmoscope.

adjunct technique of **scleral depression** (Figure 2–17) can be used to enhance examination of the peripheral retina. A smooth, thin metal probe is used to gently indent the globe externally through the lids at a point just behind the corneoscleral junction (limbus). As this is done, the ora serrata and peripheral retina are pushed internally into the examiner's line of view. By depressing around the entire circumference, the peripheral retina can be viewed in its entirety.

Because of all of these advantages, indirect ophthalmoscopy is used preoperatively and intraoperatively in the evaluation and surgical repair of retinal detachments. A disadvantage of indirect ophthalmoscopy, which also applies to the Volk-style of lenses for examination of the posterior segment with a slitlamp, is that it provides an inverted image of the fundus, which requires a mental adjustment on the examiner's part. Its brighter light source can also be more uncomfortable for the patient.

OPHTHALMIC EXAMINATION BY THE NONOPHTHALMOLOGIST

The preceding sequence of tests would compose a complete routine or diagnostic ophthalmologic evaluation. A general medical examination would often include many of these same testing techniques.

Assessment of pupils, extraocular movements, and confrontation visual fields is part of any complete neurologic assessment. Direct ophthalmoscopy should always be performed to assess the appearance of the disk and retinal vessels. Separately testing the visual acuity of each eye (particularly with children) may uncover either a refractive or a medical cause of decreased vision. The three most common preventable causes of permanent visual loss in developed nations are amblyopia, diabetic retinopathy, and glaucoma. All can remain asymptomatic while the opportunity for preventive measures is gradually lost. During this time, the pediatrician or general medical practitioner may be the only physician the patient visits.

By testing children for visual acuity in each eye, examining and referring diabetics for regular dilated fundus ophthalmoscopy, and referring patients with suspicious disks to the ophthalmologist, the nonophthalmologist may indeed be the one who truly "saves" that patient's eyesight. This represents both an important opportunity and responsibility for every primary care physician.

III. SPECIALIZED OPHTHALMOLOGIC EXAMINATIONS

This section will discuss ophthalmologic examination techniques with more specific indications that would not be performed on a routine basis. They will be grouped according to the function or anatomic area of primary interest.

DIAGNOSIS OF VISUAL ABNORMALITIES

1. PERIMETRY

Perimetry is used to examine the central and peripheral visual fields. Usually performed separately for each eye, it assesses the combined function of the retina, the optic nerve, and the intracranial visual pathway. It is used clinically to

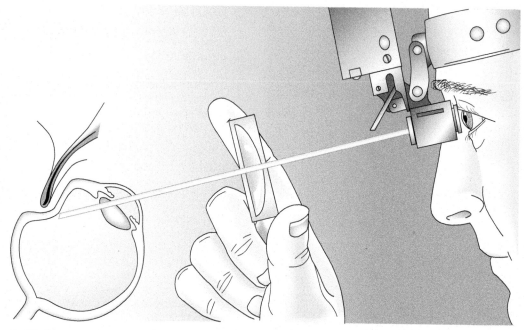

▲ **Figure 2–17.** Diagrammatic representation of indirect ophthalmoscopy with scleral depression to examine the far peripheral retina. Indentation of the sclera through the lids brings the peripheral edge of the retina into visual alignment with the dilated pupil, the hand-held condensing lens, and the head-mounted ophthalmoscope.

detect or monitor field loss due to disease at any of these locations. Damage to specific parts of the neurologic visual pathway may produce characteristic patterns of change on serial field examinations.

The visual field of the eye is measured and plotted in degrees of arc. Measurement of degrees of arc remains constant regardless of the distance from the eye that the field is checked. The sensitivity of vision is greatest in the center of the field (corresponding to the foveola) and least in the periphery. Perimetry relies on subjective patient responses, and the results will depend on the patient's psychomotor as well as visual status. Perimetry must always be performed and interpreted with this in mind.

▶ The Principles of Testing

Although perimetry is subjective, the methods discussed below have been standardized to maximize reproducibility and permit subsequent comparison. Perimetry requires (1) steady fixation and attention by the patient; (2) a set distance from the eye to the screen or testing device; (3) a uniform, standard amount of background illumination and contrast; (4) test targets of standard size and brightness; and (5) a universal protocol for administration of the test by examiners.

As the patient's eye fixates on a central target, test objects are randomly presented at different locations throughout the field. If they are seen, the patient responds either verbally or with a hand-held signaling device. Varying the target's size or brightness permits quantification of visual sensitivity of different areas in the field. The smaller or dimmer the target seen, the higher is the sensitivity of that location.

There are two basic methods of target presentation—static and kinetic—that can be used alone or in combination during an examination. In **static perimetry**, different locations throughout the field are tested one at a time. A dim stimulus, usually a white light, is first presented at a particular location. If it is not seen, the size or intensity is incrementally increased until it is just large enough or bright enough to be detected. This is called the "threshold" sensitivity level of that location. This sequence is repeated at a series of other locations, so that the sensitivity of multiple points in the field can be evaluated and combined to form a profile of the visual field.

In **kinetic perimetry**, the sensitivity of the entire field to one single test object (of fixed size and brightness) is first tested. The object is slowly moved toward the center from a peripheral area until it is first spotted. By moving the same object inward from multiple directions, a boundary called an "**isopter**" can be mapped out that is specific for that target. The isopter outlines the area within which the target can be seen and beyond which it cannot be seen. Thus, the larger the isopter, the better is the visual field of that eye. The boundaries of the isopter are measured and plotted in degrees of arc.

By repeating the test using objects of different size or brightness, multiple isopters can then be plotted for a given eye. The smaller or dimmer test objects will produce smaller isopters.

Methods of Perimetry

The **tangent screen** is the simplest apparatus for standardized perimetry. It uses different-sized pins on a black wand presented against a black screen and is used primarily to test the central 30° of visual field. The advantages of this method are its simplicity and rapidity, the possibility of changing the subject's distance from the screen, and the option of using any assortment of fixation and test objects, including different colors.

The more sophisticated **Goldmann perimeter** (Figure 2–18) is a hollow white spherical bowl positioned a set distance in front of the patient. A light of variable size and intensity can be presented by the examiner (seated behind the **perimeter**) in either static or kinetic fashion. This method can test the full limit of peripheral vision and was for years the primary method for plotting fields in glaucoma patients.

Computerized automated perimeters (Figure 2–19) now constitute the most sophisticated and sensitive equipment available for visual field testing. Using a bowl similar to the Goldmann perimeter, these instruments display test lights of varying brightness and size but use a quantitative static threshold testing format that is more precise and comprehensive

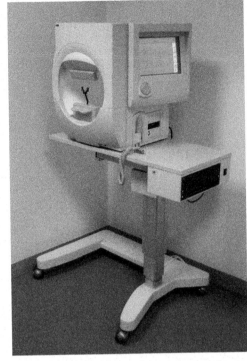

▲ **Figure 2–19.** Computerized automated perimeter.

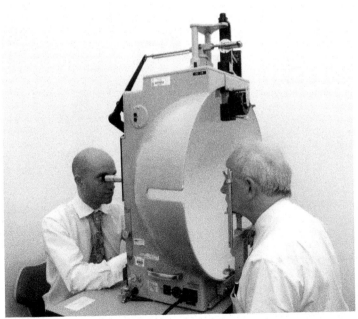

▲ **Figure 2–18.** Goldmann perimeter. (Photo by Richard Leung and Matthew Richardson. Used with permission from King's College Hospital, London.)

than other methods. Numerical scores (Figure 2–20) corresponding to the threshold sensitivity of each test location can be stored in the computer memory and compared statistically with results from previous examinations or from other normal patients. The higher the numerical score, the better is the visual sensitivity of that location in the field. Another important advantage is that the test presentation is programmed and automated, eliminating any variability on the part of the examiner. Analysis of the results provides information on whether visual field loss is diffuse or focal and on the patient's ability to perform the test reliably.

2. AMSLER GRID

The **Amsler grid** is used to test the central 20° × 20° of the visual field. The grid (Figure 2–21) is viewed by each eye separately at normal reading distance and with reading glasses on if the patient uses them. It is most commonly used to test macular function.

While fixating on the central dot, the patient checks to see that the lines are all straight, without distortion, and that no spots or portions of the grid are missing. One eye is compared with the other. A scotoma or blank area—either

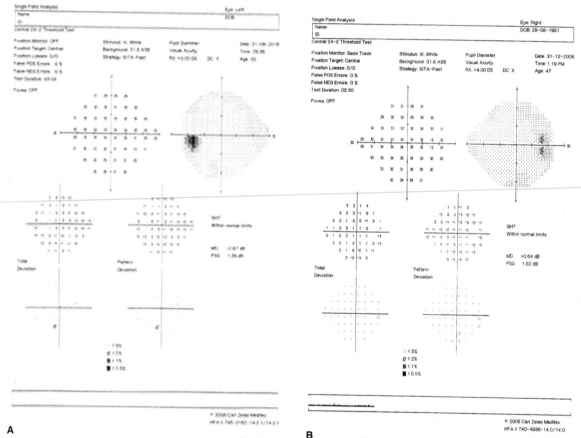

A

B

▲ **Figure 2–20.** Printouts of computerized static threshold perimetry of central 24° (radius). **A** and **B:** Normal left eye (**A**) and right eye (**B**). At the top are demographic data and test parameters including the power of any corrective lens. Each numerical plot is accompanied by a gray scale showing the probability of deviation from the normal range of the result at each test point; the darker the square, the greater is the deviation. The top field plot shows the threshold sensitivity in decibels at each of the test locations; the higher the number, the greater is the sensitivity. The lower field plots are comparisons with age-matched controls, with pattern deviation being derived from total deviation by removal of any generalized reduction such as due to cataract. Mean deviation (MD) and pattern standard deviation (PSD) are global measures of visual field abnormality. By various means, the computer determines the reliability of the test by measuring fixation, false positives, and false negatives. **C** and **D:** Advanced glaucoma with less marked abnormality in the left eye (**C**) than in the right eye (**D**). E and F: Right lower congruous homonymous hemianopia with similar abnormality in the left eye (**E**) and the right eye (**F**). (Used with permission from Carl Zeiss Meditec, Inc.)

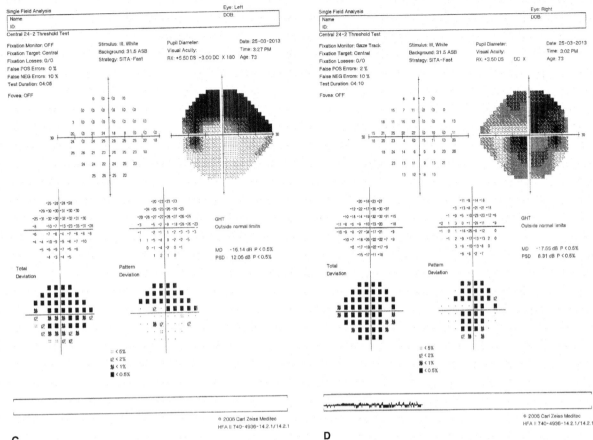

▲ Figure 2–20. (*Continued*)

central or paracentral—can indicate disease of the macula or optic nerve. Wavy distortion of the lines (metamorphopsia) can indicate macular edema or submacular fluid.

The grid can be used by patients at home to test their own central vision. For example, patients with age-related macular degeneration (see Chapter 10) can use the grid to monitor for sudden metamorphopsia. This often is the earliest symptom of acute fluid accumulation beneath the macula arising from leaking subretinal neovascularization. Because these abnormal vessels may respond to prompt treatment, early detection is important.

3. BRIGHTNESS ACUITY TESTING

The visual abilities of patients with media opacities may vary depending on conditions of lighting. For example, bright lights may cause disabling glare in patients with corneal edema or cataract due to light scattering.

Because the darkened examining room may not accurately elicit the patient's functional difficulties in real life,

instruments have been developed to test the effect of varying levels of brightness or glare on visual acuity. Distance acuity with the Snellen chart is usually tested under standard levels of incrementally increasing illumination, and the information may be helpful in making therapeutic or surgical decisions.

4. COLOR VISION TESTING

Normal color vision requires healthy function of the macula and optic nerve. The most common congenital abnormality is red-green color deficiency due to an X-linked abnormality of either the red or green retinal photoreceptors. It affects approximately 8% of males and less than 0.05% of females. Congenital blue-yellow color deficiency is caused by abnormality of the blue photoreceptors and is not sex-linked, occurring equally in less than 1% of males and females. Impaired color vision also occurs in acquired optic nerve and macular conditions. For example, in optic neuritis or optic nerve compression (eg, by a mass), red-green color

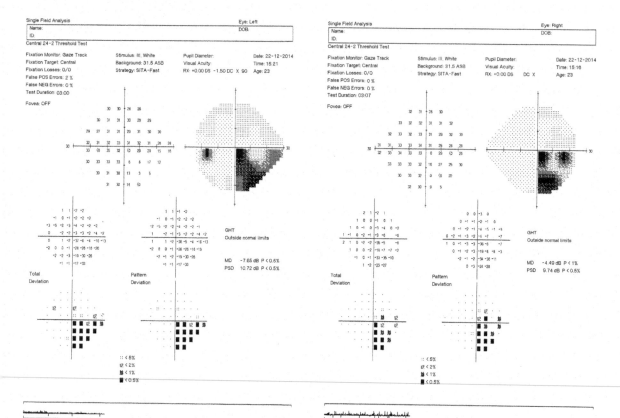

E   © 2006 Carl Zeiss Meditec   HFA II 740-4936-14.2.1/14.2.1

F   © 2006 Carl Zeiss Meditec   HFA II 740-4936-14.2.1/14.2.1

▲ **Figure 2–20.** *(Continued)*

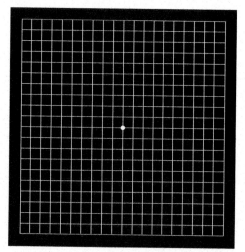

▲ **Figure 2–21.** Amsler grid. When viewed at the normal reading distance (28–30 cm), each square represents 1° × 1° field of vision.

deficiency is often an earlier indication of disease than visual acuity, which may still be 20/20. Other types of optic nerve disease such as glaucoma and macular disease tend to cause blue-yellow color deficiency.

The most common testing technique uses dots of the primary colors printed on a background mosaic of similar dots in a confusing variety of secondary colors. The primary dots are arranged in simple patterns (numbers, trails, or geometric shapes) that are interpreted incorrectly by patients with color deficiency. Examples are Ishihara (Figure 2–22) and Hardy-Rand-Rittler pseudoisochromatic plates (Figure 2–23), of which the former detect red-green and the latter detect red-green and blue-yellow color deficiency. The City University Color Vision Test (Figure 2–23) uses color comparison to test for red-green and blue-yellow color deficiency.

5. CONTRAST-SENSITIVITY TESTING

Contrast sensitivity is the ability of the eye to discern subtle degrees of contrast. Retinal and optic nerve disease and clouding of the ocular media (eg, cataracts) can impair this

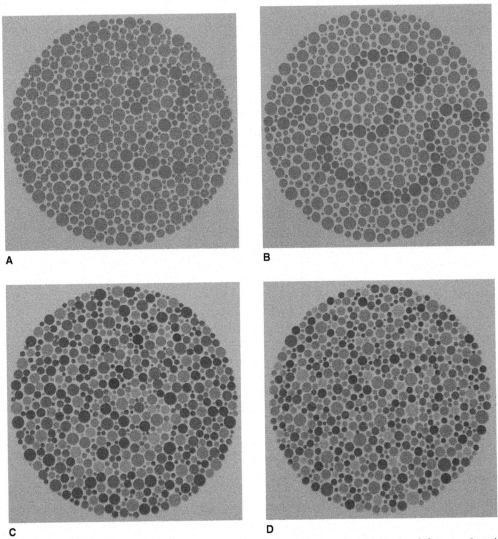

▲ **Figure 2–22.** Examples of Ishihara pseudoisochromatic plates that detect red-green color deficiency. **A** and **B:** Control plates that are interpreted correctly by all individuals unless visual acuity is severely reduced, cognition is impaired, or performance is unreliable. **C** and **D:** In red-green deficiency, the number is seen as 5 rather than 3 and the trail is not followed correctly. **E:** In red-green deficiency, the number is seen as 2 or 4. **F:** In red-green deficiency, 45 is seen, whereas no number is seen by individuals with normal color vision.

ability. Like color vision, contrast sensitivity may be reduced despite normal visual acuity.

Contrast sensitivity is best tested by using standard preprinted charts with a series of test targets (Figure 2–24). Since illumination greatly affects contrast, it must be standardized and checked with a light meter. Each separate target consists of a series of dark parallel lines in one of three different orientations. They are displayed against a lighter, contrasting gray background. As the contrast between the lines and their background is progressively reduced from one target to the next, it becomes more difficult for the patient to judge the orientation of the lines. The patient can be scored according to the lowest level of contrast at which the pattern of lines can still be discerned.

6. ASSESSING POTENTIAL VISION

When opacities of the cornea or lens coexist with disease of the macula or optic nerve, the visual potential of the eye may be difficult to determine by clinical examination.

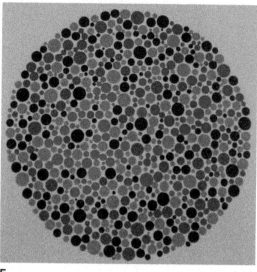

E

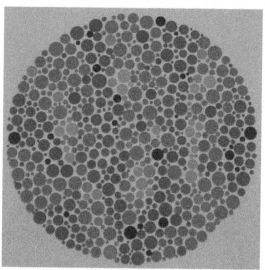

F

▲ Figure 2–22. (Continued)

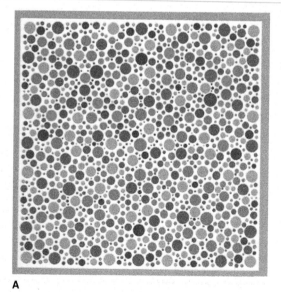

A

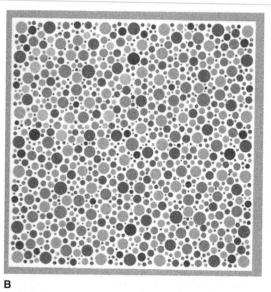

B

▲ Figure 2–23. Example plates of color vision tests that detect blue-yellow as well as red-green color deficiency. A–D: Hardy-Rand-Rittler pseudoischromatic plates have shapes that have to be identified and traced, with a demonstration plate (A), a screening plate (B), and plates that identify red-green deficiency (C) or blue-yellow deficiency (D). E and F: In the City University Color Vision Test, the individual identifies the peripheral disk most closely matching the central disk. With these example plates, normal individuals pick the right (C) and left (D) peripheral disks, whereas individuals with red-green color deficiency pick the left or bottom disk (A) and top or right disk (B) and individuals with blue-yellow-deficiency pick the top (C) and bottom (D) disks.

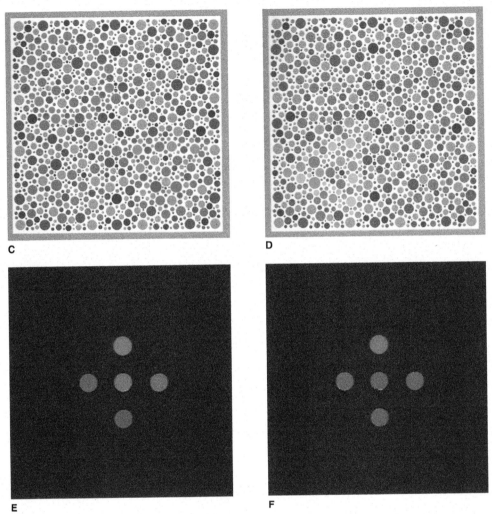

C   D

E   F

▲ **Figure 2–23.** (*Continued*)

The **potential acuity meter** projects a Snellen acuity chart through any relatively clear portion of the media (eg, through a less-dense region of a cataract) onto the retina. A limitation of this test is that false-positive and false-negative results do occur, depending on the type of disease present. Thus, these methods are helpful but not completely reliable.

7. TESTS FOR FUNCTIONAL VISUAL LOSS

The measurement of vision requires reliable responses by the patient, and the validity of a test may be affected by the alertness or cooperation of the patient. Functional, also known as nonorganic or medically unexplained, visual loss is impaired vision without any organic explanation whether or not it is purposeful (malingering).

Functional visual loss may be detected by inconsistent or contradictory performance on vision testing, such as tunnel visual field on testing with a tangent screen. The patient's visual field is plotted at the standard distance of 1 m. Typically there is a central area of intact vision beyond which even large object—such as a hand—are reported as not being seen. The visual field is retested at a distance of 2 m. The diameter of the visual field should be twice the diameter when tested at 1 m. If the patient reports an area of the same size or smaller when tested at 2 m compared to when tested at 1 m, functional visual loss is likely, but a number of conditions, such as advanced glaucoma, severe retinitis pigmentosa, and cortical blindness, need to be excluded. Testing of visual acuity at different distances also is helpful. Typically, in functional visual loss, the patient

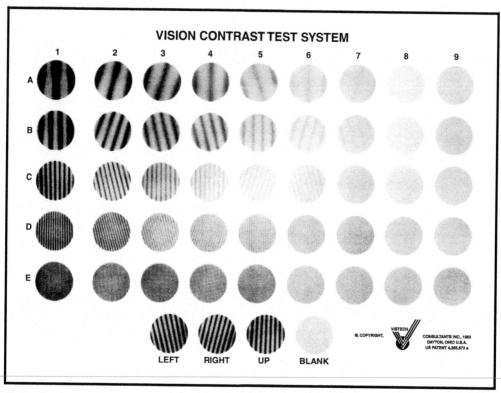

VISION CONTRAST TEST SYSTEM

LEFT   RIGHT   UP   BLANK

© COPYRIGHT, VISTECH CONSULTANTS INC., 1983 DAYTON, OHIO U.S.A. US PATENT 4,365,873 ∗

▲ **Figure 2–24.** Contrast-sensitivity test chart. (Used with permission from Vistech Consultants, Inc.)

reads correctly the same number of lines at each of the test distances, whereas more lines should be read correctly as testing distance is reduced whether vision is normal or reduced due to organic disease.

DIAGNOSIS OF OCULAR ABNORMALITIES

1. MICROBIOLOGY & CYTOLOGY

Like any mucous membrane, the conjunctiva can be cultured with swabs for the identification of bacterial infection. Specimens for cytologic examination are obtained by lightly scraping the palpebral conjunctiva (ie, lining the inner aspect of the lid), such as with a small platinum spatula, following topical anesthesia. For the cytologic evaluation of conjunctivitis, Giemsa's stain is used to identify the types of inflammatory cells present, while Gram's stain may demonstrate the presence (and type) of bacteria. These applications are discussed at length in Chapter 5.

The cornea is normally sterile. The base of any suspected infectious corneal ulcer should be scraped with the platinum spatula or other device for Gram staining and culture. This procedure is performed at the slitlamp. Because in many cases only trace quantities of bacteria are recoverable, the scrapings should be transferred directly onto culture plates without the

intervening use of transport media. Any amount of culture growth, no matter how scant, is considered significant, but many cases of infection may still be "culture-negative."

Culture of intraocular fluids is the standard method of diagnosing or ruling out bacterial endophthalmitis. Aqueous can be tapped by inserting a short 25-gauge needle on a tuberculin syringe through the limbus parallel to the iris. Care must be taken not to traumatize the lens. The diagnostic yield is better if vitreous is cultured. Vitreous specimens can be obtained by a needle tap through the pars plana or by doing a surgical vitrectomy. Polymerase chain reaction of vitreous samples has become the standard method of diagnosing viral retinitis. In the evaluation of noninfectious intraocular inflammation, cytology specimens are occasionally obtained using similar techniques.

2. TECHNIQUES FOR CORNEAL EXAMINATION

Several additional techniques are available for more specialized evaluation of the cornea. The **keratometer** is a calibrated instrument that measures the radius of curvature of the cornea in two meridians 90° apart. If the cornea is not perfectly spherical, the two radii will be different. This results in **corneal astigmatism**, which is quantified by the difference between the two radii of curvature. Keratometer measurements are used in contact lens fitting and for intraocular lens power calculations prior to cataract surgery.

Many corneal diseases result in distortion of the otherwise smooth surface of the cornea, which impairs its optical quality. The **photokeratoscope** is an instrument that assesses the uniformity and evenness of the surface by reflecting a pattern of concentric circles onto it. This pattern, which can be visualized and photographed through the instrument, should normally appear perfectly regular and uniform. Focal corneal irregularities will instead distort the circular patterns reflected from that particular area.

Computerized corneal topography is an advanced technique of mapping the anterior corneal surface. Whereas keratometry provides only a single corneal curvature measurement and photokeratoscopy provides only qualitative information, these computer systems combine and improve on the features of both. A real-time video camera records the concentric keratoscopic rings reflected from the cornea. A computer digitizes the data from thousands of locations across the corneal surface and displays the measurements in a color-coded map (Figure 2–25). This enables quantification and analysis of minute changes in shape and refractive power across the entire cornea due to disease or surgery. Wavefront aberrometry measures the quality of the eye's optics and may be combined together with corneal topography in a single instrument (Figure 2–25). By recording the path of diagnostic laser beams bouncing off of the retina, these devices can diagnose optical distortions called higher-order aberrations that are caused either by the cornea or the lens. Higher-order aberrations can result in blurred vision, halos, glare, and starbursts that are most symptomatic at night due to larger pupil size. These optical distortions are not corrected by eyeglasses.

The endothelium is a monolayer of cells lining the posterior corneal surface, which function as fluid pumps and are responsible for keeping the cornea thin and dehydrated, thereby maintaining its optical clarity. If these cells become impaired or depleted, corneal edema and thickening result, ultimately decreasing vision. The endothelial cells themselves can be photographed with a special slitlamp camera, enabling one to study cell morphology and perform cell counts. Central corneal thickness can be accurately measured with an ultrasonic pachymeter. These measurements are useful for monitoring increasing corneal thickness due to edema caused by progressive endothelial cell loss and, as discussed earlier, in determining the validity of intraocular pressure measurements obtained by applanation tonometry.

3. LACRIMAL SYSTEM EVALUATION

Evaluation of Tear Production

Tears and their components are produced by the lacrimal gland and accessory glands in the lid and conjunctiva (see Chapter 5). The **Schirmer test** is a simple method for assessing gross tear production. Schirmer strips are disposable 35-mm-length dry strips of filter paper. The tip of one end is folded at the preexisting notch so that it can drape over the lower lid margin just lateral to the cornea (Figure 2–26).

Tears in the conjunctival sac will cause progressive wetting of the paper strip. The distance between the leading edge of wetness and the initial fold can be measured after 5 minutes using a millimeter ruler. The ranges of normal measurements vary depending on whether topical anesthetic is used. Without anesthesia, irritation from the Schirmer strip itself will cause reflex tearing, thereby increasing the measurement. With anesthesia, less than 5 mm of wetting after 5 minutes is considered abnormal.

Significant degrees of chronic dryness cause surface changes in the exposed areas of the cornea and conjunctiva. **Fluorescein** will stain punctate areas of epithelial loss on the cornea. Another dye, **rose bengal**, is able to stain devitalized cells of the conjunctiva and cornea before they actually degenerate and drop off.

Evaluation of Lacrimal Drainage

The anatomy of the lacrimal drainage system is discussed in Chapters 1 and 4. The pumping action of the lids draws tears nasally into the upper and lower canalicular channels through the medially located "punctal" openings in each lid margin. After collecting in the lacrimal sac, the tears then drain into the nasopharynx via the nasolacrimal duct. Symptoms of watering are frequently due to increased tear production as a reflex response to some type of ocular irritation. However, the patency and function of the lacrimal drainage system must be checked in the evaluation of otherwise unexplained tearing.

The **Jones I** test evaluates whether the entire drainage system as a whole is functioning. Concentrated fluorescein dye is instilled into the conjunctival sac on the side of the suspected obstruction. After 5 minutes, a cotton Calgiswab is used to attempt to recover dye from beneath the inferior nasal turbinate. Alternatively, the patient blows his or her nose into a tissue, which is checked for the presence of dye. Recovery of any dye indicates that the drainage system is functioning.

The **Jones II** test is performed if no dye is recovered, indicating some abnormality of the system. Following topical anesthesia, a smooth-tipped metal probe is used to gently dilate one of the puncta (usually lower). A 3-mL syringe with sterile water or saline is prepared and attached to a special lacrimal irrigating cannula. This blunt-tipped cannula is used to gently intubate the lower canaliculus, and fluid is injected as the patient leans forward. With a patent drainage system, fluid should easily flow into the patient's nasopharynx without resistance.

If fluorescein can now be recovered from the nose following irrigation, a partial obstruction might have been present. Recovery of clear fluid without fluorescein, however, may indicate inability of the lids to initially pump dye into the lacrimal sac with an otherwise patent drainage apparatus. If

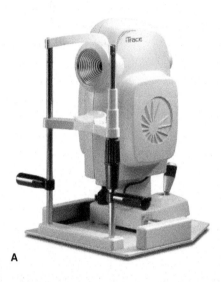

A

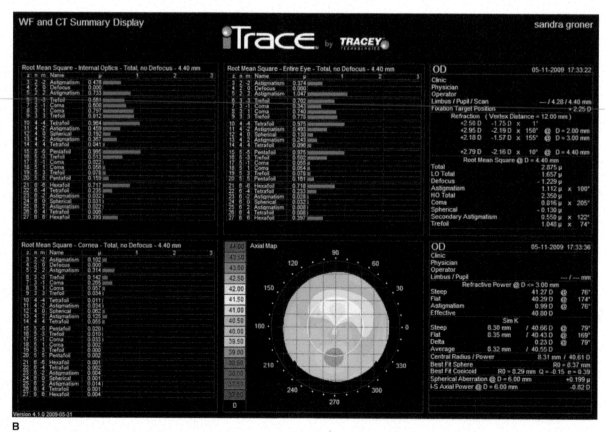

B

▲ Figure 2–25. **A:** Computerized corneal topography and wavefront aberrometry system. **B:** Color-coded corneal topographic display of curvature across the entire corneal surface, combined with quantitative measurements of higher-order aberrations from the total eye (top right), lens (top left), and cornea (bottom left). (Used with permission from Tracey Technologies, Inc.)

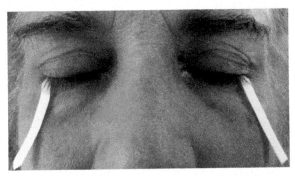

▲ **Figure 2–26.** Schirmer test with wetting of the filter strips.

no fluid can be irrigated through to the nasopharynx using the syringe, total occlusion is present. Finally, some drainage problems may be due to stenosis of the punctal lid opening, in which case the preparatory dilation may be therapeutic.

4. ORBITAL EVALUATION

▶ **Exophthalmometry**

A method is needed to measure the anteroposterior location of the globe with respect to the bony orbital rim. The lateral orbital rim is a discrete, easily palpable landmark and is used as the reference point. The Hertel exophthalmometer (Figure 2–27) is a hand-held instrument with two identical measuring devices (one for each eye), connected by a horizontal bar. The distance between the two devices can be varied by sliding one toward or away from the other, and each has a notch that fits over the edge of the corresponding lateral orbital rim. When properly aligned, an attached set of mirrors reflects a side image of each eye profiled alongside a measuring scale, calibrated in millimeters. The tip of the corneal image aligns with a scale reading representing its distance from the orbital rim.

The patient is seated facing the examiner. The distance between the two measuring devices is adjusted so that each aligns with and abuts against its corresponding orbital rim. To allow reproducibility for repeat measurements in the future, the distance between the two devices is recorded from an additional scale on the horizontal bar. Using the first mirror scale, the patient's right eye position is measured as it fixates on the examiner's left eye. The patient's left eye is measured while fixating on the examiner's right eye.

The distance from the cornea to the orbital rim typically ranges from 12 to 20 mm, and the two eye measurements are normally within 2 mm of each other. A greater distance is seen in exophthalmos, which can be unilateral or bilateral. This abnormal forward protrusion of the eye can be produced by any significant increase in orbital mass, because of the fixed size of the bony orbital cavity. Causes might include orbital hemorrhage, neoplasm, inflammation, or edema.

5. FUNDUS PHOTOGRAPHY

Special retinal cameras are used to document details of the fundus for study and future comparison. In the past, standard film was used for 35-mm color slides. Digital photography is now more common. As with any form of ophthalmoscopy, a dilated pupil and clear ocular media provide the most optimal view. All of the fundus photographs in this textbook were taken with such a camera.

One of the most common applications is disk photography, used in the evaluation for glaucoma. Since the slow progression

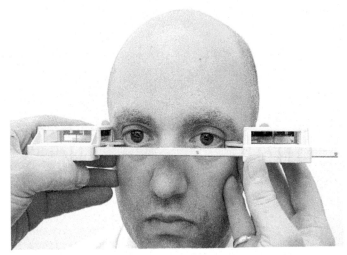

▲ **Figure 2–27. Hertel exophthalmometer.** (Photo by Richard Leung and Matthew Richardson. Used with permission from King's College Hospital, London.)

of glaucomatous optic nerve damage may be evident only by subtle alteration of the disk's appearance over time (see Chapter 11), precise documentation of its morphology is needed. By slightly shifting the camera angle on two consecutive shots, a "stereo" pair of slides can be produced that will provide a three-dimensional image when studied through a stereoscopic slide viewer. Stereo disk photography thus provides the most sensitive means of detecting increases in glaucomatous cupping.

6. FLUORESCEIN AND INDOCYANINE GREEN ANGIOGRAPHY

The capabilities of fundus photographic imaging are enhanced by fluorescein, a dye whose molecules emit green light when stimulated by blue light. The dye highlights vascular and anatomic details of the fundus, making **fluorescein angiography** invaluable in the diagnosis and evaluation of many retinal conditions. Because it can so precisely delineate areas of abnormality, it is an essential guide for planning laser treatment of retinal vascular disease.

Technique

The patient is seated in front of the retinal camera following pupillary dilation. After a small amount of fluorescein is injected into a vein in the arm, it circulates throughout the body before eventually being excreted by the kidneys. As the dye passes through the retinal and choroidal circulation, it can be visualized and photographed because of its properties of fluorescence. Two special filters within the camera produce this effect. A blue "**excitatory**" filter bombards the fluorescein molecules with blue light from the camera flash, causing them to emit a green light. The "**barrier**" filter allows only this emitted green light to reach the photographic film, blocking out all other wavelengths of light. A digital black and white photograph results, in which only the fluorescein image is seen.

Because the fluorescein molecules do not diffuse out of normal retinal vessels, the latter are highlighted photographically by the dye (Figure 2–28). The diffuse background "ground glass" appearance results from fluorescein filling of the separate underlying choroidal circulation. The choroidal and retinal circulations are anatomically separated by a thin, homogeneous monolayer of pigmented cell—the "retinal pigment epithelium." Denser pigmentation located in the macula obscures more of this background choroidal fluorescence, causing the darker central zone on the photograph. In contrast, focal atrophy of the pigment epithelium causes an abnormal increase in visibility of the background fluorescence (Figure 2–29).

Applications

A high-speed motorized frame advance allows for rapid sequence photography of the dye's transit through the retinal and choroidal circulations over time. A fluorescein study or "angiogram" therefore consists of multiple

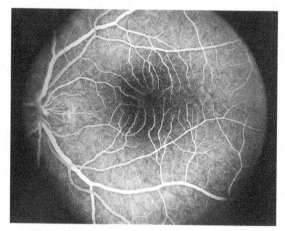

▲ **Figure 2–28.** Normal fluorescein angiogram of the central retina. The photo has been taken after the dye (appearing white) has already sequentially filled the choroidal circulation (seen as a diffuse, mottled, whitish background), the arterioles, and the veins. The macula appears dark due to heavier pigmentation, which obscures the underlying choroidal fluorescence that is visible everywhere else. (Used with permission from R. Griffith and T. King.)

sequential black and white photos of the fundi taken at different times following dye injection (Figure 2–30). Early-phase photos document the dye's initial rapid, sequential perfusion of the choroid, the retinal arteries, and the retinal

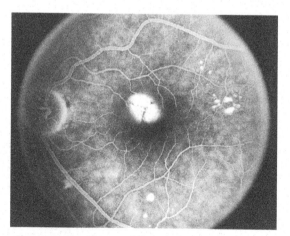

▲ **Figure 2–29.** Abnormal fluorescein angiogram in which dye-stained fluid originating from the choroid has pooled beneath the macula. This is one type of abnormality associated with age-related macular degeneration (see Chapter 10). Secondary atrophy of the overlying retinal pigment epithelium in this area causes heightened, unobscured visibility of this increased fluorescence. (Used with permission from R. Griffith and T. King.)

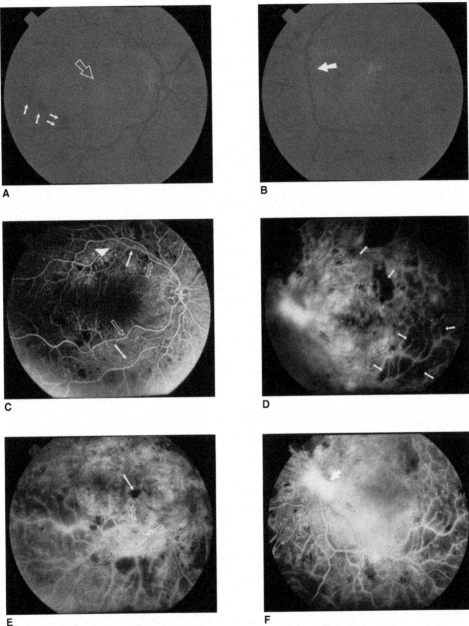

▲ **Figure 2–30.** Fluorescein angiogram of diabetic retinopathy. Fundus photographs (before fluorescein). **A:** Right eye showing poorly defined (edematous) macula **(unfilled arrow)** with scanty exudates and multiple large dark blot hemorrhages **(filled arrows)** suggesting retinal ischemia. **B:** Left eye neovascularization (abnormal new vessels) on the disk **(unfilled arrow)**. **C:** Right eye arteriovenous phase when fluorescein (seen as white) has filled the arterioles **(unfilled arrows)** and almost completely filled the veins **(filled arrows)**. The multiple hyperfluorescent spots **(arrowhead)** are microaneurysms. **D:** Left eye late phase showing extensive retinal nonperfusion (hypofluorescence) **(arrows)**. **E:** Right eye late phase showing enlargement of the foveal avascular (nonfluorescent) zone **(filled arrow)** and leakage of fluorescein (edema) in the surrounding retina **(unfilled arrows)**. **F:** Left eye later phase showing increasing leakage of fluorescein **(arrow)** from the new vessels on the optic disk. (Photos used with permission from St. Thomas' Hospital, London.)

veins. Later-phase photos may, for example, demonstrate the gradual, delayed leakage of dye from abnormal vessels. This extravascular dye-stained edema fluid will persist long after the intravascular fluorescein has exited the eye.

The dye delineates structural vascular alterations, such as aneurysms or neovascularization. Changes in blood flow such as ischemia and vascular occlusion are seen as an interruption of the normal perfusion pattern. Abnormal vascular permeability is seen as a leaking cloud of dye-stained edema fluid increasing over time. Hemorrhage does not stain with dye but rather appears as a dark, sharply demarcated void. This is due to blockage and obscuration of the underlying background fluorescence.

Indocyanine green angiography is superior for imaging the choroidal circulation, particularly when there is surrounding or overlying blood, exudate, or serous fluid. As opposed to fluorescein, indocyanine green is a larger molecule that binds completely to plasma proteins, causing it to remain in the choroidal vessels. Unique photochemical properties allow the dye to be transmitted better through melanin (eg, in the retinal pigment epithelium), blood, exudate, and serous fluid. This technique may serve as a useful adjunct to fluorescein angiography for imaging occult choroidal neovascularization.

7. OTHER IMAGING TECHNIQUES

Optical coherence tomography (OCT) is a computerized, cross-sectional tomographic imaging modality used to examine and measure intraocular structures in three dimensions. The operational principle of OCT is analogous to ultrasound, except that it uses 840-nm-wavelength light instead of sound. The OCT interferometer measures the echo delay time of light that is projected from a superluminescent diode and then reflected from different structures within the eye, so as to provide tomographic coronal sections perpendicular to the optical axis that are processed to provide a three-dimensional topographic image. Because the speed of light is nearly 1 million times faster than the speed of sound, OCT can image and measure structures on a 5-μm scale, compared to the 100-μm image resolution for ultrasound. OCT can be performed through an undilated pupil and, unlike ultrasound, does not require contact with the tissue examined. The instrumentation is similar to a fundus camera and is used in the office.

Posterior segment OCT enables detailed analysis of the optic disk, retinal nerve fiber layer, and macula. Microscopic changes in the macula, such as edema (Figure 2–31), can be imaged and measured. OCT angiography allows retinal and choroidal vascular imaging without intravenous dye injection. Imaging of the optic disk and the peripapillary retinal nerve fiber layer, with comparison to data from normal individuals and from prior examinations, facilitates early detection and monitoring of optic nerve damage (Figure 2–32). OCT changes often precede the appearance of visual field abnormalities and provide objective evidence of progression, with both features being particularly important in the management of glaucoma. Confocal **scanning laser tomography**, which analyzes reflections from a scanning laser beam at different tissue depths, provides similar information to optic disk and retinal nerve fiber layer OCT.

For the anterior segment, a different OCT instrument projecting a longer-wavelength infrared light beam (1300 nm) is used. This can provide high-resolution images and measurements of the cornea, iris, and intraocular devices and lenses.

Fundus autofluorescence depends on the autofluorescence of lipofuscin, which is a naturally occurring byproduct of phagocytosis of photoreceptor outer segments, but abnormalities of its distribution and concentration are useful indicators of retinal damage (Figure 2–33).

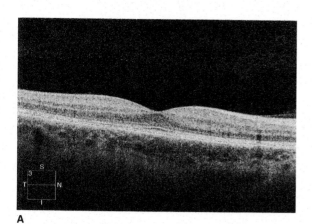
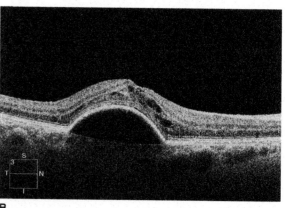

A   B

▲ **Figure 2–31.** Optical coherence tomography cross-section image of a normal macula **(A)** and a macula with pigment epithelial detachment showing fluid beneath the retinal pigment epithelium **(B)**. (Images taken with Cirrus Spectral Domain OCT, Carl Zeiss Meditec, Inc.)

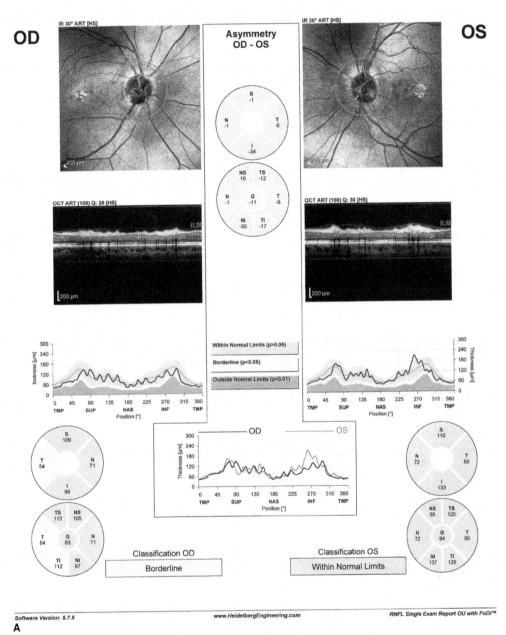

▲ **Figure 2–32.** Retinal nerve fiber layer optical coherence tomography scans showing borderline thinning in one eye **(A)**, predominantly temporal thinning in both eyes **(B)**, and global thinning in both eyes **(C)**. (Images taken with Spectralis OCT, Heidelberg Engineering Inc. Used with permission from Heidelberg Engineering Inc., Franklin, MA.)

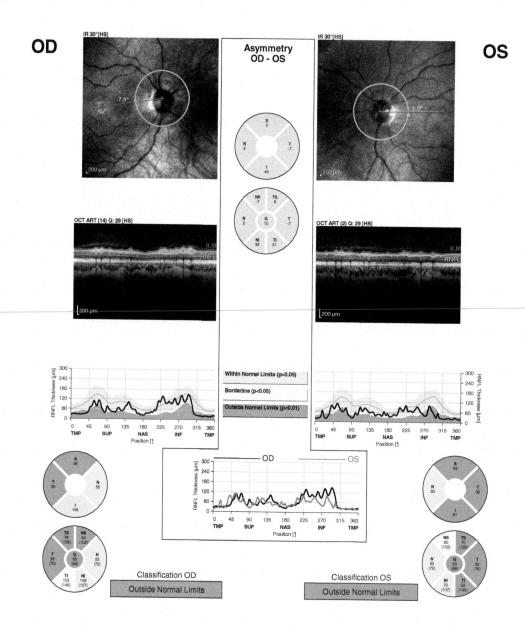

▲ **Figure 2–32.** (*Continued*)

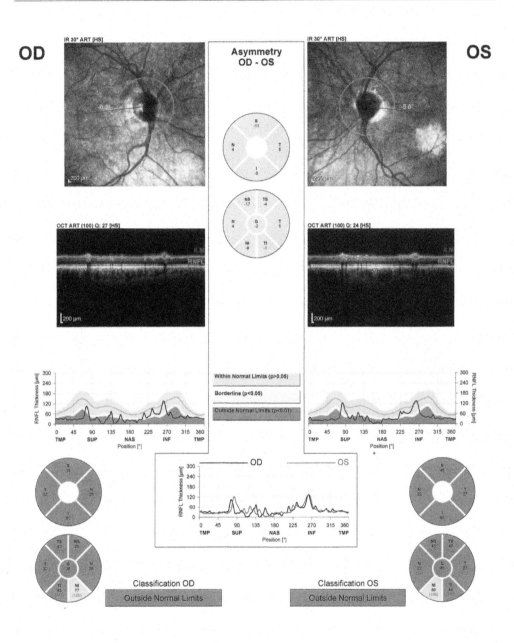

C

▲ **Figure 2–32.** (*Continued*)

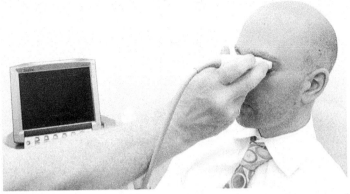

▲ **Figure 2–34.** Ultrasonography using B scan probe. The image will appear on the screen, visible in the background. (Photo by Richard Leung and Matthew Richardson. Used with permission from King's College Hospital, London.)

▶ Ultrasonography

Ultrasonography uses the principle of sonar to study structures that may not be directly visible. It can be used to evaluate either the globe or the orbit. High-frequency sound waves are emitted from a special transmitter toward the target tissue. As the sound waves bounce back off the various tissue components, they are collected by a receiver that amplifies and displays them on an oscilloscope screen.

A single probe that contains both the transmitter and receiver is placed against the eye and used to aim the beam of sound (Figure 2–34). Various structures in its path will reflect separate echoes (which arrive at different times) back toward the probe. Those derived from the most distal structures arrive last, having traveled the farthest.

There are two methods of clinical ultrasonography: A scan and B scan. In **A scan ultrasonography**, the sound beam is aimed in a straight line. Each returning echo is displayed as a spike whose amplitude is dependent on the density of the reflecting tissue. The spikes are arranged in temporal sequence, with the latency of each signal's arrival correlating with that structure's distance from the probe (Figure 2–35). If the same probe is now swept across the eye, a continuous series of individual A scans is obtained. From spatial summation of these multiple linear scans, a two-dimensional image, or **B scan**, can be constructed.

Both A and B scans can be used to image and differentiate orbital disease or intraocular anatomy concealed by opaque media. In addition to defining the size and location of intraocular and orbital masses, A and B scans can provide

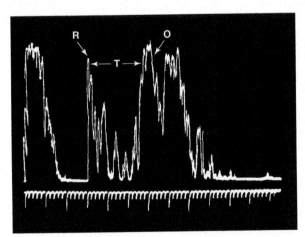

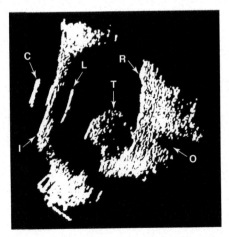

▲ **Figure 2–35.** Ultrasonography: A scan **(left)** and B scan **(right)** of an intraocular tumor (melanoma). C = cornea; I = iris; L = posterior lens surface; O = optic nerve; R = retina; T = tumor. (Used with permission from R.D. Stone.)

clues to the tissue characteristics of a lesion (eg, solid, cystic, vascular, calcified).

For purposes of measurement, the A scan is the most accurate method. Sound echoes reflected from two separate locations will reach the probe at different times. This temporal separation can be used to calculate the distance between the points, based on the speed of sound in the tissue medium. The most commonly used ocular measurement is the axial length (cornea to retina). This is important in cataract surgery in order to calculate the power for an intraocular lens implant. A scan can also be used to quantify tumor size and monitor growth over time.

The application of pulsed ultrasound and spectral Doppler techniques to orbital ultrasonography provides information on the orbital vasculature. It is certainly possible to determine the direction of flow in the ophthalmic artery and the ophthalmic veins and reversal of flow in these vessels occurring in internal carotid artery occlusion and carotid-cavernous fistula, respectively. As yet, the value of measuring flow velocities in various vessels, including the posterior ciliary arteries, without being able to measure blood vessel diameter is not fully established.

Ophthalmic Radiology (X-Ray, Computed Tomography, Magnetic Resonance Imaging)

Computed tomography (CT) and magnetic resonance imaging (MRI) scans and, to a much lesser extent, plain x-rays are vital to the evaluation of **orbital** and **intracranial** conditions (see Chapters 13 and 14). For orbital disease, CT can be as or more informative than MRI particularly for bony abnormalities and is quicker and more easily accessed. MRI does not expose the patient to ionizing radiation and is particularly useful for intracranial and intrinsic optic nerve disease especially due to inflammation or neoplasia.

The **intraocular** applications of radiology are primarily in the detection of foreign bodies following trauma and the demonstration of intraocular calcium in tumors such as retinoblastoma. CT scan is useful for foreign body localization because of its multidimensional reformatting capabilities and its ability to image the ocular walls. MRI is contraindicated if a metallic foreign body is suspected.

8. ELECTROPHYSIOLOGY

Physiologically, "vision" results from a series of electrical signals initiated in the retina and ending in the occipital cortex. Electroretinography, electro-oculography, and visual evoked response testing are methods of evaluating the performance of the neural circuitry.

Electroretinography & Electro-Oculography

Electroretinography (ERG) measures the electrical response of the retina to flashes of light, the **flash electroretinogram**, or to a reversing checkerboard stimulus, the **pattern ERG (PERG)**. The recording electrode is placed on the surface of the eye, and a reference electrode is placed on the skin of the face. The amplitude of the electrical signal is less than 1 mV, and amplification of the signal and computer averaging of the response to repeated trials are thus necessary to achieve reliable results.

The flash ERG has two major components: the "a wave" and the "b wave." An early receptor potential preceding the "a wave" and oscillatory potentials superimposed on the "b wave" may be recorded under certain circumstances. The early part of the flash ERG reflects photoreceptor function, whereas the later response particularly reflects the function of the Müller cells, which are glial cells within the retina. Varying the intensity, wavelength, and frequency of the light stimulus and recording under conditions of light or dark adaptation modulates the waveform of the flash ERG and allows examination of rod and cone photoreceptor function. The flash ERG is a diffuse response from the whole retina and is thus sensitive only to widespread, generalized diseases of the retina, eg, inherited retinal degenerations (retinitis pigmentosa), in which flash ERG abnormalities precede visual loss; congenital retinal dystrophies, in which flash ERG abnormalities may precede ophthalmoscopic abnormalities; and toxic retinopathies from drugs or chemicals (eg, iron intraocular foreign bodies). It is not sensitive to focal retinal disease, even when the macula is affected, and is not sensitive to abnormalities of the retinal ganglion cell layer, such as in optic nerve disease.

The PERG also has two major components: a positive wave at about 50 ms (P50) and a negative wave at about 95 ms (N95) from the time of the pattern reversal. The P50 reflects macular retinal function, whereas the N95 appears to reflect ganglion cell function. Thus, the PERG is useful in distinguishing retinal and optic nerve dysfunction and in diagnosing macular disease.

Electro-oculography (EOG) measures the standing corneoretinal potential. Electrodes are placed at the medial and lateral canthi to record the changes in electrical potential while the patient performs horizontal eye movements. The amplitude of the corneoretinal potential is least in the dark and maximal in the light. The ratio of the maximum potential in the light to the minimum in the dark is known as the **Arden index**. Abnormalities of the EOG principally occur in diseases diffusely affecting the retinal pigment epithelium and the photoreceptors and often parallel abnormalities of the flash ERG. Certain diseases, such as Best's vitelli-form dystrophy, produce a normal ERG but a characteristically abnormal EOG. EOG is also used to record eye movements.

Visual Evoked Response

Like electroretinography, the visual evoked response (VER) measures the electrical potential resulting from a visual stimulus. However, because it is measured by scalp electrodes placed over the occipital cortex, the entire visual pathway from retina to cortex must be intact in order to produce a

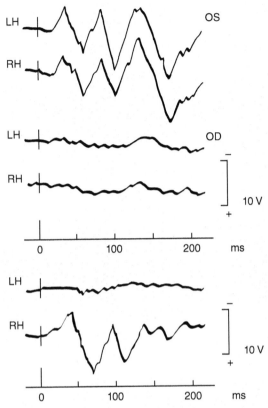

Figure 2–36. Top: Normal VER generated by stimulating the left eye (OS) is contrasted with the absent response from the right eye (OD), which has a severe optic nerve lesion. LH and RH signify recordings from electrodes over the left and right hemispheres of the occipital lobe. **Bottom:** VER with right homonymous hemianopia. No response is recorded from over the left hemisphere. (Used with permission from M. Feinsod.)

normal electrical waveform reading. Like the ERG wave, the VER pattern is plotted on a scale displaying both amplitude and latency (Figure 2–36).

Interruption of neuronal conduction by a lesion will result in reduced amplitude of the VER. Reduced speed of conduction, such as with demyelination, abnormally prolongs the latency of the VER. Unilateral prechiasmatic (retinal or optic nerve) disease can be diagnosed by stimulating each eye separately and comparing the responses. Postchiasmatic disease (eg, homonymous hemianopia) can be identified by comparing the electrode responses measured separately over each hemisphere.

Proportionately, the majority of the occipital lobe area is devoted to the macula. This large cortical area representing the macula is also in close proximity to the scalp electrode, so that the clinically measured VER is primarily a response generated by the macula and optic nerve. Thus the VER can be used to assess visual acuity, making it a valuable objective test in situations where subjective testing is unreliable, such as in infants, unresponsive individuals, and suspected malingerers.

9. DARK ADAPTATION

In going from conditions of bright light to darkness, a certain period of time must pass before the retina regains its maximal sensitivity to low amounts of light. This phenomenon is called dark adaptation. It can be quantified by measuring the recovery of retinal sensitivity to low-light levels over time following a standard period of bright-light exposure. Dark adaptation is often abnormal in retinal diseases characterized by rod photoreceptor dysfunction and impaired night vision.

REFERENCES

Alward WLM: Gonisocopy. Available at: http://www.gonioscopy.org/.
Barton JJS et al: *Field of Vision. A Manual and Atlas of Perimetry.* Humana Press, 2003.
Blomquist PH et al: *Practical Ophthalmology: A Manual for Beginning Residents,* 7th ed. American Academy of Ophthalmology, 2015.
Cavas-Martínez F et al: Corneal topography in keratoconus: State of the art. Eye Vis (Lond) 2016;3:5. [PMID: 26904709]
DiBernardo CW et al: *Ophthalmic Ultrasound: A Diagnostic Atlas,* 2nd ed. Thieme, 2006.
Dithmar S et al. *Fluorescence Angiography in Ophthalmology.* Springer Medizin Verlag, 2008.
Fairbanks A et al: Ocular Ultrasound: A Quick Reference Guide for the On-Call Physician, 2016. Available at: http://www.EyeRounds.org/tutorials/ultrasound/.
Faschinger C et al. *Gonioscopy.* Springer-Verlag, 2012.
Girach A et al: *Optical Coherence Tomography.* Springer, 2016.
Givre SJ et al: *Ancillary Testing in Neuro-ophthalmology (Focal Points 2015 Module).* American Academy of Ophthalmology, 2015.
Goins KM et al: *Imaging the Anterior Segment.* Vol 27, No. 11, in: *Focal Points 2009. Clinical Modules for Ophthalmologists.* American Academy of Ophthalmology, 2009.
Gundogan FC et al: Pattern visual evoked potentials in the assessment of visual acuity in malingering. Ophthalmology 2007;114: 2332. [PMID: 17618689]
Harrie RP et al: *Clinical Ophthalmic Echography,* 2nd ed. Springer, 2014.
Holder GE et al: Electrodiagnostic assessment in optic nerve disease. Curr Opin Neurol 2009;22:3. [PMID: 19155758]
Hoyt CS et al: *How to Examine the Eye of the Neonate.* Vol 7, Module 1, in: *Focal Points 1989: Clinical Modules for Ophthalmologists.* American Academy of Ophthalmology, 1989.
Huang D et al: *Retinal Imaging.* Mosby, 2006.
Kim JD et al: Neuroimaging in ophthalmology. Saudi J Ophthalmol 2012;26:401. [PMID: 23961025]
Krachmer J et al: *Cornea Atlas.* Saunders, 2013.
Lee MS: *Diplopia: Diagnosis and Management.* Vol 25, No. 12, in: *Focal Points 2007. Clinical Modules for Ophthalmologists.* American Academy of Ophthalmology, 2007.
Lin SC et al: Optic nerve head and retinal nerve fiber layer analysis: A report by the American Academy of Ophthalmology. Ophthalmology 2007;114:1937. [PMID: 17908595]

Lumbroso B et al: *Practical Handbook of Fluorescein Angiography*. Jaypee Brothers Medical Publishers Ltd., 2014.

Ly A et al: Fundus autofluorescence in age-related macular degeneration. Optom Vis Sci 2017;94:246. [PMID: 27668639]

McBain VA et al: Assessment of patients with suspected non-organic visual loss using pattern appearance visual evoked potentials. Graefes Arch Clin Exp Ophthalmol 2007;245:502. [PMID: 17111152]

Miller BW: A review of practical tests for ocular malingering and hysteria. Surv Ophthalmol 1973;17:241. [PMID: 4802377]

Miller NR: Functional neuro-ophthalmology. Handb Clin Neurol 2011;102:493. [PMID: 21601078]

Newman SA: *Automated Perimetry in Neuro-Ophthalmology*. Vol 13, No. 6, in: *Focal Points 1995: Clinical Modules for Ophthalmologists*. American Academy of Ophthalmology, 1995.

Odom JV et al: ISCEV standard for clinical visual evoked potentials: 2016 update. Doc Ophthalmol 2016;133:1. [PMID: 27443562]

Parmar H et al: A "first cut" at interpreting brain MRI signal intensities: What's white, what's black, and what's gray. J Neuro-Ophthalmol 2010;30:91. [PMID: 20182216]

Puech B et al. *Inherited Chorioretinal Dystrophies: A Textbook and Atlas*. Springer-Verlag, 2014.

Rosenthal ML et al: The technique of binocular indirect ophthalmoscopy. Highlights Ophthalmol 1966;9:179. (Reprinted as Appendix in: Hilton GF et al: *Retinal Detachment*, 2nd ed. American Academy of Ophthalmology, 1995.)

Schuman JS et al: *Optical Coherence Tomography of Ocular Diseases*, 3rd ed. Slack, 2013.

Schwartz GS: *The Eye Exam: A Complete Guide*. Slack, 2006.

Skalicky SE: *Ocular and Visual Physiology: Clinical Application*. Springer, 2016.

Stein HA et al: *The Ophthalmic Assistant: A Guide for Ophthalmic Medical Personnel*, 9th ed. Saunders, 2012.

Steinert RF et al: *Anterior Segment Optical Coherence Tomography*. Slack, 2008.

Thompson HS et al: *Clinical Importance of Pupillary Inequality*. Vol 10, No. 10, in: *Focal Points 1992: Clinical Modules for Ophthalmologists*. American Academy of Ophthalmology, 1992.

Wang M: *Corneal Topography in the Wavefront Era: A Guide for Clinical Application*, 2nd ed. Slack, 2011.

Yap GH et al: Clinical value of electrophysiology in determining the diagnosis of visual dysfunction in neuro-ophthalmology patients. Doc Ophthalmol 2015;131:189. [PMID: 26471028]

Young B et al: Current electrophysiology in ophthalmology: A review. Curr Opin Ophthalmol 2012;23:497. [PMID: 23047167]

Ophthalmic Emergencies

3

Paul Riordan-Eva, FRCOphth

INTRODUCTION

Prompt recognition and treatment of ophthalmic emergencies are crucial to prevention of unnecessary visual impairment. Using simple guidelines, patients requiring emergency or urgent ophthalmologic evaluation can be identified. Intensity and duration of pain, rapidity of onset and severity of visual loss (primarily assessed by visual acuity, which should be measured for each eye in all patients presenting with ophthalmic emergencies), gross appearance of the globe, and abnormalities on ophthalmoscopy are particularly important parameters.

Excluding ocular and orbital trauma, which is covered in Chapter 19, this chapter reviews the common ophthalmic emergencies, for the most part grouped according to the predominant symptom. For each group, the section on triage highlights the features that are crucial during initial assessment such as on presentation to an emergency department. The section on clinical assessment emphasizes what is important during ophthalmologic evaluation. The management of the more common or important entities is then briefly discussed, principally to provide reference to discussion in other chapters.

ACUTE RED EYE

The majority of patients with acute red eye have a relatively benign condition, such as bacterial, viral, or allergic conjunctivitis, subconjunctival hemorrhage, or blepharitis, which poses little or no threat to vision. Conversely a few are at risk of rapid progression within a few hours or days to severe visual impairment, even blindness, such as from acute angle-closure glaucoma, intraocular infection (endophthalmitis), bacterial, viral, amebic, or fungal corneal infection, acute uveitis, or scleritis.

▶ Triage

(See Differential Diagnosis of Common Causes of the Inflamed Eye on Inside Front Cover)

Emergency or urgent ophthalmologic evaluation should be arranged for any patient with acute red eye and a history within the past few weeks of intraocular surgery, which predisposes to endophthalmitis; contact lens wear, which predisposes to corneal infection; recent or distant history of corneal transplantation because of the possibility of graft rejection; previous episodes of acute uveitis or scleritis; or systemic diseases predisposing to uveitis or scleritis, such as ankylosing spondylitis and rheumatoid arthritis. In acutely ill patients, particularly those with sepsis or requiring prolonged intravenous cannulation such as in intensive therapy units or for parenteral nutrition, an acute red eye may be due to bacterial or fungal endophthalmitis. Ocular involvement in toxic epidermal necrolysis, Stevens-Johnson syndrome, or erythema multiforme requires urgent ophthalmologic assessment.

Pain, rather than discomfort, should be regarded as inconsistent with conjunctivitis, episcleritis, or blepharitis. It is suggestive of keratitis, intraocular or scleral inflammation, or raised intraocular pressure, with the likelihood of a serious cause increasing with increasing severity. Associated nausea and vomiting are particularly suggestive of markedly raised intraocular pressure. Deep, boring pain, typically waking the patient at night, is characteristic of scleritis. Photophobia characteristically occurs in keratitis and anterior uveitis.

Reduced vision, whether reported by the patient or identified by measurement of visual acuity, in the absence of a pre-existing explanation, should also be regarded as inconsistent with conjunctivitis, episcleritis, or blepharitis, and as with pain, the greater the severity, the greater is the likelihood of a serious cause.

Severity of redness is not necessarily a guide to the seriousness of the underlying condition for example, despite its bright red appearance, subconjunctival hemorrhage is a benign entity. Distribution of redness can be helpful; predominance around the limbus (circumcorneal) is indicative of intraocular disease, diffuse redness involving the tarsal and bulbar conjunctiva is indicative of conjunctivitis, focal

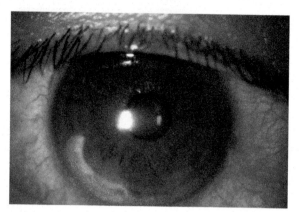

▲ **Figure 3–1.** Acute red eye with peripheral corneal ulceration.

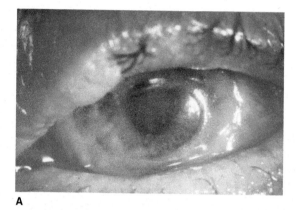

A

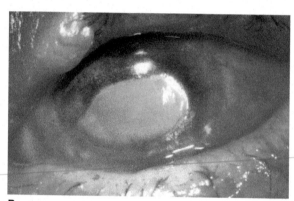

B

▲ **Figure 3–3.** Large corneal epithelial defect. **A:** Before instillation of fluorescein. **B:** After instillation of fluorescein.

or diffuse redness of the globe is consistent with episcleritis, and redness of the eyelid margins is indicative of blepharitis. Bluish redness (violaceous discoloration) of the globe, best identified in natural rather than artificial light, is characteristic of scleritis. Vesicles or ulcerations of the lids or periocular skin are typical of ophthalmic zoster (shingles) and less commonly varicella or primary herpes simplex virus infection.

Conjunctivitis usually causes purulent, mucoid, or watery discharge, and allergic conjunctivitis typically causes itching. Profuse purulent discharge is characteristic of gonococcal conjunctivitis, which requires emergency treatment (see later in the chapter).

Any abnormality of the cornea apparent on gross examination, such as ulceration (Figure 3–1) or focal opacity (Figure 3–2), which may be due to infection, or diffuse cloudiness, which may be due to markedly raised intraocular pressure when it is usually associated with a semi-dilated unreactive pupil, warrants emergency ophthalmologic assessment unless it is known to be longstanding (eg, pterygium).

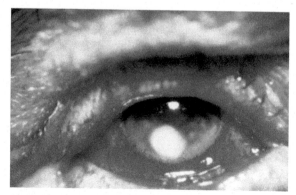

▲ **Figure 3–2.** Acute red eye with focal corneal opacity.

Instillation of fluorescein facilitates identification of an epithelial defect (Figure 3–3), including dendritic ulceration due to herpes simplex virus keratitis. A constricted pupil is suggestive of intraocular inflammation, typically due to anterior uveitis. Hypopyon (pus within the anterior chamber), a feature of corneal infection, intraocular infection, or acute anterior uveitis (iritis) (Figure 3–4), necessitates emergency ophthalmologic assessment.

▶ **Clinical Assessment**

Slitlamp examination facilitates assessment of distribution of redness; identification of conjunctival abnormalities, including examination of the superior tarsal conjunctiva following eversion of the upper eyelid; diagnosis of episcleritis and scleritis; characterization of corneal lesions; and detection of corneal keratic precipitates, anterior chamber flare and cells, and possibly hypopyon indicative of anterior chamber inflammation due to anterior uveitis, intraocular infection, or secondary to corneal inflammation, including

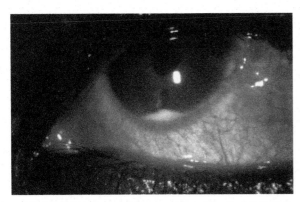

▲ **Figure 3–4.** Hypopyon in acute anterior uveitis (iritis).

Management

There are many causes of acute conjunctivitis, which in most cases is a benign, often self-limiting, condition (see Chapter 5). However, care needs to be exercised in neonates (**ophthalmia neonatorum**) (see Chapter 17) because of the possibility of infection with **chlamydia** or **gonococcus**, both of which are associated with nonocular disease that requires systemic therapy, or **herpes simplex virus**, which may be associated with encephalitis and requires hospitalization and parenteral antiviral therapy. Gonococcal conjunctivitis at all ages, characteristically causing profuse purulent discharge as well as severe conjunctival inflammation, necessitates emergency investigation by microscopy and culture of the discharge and parenteral antibiotic therapy with ceftriaxone to avoid progression to severe corneal damage. Treatment with parenteral antiviral therapy within 72 hours of the appearance of the rash reduces the likelihood of ocular complications in ophthalmic zoster (shingles) (see Chapters 5 and 6). Skin lesions on the tip of the nose (Hutchinson's sign) or the eyelid margins are predictive of ocular complications.

Management of acute **keratitis** primarily involves identification and treatment of infection, for which contact lens wear, pre-existing ocular surface disease, and corneal anesthesia or exposure are the common predisposing factors (see Chapter 6). Occasionally it is apparent straightaway that there is a noninfectious inflammatory process that requires other therapy, possibly topical or systemic steroids, but steroid therapy should not be started without ophthalmologic assessment.

Management of acute intraocular inflammation (**uveitis**) also primarily involves identification and treatment of

infection. In cases of intraocular inflammation, dilated fundal examination is essential to determine whether there is involvement of the vitreous, retina, or choroid, which is important to diagnosis as well as assessment of severity (see Chapters 7 and 15).

infection, particularly if there is posterior segment involvement (vitritis, retinitis, or choroiditis) or recent history of intraocular surgery, but a noninfectious inflammatory process is more common than in acute keratitis (see Chapter 7). Topical or systemic steroid therapy should not be started without ophthalmologic assessment. Scleritis is infrequently caused by infection, with autoimmune disease being more commonly responsible, and can often be managed in the first instance by oral nonsteroidal anti-inflammatory drugs (NSAIDs), but ophthalmologic assessment is necessary to make the diagnosis and exclude other entities.

In **acute angle-closure glaucoma**, prompt recognition and treatment are required if severe visual loss is to be avoided (see Chapter 11). The mainstay of initial treatment is intravenous and oral acetazolamide, as well as topical agents, to reduce intraocular pressure, supplemented by topical steroids to reduce inflammation and topical pilocarpine to constrict the pupil. Definitive treatment is usually laser peripheral iridotomy with prophylactic treatment to the fellow eye. Emergency ophthalmologic assessment is essential to establish the diagnosis, including exclusion of other causes of markedly raised intraocular pressure that may require distinctly different treatment.

ACUTE ORBITAL DISEASE

Acute orbital disease is uncommon, but a few entities need to be recognized promptly to avoid the severe visual loss, or even nonocular morbidity and possibly mortality, that may result from delay in treatment (see Chapter 13).

Triage

Orbital cellulitis is usually a disease of childhood and due to spread of infection from the ethmoid sinuses. It is characterized by fever, pain, eyelid swelling and erythema, proptosis, limitation of extraocular movements, and systemic upset with leukocytosis. **Pre-septal cellulitis**, in which there is no proptosis or limitation of eye movement, may be due to a localized infection in the anterior (pre-septal) portion of the eyelid or may be the early manifestation of orbital cellulitis. In adolescents and young adults, orbital signs may be indicative of extension of infection from the fronto-ethmoidal sinus complex. In diabetics and the immunocompromised, acute orbital disease may be due to fungal infection (**mucormycosis**), with a high risk of death even with early treatment.

Usually occurring in patients with autoimmune hyperthyroidism (Graves' disease), which may or may not have been diagnosed previously, acute Graves' ophthalmopathy may lead to marked proptosis, with the possibility of corneal exposure or optic nerve compression, and limitation of eye movements. Pseudotumor, another inflammatory orbital disease, and carotid artery–cavernous sinus fistula, due to dural shunts that typically occur in patients with diabetes and/or systemic hypertension or due to spontaneous rupture of an intracavernous internal carotid artery aneurysm, may present in a similar manner.

► Clinical Assessment

Reduced vision unexplained by corneal exposure, especially if associated with impaired color vision and/or a relative afferent pupillary defect, indicates optic nerve dysfunction. In orbital cellulitis, nonaxial proptosis implies abscess formation. Other complications include cavernous sinus thrombosis and intracranial infection, the latter being more likely if there is infection in the frontal sinus.

► Management

Orbital cellulitis is a clinical diagnosis and requires immediate institution of antibiotic therapy, usually intravenously, together with early ophthalmologic and otolaryngologic assessments. Orbital imaging may be undertaken in all cases or reserved for those in whom orbital abscess or another complication is suspected.

Orbital imaging, usually computed tomography (CT) but possibly magnetic resonance imaging (MRI), is generally sufficient to differentiate between Graves' ophthalmopathy, orbital pseudotumor, and carotid artery–cavernous sinus fistula, but orbital ultrasound blood flow studies are particularly helpful in diagnosing the third.

ACUTE PAINLESS VISUAL LOSS

Sudden-onset painless visual loss is a very important symptom, because it may be due to ophthalmic disease that requires emergency or urgent treatment, ocular vascular disease with immediate or early threat to the patient's life or remaining vision, or acute intracranial disease.

► Triage

It is essential to determine from the outset whether the reported visual loss involves one or both eyes, including clearly distinguishing monocular visual loss from loss of vision to one side in both eyes (ie, homonymous hemianopia). Patients often will not have checked, by closing one eye and then the other, and if necessary, they should be asked to carry out this simple test. Monocular visual loss indicates disease of the globe or optic nerve, whereas bilateral visual loss, including homonymous hemianopia, indicates a lesion at or posterior to the optic chiasm.

Also it is essential to determine whether the visual loss that has been noticed is definitely of recent onset or whether it may have been longstanding and only recently identified. This requires establishing when the patient was last aware that vision in the affected eye(s) was unaffected, such as when last tested by an optometrist.

History of recent onset of black spots or shapes ("floaters") with flashing lights (photopsia) followed by a field defect progressing upward from below in one eye is characteristic of retinal detachment (see Chapter 9). Preservation of good central vision, implying that the central retina (macula) has not yet detached, warrants emergency ophthalmologic referral. Sudden onset of floaters may also be caused by vitreous hemorrhage, of which the main causes are retinal tear and proliferative retinopathy due to diabetes or retinal vein occlusion. Any patient with sudden-onset floaters and/or flashes, even with otherwise normal vision, requires urgent ophthalmologic assessment. Unless another cause is apparent, patients age 55 or older with acute or subacute unilateral central visual loss, particularly if associated with distortion of images, should be assumed to have wet (neovascular) age-related macular degeneration, and urgent ophthalmologic referral should be arranged.

A reliable account of the rapidity of progression of visual loss can be a very helpful clue to diagnosis, with an abrupt onset being very suggestive of an arterial vascular event. Whether there has been any recovery of vision is important; full recovery after a short period of impairment suggests an embolic arterial event. All patients with possible ocular vascular disease should be asked about vascular risk factors, such as diabetes mellitus, systemic hypertension, and hyperlipidemia. Patients age 55 or older with suspected arterial disease must be questioned about symptoms of giant cell arteritis and have their erythrocyte sedimentation rate (ESR) and/or C-reactive protein (CRP) checked.

Ophthalmoscopy (see Chapter 2) often provides the diagnosis in acute painless visual loss. Lack of a red reflex with abnormal or absent view of the retina is suggestive of vitreous hemorrhage or retinal detachment, for which urgent or emergency ophthalmologic referral is required (see Chapter 10). Widespread or sectoral retinal hemorrhages indicate central or branch retinal vein occlusion for which urgent ophthalmologic assessment is indicated. Widespread retinal whitening with a cherry-red spot indicates central retinal artery occlusion for which emergency ophthalmologic assessment must be arranged, and giant cell arteritis and embolic disease need to be excluded. Sectoral retinal whitening indicates branch retinal artery occlusion, for which urgent ophthalmologic assessment is important to confirm the diagnosis, but prompt investigations for embolic disease need to be undertaken. Optic disk swelling in an eye with recent acute or subacute visual loss is commonly due to anterior ischemic optic neuropathy (see Chapter 14), for which giant cell arteritis must be excluded in patients age 55 or older.

► Clinical Assessment

The ophthalmologist must clarify whether the visual loss is monocular or binocular, not only by reviewing the history but also by assessment of visual acuity and visual field in each eye, the latter initially by confrontation testing but, if necessary, by perimetry. Detection of bilateral visual field loss, including abnormality in a subjectively unaffected fellow eye, may establish that the disease process involves the optic chiasm, when there is a bitemporal hemianopia or a temporal hemianopia in the subjectively unaffected fellow eye, or the retrochiasmal visual pathways, when there is homonymous hemianopia. Assessment of color vision and pupillary reactions to light, particularly looking for a relative afferent pupillary defect, is important in detection of optic nerve disease (see Chapter 14).

Fundal examination following pupillary dilation provides the best means of diagnosing retinal tears with or without retinal detachment; vitreous hemorrhage and its cause if the hemorrhage is not too dense (otherwise ultrasound examination is necessary); age-related macular degeneration, including whether it has features of the wet type; retinal vein or artery occlusion; and anterior ischemic optic neuropathy. In giant cell arteritis, fundal examination may be normal when visual loss is due to choroidal ischemia or posterior ischemic optic neuropathy.

Management

Retinal detachment is usually treated surgically, with urgency primarily being determined by whether the macula is detached but also the underlying cause (see Chapter 10). Management of vitreous hemorrhage is determined by the underlying cause (see Chapters 9 and 10). Repeated intravitreal injection of inhibitors of vascular endothelial growth factor (VEGF) has become the standard treatment for wet age-related macular degeneration (see Chapter 10).

All patients with transient monocular visual loss ("amaurosis fugax") likely to be due to retinal emboli should undergo investigations for carotid and cardiac sources (see Chapters 14 and 15) with consideration of urgent carotid revascularization if there is 70% or greater ipsilateral internal carotid artery stenosis. Transient visual loss can also be due to giant cell arteritis or optic disk swelling due to raised intracranial pressure (see later in the chapter).

No treatment in the acute stage is established to alter visual outcome in central or branch retinal vein occlusion, but various treatments, including intravitreal injections of vascular endothelial growth factor (VEGF) inhibitors or triamcinolone, retinal laser photocoagulation, and various surgical techniques, are effective for the long-term complications (see Chapter 10). Various treatments, including intra-arterial thrombolytic therapy, are advocated in the acute stage of central retinal artery occlusion, but evidence for their usefulness is lacking, particularly in view of the risk of adverse events in the case of intra-arterial thrombolysis (see Chapters 10 and 14). No treatment in the acute stage is established to alter visual outcome in nonarteritic anterior ischemic optic neuropathy (see Chapters 14 and 15), but failure to promptly treat giant cell arteritis causing anterior ischemic optic neuropathy or central retinal artery occlusion is likely to lead rapidly to complete bilateral blindness (see Chapters 14 and 15).

Sudden visual loss due to optic chiasmal or retrochiasmal disease necessitates emergency imaging and appropriate management thereafter, which may involve neurology or neurosurgery referral.

ACUTE PAINFUL VISUAL LOSS WITHOUT A RED EYE

A number of relatively uncommon but important conditions present with painful visual loss without a red eye because, for the most part, they are retrobulbar in location.

▶ Triage

There are many causes of optic nerve inflammation ("**optic neuritis**") (see Table 14–1). The most common is the acute demyelinative optic neuropathy associated with multiple sclerosis, occurring as the initial manifestation or part of a subsequent relapse. It characteristically presents as subacute monocular visual loss with peri- or retro-ocular discomfort exacerbated by eye movements (see Chapter 14).

Pituitary apoplexy, usually due to hemorrhagic infarction of a pituitary tumor, is rare but requires prompt recognition and treatment to reduce the risk of severe morbidity, possibly death, as well as severe visual loss, possibly complete blindness. Characteristically, it presents with sudden-onset headache, unilateral or bilateral visual loss, sometimes impaired eye movements, and metabolic and circulatory derangement due to pituitary failure, particularly resulting in adrenal insufficiency. **Sphenoid sinusitis** also presents with headache, typically localized to the vertex, and acute unilateral or bilateral visual loss. Diagnosis of **posterior scleritis** is often delayed because of the frequent lack of specific diagnostic features, including the absence of apparent inflammation of the globe to suggest an inflammatory condition (see Chapter 7).

▶ Clinical Assessment

In acute demyelinative optic neuropathy, there are features of optic nerve dysfunction (impaired color vision, visual field loss, and a relative afferent pupillary defect), with progression of visual loss over a few days, and usually no ophthalmoscopic abnormality, but mild optic disk swelling is present in one-third of cases.

The ophthalmic manifestations of pituitary apoplexy are unilateral or bilateral often severe visual loss with impaired pupillary light reactions, sometimes impaired eye movements (external ophthalmoplegia) due to ocular motor cranial nerve palsies, and normal or pale optic disks depending on whether the pituitary tumor previously has caused anterior visual pathway compression.

In sphenoid sinusitis, the visual loss also has features of optic nerve dysfunction, with normal or pale optic disks depending on whether there has been chronic optic nerve compression from a pre-existing sphenoid sinus mucocele (see Chapter 13). The clinical signs in posterior scleritis include proptosis, limitation of eye movements, induced refractive error, choroidal folds, fundal mass, exudative retinal detachment, and optic disk swelling (see Chapter 7). Ultrasound is the best diagnostic test.

Management

In most cases of acute demyelinative optic neuropathy, the vision recovers spontaneously, and management centers on investigation of the likelihood of multiple sclerosis and the need for disease-modifying therapy, but the crucial issue in the acute management is excluding other entities that require urgent treatment. Pituitary apoplexy is an endocrine and neurosurgical emergency. The patient may require emergency resuscitation. Intravenous hydrocortisone should be given to all patients prior to investigation with MRI, or CT if the patient's condition is unstable. Urgent neurosurgery is frequently required, particularly in patients with visual loss. Sphenoid sinusitis causing visual loss requires surgical drainage as well as antibiotic therapy. Posterior scleritis may respond to oral NSAIDs, but oral steroid therapy may be required.

DOUBLE VISION AND EYE MOVEMENT ABNORMALITIES

Double vision has many causes, ranging from the benign entity of an incorrect spectacle prescription to the life-threatening expansion of a posterior communicating artery aneurysm. Ocular, orbital, intracranial, generalized neurologic, and systemic diseases can all present with double vision.

Triage

Assessment of double vision is complex and can cause great difficulty. In oculomotor (third cranial) nerve palsy, there may be clues from associated ptosis or pupillary abnormality. Otherwise, unless the pattern of double vision reported by the patient or the examination of the range of eye movements quickly leads to identification of a specific entity such as an abducens (sixth cranial) nerve (lateral rectus) palsy, more useful guidance to the clinical urgency is derived from other features, such as whether there is also impairment of vision, orbital signs such as lid swelling or proptosis, periocular pain or headache, nonocular neurologic abnormalities, or systemic illness. In general, patients with multiple cranial nerve palsies or other neurologic features, severe headache, associated systemic illness, or age under 50 with single or multiple cranial nerve palsy are most likely to have a serious underlying condition.

Clinical Assessment

Double vision is usually due to ocular misalignment, but the first step in its evaluation is to determine whether it is monocular or binocular. If double vision, or even more than two images, is present when the patient is viewing with only one eye (monocular), whether it is just with one eye or with each eye alone, the visual disturbance is not due to ocular misalignment. Instead, it is likely to be due to refractive error, lens opacity, or possibly macular disease. Unless there are other features to clearly implicate cerebral disease, multiple images on monocular viewing can be assumed not to be due to intracranial disease.

Effectively every episode of double vision has an acute onset because double vision is either present or not. What needs to be established is for how long double vision has been noticed and whether, during the one or many episodes that have occurred, there has been change in the pattern, as judged by the direction of separation of images and the directions of gaze in which double vision has been present, or severity, as judged by the distance separating the two images. It is also helpful to establish whether the double vision can be overcome with voluntary effort, because this implies a longstanding abnormality that has become more difficult to overcome (decompensated).

Whenever an ocular motor cranial nerve palsy is diagnosed, it is essential to determine whether it is isolated or part of multiple cranial nerve dysfunction, including assessment of trigeminal nerve as well optic nerve function, not only to provide anatomical localization of the disease process but also as a guide to the likelihood of a serious underlying condition.

In oculomotor nerve palsy, the presence of pupillary dysfunction, either anisocoria or particularly an impaired response to light, provides an important clue to the possibility of a compressive lesion such as a posterior communicating artery aneurysm (see Chapter 14). Severe pain is another important clue to the presence of an aneurysm, but it also may occur in pituitary apoplexy (see earlier in the chapter).

In all cases of double vision, careful attention needs to be paid to identification of any orbital signs, not least to avoid unnecessary investigation for a possible intracranial lesion. Specific eye movement abnormalities provide precise anatomical localization. Internuclear ophthalmoplegia, in which there is impairment of adduction of one or both eyes, localizes to the medial longitudinal fasciculus within the brainstem (see Chapter 14). Horizontal gaze palsy, in which there is loss of conjugate horizontal gaze to one or both sides, localizes to the pons, whereas vertical gaze palsy localizes to the midbrain (see Chapter 14). Variability of double vision, during or between episodes, typically with increasing severity with fatigue that may also manifest as increasing ptosis, is suggestive of myasthenia gravis (see Chapter 14).

Management

Investigation of patients with binocular double vision depends on the clinical assessment. Many cases of isolated ocular motor cranial nerve palsy in patients over 50 are due to ischemic (microvascular) disease, which requires little investigation apart from exclusion of giant cell arteritis and review of vascular risk factors, and in which spontaneous recovery is the rule. In contrast, in isolated oculomotor nerve palsy, suspicion of posterior communicating artery aneurysm due to pupillary involvement, severity of pain, or age under 50 necessitates emergency imaging, with the outcome being much better if treatment can be undertaken prior to subarachnoid hemorrhage due to aneurysm rupture. Similarly, multiple cranial nerve dysfunction requires urgent investigation, usually guided primarily by a neurologist, who will also guide investigations when the disease process localizes to the brainstem. Management of orbital disease usually depends on the outcome of imaging with CT or MRI. When clinical evaluation suggests decompensation of a longstanding abnormality, such as a congenital superior oblique (trochlear) palsy, further investigation may not be required, and initial treatment will be with prisms (see Chapter 14).

In any patient with suspected myasthenia gravis, it is important to establish whether there is nonocular weakness suggesting generalized disease, especially impairment of breathing or swallowing, for which emergency neurologic assessment is essential.

PUPIL ABNORMALITIES

Abnormalities of pupil size and/or reactions result from a wide variety of causes, including structural abnormalities of the iris, which also usually cause pupillary distortion; miosis in intraocular inflammation; mydriasis in markedly raised intraocular pressure; tonic pupil; oculomotor nerve palsy; Horner's syndrome; and midbrain dysfunction.

▶ Triage

Acute isolated, dilated, unreactive pupil in an otherwise well individual is rarely due to a serious underlying condition, with the likely possibilities being the benign entity of tonic pupil (see Chapter 14) or pharmacologic mydriasis, such as from accidental ocular inoculation with an anticholinergic agent in travel sickness medication. In contrast, isolated, dilated, unreactive pupil in a patient with depressed conscious level due to head injury or other acute intracranial disease is an ominous sign, being suggestive of tentorial herniation. As discussed earlier, pupil involvement in oculomotor nerve palsy is an important clue to the possibility of a compressive lesion, including posterior communicating artery aneurysm. Miosis with ptosis is characteristic of Horner's syndrome (see Chapter 14). Acute painful Horner's syndrome, possibly following neck trauma, requires urgent exclusion of carotid dissection. Pupillary light-near dissociation (impaired pupillary constriction to light with better constriction to near) is traditionally associated with central nervous system syphilis (Argyll Robertson pupils), but can be due to midbrain dysfunction, typically compression from a pineal tumor or

dilated third ventricle in hydrocephalus, when usually there is also impairment of vertical eye movements.

▶ Clinical Assessment

Besides confirming a suspected diagnosis of oculomotor nerve palsy or Horner's syndrome, the ophthalmologist's particular role in assessment of acute pupil abnormalities is the identification of benign entities, such as tonic pupil and pharmacologic mydriasis, to avoid unnecessary investigation, and ophthalmic entities, such as acute angle-closure glaucoma, to direct management. In all three instances, there will be no related ptosis or impairment of eye movements. Tonic pupil may be identified by the delayed dilation following a near response from which it derives its name; abnormal spiraling ("vermiform") movements of the iris when constricting to a light stimulus, best seen on slitlamp examination; or constriction to dilute (0.125%) pilocarpine eye drops. Pharmacologic mydriasis is characterized by lack of pupil constriction to bright light and standard-strength (2%) pilocarpine eye drops.

BILATERAL OPTIC DISK SWELLING

There are many causes of optic disk swelling, including inflammatory or ischemic optic neuropathy, central retinal vein occlusion, uveitis, posterior scleritis, and intra-orbital optic nerve compression, all of which are usually unilateral. Bilateral optic disk swelling is a characteristic feature of raised intracranial pressure and malignant (accelerated) systemic hypertension, both of which require emergency or urgent investigation and treatment (see Chapters 14 and 15).

▶ Triage

Papilledema (optic disk swelling due to raised intracranial pressure) is usually identified as part of the examination of a patient with neurologic symptoms, particularly headache. It may be identified incidentally, such as during routine optometric examination, but even then, it still requires urgent head imaging to exclude an intracranial mass lesion. Blood pressure should be checked in every patient with bilateral optic disk swelling, even a child.

▶ Clinical Assessment

When the abnormalities are florid, recognition of optic disk swelling is straightforward. When the abnormalities are less marked (see Figure 14–9), ophthalmologic assessment may be crucial, particularly to identify other entities such as myelinated nerve fibers, optic nerve head drusen, or congenitally small and crowded optic disks (pseudopapilledema) (Figure 3–5) that mimic optic disk swelling, so that unnecessary investigations and anxiety can be avoided. In individuals with papilledema, particularly when it is acute with retinal exudates or atrophic, assessment of vision by an

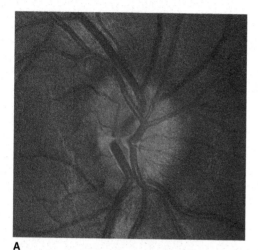

A

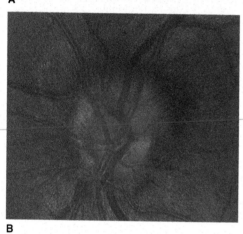

B

▲ **Figure 3–5.** Congenitally small and crowded optic disks (pseudopapilledema). **A:** Right eye. **B:** Left eye.

ophthalmologist, including visual fields, is a crucial guide to urgency of treatment. In malignant hypertension, optic disk swelling is usually accompanied by retinal and choroidal abnormalities and is an indication for urgent reduction in blood pressure, although precipitous reduction should be avoided to reduce the risk of optic nerve infarction.

REFERENCES

Adam MK et al: Inpatient ophthalmology consultation for fungemia: Prevalence of ocular involvement and necessity of funduscopic screening. Am J Ophthalmol 2015;160:1078. [PMID: 26235339]

Adoni A et al: The pupillary response in traumatic brain injury: A guide for trauma nurses. J Trauma Nurs 2007;14:191. [PMID: 18399377]

Akal A et al: Do we really need to panic in all acute vision loss in ICU? Acute angle-closure glaucoma. J Pak Med Assoc 2014;64:960. [PMID: 25252529]

Al-Dhibi HA et al: A systematic approach to emergencies in uveitis. Middle East Afr J Ophthalmol 2014;21:251. [PMID: 25100911]

Amin N et al: Assessment and management of orbital cellulitis. Br J Hosp Med (Lond) 2016;77:216. [PMID: 27071427]

Andreola B et al: Unilateral mydriasis due to Angel's trumpet. Clin Toxicol (Phila) 2008;46:329. [PMID: 18363132]

Arif M et al: Sudden loss of vision in an Acute Medical Unit. Acute Med 2014;13:26. [PMID: 24616901]

Atfeh MS et al: Orbital infections: Five-year case series, literature review and guideline development. J Laryngol Otol 2015;129:670. [PMID: 26059425]

Azari AA et al: Conjunctivitis: A systematic review of diagnosis and treatment. JAMA 2013;310:1721. [PMID: 24150468]

Biousse V et al: Retinal and optic nerve ischemia. Continuum (Minneap Minn) 2014;20:838. [PMID: 25099097]

Biousse V, Newman NJ: Ischemic optic neuropathies. N Engl J Med 2015;372:2428. [PMID: 26083207]

Brown GC et al: Photopsias: A key to diagnosis. Ophthalmology 2015;122:2084. [PMID: 26249730]

Caglayan HZ et al: A diagnostic challenge: Dilated pupil. Curr Opin Ophthalmol 2013;24:550. [PMID: 24100369]

Callizo J et al: Cardiovascular risk factors in central retinal artery occlusion: Results of a prospective and standardized medical examination. Ophthalmology 2015;122:1881. [PMID: 26231133]

Capatina C et al: Management of endocrine disease: Pituitary tumour apoplexy. Eur J Endocrinol 2015;172:R179-90. [PMID: 25452466]

Carlisle RT et al: Differential diagnosis of the swollen red eyelid. Am Fam Physician 2015;92:106. [PMID: 26176369]

Chan JW et al: Causes of isolated recurrent ipsilateral sixth nerve palsies in older adults: a case series and review of the literature. Clin Ophthalmol 2015;9:373. [PMID: 25750515]

Chaudhry P et al: Unilateral pupillary mydriasis from nebulized ipratropium bromide: A false sign of brain herniation in the intensive care unit. Indian J Crit Care Med 2014;18:176. [PMID: 24701070]

Chen KJ et al: Risk factors predictive of endogenous endophthalmitis among hospitalized patients with hematogenous infections in the United States. Am J Ophthalmol 2015;160:391. [PMID: 26187877]

Cho HJ et al: Prognostic factors for survival in patients with acute invasive fungal rhinosinusitis. Am J Rhinol Allergy 2015;29:48. [PMID: 25590320]

Cohen EJ: Management and prevention of herpes zoster ocular disease. Cornea. 2015;34(Suppl 10):S3. [PMID: 26114827]

Cohen E et al: Persistent dilemmas in zoster eye disease. Br J Ophthalmol 2016;100:56. [PMID: 25966739]

Cornblath WT: Diplopia due to ocular motor cranial neuropathies. Continuum (Minneap Minn) 2014;20:966. [PMID: 25099103]

Coronica R et al: Ocular emergencies: Screening tool and alert protocol. Insight 2015;40:5. [PMID: 26638251]

Cortina G et al: Severe visual loss caused by unrecognized malignant hypertension in a 15-year-old girl. Pediatr Int 2015;57:e42. [PMID: 25868960]

De Smit E et al: Giant cell arteritis: ophthalmic manifestations of a systemic disease. Graefes Arch Clin Exp Ophthalmol 2016;254:2291. [PMID: 27495301]

Egan RA et al: Should patients with acute central retinal artery occlusion be treated with intra-arterial t-PA? J Neuroophthalmol 2015;35:205. [PMID: 25985436]

Epling J: Bacterial conjunctivitis. BMJ Clin Evid 2012;2012:0704. [PMID: 22348418]

Friedman DI: The eye and headache. Continuum (Minneap Minn) 2015;21:1109. [PMID: 26252594]

Gelston CD: Common eye emergencies. Am Fam Physician 2013;88:515. [PMID: 24364572]

Goudie C et al: The accuracy of the Edinburgh visual loss diagnostic algorithm. Eye (Lond) 2015;29:1483. [PMID: 26293143]

Gower EW et al: Characteristics of endophthalmitis after cataract surgery in the United States Medicare population. Ophthalmology 2015;122:1625. [PMID: 26045364]

Gupta S et al: Clinical presentation and outcome of the orbital complications due to acute infective rhino sinusitis. Indian J Otolaryngol Head Neck Surg 2013;65(Suppl 2):431. [PMID: 24427692]

Handor H et al: Images in clinical medicine. Hypertensive retinopathy associated with preeclampsia. N Engl J Med 2014;370:752. [PMID: 24552322]

Hayreh SS: Ocular vascular occlusive disorders: natural history of visual outcome. Prog Retin Eye Res 2014;41:1. [PMID: 24769221]

Huff JS et al: Neuro-ophthalmology in emergency medicine. Emerg Med Clin North Am 2016;34:967. [PMID: 27741997]

Iijima K et al: A study of the causes of bilateral optic disc swelling in Japanese patients. Clin Ophthalmol 2014;8:1269. [PMID: 25031527]

Johnston PC et al: Pituitary tumor apoplexy. J Clin Neurosci 2015;22:939. [PMID: 25800143]

Kahloun R et al: Ocular involvement and visual outcome of herpes zoster ophthalmicus: Review of 45 patients from Tunisia, North Africa. J Ophthalmic Inflamm Infect 2014;4:25. [PMID: 25246984]

Kahawita S et al: Flashes and floaters: A practical approach to assessment and management. Aust Fam Physician 2014;43:201. [PMID: 24701623]

Kikushima W et al: Quick referral and urgent surgery to preempt foveal detachment in retinal detachment repair. Asia Pac J Ophthalmol (Phila) 2014;3:141. [PMID: 26107583]

Lawlor M et al: Strokes and vision: The management of ischemic arterial disease affecting the retina and occipital lobe. Surv Ophthalmol 2015;60:296. [PMID: 25937273]

Lizé F et al: Septic cavernous sinus thrombosis secondary to acute bacterial sinusitis: A retrospective study of seven cases. Am J Rhinol Allergy 2015;29:e7. [PMID: 25590307]

Lumi X et al: Ageing of the vitreous: From acute onset floaters and flashes to retinal detachment. Ageing Res Rev 2015;21:71. [PMID: 25841656]

Mascarenhas J et al: Acanthamoeba, fungal, and bacterial keratitis: A comparison of risk factors and clinical features. Am J Ophthalmol 2014;157:56. [PMID: 24200232]

Mayor MT et al: Diagnosis and management of gonococcal infections. Am Fam Physician 2012;86:931. [PMID: 23157146]

McAnena L et al: Prevalence of gonococcal conjunctivitis in adults and neonates. Eye 2015;29:875. [PMID: 25907207]

McDonald EM et al: Antivirals for management of herpes zoster including ophthalmicus: A systematic review of high-quality randomized controlled trials. Antivir Ther 2012;17:255. [PMID: 22300753]

McDonald EM et al: Topical antibiotics for the management of bacterial keratitis: An evidence-based review of high quality randomised controlled trials. Br J Ophthalmol 2014;98:1470. [PMID: 24729078]

Mercier J et al: Interest of local intra-arterial fibrinolysis in acute central retinal artery occlusion: Clinical experience in 16 patients. J Neuroradiol 2015;42:229. [PMID: 25451669]

Mukhi SV et al: MRI in the evaluation of acute visual syndromes. Top Magn Reson Imaging 2015;24:309. [PMID: 26636637]

Mustafa S et al: Approach to diagnosis and management of optic neuropathy. Neurol India 2014;62:599. [PMID: 25591670]

Nagendran ST et al: Flashes, floaters and fuzz. Br J Hosp Med (Lond) 2013;74:91. [PMID: 23411978]

Ng J et al: Accidental unilateral mydriasis from hyoscine patch in a care provider. Semin Ophthalmol 2015;30:462. [PMID: 24460454]

Ossorio A: Red eye emergencies in primary care. Nurse Pract 2015;40:46. [PMID: 26545092]

Peña MT et al: Orbital complications of acute sinusitis: Changes in the post-pneumococcal vaccine era. JAMA Otolaryngol Head Neck Surg 2013;139:223. [PMID: 23429877]

Pielen A et al: Predictors of prognosis and treatment outcome in central retinal artery occlusion: local intra-arterial fibrinolysis vs. conservative treatment. Neuroradiology 2015;57:1055. [PMID: 26349479]

Polomský M et al: Unilateral mydriasis due to hemorrhoidal ointment. J Emerg Med 2012;43:e11-5. [PMID: 19596177]

Santana-Cabrera L et al: Unilateral mydriasis secondary to ipratropium bromide in a critically ill patient. J Emerg Trauma Shock 2012;5:199. [PMID: 22787356]

Schrag M et al: Intravenous fibrinolytic therapy in central retinal artery occlusion: A patient-level meta-analysis. JAMA Neurol 2015;72:1148. [PMID: 26258861]

Schröder T et al: A hypertensive emergency with acute visual impairment due to excessive licorice consumption. Neth J Med 2015;73:82. [PMID: 25753073]

Shenoy SB et al: Endogenous endophthalmitis in patients with MRSA septicemia: A case series and review of literature. Ocul Immunol Inflamm 2016;24:515. [PMID: 26222985]

Spierer O et al: Amaurosis fugax, anterior ischemic optic neuropathy and cilioretinal artery occlusion secondary to giant cell arteritis. Isr Med Assoc J 2015;17:392. [PMID: 26234004]

Stacey AW et al: Hypertensive emergency presenting as blurry vision in a patient with hypertensive chorioretinopathy. Int J Emerg Med 2015;8:13. [PMID: 25932053]

Suzuki T et al: Conjunctivitis caused by Neisseria gonorrhoeae isolates with reduced cephalosporin susceptibility and multidrug resistance. J Clin Microbiol 2013;51:4246. [PMID: 24025911]

Szent-Ivanyi J et al: Herpes zoster ophthalmicus: Is the globe involved? BMJ Case Rep 2014;2014:bcr2014204566. [PMID: 24744079]

Tamhankar MA et al: Isolated third, fourth, and sixth cranial nerve palsies from presumed microvascular versus other causes: A prospective study. Ophthalmology 2013;120:2264. [PMID: 23747163]

Thurtell MJ et al: Third nerve palsy as the initial manifestation of giant cell arteritis. J Neuroophthalmol 2014;34:243. [PMID: 24667773]

Timlin H et al: The accuracy of the Edinburgh Red Eye Diagnostic Algorithm. Eye (Lond) 2015;29:619. [PMID: 25697458]

Tsai TH et al: Metastatic endophthalmitis combined with subretinal abscess in a patient with diabetes mellitus: A case report. BMC Ophthalmol 2015;15:105. [PMID: 26272662]

Varma DD et al: A review of central retinal artery occlusion: Clinical presentation and management. Eye 2013;27:688. [PMID: 23470793]

Vasselon P et al: Unilateral mydriasis due to scopolamine patch. Int J Clin Pharm 2011;33:737. [PMID: 21870093]

Watkinson S: Assessment and management of patients with acute red eye. Nurs Older People 2013;25:27. [PMID: 23914708]

Weinreb RN et al: The pathophysiology and treatment of glaucoma: a review. JAMA 2014;311:1901. [PMID: 24825645]

Welch JF et al: Red Alert: diagnosis and management of the acute red eye. J R Nav Med Serv 2014;100:42. [PMID: 24881426]

Welman T et al: Assessment of Emergency Department eye examinations in patients presenting with mid-face injury. J Emerg Med 2016;50:422. [PMID: 26443644]

Weyand CM et al: Clinical practice. Giant-cell arteritis and polymyalgia rheumatica. N Engl J Med 2014;371:50. [PMID: 24988557]

Winegar BA et al: Imaging of orbital trauma and emergent non-traumatic conditions. Neuroimaging Clin N Am 2015;25:439. [PMID: 26208419]

Wiswell JL et al: Images in emergency medicine. Young boy with eye pain. Herpes zoster ophthalmicus, varicella zoster stromal keratitis, episcleritis and iritis. Ann Emerg Med 2012;60:554. [PMID: 23089088]

Wyatt K: Three common ophthalmic emergencies. JAAPA 2014;27:32. [PMID: 24853153]

Yawn BP et al: Herpes zoster eye complications: Rates and trends. Mayo Clin Proc 2013;88:562. [PMID: 23664666]

Yildirim A et al: Diagnosis of malignant hypertension with ocular examination: A child case. Semin Ophthalmol 2014;29:32. [PMID: 24168178]

Lids & Lacrimal Apparatus

4

M. Reza Vagefi, MD

4.1. Lids

▼ ANATOMY OF THE LIDS

The lids are thin structures comprised of skin, muscle, and fibrous tissue that serve to protect the eye (see Figure 1–22). The great mobility of the lids is possible because the skin is among the thinnest of the body. Beneath the skin lies a very thin fibroadipose layer through which septa pass and closely adhere to the orbicularis oculi muscle. The orbicularis oculi muscle consists of striated muscle innervated on its deep surface by the facial nerve (cranial nerve [CN] VII). The muscle functions to close the lids and is divided into orbital, preseptal, and pretarsal divisions. The orbital portion is a circular muscle with no temporal insertion and is thought to function primarily in forcible closure. The preseptal and pretarsal muscles are believed to be involved in involuntary blink. They have superficial and deep medial heads that participate in lacrimal pump function (see Section 4.3 Lacrimal Apparatus).

The lids are supported by the tarsi, rigid collagenous plates that are attached to the orbital rim via the medial and lateral canthal tendons. The lateral canthus lies 1–2 mm higher than the medial. The orbital septum originates from the orbital rim and functions as an important barrier between the lids and the orbit. In the upper lid, the septum attaches to the levator aponeurosis, which then joins the tarsus. Behind the septum lies the medial and the central or preaponeurotic fat pad, a helpful surgical landmark. In the lower lid, the septum joins the inferior border of the tarsus. The lower lid has three anatomically distinct fat pads beneath the orbital septum.

Deep to the fat in the upper lid lies the levator palpebrae superioris (LPS)—the principal retractor of the upper lid—and its equivalent, the capsulopalpebral fascia in the lower lid. The LPS is a striated muscle that originates in the apex of the orbit and is innervated by the oculomotor nerve (CN III). As it enters the lid, it forms an aponeurosis that attaches to the lower third of the superior tarsal plate. A crease usually present in the mid position of the upper lid in Caucasians represents an attachment of levator aponeurosis fibers to the more superficial layers. The crease is much lower or is absent in the Asian lid. In the lower lid, the capsulopalpebral fascia originates from the inferior rectus muscle and inserts on the inferior border of the tarsus. It serves to retract the lower lid in downgaze.

The superior (Müller's) and inferior tarsal muscle form the next layer, which is adherent to the conjunctiva. These sympathetically innervated smooth muscles are also lid retractors. Conjunctiva lines the inner surface of the lids and forms the blind cul-de-sacs of the upper and lower fornices as it reflects onto the eye. The conjunctiva contains glands essential for lubrication of the ocular surface.

▼ INFECTIONS & INFLAMMATIONS OF THE LIDS

HORDEOLUM

A hordeolum is an infection of one or more glands of the lid. When the meibomian glands are involved, it is called an internal hordeolum. An external hordeolum (stye) is an infection of a gland of Zeis or Moll.

Pain, redness, and swelling are the principal symptoms. The intensity of the pain is a function of the amount of lid swelling. An internal hordeolum may point to the skin or to the conjunctival surface. An external hordeolum always points to the skin.

Most hordeola are caused by staphylococcal infections, usually *Staphylococcus aureus*. Culture is seldom required.

Treatment consists of warm compresses several times a day for 10–15 minutes. If the process does not begin to resolve within 48 hours, incision and drainage of the purulent material is indicated. A vertical incision should be made on the conjunctival surface to avoid cutting across the meibomian glands. If the hordeolum is pointing externally, a horizontal incision adjacent and parallel to the eyelash line should be made on the skin to conceal the incision. Antibiotic ointment is routinely applied to the site. Systemic antibiotics are indicated if cellulitis develops.

CHALAZION

A chalazion is a sterile, focal, chronic inflammation of the lid that results from obstruction of a meibomian gland (Figure 4–1). It is commonly associated with rosacea and posterior blepharitis. Symptoms begin with mild inflammation and tenderness that persists over a period of weeks to months. It is differentiated from a hordeolum by the absence of acute inflammatory signs. Most chalazia point toward the conjunctival surface, which may be slightly reddened or elevated. If sufficiently large, a chalazion may press on the globe and cause astigmatism. Intervention is indicated if the lesion is not amenable to a warm compress regimen, distorts the vision, or is aesthetically unacceptable.

Pathology studies are seldom indicated, but on histologic examination, there is proliferation of the endothelium of the acinus and a granulomatous inflammatory response that includes Langerhans-type giant cells. Biopsy is, however, indicated for recurrent chalazion, since sebaceous cell carcinoma may mimic the appearance of chalazion.

Surgical incision and drainage is performed via a vertical incision into the tarsus from the conjunctival surface followed by curettement of the gelatinous material and glandular epithelium. Intralesional steroid injections alone may be useful for small lesions and in combination with excision for more chronic cases.

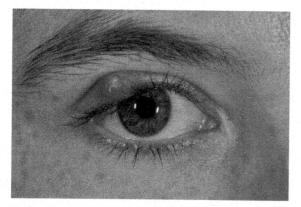

▲ Figure 4–1. Chalazion of right upper lid.

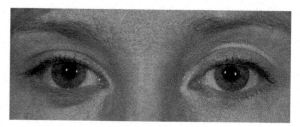

▲ Figure 4–2. Severe anterior blepharitis.

ANTERIOR BLEPHARITIS

Anterior blepharitis is a common, chronic bilateral inflammation of the lid margins (Figure 4–2). There are two main types: staphylococcal and seborrheic. Staphylococcal blepharitis may be due to infection with *S aureus, Staphylococcus epidermidis,* or coagulase-negative staphylococci. Seborrheic blepharitis is usually associated with the presence of *Malassezia furfur* (formerly known as *Pityrosporum ovale*), although this organism has not been shown to be causative. Often, both types of blepharitis are present (mixed).

The chief symptoms are irritation, burning, and itching of the eyes and lid margins. The eyes are "red-rimmed." Many scales or scurf can be seen clinging to the lashes of both the upper and lower lids. In the staphylococcal type, the scales are dry, the lids are erythematous, the lid margins may be ulcerated, and the lashes tend to fall out. In the seborrheic type, the scales are greasy, ulceration does not occur, and the lid margins are less inflamed. Seborrhea of the scalp, brows, and ears is also frequently found. In the more common mixed type, both dry and greasy scales are present with lid margin inflammation. Staphylococcal species and *M furfur* can be seen together or singly in stained material scraped from the lid margins.

Staphylococcal blepharitis may be complicated by hordeola, chalazia, epithelial keratitis of the lower third of the cornea, and marginal keratitis (see Chapter 6). Both forms of anterior blepharitis predispose to recurrent conjunctivitis.

Treatment consists of lid hygiene, particularly in the seborrheic type of blepharitis. Scales must be removed daily from the lid margins by gentle mechanical scrubbing with a damp cotton applicator and a mild soap such as baby shampoo. Staphylococcal blepharitis is treated with antistaphylococcal antibiotic or sulfacetamide ointment applied on a cotton applicator once daily to the lid margins. Both types may run a chronic course over a period of months or years if not treated adequately. Associated staphylococcal conjunctivitis or keratitis usually disappears promptly following local antistaphylococcal medication.

POSTERIOR BLEPHARITIS

Posterior blepharitis is inflammation of the lids secondary to dysfunction of the meibomian glands (Figure 4–3). Like anterior blepharitis, it is a bilateral, chronic condition.

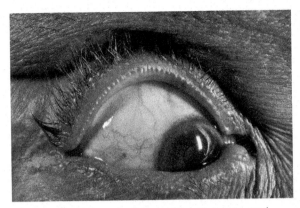

▲ **Figure 4–3.** Posterior blepharitis with inspissated meibomian glands.

Anterior and posterior blepharitis may coexist. Seborrheic dermatitis is commonly associated with meibomian gland dysfunction. Colonization or frank infection with strains of staphylococci is frequently associated with meibomian gland disease and may represent one reason for the disturbance of meibomian gland function. Bacterial lipases may cause inflammation of the meibomian glands and conjunctiva and disruption of the tear film.

Posterior blepharitis is manifested by a broad spectrum of symptoms involving the lids, tear film, conjunctiva, and cornea. Meibomian gland changes include inflammation of the meibomian orifices (meibomianitis), plugging of the orifices with inspissated secretions, dilatation of the meibomian glands in the tarsal plates, and production of abnormal soft, cheesy secretion upon pressure over the glands. Hordeola and chalazia may also occur. The lid margin demonstrates hyperemia and telangiectasia and may become rounded and rolled inward as a result of scarring of the tarsal conjunctiva, causing an abnormal relationship between the precorneal tear film and the meibomian gland orifices. The tears may be frothy or filled with debris. Posterior blepharitis is often associated with rosacea (see Chapter 15).

Primary therapy is application of warm compresses to the lids, with periodic meibomian gland expression. Further treatment is determined by the associated conjunctival and corneal changes. Topical therapy with antibiotics is guided by results of bacterial cultures from the lid margins. Frank inflammation of the lids calls for anti-inflammatory treatment, including long-term therapy with topical Metrogel (metronidazole, 0.75% daily), oral doxycycline (50–100 mg twice daily), or oral azithromycin (1 g weekly for 3 weeks). Short-term treatment with weak topical steroids (eg, prednisolone acetate, 0.125% twice daily) can be considered. Tear film dysfunction may necessitate artificial tears with a preference for preservative free formulations to avoid toxic reactions. Hordeola and chalazia should be treated appropriately.

ENTROPION

Entropion is an inward turning of the lid margin (Figure 4–4). It may be involutional, spastic, cicatricial, or congenital. Involutional entropion is the most common and by definition occurs as a result of aging. It always affects the lower lid and is the result of a combination of horizontal lid laxity, disinsertion of the lower lid retractors, and overriding of the preseptal orbicularis muscle.

Cicatricial entropion may involve the upper or lower lid and is the result of conjunctival and tarsal scar formation. It is most often found with chronic inflammatory diseases such as trachoma or ocular cicatricial pemphigoid.

Congenital entropion is rare and should not be confused with congenital **epiblepharon**, which often presents in Asians. In congenital entropion, the lid margin is rotated toward the cornea, whereas in epiblepharon, the pretarsal skin and orbicularis muscle cause the lashes to rotate around the tarsal border.

Trichiasis is misdirection of eyelashes toward the cornea and may be due to epiblepharon or simply misdirected growth. Chronic inflammatory lid diseases such as blepharitis may also cause scarring of the lash follicles and subsequent misdirected growth. It causes corneal irritation and may result in corneal ulceration.

Distichiasis is a condition manifested by accessory eyelashes, often growing from the orifices of the meibomian glands. It may be congenital or the result of inflammatory, metaplastic changes in the glands of the lid margin.

Correction of involutional entropion may be achieved by a number of approaches with consideration for horizontal lid tightening, repair of the lower lid retractors, or rotation of the lid margin. Useful temporary measures include taping the lower lid to the cheek, injection of botulinum toxin in the pretarsal orbicularis, or performing rotational lid sutures. Cicatricial entropion repair depends on the degree of severity with the option of skin resection for mild

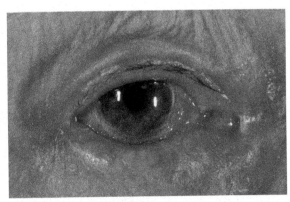

▲ **Figure 4–4.** Involutional entropion of right lower lid.

disease, tarsal infracture or margin rotation for moderate disease, and scar tissue release with grafting of the posterior lid for severe disease. Trichiasis without entropion can be temporarily relieved by epilating the offending eyelashes. Permanent relief may be achieved with electrolysis, laser, cryotherapy, or lid surgery.

ECTROPION

Ectropion is an outward turning of the lid margin (Figure 4–5). It may be involutional, paralytic, cicatricial, mechanical, or congenital. Involutional ectropion is the result of horizontal lid laxity from aging. Paralytic ectropion follows facial nerve palsy. Cicatricial ectropion is caused by contracture of the skin of the lid from trauma or inflammation. Mechanical ectropion usually occurs because of bulky tumors of the lid. Symptoms of tearing and irritation resulting in exposure keratitis may occur with any type.

Involutional and paralytic ectropion can be treated surgically by horizontal shortening of the lid. Treatment of cicatricial ectropion requires surgical revision of the scar and often skin grafting. Correction of mechanical ectropion requires removal of the neoplasm followed by lid reconstruction.

COLOBOMA

Congenital coloboma is the result of incomplete fusion of fetal maxillary processes. The consequence is a lid margin cleft of variable size. The medial aspect of the upper lid is most often involved, and there can be associated limbal dermoid tumors as in **Goldenhar syndrome**. Surgical reconstruction can usually be delayed for years but should be done immediately if the cornea is at risk. Coloboma may also refer to a full-thickness lid defect from any cause.

EPICANTHUS

Epicanthus is characterized by a vertical fold of skin over the medial canthus. It is typical of Asians and is present to some degree in most children of all races. The skinfold is often large enough to cover part of the nasal sclera and cause "pseudoesotropia" where the eye appears to be crossed. The most frequent type is **epicanthus tarsalis**, in which the superior lid fold is continuous medially with the epicanthal fold. In **epicanthus inversus**, the skinfold blends into the lower lid. Epicanthal skinfolds may also be acquired after surgery or trauma to the medial lid and nose. The cause of epicanthus is vertical shortening of the skin between the canthus and the nose. Surgical correction is directed at vertical lengthening and horizontal shortening. In children without congenital abnormalities, epicanthal folds diminish gradually by puberty and seldom require surgery.

TELECANTHUS

The normal distance between the medial canthus of each eye, the intercanthal distance, is equal to the length of each palpebral fissure (approximately 30 mm in adults). A wide intercanthal distance may be the result of trauma or congenital disorders (eg, Down syndrome, fetal alcohol syndrome, blepharophimosis syndrome). Minor degrees can be corrected with skin and soft tissue surgery. Larger reconstruction, however, is required in instances of trauma (see Chapter 17). Telecanthus should be distinguished from **hypertelorism** in which the overall distance between the two orbits is increased where both the intercanthal and the interpupillary distances are elongated. This finding is seen in syndromes of craniofacial dysgenesis such as **Crouzon's disease**.

▼ BLEPHAROCHALASIS

Blepharochalasis is a rare condition of unknown cause, sometimes familial, which resembles angioneurotic edema (Figure 4–6). Repeated attacks begin near puberty, diminish

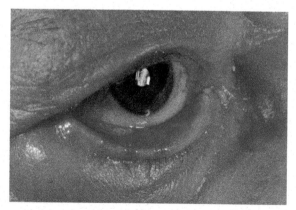

▲ **Figure 4–5.** Involutional ectropion of right lower lid.

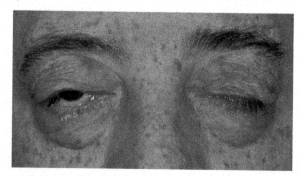

▲ **Figure 4–6.** Blepharochalasis.

during adulthood, and cause atrophy of periorbital structures. Lid skin appears thin, wrinkled, and redundant and is described as resembling crepe paper. A sunken appearance is the result of fat atrophy. Involvement of the levator aponeurosis produces moderate to severe ptosis. Medical management is limited to symptomatic treatment of edema. Surgical repair of levator dehiscence and excision of redundant skin are most likely to be successful after attacks have abated.

DERMATOCHALASIS

Dermatochalasis is lid skin redundancy and loss of elasticity as a result of aging (Figure 4–7). In the upper lid, the preseptal skin and orbicularis muscle hang over the pretarsal portion of the lid. When dermatochalasis is severe, the superior and peripheral visual fields are obstructed. Weakness of the orbital septum may result in prolapse of the medial and preaponeurotic fat pads. Similarly, "bags" in the preseptal region of the lower lid represent herniated orbital fat.

Blepharoplasty may be indicated for visual or aesthetic reasons. In the upper lid, superfluous lid skin is removed with or without the orbicularis muscle, and prominent orbital fat may be sculpted for optimum aesthetics. Lower lid blepharoplasty is considered cosmetic surgery unless extreme redundancy contributes to ectropion of the lid margin. Fat excision

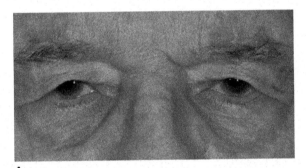

A

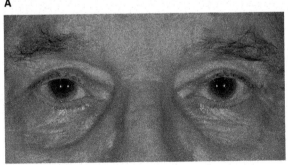

B

▲ **Figure 4–7.** Blepharoplasty. **(A)** Dermatochalasis of upper lids. **(B)** Upper lid blepharoplasty surgery results in removal of excess skin and improved peripheral vision.

and/or repositioning can be considered from a transconjunctival or subciliary approach in conjunction with conservative skin removal when necessary. Pulsed CO_2 and erbium lasers, while effective for facial aesthetic surgery, must be used with extreme caution in the periocular area.

BLEPHAROSPASM

Benign essential blepharospasm (BEB) is focal dystonia characterized by bilateral, synchronous, involuntary spasms of the lids. Onset is typically during adulthood, with a 3:1 female predominance. The spasms tend to progress in force and frequency, incapacitating patients with only brief intervals of vision between spasms. Early diagnosis is frequently missed or delayed. BEB may present with oromandibular dystonia and is then denoted a segmental dystonia because of involvement of two or more contiguous regions.

The cause of BEB is not known, but studies have implicated dysfunction of the basal ganglia and a number of cortical and subcortical centers that control blinking. However, current understanding of BEB implicates a defect in circuit activity, rather than that of a particular locus. Emotional stress and fatigue sometimes make the condition worse.

The primary treatment of BEB is directed at addressing the motor output with routine injections of botulinum toxin to produce temporary neuromuscular paralysis of the orbicularis oculi muscle. If intolerance or unresponsiveness to botulinum toxin develops, selective extirpation of the orbicularis muscles or surgical ablation of the facial nerve can be considered. Modification of the sensory input has also been shown to be beneficial with reduction of triggering, noxious stimuli by addressing light sensitivity and ocular surface disease. Central neuronal control using systemic medications has been less promising with no one drug being more efficacious and most patients responding incompletely or not at all.

It is important to differentiate BEB from **hemifacial spasm** (HFS). The latter is characterized by involuntary, irregular, tonic and clonic synchronous contractions of the muscles innervated by the ipsilateral facial nerve. HFS can result from compression of the facial nerve root exit zone by an aberrant vascular loop or, less frequently, a posterior fossa tumor. Microvascular decompression is the definitive mode of treatment; however, chemical denervation with botulinum toxin is less invasive and more frequently employed.

Other types of involuntary lid movements include **myokymia**, which is characterized by involuntary, fine, continuous, undulating contractions that spread across the lid. It is typically unilateral, involves the lower lid, and is rarely an early manifestation of BEB or HFS. **Aberrant facial nerve regeneration** is a recognized complication of peripheral facial nerve palsy. It is believed to arise when regenerating nerve fibers from facial subnucleus motoneurons are misdirected to other facial muscles and result in spasms.

BLEPHAROPTOSIS

The upper lid normally rests approximately midway between the superior limbus and the pupillary margin. Some variation in lid height may exist, but symmetry between the two sides is maintained. Blepharoptosis, or "ptosis" as it is more commonly called, is the condition in which one or both upper lids assume an abnormally low position.

▶ Classification

Blepharoptosis may be congenital or acquired (Table 4–1). Classification is important for selection of appropriate treatment.

CONGENITAL PTOSIS

1. Congenital Myogenic Ptosis

Congenital myogenic ptosis is the result of an isolated dystrophy of the levator muscle affecting both contraction and relaxation of the fibers. Ptosis is present in the primary position of gaze, and there is decreased lid excursion from upgaze to downgaze. In addition, lid lag on downgaze is an important clue to diagnosis of levator maldevelopment. Other ocular abnormalities, such as strabismus, may be present. In 25% of cases, the superior rectus muscle shares the same dystrophic changes as the levator, resulting in weakness of upgaze (**monocular elevation deficiency**).

    Blepharophimosis syndrome accounts for 5% of cases of congenital ptosis. Severe ptosis with poor levator function is accompanied by telecanthus, epicanthus inversus, and sometimes ectropion of the lower lids. It can also be associated with premature ovarian failure in females. The condition is autosomal dominant and caused by a mutation in the *FOXL2* gene on chromosome 3.

2. Congenital Neurogenic Ptosis

Congenital oculomotor nerve palsy may be partial or complete and manifests as blepharoptosis associated with the inability to elevate, depress, or adduct the globe. Mydriasis may also be observed. If the lid is completely closed, deprivational amblyopia will develop unless the ptosis is corrected.

    Congenital Horner's syndrome manifests as mild ptosis, miosis with decreased pigmentation of the iris resulting in heterochromia, and anhidrosis of the ipsilateral face. In most cases, no etiology is identified, and failure of development of the sympathetic nervous chain may be responsible. Birth trauma is the most commonly identified etiology, but neuroblastoma is responsible in a few cases and urine testing for catecholamines may be required. Unexplained acquired Horner's in infants necessitates imaging for neuroblastoma.

Table 4–1. Classification of Blepharoptosis

Congenital ptosis
Myogenic
Simple
With monocular elevation deficiency
Blepharophimosis syndrome
Neurogenic
Congenital oculomotor nerve palsy
Congenital Horner syndrome
Marcus Gunn jaw-winking syndrome
Congenital fibrosis of the extraocular muscles
Mechanical
Eyelid mass (eg, capillary hemangioma)
Acquired ptosis
Aponeurotic
Senescent (involutional)
Trauma
Blepharochalasis
Pregnancy
Graves ophthalmopathy
Myogenic
Chronic progressive external ophthalmoplegia
Oculopharyngeal muscular dystrophy
Myotonic dystrophy
Myasthenia gravis
HIV associated
Neurogenic
Acquired oculomotor nerve palsy
Ischemia (microvascular disease)
Trauma
Compression
Acquired Horner syndrome
Chemodenervation secondary to botulinum toxin injection
Mechanical
Edema
Eyelid mass (eg, chalazion or cutaneous carcinoma)
Scar tissue
Pseudoptosis
Dermatochalasis
Contralateral upper eyelid retraction
Vertical strabismus
Reduced orbital volume
Anophthalmos
Enophthalmos
Microphthalmos
Phthisis bulbi

    In **Marcus Gunn jaw-winking syndrome**, aberrant innervation of the levator muscle by the motor division of the trigeminal nerve (CN V) results in a synkinesis, manifesting as elevation of the ptotic lid with movement of the mandible.

    Congenital fibrosis of the extraocular muscles (CFEOM) is a rare genetic disorder manifesting as ptosis and restrictive ophthalmoplegia. The name of the disease is a misnomer as recent studies support a defect in neuronal differentiation. Several types exist and are classified according to genotype and phenotype. Inheritance is usually in an autosomal dominant pattern. Mutations of *KIF21A* (chromosome 12), *PHOX2A* (chromosome 11), and *TUBB3* (chromosome 16) genes have been identified.

ACQUIRED PTOSIS

1. Aponeurotic Ptosis

Senescent or involutional ptosis is the most common type of acquired ptosis. It results from partial disinsertion or dehiscence of the levator aponeurosis from the tarsal plate with age. Typically, there are sufficient residual attachments to the tarsus to maintain full excursion of the lid from upgaze to downgaze. Upward displacement or loss of insertion of the levator fibers into the skin and orbicularis muscle results in an unusually high lid crease. Thinning of the lid may also occur. Ptosis due to trauma (including ocular surgery or birth trauma) or blepharochalasis or associated with pregnancy is also usually due to disinsertion of the levator aponeurosis. Ptosis in Graves' disease may be aponeurotic, but myasthenia gravis should also be considered.

2. Acquired Myogenic Ptosis

Chronic progressive external ophthalmoplegia (CPEO), one form of mitochondrial cytopathy, is a slowly progressive neuromuscular disease that usually begins in mid-life. Although it is associated with deletions in mitochondrial DNA, the disease is usually sporadic because of new mutations rather than inherited. All extraocular muscles, including the levator, and the muscles of facial expression gradually become affected. A wide range of other neurodegenerative disorders may be present. In **Kearns-Sayre syndrome**, ophthalmoplegia, pigmentary retinopathy, and heart block manifest before age 15.

Oculopharyngeal muscular dystrophy, an autosomal dominant disease affecting individuals usually of French-Canadian ancestry, predominantly manifests as dysphagia but also as facial weakness, ptosis, and usually mild ophthalmoplegia. Ptosis and facial weakness also occur in **myotonic dystrophy**. Other findings include cataract, pupillary abnormalities, frontal baldness, testicular atrophy, and diabetes.

Myasthenia gravis (MG) (see Chapter 14) is an autoimmune disorder in which circulating antibodies impair binding of acetylcholine at the postsynaptic neuromuscular junction and thus muscle contraction. Ptosis and/or diplopia are commonly the initial manifestation of both the ocular and generalized forms. Lid fatigue with increasing ptosis on prolonged upgaze is a consistent sign. Rest or the local application of ice may transiently reverse ptosis. The orbicularis oculi muscles are also frequently involved. Cogan's lid twitch, in which the upper lid twitches upward on rapid movements

of the eyes from downward gaze to primary position, is sometimes present but is not specific. Testing for circulating antibodies to acetylcholine receptors, which can be divided into binding, blocking and modulating, or muscle-specific kinase is not sensitive for ocular MG (50–70%) but is very specific. Electromyography (EMG), particularly single-fiber studies of orbicularis oculi in ocular myasthenia, may be diagnostic (sensitivity of 88–99%). The diagnosis can also be confirmed by the reversal of muscle weakness following administration of intravenous edrophonium or intramuscular neostigmine, which prevents the breakdown of acetylcholine by inhibiting cholinesterase. Medical management with anticholinesterase agents, systemic steroids, or other immunosuppressants is usually effective. Screening for thymoma is necessary because about 10% of patients with MG will have this benign tumor.

3. Acquired Neurogenic Ptosis

Although the majority of **acquired oculomotor nerve palsies** are caused by ischemia (microvascular disease), usually secondary to arteriosclerosis, some are due to serious intracranial disease such as aneurysm or tumor (see Chapter 14). Typically there is lid ptosis and impairment of adduction, depression, and elevation of the globe, but the severity of each component varies. Pupillary abnormalities are common in traumatic palsies and compressive lesions. For acute, painful, isolated oculomotor nerve palsy with pupil involvement, aneurysmal compression should be considered until proven otherwise. Oculomotor palsy due to trauma, acute aneurysmal compression, or chronic compression, typically cavernous sinus lesion, may be complicated by oculomotor synkinesis (aberrant regeneration), resulting in inappropriate movements of the globe, lid, or pupil (eg, lid elevation on downgaze).

Acquired Horner's syndrome results from disruption of sympathetic innervation. It results in mild ptosis, due to paralysis of Müller's muscle in the upper lid, and mild elevation of the lower lid, due to paralysis of the inferior tarsal muscle, the combination giving a false impression of enophthalmos and miosis. If the lesion of the sympathetic pathway is proximal to the superior cervical ganglion, there is absence of sweating (anhidrosis) of the ipsilateral face and neck (see Chapter 14).

Lastly, neurogenic ptosis can be induced by injection of botulinum toxin into the levator muscle. This may be intentional, such as to treat severe exposure keratopathy, or accidental, with migration of the toxin in the treatment of lid spasms or periocular rhytids.

4. Mechanical Ptosis

The upper lid may be prevented from opening completely because of a lid lesion such as a neoplasm, mass effect from edema, or the tethering effect of scar formation. Excessive horizontal shortening of the upper lid is a common cause of mechanical ptosis. Another form is seen following enucleation, in which absence of support from the globe allows the lid to drop.

PSEUDOPTOSIS

In severe dermatochalasis, excess skin of the upper lid may conceal the lid margin and give the appearance of ptosis. Alternatively, contralateral upper lid retraction may be mistakenly interpreted as ipsilateral ptosis. Vertical strabismus may also give the appearance of ptosis. When fixating with the hypotropic eye, the upper lid of the hypertropic eye will appear to have a lower resting position on the cornea, giving the appearance of ptosis. Alternatively, when the hypertropic eye is used for fixation, the contralateral, hypotropic eye will assume a downward gaze position and a lower resting position of the upper lid, giving the appearance of ptosis on the hypotropic side. Evaluating each eye separately through cross cover testing will unmask the pseudoptosis. Conditions in which orbital volume is reduced, such as anophthalmos, enophthalmos, microphthalmos, and phthisis bulbi, can create the appearance of ptosis.

▶ Treatment

Surgical treatment of blepharoptosis is dependent on the degree of levator function. In patients with good function, surgery can be directed to the retractors of the lid and may by approached from the skin or conjunctiva with resection of the levator aponeurosis or Müller's muscle, respectively (Figure 4–8). The superior portion of the tarsus may be resected for additional elevation, especially in congenital ptosis. Successful surgical outcome for congenital ptosis in the presence of superior rectus weakness often requires resection of an additional length of levator muscle. With myasthenia gravis, treatment is first directed at medical management of the autoimmune disease. Should this fail or there be an incomplete response, surgical correction may be considered.

Patients with little or no levator function, as in severe congenital or acquired neurogenic or myogenic ptosis, require an alternative source for elevation. Suspension of the lids to the brow via a sling allows the patient to elevate the lids with the natural movement of the frontalis muscle. A number of materials may be used, each with its own advantages and disadvantages. These include autogenous fascia lata, allogeneic fascia lata, silicone tubing or rod, Mersilene mesh, or Gore-Tex suture. When lid closure, Bell's phenomenon, and other extraocular movements are impaired, ptosis correction must be undertaken with caution because of the risk of exposure keratitis.

One of the main goals of surgery is symmetry of the lid heights. This is only possible in all positions of gaze if the levator function is unimpaired. In some cases, the best result that can be achieved is to balance the lids in the primary position. With unilateral ptosis, achievement of symmetry in other positions of gaze is proportionate to levator function.

In children, the timing of congenital ptosis correction can be critical. The position of the upper lid may result in obstruction of the visual axis, leading to deprivational amblyopia especially in cases of severe, unilateral ptosis. Refractive error and strabismus are also associated with congenital ptosis. Thus careful monitoring of the child for visual development is important. Observation is typically elected for mild ptosis with surgery considered once a more accurate evaluation can be obtained with cooperation of the child, usually at 4 or 5 years of age. With evidence of amblyopia or worsening head position (chin-up posture), early surgical intervention is indicated.

4.2. Lid Tumors

This section presents an overview of the most common and most important neoplasms, choristomas, and hamartomas of the lid. Simulating lesions of inflammatory, infectious, or degenerative nature (eg, chalazion, hordeolum) are discussed in other sections of this chapter.

BENIGN TUMORS OF THE LIDS

Benign neoplasms are acquired cellular tumors of cells that are atypical but not sufficient to be classified as malignant. They may enlarge slowly but have little or no invasive potential

and no metastatic capability. **Hamartomas** are congenital tumors composed of normal or near-normal cells and tissues for the anatomic site but in excessive amounts. **Choristomas** are congenital tumors consisting of normal cells and tissue elements but not occurring normally at the anatomic site.

▶ Benign Epidermal Neoplasms

The epidermis and dermis of the lid may be affected by a variety of acquired neoplasms that range from benign to precancerous. Each type of epithelial tumor exhibits some

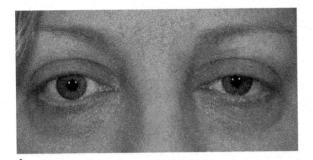

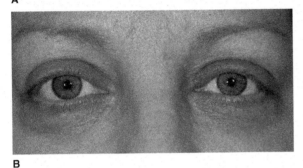

A

B

▲ **Figure 4–8.** Blepharoptosis correction. **(A)** Blepharoptosis of the left upper lid. **(B)** External levator resection on left side results in improvement of upper lid height.

variation in its clinical features such that clinical diagnosis may not be reliable and definitive diagnosis requires histopathologic examination.

Squamous papilloma of the skin (skin tag) is a focal hyperplasia of the stratified squamous epithelium of the epidermis (Figure 4–9). Single or multiple, with a fleshy color and irregular surface, squamous papillomas may be sessile or pedunculated. Growths may be observed or excised.

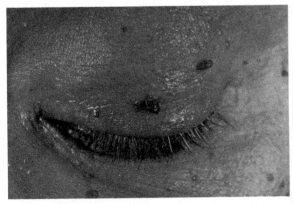

▲ **Figure 4–9.** Squamous papillomas (skin tags) of the right upper and lower lids.

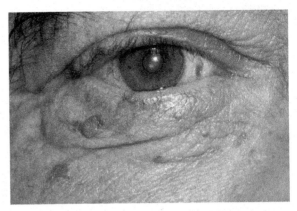

▲ **Figure 4–10.** Seborrheic keratosis of the right lower lid and lid margin.

Seborrheic keratosis predominantly occurs in middle-aged and older adults (Figure 4–10). It manifests as a dome-shaped to verrucoid (wart-like) adherent papule that is fleshy to gray-brown in color, with a crusty surface due to hyperkeratosis. Treatment of an aesthetically bothersome growth is surgical excision.

Keratoacanthoma (KA) is a low-grade tumor that is believed to originate from the pilosebaceous unit. It closely resembles squamous cell carcinoma, and some experts now consider KA a variant of it. The neoplasm usually manifests as a rapidly growing single nodule in a middle-aged individual. Umbilicated, with a distinctive crater filled with a keratin plug, the lesion develops over a few weeks but typically undergoes spontaneous involution within 6 months, leaving an atrophic scar. Multiple KAs are a common feature of the **Muir-Torre syndrome**, an autosomal dominant disease that manifests with neoplasms of the skin and viscera, most commonly colorectal cancer (47%) and genitourinary malignancies (21%). Most experts agree that surgical excision of KA is the treatment of choice.

Actinic keratosis (solar keratosis) manifests as an erythematous, scaly flat lesion, developing in a middle-aged or older person. The frequency of malignant transformation to squamous cell carcinoma has been estimated to be as high as 20%. Treatment options include topical therapy, chemical peeling, photodynamic therapy, cryosurgery, and excision.

▶ **Benign Melanocytic Neoplasms**

Melanocytic skin lesions may arise from epidermal (dendritic) melanocytes, nevus cells in the epidermis, or dermal (fusiform) melanocytes (Figure 4-11). Most benign melanocytic neoplasms are melanocytic nevi, of which the three principal subtypes are termed junctional, compound, and intradermal. A junctional nevus typically appears as a small, flat, tan macule that first becomes apparent in childhood

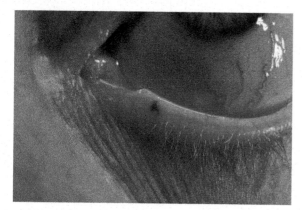

▲ **Figure 4–11.** Nevus of the left lower lid margin lateral to puncta. Note the associated cysts within the lesion.

and gradually increases in size but only to a limited extent. It represents nests of melanocytes within the epidermis at the dermal-epidermal junction. As the lesion stops growing, some of the nests of melanocytes migrate into the dermis, forming a compound nevus, which clinically is slightly elevated and melanotic. Further evolution of the lesion, with the remaining epidermal nests migrating into the dermis, produces an intradermal nevus, which may be dome-shaped, pedunculated, or papillomatous. Intradermal nevi are commonly present in adults and usually are hypomelanotic or amelanotic. Diagnosis of melanocytic nevi is based on clinical appearance. Although malignant transformation is rare, it may occur in the junctional or compound stages. Suspicious-looking lesions that demonstrate significant growth should be biopsied or excised.

Adnexal Neoplasms

Adnexal tumors of the lid are benign neoplasms arising from tissues such as hair follicle epithelium, sweat glands (glands of Moll), and sebaceous glands (Meibomian glands in the tarsus and glands of Zeiss in the eyelashes). Two noteworthy categories are **sebaceous adenoma**, which arises from Meibomian glands of the tarsus and therefore develops close to or contiguous with a hair follicle, and the **trichoepithelioma**, which arises from the hair follicle epithelium and therefore develops adjacent to hair shafts, including the eyelashes. These tumors typically appear as solitary, well-circumscribed, superficial nodules. Treatment is surgical excision.

Hamartomas

Vascular hamartomas of the lid comprise a spectrum of benign blood vessel tumors that includes **nevus flammeus** (congenital telangiectatic hemangioma) associated with Sturge-Webber syndrome, **capillary hemangioma** (strawberry nevus), **varix**, and **glomus tumor**. Capillary hemangioma is composed of a hamartomatous proliferation of vascular endothelial cells. It is sometimes evident at birth but usually becomes apparent during the first few months of life. It progressively enlarges and becomes more elevated for several months and stabilizes around 1 year of age. It is estimated that 30% completely involute by the age of 3 years and 75–90% by the age of 7 years. Clinically, the superficial lesion typically manifests as a red vascular macule that may become large enough to cause ptosis, indentational astigmatism, and amblyopia (Figure 4–12). A deeper lesion has a blue-gray color, is soft to palpation, and becomes more evident when the child cries or strains. Tumor extension into the orbit may cause proptosis and/or strabismus. Since most capillary hemangiomas regress spontaneously, the principal indications for treatment are amblyopia, compressive optic neuropathy, and/or exposure keratopathy. In the past, systemic or intralesional steroids were considered the first line of therapy to hasten tumor regression. The systemic beta-blocker propranolol has been newly employed with promising results. Treatment requires close monitoring for potential side effects including shortness of breath, bradycardia, and hypoglycemia and is initiated in the hospital. Topical application of timolol maleate gel, another beta-blocker, has shown efficacy for superficial lesions. Surgical excision is now typically reserved for lesions that are refractory and result in visual compromise.

Lymphangioma of the lid is a congenital overgrowth of lymph channels. More than half are evident at birth, and approximately 90% are clinically apparent by age 2. It usually lies deep to the epidermis and manifests as a dark blue, soft, fluctuant mass. There may also be conjunctival or orbital involvement. Spontaneous or posttraumatic bleeding may occur. Management options include observation of small lesions, surgical resection of aesthetically bothersome circumscribed lesions, and surgical debulking of diffuse lesions.

Choristomas

Choristomas of the lid are rare. Present at birth, they slowly enlarge. Several types are recognized, including phakomatous choristoma (Zimmerman tumor) consisting of lens material; odontogenic choristoma consisting of dental tissue; osseous choristoma consisting of bone tissue; **epidermoid cyst** consisting of a stratified squamous epithelium and filled with

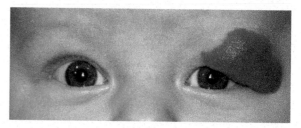

▲ **Figure 4–12.** Capillary hemangioma of the left upper lid in an infant causing ptosis. (Used with permission from William R. Katowitz, MD.)

desquamated keratin; and **dermoid cyst** consisting of adnexal structures such as sebaceous glands, eccrine sweat glands, and hair follicles, in addition to the keratinizing epithelium. Lid choristomas can develop in the superficial or deep tissues of the lid and orbit and are found in almost any location (see Chapter 13). Clinically, they manifest as a solitary, firm, slowly enlarging, nontender masses, most commonly in the lateral upper lid and brow. Treatment is complete surgical removal.

MALIGNANT TUMORS OF THE LIDS

Primary Malignant Epidermal Neoplasms

Basal cell carcinoma and squamous cell carcinoma comprise the majority of malignant lid neoplasms. Risk factors for cutaneous carcinomas include ultraviolet light exposure, radiation exposure, carcinogen exposure, fair skin, age greater than 50, personal or family history of skin cancer, arsenic exposure, immunosuppressants, and genetic disorders such as xeroderma pigmentosum. Patients with cutaneous carcinomas require routine surveillance of sun-exposed skin in conjunction with a dermatologist.

Basal cell carcinoma (BCC) arises from pluripotent stem cells within the basal layers of the epidermis and external root sheaths of hair follicles. It does not appear to arise from mature differentiated basal cells. It comprises about 90% of all lid malignancies. The incidence of BCC of the lid skin increases with age, and there is a slight male preponderance (3:2 male-to-female ratio). Clinically, it typically manifests as a firm painless indurated nodule with a pearly, rolled border and fine (small) telangiectatic surface vessels (Figure 4–13). Sixty-five percent of cases occur in the lower lid. Treatment consists of surgical excision with margin control or Mohs micrographic surgery. Incisional biopsy is recommended to confirm the diagnosis prior to a wide surgical excision

that may require a complex lid reconstruction. For locally advanced or metastatic BCC that cannot be treated with surgery or radiation, vismodegib, a hedgehog pathway inhibitor, is a new therapeutic option.

Squamous cell carcinoma arises from the stratified squamous epithelium. It tends to be locally invasive and may metastasize to regional lymph nodes. It comprises 5–10% of all lid malignancies, being much less common than basal cell carcinoma. Although typically observed in elderly patients, squamous cell carcinoma may be seen in younger patients with a history of radiotherapy or systemic immunosuppression. Clinically, lid squamous cell carcinoma typically appears as a slow-growing, painless, hyperkeratotic nodule that eventually becomes ulcerated (Figure 4–14). Subsequently there is shallow ulceration with a granular, red base surrounded by an elevated, hard border. Treatment is surgical excision of the entire lesion either by conventional methods or Mohs micrographic surgery, followed by reconstruction of the defect. Focal radiation therapy is used occasionally to treat perineural invasion into bone or the orbit, and exenteration is reserved for cases with orbital invasion.

Sebaceous cell carcinoma of the lid arises from sebaceous glands in the skin. Clinically, it can appear as a painless nodule arising from the tarsus or diffuse thickening of the lid. Lash loss in involved areas is common. Initially, sebaceous carcinoma of the lid is frequently misdiagnosed as a benign condition such as recurrent chalazia and chronic blepharitis, leading to delay in effective treatment. Histopathologically, there are four recognized patterns of growth the tumor may exhibit including lobular, comedocarcinoma, papillary, and mixed. Tumor cells tend to have vacuolated cytoplasm from the lipid content. Further classification as to the degree of atypia can also be made with well, moderately, and poorly differentiated designations. Tumor cells are frequently found in the adjacent epithelia separate from the main tumor, a feature known as

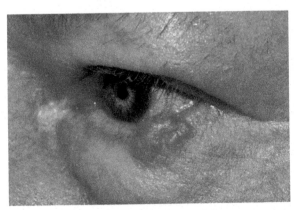

▲ **Figure 4–13.** Basal cell carcinoma of the left lower lid demonstrating pearly appearance, telangiectatic vessels, destruction of lid margin, and loss of eyelashes.

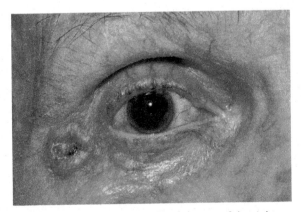

▲ **Figure 4–14.** Squamous cell carcinoma of the right lateral canthus with erythematous, raised edges, and central ulceration.

pagetoid spread. This typically occurs within the conjunctiva, but it can also occur in the skin or cornea. Special stains to confirm the histologic diagnosis are oil red-O and Sudan black (specific for cytoplasmic fat) and epithelial membrane antigen (EMA) immunoperoxidase staining (specific for sebaceous differentiation). Sebaceous cell carcinoma exhibits an aggressive clinical course, with a significant tendency for local recurrence after excision and regional or distant metastasis. Delay in diagnosis likely contributes to poorer outcomes, and thus a high degree of clinical suspicion and readiness to biopsy peculiar lesions are necessary. Map biopsies will help define the degree of conjunctival involvement. Definitive treatment is wide surgical excision. The role of radiotherapy has not been defined and has traditionally been considered palliative but not curative. Sebaceous cell carcinoma is also associated with Muir-Torre syndrome.

Cutaneous **melanoma** accounts for only 1% of all lid tumors but is associated with relatively high frequencies of metastasis and tumor-related death. It generally affects Caucasians and occurs preferentially in areas of skin exposed excessively to ultraviolet light. There are four types of primary cutaneous melanoma: lentigo maligna melanoma, superficial spreading melanoma, nodular melanoma, and acral lentiginous melanoma. The typical clinical appearance of lid melanomas is a broad, flat, tan to brown irregular macule with nodularity and possible ulceration. Lid melanomas may metastasize to regional lymph nodes of the head and neck, emphasizing the importance of examination for preauricular and submandibular lymphadenopathy. Treatment is wide surgical excision followed by reconstructive surgery. Exenteration of the orbit is performed for some patients with massive orbital invasion, although there is little evidence that such surgery improves survival. The prognosis in lid melanoma is related to size of the tumor, depth of invasion, atypical features of tumor cells, and completeness of initial excision.

▶ Other Malignant Tumors

In cutaneous **lymphoma** of the lid, there is infiltration by malignant lymphocytic cells, resulting in thickening or edema of the tissue bed. Usually it is not tender or painful, but severe pruritus is common. Unlike conjunctival, intraocular, and orbital lymphomas, which are almost always disorders of B-cell–derived lymphocytes, a high proportion of lid lymphomas are cutaneous T-cell lymphomas. **Mycosis fungoides** is the most common type observed and often presents with cicatricial ectropion. Cutaneous B-cell lymphomas are less frequently seen but can also involve the lid. Diagnosis is usually based on tissue biopsy. In general, management of patients with ocular adnexal lymphomas begins with a thorough examination with baseline systemic staging using the World Health Organization classification (fourth edition, 2008). Treatment of disseminated cutaneous lymphoma is usually intravenous chemotherapy. However, radiation therapy can be used for treatment of limited disease, including lid involvement. Intralesional chemotherapy is also an option. Prognostic factors for survival in patients with cutaneous lymphoma include tumor classification, staging, age at the time of diagnosis, and tumor-specific genetic markers.

Kaposi's sarcoma (KS) is a malignant mesenchymal neoplasm. It was relatively rare and encountered mainly in southern Europe in persons over 40 years of age. KS became more widely recognized as one of the acquired immunodeficiency syndrome (AIDS)-defining illnesses in the 1980s. The tumor is caused by an infection with human herpes virus 8. The extremities are involved most frequently, but any region of the skin can be affected. KS of the lid manifests as a red to purple subcutaneous lesion that can be circumscribed, diffuse, nodular, or pedunculated. Histopathologically, KS comprises a network of proliferating endothelial cells that form a channel-like structure filled with blood. Treatment for KS of the lid consists of intravenous chemotherapy (especially if the patient has multiple skin lesions in various anatomic sites) or focal palliative radiotherapy.

Lid metastasis, due to occasional hematogenous spread from nonophthalmic primary cancer, typically manifests as an abruptly enlarging subepidermal mass, with metastases at various other anatomic sites also usually being detectable. In general, survival of a patient with a lid metastasis is poor. Treatment is typically dictated by therapy for the primary tumor. Surgical excision or radiotherapy can be considered for palliation.

4.3. Lacrimal Apparatus

The lacrimal apparatus comprises structures involved in the production and drainage of tears (also see Chapter 5). The secretory system consists of the glands that produce the various components of the tear film, which is distributed over the surface of the eye by the action of blinking. The lacrimal puncta, canaliculi, and sac and the nasolacrimal duct form the drainage system that ultimately empties into the nose.

LACRIMAL SECRETORY SYSTEM

The tear film is composed of three layers. Unicellular goblet cells, which are scattered throughout the conjunctiva, secrete glycoprotein in the form of mucin that comprises the inner-most layer of the tear film. The main and accessory lacrimal glands provide the intermediate aqueous layer. The lipid layer is the final layer of the tear film that is produced by the meibomian glands of the tarsus.

The lacrimal gland is located in the lacrimal fossa in the superior temporal quadrant of the orbit. This almond-shaped gland is divided by the lateral horn of the levator aponeurosis into a larger orbital lobe and a smaller palpebral lobe. Ducts from the orbital lobe join those of the palpebral lobe and empty into the superior temporal fornix (see Chapter 1). The palpebral lobe can sometimes be visualized by everting the upper lid. The accessory lacrimal glands are comprised of the glands of Krause and Wolfring and are located in the conjunctiva mainly in the superior fornix and superior tarsal border. Traditionally, basal tear production has been attrib-uted to the accessory glands. This belief, however, has been questioned because tear production diminishes during sleep and under general or local anesthesia. Some experts thus believe that all tearing is reflexive in nature and is initiated by some external or internal stimuli.

Noxious stimuli or emotional distress triggers secretions from the lacrimal gland and results in tears flowing copi-ously over the lid margin (epiphora). The afferent pathway of the reflex arc is the ophthalmic branch of the trigeminal nerve. The efferent pathway is comprised of parasympathetic and sympathetic contributions. Parasympathetic innerva-tion originates from the pontine lacrimal (superior salivary) nucleus and joins general somatic sensory and special sensory fibers to form the nervus intermedius. The pregan-glionic parasympathetic fibers pass through the geniculate ganglion where they do not synapse and exit as the greater petrosal nerve. They then enter the middle cranial fossa and proceed to the foramen lacerum to join the deep petrosal nerve and form the nerve of the pterygoid canal (Vidian nerve). The parasympathetic fibers then synapse in the pterygopalatine ganglion and, via the maxillary nerve, join the zygomatic nerve to enervate the lacrimal gland. The sympathetic pathway is less well characterized.

DISORDERS OF THE SECRETORY SYSTEM

Alacrima

Congenital absence of tearing occurs in Riley-Day syn-drome (familial dysautonomia) and anhidrotic ectodermal dysplasia. Although initially asymptomatic, patients usually develop signs of keratoconjunctivitis sicca. Reduced tear production may occur after damage to the nervus interme-dius following surgery in the cerebellopontine angle, such as for vestibular schwannoma (acoustic neuroma), or due to tumors or inflammation of the lacrimal gland.

Lacrimal Hypersecretion

Primary hypersecretion may occur as a result of tumor or inflammation of the lacrimal gland and is a rare cause of tearing. Secondary hypersecretion may be of supranuclear, infranuclear, or reflex etiologies. The most common cause of hypersecretion is reflex lacrimation resulting from ocular surface disease or tear film instability or deficiency. Treat-ment is therefore directed at stabilizing the underlying disease process. Hypersecretion always needs to be distin-guished from tearing due to obstruction of the lacrimal drainage system.

Paradoxical Lacrimation ("Crocodile Tears")

This condition is characterized by tearing while eating. Although it may be congenital, it is usually acquired after Bell's palsy and is the result of aberrant regeneration of the facial nerve. Injecting botulinum toxin into the lacrimal gland can treat unnecessary tear production.

Bloody Tears

Hemolacria is a rare clinical entity attributed to a variety of causes, including conjunctivitis, trauma, blood dyscrasias, vascular tumors, and tumors of the lacrimal sac.

Dacryoadenitis

Inflammation of the lacrimal gland can be acute or chronic and due to infection or systemic disease. **Acute dacryoad-enitis** is less common and usually seen in children as a com-plication of a viral infection including mumps, Epstein-Barr virus, measles, or influenza. It is, however, sometimes due to bacterial or fungal infection. In adults, *Neisseria gonorrhoeae* may be responsible. Symptoms typically evolve over hours or days. There is marked pain, with swelling and redness of the outer portion of the upper lid, which often assumes an S-shaped curve. If there is purulent discharge, a Gram stain and culture can be performed. Bacterial infections usually respond to systemic antibiotics, without the need for surgi-cal drainage.

Chronic dacryoadenitis, defined as inflammation for longer than 1 month, is more common. It can be bilateral and often is painless. It may be associated with systemic inflam-matory diseases such as sarcoidosis, Graves' disease, Sjögren's syndrome, systemic lupus erythematosus, or IgG4-related disease. Infectious causes are rare but include syphilis, tuberculosis, leprosy, and trachoma. Lymphoma involving the lacrimal gland may mimic chronic dacryoadenitis (see Chapter 13). Often laboratory workup for inflammatory etiologies reveals little; however, biopsy of the gland may be useful, especially to differentiate from a neoplastic process.

LACRIMAL DRAINAGE SYSTEM

The drainage system is composed of the puncta, canaliculi, lacrimal sac, and nasolacrimal duct (see Chapter 1). With each blink, the lids close like a zipper—beginning laterally, distributing tears evenly across the cornea, and delivering them to the drainage system on the medial aspect of the lids. Under normal circumstances, tears are produced at about their rate of evaporation, and thus, few pass through the drainage system. When tears flood the conjunctival sac, they enter the puncta partially by capillary attraction. With lid closure, the specialized portion of pretarsal orbicularis surrounding the ampulla tightens to prevent their escape. Simultaneously, the lid is drawn toward the posterior lacrimal crest and traction is placed on the fascia surrounding the lacrimal sac, causing the canaliculi to shorten and creating negative pressure within the sac. This dynamic pumping action draws tears into the sac. The tears then pass by gravity and tissue elasticity through the nasolacrimal duct to exit beneath the inferior meatus of the nose. Valve-like folds of the epithelial lining of the duct tend to resist the retrograde flow of tears and air. The most developed of these flaps is the valve of Hasner at the distal end. This structure is important because when imperforate, it is the most common cause of congenital nasolacrimal duct obstruction, resulting in epiphora and chronic dacryocystitis.

DISORDERS OF THE DRAINAGE SYSTEM

1. NASOLACRIMAL DUCT OBSTRUCTION AND DACRYOCYSTITIS

Infection of the lacrimal sac is common, most often unilateral, and secondary to obstruction of the nasolacrimal duct.

In **infantile dacryocystitis** the site of obstruction is usually a persistent membrane covering the valve of Hasner. Failure of canalization of the nasolacrimal duct occurs in up to 87% of newborns, but it usually becomes patent at the end of the first month of life in 90% of neonates. Chronic dacryocystitis is more common than acute dacryocystitis, but prompt and aggressive treatment of acute dacryocystitis should be instituted because of the risk of orbital cellulitis. Microorganisms involved in chronic and acute infantile dacryocystitis include *Streptococcus pneumoniae*, *Staphylococcus* species, *Haemophilus influenzae*, and Enterobacteriaceae species.

In adults, nasolacrimal duct obstruction typically occurs in postmenopausal women. The cause is often uncertain but generally is attributed to chronic inflammation resulting in fibrosis within the duct. Stasis of tears within the sac may lead to secondary infections. Acute and chronic dacryocystitis are usually caused by *S aureus*, *S epidermidis*, *Pseudomonas aeruginosa*, or anaerobic organisms such as *Peptostreptococcus* and *Propionibacterium* species. Dacryocystitis is otherwise uncommon unless it follows trauma or is caused by formation of a cast (dacryolith) within the lacrimal sac.

Clinical Findings

The chief symptoms of dacryocystitis are tearing and discharge. In the acute form, there is inflammation, pain, swelling, and tenderness beneath the medial canthal tendon in the area of the lacrimal sac (Figure 4–15). Purulent material can be expressed through the lacrimal puncta by direct pressure on the sac. In the chronic form, tearing and matting of lashes are usually the only symptoms, but mucoid material usually can be expressed from the sac.

Dilation of the lacrimal sac (mucocele) indicates obstruction of the nasolacrimal duct. Regurgitation of mucus or pus through the puncta can be demonstrated on compression of the enlarged sac. It is also important to examine within the nose to determine whether there is adequate drainage space between the inferior turbinate and the lateral nasal wall.

Treatment

Acute dacryocystitis usually responds to appropriate systemic antibiotics. The infectious agent can be identified by Gram stain and culture of material expressed from the tear sac. Occasionally, incision and drainage of the lacrimal sac may be necessary. Chronic infections can often be kept latent with antibiotic drops. In either case, correction of the obstruction is the definitive cure.

In infants (see Chapter 17), forceful compression of the lacrimal sac will sometimes rupture the membrane and establish patency. If stenosis persists for more than 6 months or if there is an episode of acute dacryocystitis, nasolacrimal probing is indicated. One probing is effective in 75% of cases. In the remainder, cure can almost always be achieved by repeated probing, by inward fracture of the inferior turbinate, or by temporary silicone stent intubation or balloon catheter dilation of the lacrimal system. Lacrimal surgery is rarely required. Probing should not be attempted in the presence of acute infection.

In **adults**, surgical correction of nasolacrimal duct obstruction is usually achieved by **dacryocystorhinostomy**, in which a permanent fistula is formed between the lacrimal sac and the nose. With the traditional approach, exposure

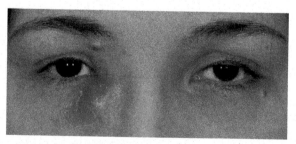

▲ **Figure 4–15.** Acute dacryocystitis.

is gained by an external incision over the anterior lacrimal crest. Bone is removed from the lateral wall of the nose and incisions are made in the lacrimal sac and adjacent nasal mucosa followed by anastomosis of the mucosal flaps with suture placement. Various endonasal endoscopic techniques to create the fistula have been developed, with the advantage of avoiding an external incision. Balloon catheter dilation of the distal nasolacrimal duct may be useful for patients with partial obstruction but is ineffective in resolving a complete obstruction. Patients with chronic dacryocystitis should undergo lacrimal surgery prior to elective intraocular surgery to reduce the risk of endophthalmitis.

2. CANALICULAR DISORDERS

Congenital anomalies of the canalicular system include imperforate puncta, accessory puncta, canalicular fistulas, and, rarely, agenesis of the canalicular system.

Most cases of canalicular stenosis are acquired and are due to viral infections, usually varicella-zoster, herpes simplex, or adenovirus infection, trauma, conjunctival inflammatory diseases such as Stevens-Johnson syndrome, toxic epidermal necrolysis, erythema multiforme, and ocular cicatricial pemphigoid. Alternatively, it may result from drug therapy, either systemic chemotherapy with fluorouracil or topical idoxuridine.

Canaliculitis is an uncommon chronic unilateral infection caused by *Actinomyces* species, *Candida albicans*, *Aspergillus* species, anaerobic streptococci, or staphylococci (Figure 4–16). The patient typically complains of a mildly red and irritated eye with a slight discharge that is often incorrectly diagnosed as conjunctivitis. It affects the lower canaliculus more often than the upper, usually occurs in adults, and causes a secondary conjunctivitis. If untreated, it can result in canalicular stenosis.

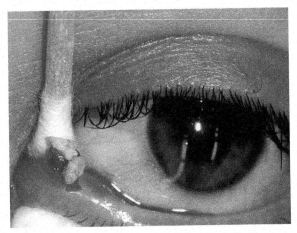

▲ **Figure 4–16.** Canaliculitis secondary to *Actinomyces israelii.*

▶ Clinical Findings

Canalicular probing and irrigation aid in identification of the location and severity of obstruction. Further evidence is provided by compression of the lacrimal sac. No regurgitation of material through the puncta will occur if there is complete obstruction of the common canaliculus or of both the upper and lower canaliculi.

In canaliculitis, the punctum usually pouts, and pus can be expressed from the canaliculus, with the organism being identifiable by Gram stain and culture.

▶ Treatment

Partial common canalicular stenosis may be amenable to intubation with a silicone stent for 3–6 months, but severe cases require dacryocystorhinostomy combined with canaliculoplasty and silicone intubation. Total canalicular obstruction necessitates formation of a fistula between the conjunctival sac and the nose (conjunctivo-dacryocystorhinostomy) with insertion of a Pyrex glass (Jones) tube to maintain its patency.

For canaliculitis, curettage of dacroliths from the involved canaliculus, followed by irrigation with antibiotic solution, may be effective in establishing patency, with ongoing antibiotic therapy dictated by microbiological results. Often, canaliculotomy is necessary to ensure removal of all stones. Recurrent infection is common.

REFERENCES

Lids

Allen RC: Genetic diseases affecting the eyelids: What should a clinician know? Curr Opin Ophthalmol 2013;24:463. [PMID: 23846188]

Allen RC et al: The current state of ptosis repair: A comparison of internal and external approaches. Curr Opin Ophthalmol 2011;22:39. [PMID: 21730839]

Andrews CV et al: Congenital fibrosis of the extraocular muscles. 2004 Apr 27 [Updated 2011 Dec 29]. In: Pagon RA, Adam MP, Ardinger HH, et al, eds. GeneReviews® [Internet]. Seattle, WA: University of Washington, Seattle; 1993-2015. Available at: http://www.ncbi.nlm.nih.gov/books/NBK1348/

Bansal RK et al: Results and complications of silicone frontalis sling surgery for ptosis. J Pediatr Ophthalmol Strabismus 2015;52:93. [PMID: 25973459]

Bernardini FP et al: Treatment of unilateral congenital ptosis: putting the debate to rest. Curr Opin Ophthalmol 2013;24:484. [PMID: 23925061]

Cahill JA et al: Eye on children: Acute work-up for pediatric Horner's syndrome. Case presentation and review of the literature. J Emerg Med 2015;48:58. [PMID: 25281181]

Chang S et al: A systematic review of comparison of upper eyelid involutional ptosis repair techniques: Efficacy and complication rates. Plast Reconstr Surg 2012;129:149. [PMID: 22186506]

Chi JJ. Management of the eye in facial paralysis. Facial Plast Surg Clin North Am 2016;24:21. [PMID: 26611698]

Demirci H et al: Marcus Gunn jaw-winking synkinesis clinical features and management. Ophthalmology 2010;117:1447. [PMID: 20188419]

Geerling G et al: The international workshop on meibomian gland dysfunction: Report of the subcommittee on management and treatment of meibomian gland dysfunction. Invest Ophthalmol Vis Sci 2011;52:2050. [PMID: 21450919]

Goold LA et al: Acute suppurative bacterial dacryoadenitis: A case series. Br J Ophthalmol 2013;97:735. [PMID: 23603486]

Hahn S et al: Upper lid blepharoplasty. Facial Plast Surg Clin North Am 2016;24:119. [PMID: 27105797]

Hallett M et al: Evidence-based review and assessment of botulinum neurotoxin for the treatment of movement disorders. Toxicon 2013;67:94. [PMID: 23380701]

Hellman A et al: Botulinum toxin in the management of blepharospasm: Current evidence and recent developments. Ther Adv Neurol Disord 2015;8:82. [PMID: 25922620]

Kakizaki H et al: Upper eyelid anatomy: An update. Ann Plast Surg 2009;63:336. [PMID: 19602949]

Kakizaki H et al: Lower eyelid anatomy: An update. Ann Plast Surg 2009;63:344. [PMID: 19602948]

Litwin AS et al: Blepharoptosis surgery in patients with myasthenia gravis. Br J Ophthalmol 2015;99:899. [PMID: 25595175]

Marcet MM et al: Involutional entropion: Risk factors and surgical remedies. Curr Opin Ophthalmol 2015;26:416. [PMID: 26154839]

Ojo OO et al: Is it time for flexibility in botulinum inter-injection intervals? Toxicon 2015;107:72. [PMID: 26440738]

Pariseau B et al: Myectomy for blepharospasm 2013. Curr Opin Ophthalmol 2013;24:488. [PMID: 23925062]

Ross AH et al: Management of upper eyelid cicatricial entropion. Clin Experiment Ophthalmol 2011;39:526. [PMID: 21819506]

Ross AH et al: Review and update of involuntary facial movement disorders presenting in the ophthalmological setting. Surv Ophthalmol 2011;56:54. [PMID: 21093885]

Serin D et al: The efficacy of the combined procedure in involutional entropion surgery: A comparative study. Korean J Ophthalmol 2013;27:405. [PMID: 24311924]

SooHoo JR et al: Congenital ptosis. Surv Ophthalmol 2014;59:483. [PMID: 24657037]

Stein A et al: Congenital eyelid ptosis: onset and prevalence of amblyopia, associations with systemic disorders, and treatment outcomes. J Pediatr 2014;165:820. [PMID: 25085522]

Young SM et al: Prospective audit of ptosis surgery at the Singapore National Eye Centre: Two-year results. Ophthal Plast Reconstr Surg 2013;29:446. [PMID: 24145906]

Yadegari S: Approach to a patient with blepharoptosis. Neurol Sci 2016;37:1589. [PMID: 27329276]

Lid Tumors

Aronow ME. Ocular adnexal lymphoma: Evidence-based treatment approach. Int Ophthalmol Clin 2015;55:97. [PMID: 25436496]

Bernardini FP. Management of malignant and benign eyelid lesions. Curr Opin Ophthalmol 2006;17:480. [PMID: 16932064]

Bianciotto C et al: Metastatic tumors to the eyelid: Report of 20 cases and review of the literature. Arch Ophthalmol 2009;127:999. [PMID: 19667336]

Boulos PR et al: Cutaneous melanomas of the eyelid. Semin Ophthalmol 2006;21:195. [PMID: 16912018]

Chan FM et al: Treatment and outcomes of malignant melanoma of the eyelid: A review of 29 cases in Australia. Ophthalmology 2007;114:187. [PMID: 17140665]

Deprez M et al: Clinicopathologcial features of eyelid skin tumors. A retrospective study of 5504 cases and review of the literature. Am J Dermatopathol 2009;31:256. [PMID: 19384066]

Esmaeli B et al: American Joint Committee on Cancer T category for eyelid sebaceous carcinoma correlates with nodal metastasis and survival. Ophthalmology 2012;119:1078. [PMID: 22330966]

Frank RC et al: Visual development in infants: Visual complications of periocular hemangiomas. J Plast Reconstr Aesthet Surg 2010;632:1. [PMID: 19097831]

Léauté-Labrèze C et al: Propranolol for severe hemangiomas of infancy. N Engl J Med 2008;358:2649. [PMID: 18550886]

Leibovitch I et al: Periocular keratoacanthoma: Can we always rely upon the clinical diagnosis? Br J Ophthalmol 2005;89:1201. [PMID: 16113382]

Marchalik RJ et al: Eyelid melanoma. N Engl J Med 2016;375:75. [PMID: 27406350]

Mendoza PR et al: Sentinel lymph node biopsy for eyelid and conjunctival tumors: What is the evidence? Int Ophthalmol Clin 2015;55:123. [PMID: 25436498]

Narayanan K et al: Mohs micrographic surgery versus surgical excision for periocular basal cell carcinoma. Cochrane Database Syst Rev 2014;12:CD007041. [PMID:25503105]

Pointdujour-Lim R et al: Cutaneous horn of the eyelid in 13 cases. Ophthal Plast Reconstr Surg 2016 Nov 2. [Epub ahead of print] [PMID: 27811637]

Prabhakaran VC et al: Basal cell carcinoma of the eyelids. Compr Ophthalmol Update 2007;8:14. [PMID: 17394754]

Schwartz SR et al: Treatment of capillary hemangiomas causing refractive and occlusional amblyopia. J AAPOS 2007;11:577. [PMID: 17720571]

Sekulic A et al. Efficacy and safety of vismodegib in advanced basal-cell carcinoma. N Engl J Med 2012;366:2171. [PMID: 22670903]

Shields JA et al: Sebaceous carcinoma of the ocular region: A review. Surv Ophthalmol 2005;50:103. [PMID: 15749305]

Shumaker PR et al: Modified Mohs micrographic surgery for periocular melanoma and melanoma in situ: Long-term experience at Scripps Clinic. Dermatol Surg 2009;35:1263. [PMID: 19438663]

Spiteri Cornish K et al: The use of propranolol in the management of periocular capillary haemangioma: A systematic review. Eye (Lond) 2011;25:1277. [PMID: 21738233]

Sullivan TJ: Squamous cell carcinoma of eyelid, periocular, and periorbital skin. Int Ophthalmol Clin 2009;49:17. [PMID: 20348855]

Swerdlow SH et al: WHO Classification of Tumours of Haematopoietic and Lymphoid Tissues, 4th ed. Lyon: IARC Press, 2008.

Tildsley J et al: Mohs surgery vs primary excision for eyelid BCCs. Orbit 2010;29:140. [PMID: 20497079]

Weiss AH et al: Reappraisal of astigmatism induced by periocular capillary hemangioma and treatment with intralesional corticosteroid injection. Ophthalmology 2008;115:390. [PMID: 17588666]

Yin VT et al: Eyelid and ocular surface carcinoma: diagnosis and management. Clin Dermatol 2015;33:159. [PMID: 25704936]

Lacrimal Apparatus

Berry-Brincat A et al: Idiopathic orbital inflammation: A new dimension with the discovery of immunoglobulin G4-related disease. Curr Opin Ophthalmol 2012;23:415. [PMID: 22729180]

Carruth BP et al: Inflammatory modulators and biologic agents in the treatment of idiopathic orbital inflammation. Curr Opin Ophthalmol 2012;23:420. PubMed [PMID: 22729181]

Casady DR et al:. Stepwise treatment paradigm for congenital nasolacrimal duct obstruction. Ophthal Plast Reconstr Surg 2006;22:243. [PMID: 16855492]

Fayers T et al: Lacrimal surgery success after external dacryocystorhinostomy: Functional and anatomical results using strict outcome criteria. Ophthal Plast Reconstr Surg 2009;25:472. [PMID: 19935252]

Freedman JR et al: Primary and secondary lacrimal canaliculitis: A review of literature. Surv Ophthalmol 2011;56:336. [PMID: 21620429]

Lee DW et al: Primary external dacryocystorhinostomy versus primary endonasal dacryocystorhinostomy: A review. Clin Experiment Ophthalmol 2010;38:418. [PMID: 20665987]

Leong SC et al: A systematic review of outcomes after dacrycystorhinostomy in adults. Am J Rhinol Allergy 2010;24:81. [PMID: 20109333]

Marcet MM et al: Evidence-based review of surgical practices in endoscopic endonasal dacryocystorhinostomy for primary acquired nasolacrimal duct obstruction and other new indications. Curr Opin Ophthalmol 2014;25:443. [PMID: 24979582]

Nelson LB: Treatment of congenital nasolacrimal duct obstruction. J Pediatr Ophthalmol Strabismus 2016;53:270. [PMID: 27637019]

Pediatric Eye Disease Investigator Group: Primary treatment of nasolacrimal duct obstruction with probing in children younger than 4 years. Ophthalmology 2008;115:577. [PMID: 17996306]

Pediatric Eye Disease Investigator Group: Primary treatment of nasolacrimal duct obstruction with nasolacrimal duct intubation in children younger than 4 years of age. J AAPOS 2008;12:445. [PMID: 18595756]

Pediatric Eye Disease Investigator Group: Primary treatment of nasolacrimal duct obstruction with balloon catheter dilation in children younger than 4 years of age. J AAPOS 2008;12:451. [PMID: 18929305]

Repka MX et al: Balloon catheter dilation and nasolacrimal duct intubation for treatment of nasolacrimal duct obstruction after failed probing. Arch Ophthalmol 2009;127:633. [PMID: 19433712]

Tsubota K. Tear dynamics and dry eye. Prog Retin Eye Res 1998; 17:565. [PMID: 9777650]

Conjunctiva & Tears

Francisco J. Garcia-Ferrer, MD, James J. Augsburger, MD, and Zélia M. Corrêa, MD, PhD

5.1. Conjunctiva
Francisco J. Garcia-Ferrer, MD

I. CONJUNCTIVITIS

Inflammation of the conjunctiva (conjunctivitis) is the most common eye disease worldwide. It varies in severity from a mild hyperemia with tearing to a severe conjunctivitis with copious purulent discharge. The cause is usually exogenous, but rarely may be endogenous.

CONJUNCTIVITIS DUE TO INFECTIOUS AGENTS

The types of conjunctivitis and their most common causes are summarized in Tables 5–1 and 5–2. Conjunctival inflammation that occurs in the setting of uveitis and scleral or episcleral inflammation are discussed in Chapter 7.

Because of its location, the conjunctiva is exposed to many microorganisms and other environmental factors. Several mechanisms protect the surface of the eye. In the tear film, the aqueous component dilutes infectious material, mucus traps debris, and a pumping action of the lids constantly flushes the tears to the tear duct. In addition, the tears contain antimicrobial substances, including lysozyme and antibodies (immunoglobulin [Ig] G and IgA).

Common pathogens that can cause conjunctivitis include *Streptococcus pneumoniae*, *Haemophilus influenzae*, *Staphylococcus aureus*, *Neisseria meningitidis*, most human adenovirus strains, herpes simplex virus type 1 and type 2, and two picornaviruses. Two sexually transmitted agents that cause conjunctivitis are *Chlamydia trachomatis* and *Neisseria gonorrhoeae*.

Cytology of Conjunctivitis

Damage to the conjunctival epithelium by a noxious agent may be followed by epithelial edema, cellular death and exfoliation, epithelial hypertrophy, or granuloma formation. There may also be edema of the conjunctival stroma (chemosis) and hypertrophy of the lymphoid layer of the stroma (follicle formation). Inflammatory cells, including neutrophils, eosinophils, basophils, lymphocytes, and plasma cells, may be seen and often indicate the nature of the damaging agent. These cells migrate from the conjunctival stroma through the epithelium to the surface. They then combine with fibrin and mucus from the goblet cells to form conjunctival exudate, which is responsible for the "mattering" on the lid margins (especially in the morning).

The inflammatory cells appear in the exudate or in scrapings taken with a sterile platinum spatula from the anesthetized conjunctival surface. The material is stained with Gram's stain (to identify the bacterial organisms) and with Giemsa's stain (to identify the cell types and morphology). Predominance of polymorphonuclear leukocytes is characteristic of bacterial conjunctivitis. Generally, a predominance of mononuclear cells—especially lymphocytes—is characteristic of viral conjunctivitis. If a pseudomembrane or true membrane is present (eg, epidemic keratoconjunctivitis or herpes simplex virus conjunctivitis), neutrophils usually predominate because of coexistent necrosis. In chlamydial conjunctivitis, neutrophils and lymphocytes are generally present in equal numbers.

In allergic conjunctivitis, eosinophils and basophils are frequently present in conjunctival biopsies, but they are less common on conjunctival smears; eosinophils or eosinophilic granules are commonly found in vernal keratoconjunctivitis.

Table 5–1. Causes of Conjunctivitis

Bacterial
  Hyperacute (purulent)
    Neisseria gonorrhoeae
    Neisseria gonorrhoeae subspecies *kochii*
    Neisseria meningitidis
  Acute (mucopurulent)
    Pneumococcus (*Streptococcus pneumoniae*)
    (temperate climates)
    Haemophilus aegyptius (Koch-Weeks bacillus)
    (tropical climates)
  Subacute
    Haemophilus influenzae (temperate climates)
  Chronic, including blepharoconjunctivitis
    Staphylococcus aureus
    Moraxella lacunata (diplobacillus of Morax-Axenfeld)
  Rare types (acute, subacute, chronic)
    Streptococci
    Moraxella catarrhalis
    Coliforms
    Proteus
    Corynebacterium diphtheriae
    Mycobacterium tuberculosis

Chlamydial
  Trachoma (*Chlamydia trachomatis* serovars A–C)
  Inclusion conjunctivitis (*C trachomatis* serovars D–K)
  Lymphogranuloma venereum (LGV) (*C trachomatis* serovars L1–3)

Viral
  Acute viral follicular conjunctivitis
    Pharyngoconjunctival fever due to adenoviruses types 3 and 7 and other serotypes
    Epidemic keratoconjunctivitis due to adenovirus types 8 and 19
    Herpes simplex virus
    Acute hemorrhagic conjunctivitis due to enterovirus type 70; rarely, coxsackievirus type A24
  Chronic viral follicular conjunctivitis
    Molluscum contagiosum virus
  Viral blepharoconjunctivitis
    Varicella, herpes zoster due to varicella-zoster virus
    Measles virus

Rickettsial (rare)
  Nonpurulent conjunctivitis with hyperemia and minimal in filtration, often a feature of rickettsial diseases
    Typhus
    Murine typhus
    Scrub typhus
    Rocky Mountain spotted fever
    Mediterranean fever
    Q fever

Fungal (rare)
  Ulcerative or granulomatous
    Candida
  Granulomatous

    Rhinosporidium seeberi
    Coccidioides immitis (San Joaquin Valley fever)
    Sporothrix schenckii

Parasitic (rare but important)
  Chronic conjunctivitis and blepharoconjunctivitis
    Thelazia californiensis
    Loa loa
    Ascaris lumbricoides
    Trichinella spiralis
    Schistosoma haematobium (bladder fluke)
    Taenia solium (cysticercus)
    Phthirus pubis (*Pediculus pubis*, public louse)
  Fly larvae (*Oestrus ovis*, etc) (ocular myiasis)

Immunologic (allergic)
  Immediate (humoral) hypersensitivity reactions
    Hay fever conjunctivitis (pollens, grasses, animal danders, etc)
    Vernal keratoconjunctivitis
    Atopic keratoconjunctivitis
    Giant papillary conjunctivitis
  Delayed (cellular) hypersensitivity reactions
    Phlyctenulosis
    Mild conjunctivitis secondary to contact blepharitis
  Autoimmune disease
    Primary and secondary Sjögren syndrome
    Mucous membrane pemphigoid

Chemical or irritative
  Iatrogenic
    Idoxuridine, brimonidine, apraclonidine, dipivefrin, and other topically applied drugs
    Preservatives in eye drops
    Contact lens solutions, particularly their preservatives
  Occupational
    Acids
    Alkalies
    Smoke
    Wind
    Ultraviolet light
  Caterpillar hair

Etiology unknown
  Folliculosis
  Chronic follicular conjunctivitis (orphan's conjunctivitis, Axenfeld conjunctivitis)
  Ocular rosacea
  Psoriasis
  Stevens-Johnson syndrome, toxic epidermal necrolysis, and erythema multiforme
  Dermatitis herpetiformis
  Epidermolysis bullosa
  Superior limbic keratoconjunctivitis
  Ligneous conjunctivitis
  Reiter syndrome
  Mucocutaneous lymph node syndrome (Kawasaki disease)

(continued)

Table 5–1. Causes of Conjunctivitis (*Continued*)

Associated with systemic disease	Secondary to dacryocystitis or canaliculitis
Graves ophthalmopathy (exposure, congestive) Gouty Carcinoid Sarcoidosis Tuberculosis Syphilis	Conjunctivitis secondary to dacryocystitis pneumococci or beta-hemolytic streptococci Conjunctivitis secondary to canaliculitis *Actinomyces israelii*, *Candida* species, *Aspergillus* species (rarely)

Symptoms of Conjunctivitis

The important symptoms of conjunctivitis include foreign body sensation, scratching or burning sensation, sensation of fullness around the eyes, itching, and photophobia. Pain rather than discomfort commonly indicates corneal involvement.

Signs of Conjunctivitis (Table 5–2)

Hyperemia is the most conspicuous clinical sign of acute conjunctivitis. The redness is most marked in the fornix and diminishes toward the limbus by virtue of the dilation of the posterior conjunctival vessels. (A perilimbal dilation or ciliary flush suggests inflammation of the cornea or deeper structures.) A brilliant red suggests bacterial conjunctivitis, whereas a milky appearance suggests allergic conjunctivitis. Hyperemia without cellular infiltration suggests irritation from physical causes, such as wind, sun, smoke, and so on, but it may occur occasionally with diseases associated with vascular instability (eg, acne rosacea).

Tearing (epiphora) is often prominent in conjunctivitis, with the tears resulting from the foreign body sensation, the burning or scratching sensation, or the itching. Mild transudation also arises from the hyperemic vessels and adds to the tearing. An abnormally scant secretion of tears and an increase in mucous filaments suggest dry eye syndrome.

Exudation is a feature of all types of acute conjunctivitis. The exudate is flaky and amorphous in bacterial conjunctivitis and stringy in allergic conjunctivitis. "Mattering" of the eyelids occurs upon awakening in almost all types of conjunctivitis, and if the exudate is copious and the lids are firmly stuck together, the conjunctivitis is probably bacterial or chlamydial.

Pseudoptosis is a drooping of the upper lid secondary to infiltration and inflammation of Müller's muscle. The condition is seen in several types of severe conjunctivitis, for example trachoma and epidemic keratoconjunctivitis.

Papillary hypertrophy is a nonspecific conjunctival reaction that occurs because the conjunctiva is bound down to the underlying tarsus or limbus by fine fibrils. When the tuft of vessels that forms the substance of the papilla (along with cellular elements and exudates) reaches the basement membrane of the epithelium, it branches over the papilla like the spokes in the frame of an umbrella. An inflammatory exudate accumulates between the fibrils, heaping the conjunctiva into mounds. In necrotizing disease (eg, trachoma),

Table 5–2. Differentiation of the Common Types of Conjunctivitis

Clinical Findings and Cytology	Viral	Bacterial	Chlamydial	Allergic
Itching	Minimal	Minimal	Minimal	Severe
Hyperemia	Generalized	Generalized	Generalized	Generalized
Tearing	Profuse	Moderate	Moderate	Moderate
Exudation	Minimal	Profuse	Profuse	Minimal
Preauricular adenopathy	Common	Uncommon	Common only in inclusion conjunctivitis	None
In stained scrapings and exudates	Monocytes	Bacteria, PMNs	PMNs, plasma cells, inclusion bodies	Eosinophils
Associated sore throat and fever	Occasionally	Occasionally	Never	Never

Abbreviation: PMN, polymorphonuclear cells.

the exudate may be replaced by granulation tissue or connective tissue.

When the papillae are small, the conjunctiva usually has a smooth, velvety appearance. A red papillary conjunctiva suggests bacterial or chlamydial disease (eg, a velvety red palpebral conjunctiva is characteristic of acute trachoma). With marked infiltration of the conjunctiva, giant papillae form. Also called "cobblestone papillae" in vernal keratoconjunctivitis because of their crowded appearance, giant papillae are flat-topped, polygonal, and milky-red in color. On the upper tarsus, they suggest vernal keratoconjunctivitis and giant papillary conjunctivitis with contact lens sensitivities; on the lower tarsus, they suggest atopic keratoconjunctivitis. Giant papillae may also occur at the limbus, especially in the area that is normally exposed when the eyes are open (between 2 and 4 o'clock and between 8 and 10 o'clock). Here they appear as gelatinous mounds that may encroach on the cornea. Limbal papillae are characteristic of vernal keratoconjunctivitis but rarely occur in atopic keratoconjunctivitis.

Chemosis of the conjunctiva strongly suggests acute allergic conjunctivitis but may also occur in acute gonococcal or meningococcal conjunctivitis and especially in adenoviral conjunctivitis. Chemosis of the bulbar conjunctiva is seen in patients with trichinosis. Occasionally, chemosis may appear before there is any gross cellular infiltration or exudation.

Follicles are seen in most cases of viral conjunctivitis, in all cases of chlamydial conjunctivitis except neonatal inclusion conjunctivitis, in some cases of parasitic conjunctivitis, and in some cases of toxic conjunctivitis induced by topical medications such as idoxuridine, brimonidine, apraclonidine, and dipivefrin, or by preservatives in eye drops or contact lens solutions. Follicles in the inferior fornix and at the tarsal margins have limited diagnostic value, but when they are located on the tarsi (especially the upper tarsus), chlamydial, viral, or toxic conjunctivitis (following topical medication) should be suspected.

The follicle consists of a focal lymphoid hyperplasia within the lymphoid layer of the conjunctiva and usually contains a germinal center. Clinically, it can be recognized as a rounded, avascular white or gray structure. On slitlamp examination, small vessels can be seen arising at the border of the follicle and encircling it.

Pseudomembranes and **membranes** are the result of an exudative process and differ only in degree. A pseudomembrane is a coagulum on the *surface* of the epithelium, and when it is removed, the epithelium remains intact. In contrast, a true membrane is a coagulum involving the *entire* epithelium, and if it is removed, a raw, bleeding surface remains. Both pseudomembranes and membranes may accompany epidemic keratoconjunctivitis, primary herpes simplex virus conjunctivitis, streptococcal conjunctivitis, diphtheria, mucous membrane pemphigoid, Stevens-Johnson syndrome, toxic epidermal necrolysis, and erythema multiforme. They may also be an aftermath of chemical exposure, especially alkali burns.

Ligneous conjunctivitis is a peculiar form of recurring membranous conjunctivitis. It is bilateral, seen mainly in children, and occurs predominantly in females. It may be associated with other systemic findings, including nasopharyngitis and vulvovaginitis.

Granulomas of the conjunctiva always affect the stroma and most commonly are chalazia. Other endogenous causes include sarcoidosis, syphilis, cat-scratch disease, and, rarely, coccidioidomycosis. Parinaud oculoglandular syndrome includes conjunctival granulomas and a prominent preauricular lymph node, and this group of diseases may require biopsy to establish the diagnosis.

Phlyctenules represent a delayed hypersensitivity reaction to microbial antigen, for example, staphylococcal or mycobacterial antigens. Phlyctenules of the conjunctiva initially consist of a perivasculitis with lymphocytic cuffing of a vessel. When they progress to ulceration of the conjunctiva, the ulcer bed has many polymorphonuclear leukocytes.

Preauricular lymphadenopathy is an important sign of conjunctivitis. A grossly visible preauricular node is seen in Parinaud oculoglandular syndrome and, rarely, in epidemic keratoconjunctivitis. A large or small preauricular node, sometimes slightly tender, occurs in primary herpes simplex conjunctivitis, epidemic keratoconjunctivitis, inclusion conjunctivitis, and trachoma. Small but nontender preauricular lymph nodes tend to occur in pharyngoconjunctival fever and acute hemorrhagic conjunctivitis. Occasionally, preauricular lymphadenopathy may be observed in children with infections of the meibomian glands.

BACTERIAL CONJUNCTIVITIS

▶ Clinical Findings

A. Symptoms and Signs

The organisms that account for most cases of bacterial conjunctivitis are listed in Table 5–1. Generally it manifests as bilateral irritation and injection, purulent exudate with sticky lids on waking, and occasionally lid edema. The infection usually starts in one eye and may be spread to the eye by direct contact from the hands. It may be spread from one person to another by fomites.

Hyperacute (purulent) bacterial conjunctivitis (caused by N gonorrhoeae, Neisseria kochii, or N meningitidis) is marked by a profuse purulent exudate (Figure 5–1). Any severe, profusely exudative conjunctivitis demands immediate laboratory investigation and treatment. Delay may result in severe corneal damage or loss of the eye or in septicemia or meningitis due to access to the bloodstream from the conjunctiva of N gonorrhoeae or N meningitidis.

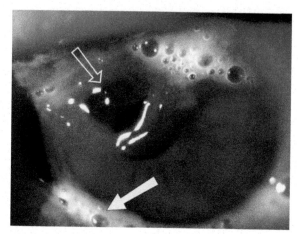

▲ **Figure 5–1.** Gonococcal conjunctivitis. Profuse purulent exudate **(filled arrow)** and severe corneal thinning **(unfilled arrow).** (Used with permission from Paulo E. C. Dantas, MD.)

Acute mucopurulent (catarrhal) conjunctivitis often occurs in epidemic form and is called "pinkeye" by most laymen. It is characterized by an acute onset of conjunctival hyperemia and a moderate amount of mucopurulent discharge. The most common causes are *S pneumoniae* in temperate climates and *Haemophilus aegyptius* in warm climates. Less common causes are staphylococci and other streptococci. The conjunctivitis caused by *S pneumoniae* and *H aegyptius* may be accompanied by subconjunctival hemorrhages. *H aegyptius* conjunctivitis in Brazil has been followed by a fatal purpuric fever produced by a plasmid-associated toxin of the bacteria.

Subacute conjunctivitis is caused most often by *H influenzae* and occasionally by *Escherichia coli* and *Proteus* species. *H influenzae* infection is characterized by a thin, watery, or flocculent exudate.

Chronic bacterial conjunctivitis occurs in patients with nasolacrimal duct obstruction and chronic dacryocystitis, which are usually unilateral. It may also be associated with chronic bacterial blepharitis or meibomian gland dysfunction. Patients with floppy lid syndrome or ectropion may develop secondary bacterial conjunctivitis.

Rarely, chronic bacterial conjunctivitis may be caused by *Corynebacterium diphtheriae* and *Streptococcus pyogenes*. Pseudomembranes or membranes caused by these organisms may form on the palpebral conjunctiva. The rare cases of chronic conjunctivitis produced by *Moraxella catarrhalis*, the coliform bacilli, *Proteus*, and other organisms are, as a rule, indistinguishable clinically.

B. Laboratory Findings

In most cases of bacterial conjunctivitis, the organisms can be identified by the microscopic examination of conjunctival scrapings stained with Gram's stain or Giemsa's stain; this reveals numerous polymorphonuclear neutrophils. Conjunctival scrapings for microscopic examination and culture are recommended for all cases and are mandatory if the disease is purulent, membranous, or pseudomembranous. Antibiotic sensitivity studies are also desirable, but initial antibiotic therapy is empirical. When the results of antibiotic sensitivity tests become available, specific antibiotic therapy can then be instituted if necessary.

▶ **Complications & Sequelae**

Chronic marginal blepharitis often accompanies staphylococcal conjunctivitis except in very young patients who are not subject to blepharitis. Conjunctival scarring may follow both pseudomembranous and membranous conjunctivitis, and in rare cases, corneal ulceration and perforation supervene.

Marginal corneal ulceration may follow infection with *N gonorrhoeae*, *N kochii*, *N meningitidis*, *H aegyptius*, *S aureus*, and *M catarrhalis*; if the toxic products of *N gonorrhoeae* diffuse through the cornea into the anterior chamber, they may cause toxic iritis.

▶ **Treatment**

Specific therapy of bacterial conjunctivitis depends on identification of the microbiologic agent. While waiting for laboratory reports, the physician can start topical therapy with a broad-spectrum antibacterial agent (eg, polymyxin-trimethoprim). In any purulent conjunctivitis in which the Gram stain shows gram-negative diplococci suggestive of *Neisseria*, both systemic and topical therapy should be started immediately. If there is no corneal involvement, a single intramuscular dose of ceftriaxone, 1 g, is usually adequate systemic therapy. If there is corneal involvement, a 5-day course of parenteral ceftriaxone, 1–2 g daily, is required.

In purulent and mucopurulent conjunctivitis, the conjunctival sac should be irrigated with saline solution as necessary to remove the conjunctival secretions. To prevent spread of the disease, the patient and family should be instructed to give special attention to personal hygiene.

▶ **Course & Prognosis**

Acute bacterial conjunctivitis is almost always self-limited. Untreated, it may last 10–14 days; if properly treated, 1–3 days. The exceptions are staphylococcal conjunctivitis that may progress to blepharoconjunctivitis and enter a chronic phase, gonococcal conjunctivitis that untreated can lead to corneal perforation and endophthalmitis, and meningococcal conjunctivitis that can be complicated by septicemia and meningitis.

Chronic bacterial conjunctivitis may become a troublesome therapeutic problem.

CHLAMYDIAL CONJUNCTIVITIS

1. TRACHOMA

Worldwide the number of individuals with profound vision loss from trachoma has dropped from 6 million to 1.3 million, but it remains one of the leading causes of preventable blindness. It is endemic in regions with poor hygiene, overcrowding, poverty, lack of clean water, and poor sanitation. Blinding trachoma occurs in many parts of Africa, in some parts of Asia, among Australian aborigines, and in northern Brazil. Nonblinding trachoma also occurs in some areas of Latin America and the Pacific Islands.

▶ Clinical Findings

A. Symptoms and Signs

Trachoma typically begins in childhood as a bilateral chronic follicular conjunctivitis that due to recurrent episodes progresses to conjunctival scarring (Figure 5–2). In severe cases trichiasis develops in early adult life. The constant abrasion by inturned lashes combined with defective tear film leads, usually after age 30 years, to corneal scarring (Figure 5–3).

The incubation period of trachoma averages 7 days but varies from 5–14 days. In an infant or child, the onset is usually insidious, and the disease may resolve with minimal or no complications. In adults, the onset is often subacute or acute, and complications may develop early. At onset, trachoma often resembles other bacterial conjunctivitis. The symptoms and signs usually consist of tearing, photophobia, pain, exudation, edema of the eyelids, chemosis of the bulbar conjunctiva, hyperemia, papillary hypertrophy, tarsal and limbal follicles, superior keratitis, pannus (corneal fibrovascular membrane) formation, and a small, tender preauricular node.

In established trachoma, there may also be superior epithelial keratitis, subepithelial keratitis, pannus, or superior limbal follicles, and ultimately the pathognomonic cicatricial remains of these follicles, known as **Herbert's pits**—small depressions

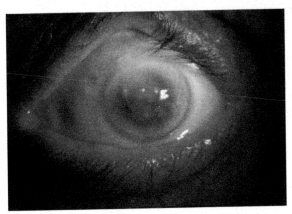

▲ **Figure 5–3.** Advanced trachoma following corneal ulceration and scarring. (Used with permission from University of California, Davis, Cornea and External Diseases.)

covered by epithelium at the limbocorneal junction. The associated pannus arises from the limbus, with vascular loops extending onto the cornea. All of the signs of trachoma are more severe in the upper than in the lower conjunctiva and cornea.

B. Laboratory Findings

Chlamydial inclusion bodies may be found in Giemsa-stained conjunctival scrapings, but they are not always present. Inclusions appear in the Giemsa-stained preparations as particulate, dark purple, or blue cytoplasmic masses that cap the nucleus of the epithelial cell. Fluorescent antibody stains and enzyme immunoassay tests are available commercially and are widely used in clinical laboratories. These and other new tests, including polymerase chain reaction (PCR), have superseded Giemsa staining of conjunctival smears and isolation of chlamydial agent in cell culture.

The agent of trachoma resembles the agent of inclusion conjunctivitis morphologically, but the two can be differentiated serologically by microimmunofluorescence. Trachoma is usually caused by *C trachomatis* serovars A, B, Ba, or C.

▶ Differential Diagnosis

1. No history of exposure to endemic trachoma speaks against the diagnosis.
2. Viral follicular conjunctivitis usually has an acute onset and is clearly resolving by 2–3 weeks.
3. Infection with genitally transmitted chlamydial strains usually has an acute onset in sexually active individuals.
4. Chronic follicular conjunctivitis due to exogenous substances resolves when the cause is removed.
5. Parinaud oculoglandular syndrome is manifested by massively enlarged preauricular or cervical lymph nodes, although the conjunctival lesion may be follicular.

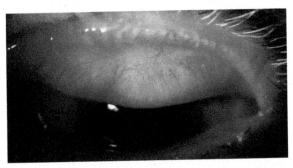

▲ **Figure 5–2.** Conjunctival scarring secondary to trachoma. The superior tarsus is the classic site for subconjunctival scarring in association with trachoma.

6. Normal young children may have conjunctival follicles (folliculosis).

7. Vernal and atopic keratoconjunctivitis are associated with giant papillae that are elevated and often polygonal, with a milky-red appearance. Eosinophils are present in smears.

8. Contact lens intolerance may lead to conjunctival scarring and pannus. Giant papillae in contact lens wearers can be confused with trachoma follicles.

▶ Complications & Sequelae

Conjunctival scarring is frequent. Destruction of accessory lacrimal glands and obliteration of ductules of the lacrimal gland reduce the aqueous component of tears, and their mucous component is reduced by loss of goblet cells. Distortion of the upper lid leads to inward deviation of individual lashes (trichiasis) or of the whole lid margin (entropion), so that the lashes constantly abrade the cornea resulting in corneal ulceration, bacterial corneal infections, and corneal scarring.

Ptosis, nasolacrimal duct obstruction, and dacryocystitis are other common complications.

▶ Treatment

Improvement is usually achieved with single-dose azithromycin, 1 g orally; doxycycline, 100 mg orally twice daily for 3 weeks; erythromycin, 1 g/d orally in four divided doses for 3–4 weeks; or tetracycline, 1–1.5 g/d orally in four divided doses for 3–4 weeks; but maximum effect is usually not achieved for 10–12 weeks, and several courses may be necessary for a cure. (Systemic tetracyclines should not be given to a child under 7 years of age or to a pregnant woman because tetracycline binds to calcium in developing teeth and in growing bone, leading to discoloration of the teeth and skeletal abnormalities.) Azithromycin has become the first choice for mass treatment campaigns, but repeated administrations may be necessary. Topical ointments or drops, including preparations of sulfonamides, tetracyclines, erythromycin, and rifampin, used four times daily for 6 weeks, also are effective.

Surgical correction of trichiasis, which can be performed by nonspecialist physicians or specially trained auxiliary personnel, is essential to prevent scarring from late trachoma.

▶ Course & Prognosis

Characteristically, trachoma is a chronic disease of long duration. Under good hygienic conditions (specifically, face-washing of young children), the disease resolves or becomes milder so that severe sequelae are avoided.

2. INCLUSION CONJUNCTIVITIS

Inclusion conjunctivitis is often bilateral and usually occurs in sexually active young people. The chlamydial agent infects the urethra of the male and the cervix of the female. Transmission to the eyes of adults is usually by oral-genital sexual practices or hand-to-eye transmission. About 1 in 300 persons with genital chlamydial infection develops the eye disease. Indirect transmission has been reported to occur in inadequately chlorinated swimming pools. In newborns, the agent is transmitted during birth by direct contamination of the conjunctiva with cervical secretions. Credé prophylaxis (1% silver nitrate) gives only partial protection against inclusion conjunctivitis.

▶ Clinical Findings

A. Symptoms and Signs

Inclusion conjunctivitis may have an acute or a subacute onset. The patient frequently complains of redness, pseudoptosis, and discharge, especially in the mornings. Newborns have papillary conjunctivitis and a moderate amount of exudate, and in hyperacute cases, pseudomembranes occasionally form and can lead to scarring. Since the newborn has no adenoid tissue in the stroma of the conjunctiva, there is no follicle formation; but if the conjunctivitis persists for 2–3 months, follicles appear, similar to the conjunctival picture in older children and adults. In the newborn, chlamydial infection may cause pharyngitis, otitis media, and interstitial pneumonitis.

In adults, the conjunctiva of both tarsi—especially the lower tarsus—have papillae and follicles (Figure 5–4). Since pseudomembranes do not usually form in the adult, scarring does not usually occur. Superficial keratitis may be noted superiorly and, less often, a small superior micropannus (<1–2 mm). Subepithelial opacities, usually marginal, often develop. Otitis media may occur as a result of infection of the auditory tube.

B. Laboratory Findings

Rapid diagnostic tests such as the direct fluorescent antibody test, enzyme-linked immunosorbent assay (ELISA),

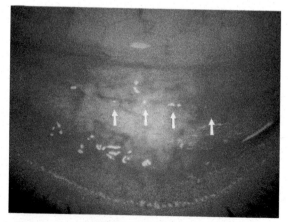

▲ **Figure 5–4.** Acute follicular conjunctivitis caused by inclusion conjunctivitis. (**Arrows** indicate follicles.) (Used with permission from Jed Rabinovitch, MD and Wills Eye Hospital Cornea Service.)

and PCR have replaced Giemsa staining in routine clinical practice. In the case of chlamydial ophthalmia neonatorum, rapid diagnosis is also imperative to prevent systemic complications such as chlamydial pneumonitis. Inclusion conjunctivitis is usually caused by *C trachomatis* serovars D–K with occasional isolations of serotype B. Serologic determinations are not useful in the diagnosis of ocular infections, but measurement of IgM antibody levels is extremely valuable in the diagnosis of chlamydial pneumonitis in infants.

Differential Diagnosis

Usually inclusion conjunctivitis can be differentiated clinically from trachoma.

1. Inclusion conjunctivitis occurs in sexually active adolescents or adults, whereas active, follicular trachoma usually occurs in young children or others living in or exposed to a community with endemic trachoma.
2. Conjunctival scarring is very rare in adult inclusion conjunctivitis.
3. Herbert's pits are a hallmark of trachoma.

Treatment

A. In Infants

Oral erythromycin suspension, 50 mg/kg/d in four divided doses for at least 14 days, is the treatment of choice. Systemic treatment is necessary because chlamydial infection also involves the respiratory and gastrointestinal tracts. Topical antibiotics do not provide any additional benefit. Both parents also should be treated (see below).

B. In Adults

In adults, cure of chlamydial disease can be achieved with azithromycin, 1 g in a single dose; doxycycline, 100 mg orally twice daily for 7 days; or erythromycin, 2 g/d for 7 days. (Systemic tetracyclines should not be given to a pregnant woman because they cause discoloration of teeth and skeletal abnormalities in the fetus.) The patient's sexual partners should be examined and treated.

If untreated, inclusion conjunctivitis runs a course of 3–9 months or longer with an average duration of 5 months.

3. CONJUNCTIVITIS CAUSED BY OTHER CHLAMYDIAL AGENTS

Lymphogranuloma venereum conjunctivitis is a rare sexually transmitted disease, manifesting as dramatic granulomatous conjunctival reaction with greatly enlarged preauricular nodes (Parinaud syndrome). It is caused by *C trachomatis* serovars L1, L2, or L3.

Chlamydia psittaci only rarely causes conjunctivitis in humans. Strains from parrots (psittacosis) and cats (feline pneumonitis) have caused follicular conjunctivitis in humans.

VIRAL CONJUNCTIVITIS

Viral conjunctivitis is common and can be caused by a wide variety of viruses. Severity ranges from mild, rapidly self-limited infection to severe, disabling disease.

1. ACUTE VIRAL CONJUNCTIVITIS

Pharyngoconjunctival Fever

Pharyngoconjunctival fever is characterized by fever of 38.3–40°C, sore throat, and a follicular conjunctivitis in one or both eyes. The follicles are often very prominent on both the conjunctiva and the pharyngeal mucosa. The disease can be either bilateral or unilateral. Injection and tearing often occur, and there may be transient superficial epithelial keratitis and occasionally some subepithelial opacities. Nontender preauricular lymphadenopathy is characteristic.

Pharyngoconjunctival fever is most frequently caused by adenovirus type 3 and occasionally by types 4 and 7. The virus can be grown on HeLa cells and identified by neutralization tests. As the disease progresses, it can be diagnosed serologically by a rising titer of neutralizing antibody. However, clinical diagnosis is usually straightforward.

Conjunctival scrapings contain predominantly mononuclear cells, and no bacteria grow in cultures. The condition is more common in children than in adults and can be transmitted in poorly chlorinated swimming pools. The conjunctivitis is self-limited, and as such, only supportive treatment is indicated, with the episode resolving in approximately 10 days.

Epidemic Keratoconjunctivitis (Figure 5–5)

The onset of epidemic keratoconjunctivitis is often unilateral, with both eyes subsequently being affected but the first eye usually being more severely affected. Initial symptoms include conjunctival injection, moderate pain, and tearing. Usually by 5–14 days, photophobia, epithelial keratitis, and round subepithelial opacities have also developed. Corneal sensation is normal. A tender preauricular node is characteristic. Edema of the eyelids, chemosis, and conjunctival hyperemia mark the acute phase, with follicles and subconjunctival hemorrhages often appearing within 48 hours. Pseudomembranes (and occasionally true membranes) may occur and may be followed by flat scars or symblepharon formation.

The conjunctivitis usually resolves by 3–4 weeks at most. The subepithelial opacities are concentrated in the central cornea, usually sparing the periphery, and may persist for months but generally heal without scars.

Epidemic keratoconjunctivitis is caused by adenovirus types 8, 19, 29, and 37 (subgroup D of the human adenoviruses).

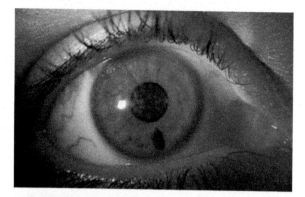

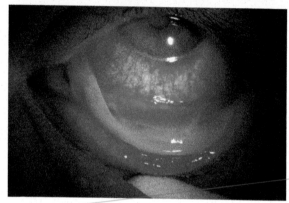

▲ **Figure 5–5.** Epidemic keratoconjunctivitis. (Used with permission from California, Davis, Cornea and External Diseases.) **A:** Uniform central round subepithelial corneal opacities. **B:** Pseudomembrane in the inferior fornix.

They can be isolated in cell culture and identified by neutralization tests. Scrapings from the conjunctiva show a primarily mononuclear inflammatory reaction; when pseudomembranes occur, neutrophils may also be prominent.

Epidemic keratoconjunctivitis in adults is confined to the external eye, but in children, there may be systemic symptoms of viral infection, such as fever, sore throat, otitis media, and diarrhea. Nosocomial transmission may occur during eye examinations, especially by use of improperly sterilized ophthalmic instruments such as tonometer tips or use of contaminated solutions, particularly topical anesthetics.

There is no specific therapy, but cold compresses and artificial tears will relieve some symptoms. Corticosteroids used during acute conjunctivitis may prolong late corneal involvement and should be avoided whenever possible. Antibacterial agents should be administered if bacterial superinfection occurs.

Herpes Simplex Virus Conjunctivitis

Herpes simplex virus (HSV) conjunctivitis, usually a disease of young children, is an uncommon entity characterized by

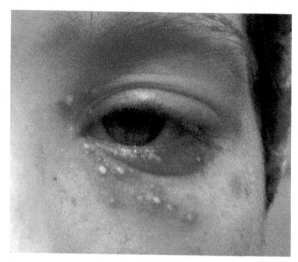

▲ **Figure 5–6.** Primary ocular herpes simplex virus infection. (Used with permission from S. Goodrich, MD.)

unilateral injection, irritation, mucoid discharge, pain, and mild photophobia. It occurs during primary infection with HSV when commonly there is also lid involvement (Figure 5–6) or during recurrent episodes of ocular herpes. It is often associated with herpes simplex keratitis, in which the cornea shows discrete epithelial lesions that usually coalesce to form single or multiple branching epithelial (dendritic) ulcers (Figure 5–7). The conjunctivitis is follicular or, less often, pseudomembranous. (Patients on topical antivirals may develop follicular conjunctivitis that can be differentiated because the herpetic follicular conjunctivitis has an acute onset.) Herpetic vesicles may sometimes appear on the eyelids and lid margins, associated

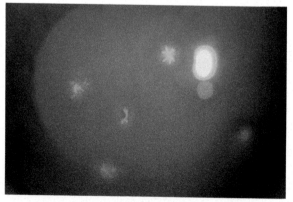

▲ **Figure 5–7.** Dendritic ulcer in herpes simplex virus keratitis. (Used with permission from California, Davis, Cornea and External Diseases.)

with severe edema of the eyelids. Typically, there is a small tender preauricular node.

No bacteria are found in scrapings or recovered in cultures. If the conjunctivitis is follicular, the predominant inflammatory reaction is mononuclear, but if it is pseudomembranous, the predominant reaction is polymorphonuclear, owing to the chemotaxis of necrosis. Intranuclear inclusions can be seen in conjunctival and corneal cells if Bouin fixation and the Papanicolaou stain are used but not in Giemsa-stained smears. The finding of multinucleated giant epithelial cells has diagnostic value. The virus can be readily isolated by gently rubbing a dry Dacron or calcium alginate swab over the conjunctiva and transferring the infected cells to a susceptible tissue culture.

HSV conjunctivitis may persist for 2–3 weeks, and if it is pseudomembranous, it may leave fine linear or flat scars. Complications consist of corneal involvement (including dendrites) and vesicles on the skin. Although type 1 herpesvirus causes the overwhelming majority of ocular cases, type 2 is the usual cause of herpetic conjunctivitis in newborns and a rare cause in adults. In the newborn, there may be generalized disease with encephalitis, chorioretinitis, hepatitis, etc. Any HSV infection in the newborn must be treated with systemic antiviral therapy (acyclovir) and monitored in a hospital setting.

If the conjunctivitis occurs in a child over 1 year of age or in an adult, it is usually self-limited and may not require therapy. Topical or systemic antivirals should be given, however, to prevent corneal involvement. For corneal ulcers, corneal debridement may be performed by gently wiping the ulcer with a dry cotton swab, applying antiviral drops, and patching the eye for 24 hours. Topical antivirals alone should be applied for 7–10 days (eg, trifluridine every 2 hours while awake or ganciclovir aqueous gel 0.15% five times daily until the ulcer heals and then three times daily). Herpetic keratitis may also be treated with 3% acyclovir ointment (not available in the United States) five times daily for 10 days, or with oral acyclovir, 400 mg five times daily for 7 days. Corticosteroid use is contraindicated since it may aggravate herpetic infections, causing a prolonged and usually more severe course.

▷ Newcastle Disease Conjunctivitis

Newcastle disease conjunctivitis is a rare disorder characterized by burning, itching, pain, redness, tearing, and (rarely) blurring of vision. It often occurs in small epidemics among poultry workers handling infected birds or among veterinarians or laboratory helpers working with live vaccines or virus.

The conjunctivitis resembles that caused by other viral agents, with chemosis, a small preauricular node, and follicles on the upper and lower tarsus. No treatment is available or necessary as the disease is self-limited.

▷ Acute Hemorrhagic Conjunctivitis

All of the continents and most of the islands of the world have had major epidemics of acute hemorrhagic conjunctivitis, which is caused by enterovirus type 70 and occasionally by coxsackievirus A24.

Characteristically, the disease has a short incubation period (8–48 hours) and course (5–7 days). The usual signs and symptoms are pain, photophobia, foreign-body sensation, copious tearing, redness, lid edema, and subconjunctival hemorrhages. Chemosis sometimes also occurs. The subconjunctival hemorrhages are usually diffuse but may be punctate at onset, beginning in the upper bulbar conjunctiva and spreading to the lower. Most patients have preauricular lymphadenopathy, conjunctival follicles, and epithelial keratitis. Anterior uveitis has been reported; fever, malaise, and generalized myalgia have been observed in 25% of cases; and motor paralysis of the lower extremities has occurred in rare cases in India and Japan.

The virus is transmitted by close person-to-person contact and by such fomites as common linens, contaminated optical instruments, and water. Recovery occurs within 5–7 days, and there is no known treatment. In the United States, closure of schools has been needed to stop epidemics.

2. CHRONIC VIRAL CONJUNCTIVITIS

▷ Molluscum Contagiosum Blepharoconjunctivitis

A molluscum skin nodule is round, waxy, and pearly-white, with an umbilicated center. Biopsy shows eosinophilic cytoplasmic inclusions that fill the entire cytoplasm of the enlarged cell, pushing its nucleus to one side. A nodule on the lid margin (Figure 5–8) or the skin of the lids or brow

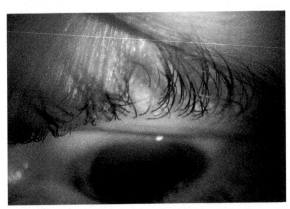

▲ **Figure 5–8.** Molluscum contagiosum nodule on the lid margin that was causing chronic follicular conjunctivitis. (Used with permission from University of California, Davis, Cornea and External Diseases.)

may produce unilateral chronic follicular conjunctivitis, superior keratitis, and superior pannus resembling trachoma. The inflammatory reaction is predominantly mononuclear (unlike the reaction in trachoma).

Excision or even incision of the nodule, thus allowing peripheral blood to permeate it, or cryotherapy cures the conjunctivitis. On very rare occasions, molluscum nodules have occurred on the conjunctiva. In these cases, excision of the nodule has also relieved the conjunctivitis. Multiple lid or facial lesions of molluscum contagiosum occur in patients with acquired immunodeficiency syndrome (AIDS).

▶ Varicella-Zoster Blepharoconjunctivitis

Hyperemia and an infiltrative conjunctivitis—associated with the typical vesicular eruption along the dermatomal distribution of the ophthalmic branch of the trigeminal nerve (Figure 5–9)—are characteristic of ophthalmic (herpes) zoster (shingles), due to reactivation of varicella-zoster virus infection. The conjunctivitis is usually papillary, but follicles, pseudomembranes, and transitory vesicles that later ulcerate have all been noted. A tender preauricular lymph node occurs early in the disease. Scarring of the lid, entropion, and the misdirection of individual lashes are sequelae.

The lid lesions of varicella, which are like the skin lesions (pox) elsewhere, may appear on both the lid margins and the lids and often leave scars. A mild exudative conjunctivitis often occurs, but discrete conjunctival lesions (except at the limbus) are very rare. Limbal lesions resemble phlyctenules and may go through all the stages of vesicle, papule,

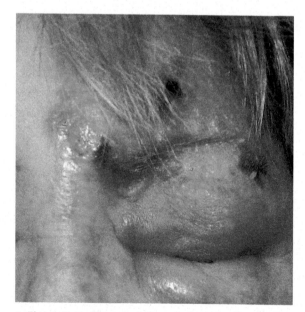

▲ **Figure 5–9.** Characteristic vesicular rash affecting the V1 dermatome in ophthalmic zoster (shingles).

and ulcer. The adjacent cornea becomes infiltrated and may vascularize.

In both zoster and varicella, scrapings from lid vesicles contain giant cells and a predominance of polymorphonuclear leukocytes; scrapings from the conjunctiva in varicella and from conjunctival vesicles in zoster may contain giant cells and monocytes. The virus can be recovered in tissue cultures of human embryo cells.

In the immunocompetent, oral antiviral therapy (acyclovir, 800 mg orally five times daily; famciclovir, 500 mg three times daily; or valacyclovir, 1 g three times daily, all for 7 days), if started within 72 hours after appearance of the rash, reduces the incidence of ocular complications but not necessarily of postherpetic neuralgia. The value of supplementary therapy with oral prednisone, initially 60 mg/d reducing over 3 weeks, is uncertain. In the immunocompromised, oral antiviral therapy should be continued for up to 2 weeks and may need to be given intravenously if there is evidence of progression of disease. Oral prednisone is contraindicated.

▶ Measles Keratoconjunctivitis

The characteristic enanthem of measles frequently precedes the skin eruption. At this early stage, the conjunctiva may have a peculiar glassy appearance, followed within a few days by swelling of the semilunar fold (Meyer's sign). Several days before the skin eruption, an exudative conjunctivitis with a mucopurulent discharge develops. At the time of the skin eruption, Koplik's spots appear on the conjunctiva and occasionally on the caruncle. At some time (early in children, late in adults), epithelial keratitis supervenes.

In the immunocompetent patient, measles keratoconjunctivitis has few or no sequelae, but in malnourished or otherwise immunocompromised patients, the ocular disease is frequently associated with a secondary HSV or bacterial infection due to *S pneumoniae*, *H influenzae*, or other organisms leading to severe visual loss.

Conjunctival scrapings show a mononuclear cell reaction unless there are pseudomembranes or secondary infection. Giemsa-stained preparations contain giant cells. Because there is no specific therapy, only supportive measures are indicated unless a secondary infection is present.

RICKETTSIAL CONJUNCTIVITIS

All rickettsiae recognized as pathogenic for humans may attack the conjunctiva, and the conjunctiva may be their portal of entry.

Q fever is associated with severe conjunctival hyperemia. Treatment with systemic tetracycline or chloramphenicol is curative.

Marseilles fever (boutonneuse fever) is often associated with ulcerative or granulomatous conjunctivitis and a grossly visible preauricular lymph node.

Endemic (murine) typhus, scrub typhus, Rocky Mountain spotted fever, and epidemic typhus have associated, variable, and usually mild conjunctival signs.

FUNGAL CONJUNCTIVITIS

▶ Candidal Conjunctivitis

Conjunctivitis caused by *Candida* species (usually *Candida albicans*) is a rare infection that usually appears as a white plaque. This may occur in diabetics or immunocompromised patients as an ulcerative or granulomatous conjunctivitis.

Scrapings show a polymorphonuclear cell inflammatory reaction. The organism grows readily on blood agar or Sabouraud's medium and can be readily identified as a budding yeast or, rarely, as pseudohyphae.

The infection responds to amphotericin B (3–8 mg/mL) in aqueous (not saline) solution or to applications of nystatin dermatologic cream (100,000 U/g) four to six times daily. The ointment must be applied carefully to ensure that it reaches the conjunctival sac and does not just build up on the lid margins.

▶ Other Fungal Conjunctivitides

Sporothrix schenckii may rarely involve the conjunctiva or the eyelids. It is a granulomatous disease associated with a visible preauricular node. Microscopic examination of a biopsy of the granuloma reveals gram-positive, cigar-shaped conidia (spores).

Rhinosporidium seeberi may rarely affect the conjunctiva, lacrimal sac, lids, canaliculi, and sclera. The typical lesion is a polypoid granuloma that bleeds after minimal trauma. Histologic examination shows a granuloma with enclosed large spherules containing myriad endospores. Treatment is by simple excision and cauterization of the base.

Coccidioides immitis may rarely cause a granulomatous conjunctivitis associated with a grossly visible preauricular node (Parinaud oculoglandular syndrome). This is not a primary disease but a manifestation of metastatic infection from a primary pulmonary infection (San Joaquin Valley fever). Disseminated disease suggests a poor prognosis.

PARASITIC CONJUNCTIVITIS

▶ *Thelazia californiensis* Infection

The natural habitat of this roundworm is the eye of the dog, but it can also infect the eyes of cats, sheep, black bears, horses, and deer. Accidental infection of the human conjunctival sac has occurred. The disease can be treated effectively by removing the worms from the conjunctival sac with forceps or a cotton-tipped applicator.

▶ *Loa loa* Infection

L loa is the eye worm of Africa. It lives in the connective tissue of humans and monkeys, and the monkey may be its reservoir. The parasite is transmitted by the bite of the horse or mango fly. The mature worm may then migrate to the lid, the conjunctiva, or the orbit.

Infection with *L loa* is accompanied by a 60–80% eosinophilia, but diagnosis is made by identifying the worm on removal or by finding microfilariae in blood examined at midday.

Diethylcarbamazine is currently the drug of choice.

▶ *Ascaris lumbricoides* Infection (Butcher's Conjunctivitis)

Ascaris may cause a rare type of violent conjunctivitis. When butchers or persons performing postmortem examinations cut tissue containing *Ascaris*, the tissue juice of some of the organisms may accidentally splash in the eye. A violent and painful toxic conjunctivitis ensues, marked by extreme chemosis and lid edema. Treatment consists of rapid and thorough irrigation of the conjunctival sac.

▶ *Trichinella spiralis* Infection

T spiralis does not cause a true conjunctivitis, but in the course of its general dissemination, there may be a doughy edema of the upper and lower eyelids, and over 50% of patients have chemosis—a pale, lemon-yellow swelling most marked over the lateral and medial rectus muscles and fading toward the limbus. The chemosis may last a week or more, and there is often pain on movement of the eyes.

▶ *Schistosoma haematobium* Infection

Schistosomiasis (bilharziasis) is endemic in Egypt, especially in the region irrigated by the Nile. Granulomatous conjunctival lesions appearing as small, soft, smooth, pinkish-yellow tumors occur, especially in males. The symptoms are minimal. Diagnosis depends on microscopic examination of biopsy material, which shows a granuloma containing lymphocytes, plasma cells, giant cells, and eosinophils surrounding bilharzial ova in various stages of disintegration.

Treatment consists of excision of the conjunctival granuloma and systemic therapy with antimonials such as niridazole.

▶ *Taenia solium* Infection

T solium rarely causes conjunctivitis but more often invades the retina, choroid, or vitreous to produce ocular cysticercosis. As a rule, the affected conjunctiva shows a subconjunctival cyst in the form of a localized hemispherical swelling, usually at the inner angle of the lower fornix, which is adherent to the underlying sclera and painful on pressure. The conjunctiva and lid may be inflamed and edematous.

Diagnosis is based on a positive complement fixation or precipitin test or on demonstration of the organism in the gastrointestinal tract. Eosinophilia is a constant feature.

The best treatment is to excise the lesion. The intestinal condition can be treated by niclosamide.

Phthirus pubis Infection (Pubic Louse Infection)

P pubis may infest the cilia and margins of the eyelids. Because of its size, the pubic louse seems to require widely spaced hair. For this reason, it has a predilection for the widely spaced cilia as well as for pubic hair. The parasites apparently release an irritating substance (probably feces) that produces a toxic follicular conjunctivitis in children and an irritating papillary conjunctivitis in adults. The lid margin is usually red, and the patient may complain of intense itching.

Finding the adult organism or the ova-shaped nits cemented to the eyelashes is diagnostic.

Lindane (Kwell) 1% or RID (pyrethrins), applied to the pubic area and lash margins after removal of the nits, is usually curative. Application of lindane or RID to the lid margins must be undertaken with great care to avoid contact with the eye. Any ointment applied to the lid margin tends to smother the adult organisms. The patient's family and close contacts should be examined and treated. All clothes and fomites should be carefully washed.

Ophthalmomyiasis

Myiasis is infection with larvae of flies. Many different species of flies may produce myiasis. The ocular tissues may be injured by mechanical transmission of disease-producing organisms and by the parasitic activities of the larvae in the ocular tissues. The larvae are able to invade either necrotic or healthy tissue. Many individuals become infected by accidental ingestion of the eggs or larvae or by contamination of external wounds or skin. Infants and young children, alcoholics, and debilitated unattended patients are common targets for infection with myiasis-producing flies.

These larvae may affect the ocular surface, the intraocular tissues, or the deeper orbital tissues.

Ocular surface involvement may be caused by *Musca domestica*, the housefly, *Fannia*, the latrine fly, and *Oestrus ovis*, the sheep botfly. These flies deposit their eggs at the lower lid margin or inner canthus, and the larvae may remain on the surface of the eye, causing irritation, pain, and conjunctival hyperemia.

Treatment of ocular surface myiasis is by mechanical removal of the larvae after topical anesthesia.

IMMUNOLOGIC (ALLERGIC) CONJUNCTIVITIS

IMMEDIATE HUMORAL HYPERSENSITIVITY REACTIONS

1. HAY FEVER CONJUNCTIVITIS

A mild, nonspecific conjunctival inflammation is commonly associated with hay fever (allergic rhinitis). In most cases, there is a history of allergy to pollens, grasses, animal danders, or other allergens. The patient complains of itching, tearing, and redness of the eyes and often states that the eyes seem to be "sinking into the surrounding tissue." There is mild injection of the palpebral and bulbar conjunctiva and, during acute attacks, often a severe chemosis, which no doubt accounts for the "sinking" description. There may be a small amount of ropy discharge, especially if the patient has been rubbing the eyes. Eosinophils are difficult to find in conjunctival scrapings. A papillary conjunctivitis may occur if the allergen persists.

Treatment consists of the instillation of topical preparations, such as emedastine and levocabastine, which are antihistamines; cromolyn, lodoxamide, nedocromil, and pemirolast, which are mast cell stabilizers; alcaftadine, azelastine, bepotastine, epinastine, ketotifen, and olopatadine, which are combined antihistamines and mast cell stabilizers; and diclofenac, flurbiprofen, indomethacin, ketorolac, and nepafenac, which are nonsteroidal anti-inflammatory drugs (see Chapter 22). Mast cell stabilization takes longer to act than antihistamine and nonsteroidal anti-inflammatory effects but is useful for prophylaxis. Topical vasoconstrictors, such as ephedrine, naphazoline, tetrahydrozoline, and phenylephrine, alone or in combination with antihistamines such as antazoline and pheniramine, are available as over-the-counter medications but are of limited efficacy in allergic eye disease and may produce rebound hyperemia and follicular conjunctivitis. Cold compresses are helpful to relieve itching, and antihistamines by mouth, such as loratadine 10 mg daily, are of some value. The immediate response to treatment is satisfactory, but recurrences are common unless the antigen is eliminated. Fortunately, the frequency of the attacks and the severity of the symptoms tend to moderate as the patient ages.

2. VERNAL KERATOCONJUNCTIVITIS

Vernal keratoconjunctivitis, also known as "spring catarrh," "seasonal conjunctivitis," or "warm weather conjunctivitis," is an uncommon bilateral allergic disease that usually begins in the prepubertal years and lasts for 5–10 years. It occurs much more often in boys than in girls. The specific allergen or allergens are difficult to identify, but patients with vernal keratoconjunctivitis usually show other manifestations of allergy known to be related to grass pollen sensitivity. The disease is less common in temperate than in warm climates and is almost nonexistent in cold climates. It is almost always more severe during the spring, summer, and fall than in the winter. It is most commonly seen in sub-Saharan Africa and the Middle East.

The patient usually complains of extreme itching and a ropy discharge. There is often a family history of allergy (hay fever, eczema, etc), and sometimes, there is a history of allergy in the young patient as well. The conjunctiva has a milky appearance with many fine papillae in the lower

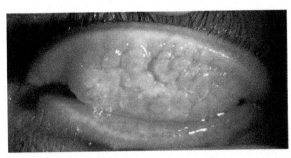

▲ **Figure 5–10.** "Cobblestone" papillae on the superior palpebral conjunctiva in vernal keratoconjunctivitis.

palpebral conjunctiva. The upper palpebral conjunctiva often has giant papillae that give a cobblestone appearance (Figure 5–10). Each giant papilla is polygonal, has a flat top, and contains tufts of capillaries.

A stringy conjunctival discharge and a fine, fibrinous pseudomembrane (Maxwell-Lyons sign) may be noted, especially on the upper tarsus on exposure to heat. In some cases, especially in persons of black African ancestry, the most prominent lesions are located at the limbus, where gelatinous swellings (papillae) are noted (Figure 5–11). A pseudogerontoxon (arcus-like haze) is often noted in the cornea adjacent to the limbal papillae. Trantas' dots are whitish dots seen at the limbus in some patients with vernal keratoconjunctivitis during the active phase of the disease. Many eosinophils and free eosinophilic granules are found in Giemsa-stained smears of the conjunctival exudate and in Trantas' dots.

Micropannus is often seen in both palpebral and limbal vernal keratoconjunctivitis, but gross pannus is unusual. Conjunctival scarring usually does not occur unless the patient has been treated with cryotherapy, surgical removal of the papillae,

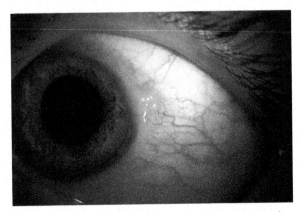

▲ **Figure 5–11.** Limbal papillae associated with vernal keratoconjunctivitis in a young male. (Used with permission from University of California, Davis, Cornea and External Diseases.)

irradiation, or other damaging procedure. Superficial corneal ("shield") ulcers (oval and located superiorly) may form and may be followed by mild corneal scarring. A characteristic diffuse epithelial keratitis frequently occurs. None of the corneal lesions respond well to standard treatment.

The disease may also be associated with keratoconus.

▶ **Treatment**

Since vernal keratoconjunctivitis is a self-limited disease, it must be recognized that the medication used to treat the symptoms may provide short-term benefit but long-term harm. Topical and systemic corticosteroids, which relieve the itching, affect the corneal disease only minimally, and their side effects (glaucoma, cataract, and other complications) can be severely damaging. Newer mast cell stabilizer-antihistamine combinations, such as epinastine, ketotifen, and olopatadine (see Chapter 22) are useful prophylactic and therapeutic agents in moderate to severe cases. Vasoconstrictors, cold compresses, and ice packs are helpful, and sleeping (and, if possible, working) in cool, air-conditioned rooms can keep the patient reasonably comfortable. Probably the best remedy of all is to relocate to a cool, moist climate. Patients able to do so benefit from a marked reduction in symptoms, if not a complete cure.

The acute symptoms of an extremely photophobic patient who is unable to function can often be relieved by a short course of topical or systemic corticosteroids followed by vasoconstrictors, cold packs, and regular use of histamine-blocking eye drops. Topical nonsteroidal anti-inflammatory agents, such as ketorolac, mast cell stabilizers, such as lodoxamide, and topical antihistamines (see Chapter 22) may provide significant symptomatic relief but may slow the reepithelialization of a shield ulcer. As has already been indicated, the prolonged use of corticosteroids should be avoided. Cyclosporine and tacrolimus eye drops are effective in severe unresponsive cases. Supratarsal injection of depot corticosteroids with or without surgical excision of giant papillae has been demonstrated to be effective for vernal shield ulcers.

Desensitization to grass pollens and other antigens has not been rewarding. Staphylococcal blepharitis and conjunctivitis are frequent complications and should be treated. Recurrences are the rule, particularly in the spring and summer; but after a number of recurrences, the papillae disappear completely, leaving no scars.

3. ATOPIC KERATOCONJUNCTIVITIS

Patients with atopic dermatitis (eczema) often also have atopic keratoconjunctivitis. The symptoms and signs are a burning sensation, mucoid discharge, redness, and photophobia. The lid margins are erythematous, and the conjunctiva has a milky appearance. There are fine papillae. Giant papillae are less developed than in vernal keratoconjunctivitis

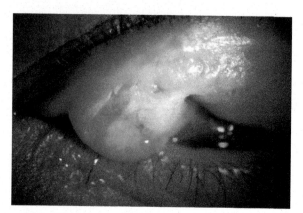

▲ **Figure 5–12.** Conjunctival scarring in atopic keratoconjunctivitis.

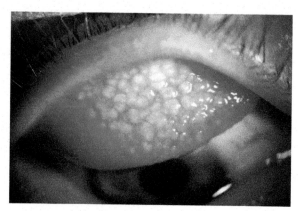

▲ **Figure 5–13.** Giant papillary conjunctivitis associated with soft contact lens wear.

and occur more frequently on the lower rather than upper palpebral conjunctiva. There may be conjunctival scarring (Figure 5–12). Severe corneal signs appear late in the disease after repeated exacerbations of the conjunctivitis. Superficial peripheral keratitis develops and is followed by vascularization. In severe cases, the entire cornea becomes hazy and vascularized, and visual acuity is reduced.

There is usually a history of allergy (hay fever, asthma, or eczema) affecting the patient or the patient's family. Most patients have had atopic dermatitis since infancy. Scarring of the flexure creases of the antecubital folds and of the wrists and knees is common. Like the dermatitis with which it is associated, atopic keratoconjunctivitis has a protracted course and is subject to exacerbations and remissions. As in vernal keratoconjunctivitis, it tends to become less active when the patient reaches the fifth decade.

Scrapings of the conjunctiva show eosinophils, though not nearly as many as are seen in vernal keratoconjunctivitis. Scarring of both the conjunctiva and cornea is often seen, and an atopic cataract, a posterior subcapsular plaque, or an anterior shield-like cataract may develop. Keratoconus, retinal detachment, and herpes simplex keratitis are all more likely than usual in patients with atopic keratoconjunctivitis, and there are many cases of secondary bacterial blepharitis and conjunctivitis, usually staphylococcal.

The management of atopic keratoconjunctivitis is often discouraging. Any secondary infection must be treated. Environmental control should be considered. Chronic topical therapy with mast cell stabilizers, antihistamines, and nonsteroidal anti-inflammatory agents (see Chapter 22) is the mainstay in treatment. Oral antihistamines are also beneficial. A short course of topical corticosteroids may also relieve symptoms. In severe cases, plasmapheresis or systemic immunosuppression may be an adjunct to therapy. In advanced cases with severe corneal complications, corneal transplantation may be needed to improve the visual acuity.

4. GIANT PAPILLARY CONJUNCTIVITIS

Giant papillary conjunctivitis with signs and symptoms resembling those of vernal conjunctivitis may develop in patients wearing plastic artificial eyes or contact lenses (Figure 5–13). It is probably a basophil-rich delayed hypersensitivity disorder (Jones-Mote hypersensitivity), perhaps with an IgE humoral component. Use of glass instead of plastic for prostheses and spectacle lenses instead of contact lenses is curative. If the goal is to maintain contact lens wear, additional therapy will be required. Careful contact lens care, including preservative-free agents, is essential. Hydrogen peroxide disinfection and enzymatic cleaning of contact lenses may also help. Alternatively, changing to a weekly disposable or daily disposable contact lens system may be beneficial. If these treatments are unsuccessful, use of contact lenses should be discontinued.

DELAYED HYPERSENSITIVITY REACTIONS

1. PHLYCTENULOSIS

Phlyctenular keratoconjunctivitis is a type IV delayed hypersensitivity response to microbial proteins, including the proteins of the tubercle bacillus, *Staphylococcus* species, *C albicans, C immitis, H aegyptius,* and *C trachomatis* serovars L1, L2, and L3. Until recently, by far the most frequent cause of phlyctenulosis in the United States was delayed hypersensitivity to the protein of the human tubercle bacillus. This is still the most common cause in regions where tuberculosis is still prevalent. In the United States, however, most cases are now associated with delayed hypersensitivity to *S aureus.*

The conjunctival phlyctenule begins as a small lesion (usually 1–3 mm in diameter) that is hard, red, elevated, and surrounded by a zone of hyperemia. At the limbus, it is often triangular in shape, with its apex toward the cornea

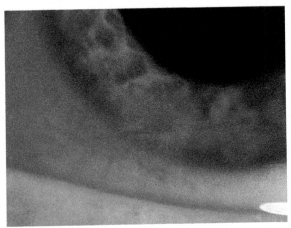

▲ **Figure 5–14.** Mild limbal phlyctenule probably secondary to *Staphylococcus* marginal disease in a 30-year-old female that improved with corticosteroid treatment.

(Figure 5–14). In this location it develops a grayish-white center that soon ulcerates and then subsides within 10–12 days. The patient's first phlyctenule and most of the recurrences develop at the limbus, but there may also be corneal, bulbar, and, very rarely, even tarsal phlyctenules.

Unlike the conjunctival phlyctenule, which leaves no scar, the corneal phlyctenule (Figure 5–15) develops as an amorphous gray infiltrate and always leaves a scar. Consistent with this difference is the fact that scars form on the corneal side of the limbal lesion and not on the conjunctival side. The result is a triangular scar with its base at the limbus—a valuable sign of old phlyctenulosis when the limbus has been involved.

Conjunctival phlyctenules usually produce only irritation and tearing, but corneal and limbal phlyctenules are usually accompanied by intense photophobia. Phlyctenulosis is often triggered by active blepharitis, acute bacterial conjunctivitis, and dietary deficiencies. Phlyctenular scarring, which may be minimal or extensive, is often followed by Salzmann's nodular degeneration.

Histologically, the phlyctenule is a focal subepithelial and perivascular infiltration of small round cells, followed by a preponderance of polymorphonuclear cells when the overlying epithelium necrotizes and sloughs—a sequence of events characteristic of the delayed tuberculin-type hypersensitivity reaction.

Phlyctenulosis induced by tuberculoprotein and the proteins of other systemic infections responds dramatically to topical corticosteroids. A major reduction of symptoms occurs within 24 hours and disappearance of the lesion in another 24 hours. Phlyctenulosis produced by staphylococcal proteins responds somewhat more slowly. Topical antibiotics should be added for active staphylococcal blepharoconjunctivitis. Treatment should be aimed at the underlying disease, and corticosteroids, when effective, should be used only to control acute symptoms and persistent corneal scarring. Severe corneal scarring may require corneal transplantation.

2. MILD CONJUNCTIVITIS SECONDARY TO CONTACT BLEPHARITIS

Contact blepharitis caused by atropine, neomycin, broad-spectrum antibiotics, and other topically applied medications, or the preservatives in them, is often followed by a mild infiltrative conjunctivitis that produces hyperemia, mild papillary hypertrophy, a mild mucoid discharge, and some irritation. Examination of Giemsa-stained scrapings often discloses only a few degenerated epithelial cells, a few polymorphonuclear and mononuclear cells, and no eosinophils.

Treatment should be directed toward finding the offending agent and eliminating it. The contact blepharitis may clear rapidly with topical corticosteroids, but their use should be limited. Long-term use of corticosteroids on the lids may lead to steroid glaucoma and to skin atrophy with disfiguring telangiectasis.

CONJUNCTIVITIS DUE TO AUTOIMMUNE DISEASE

SJÖGREN SYNDROME

Sjögren syndrome is an autoimmune disease characterized by dry eye syndrome (keratoconjunctivitis sicca) (see subsequent section on Tears) and dry mouth (xerostomia). When associated with a generalized autoimmune disease, usually

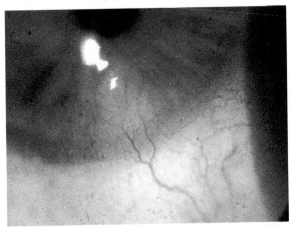

▲ **Figure 5–15.** Corneal phlyctenule. (Used with permission from Paulo E. C. Dantas, MD.)

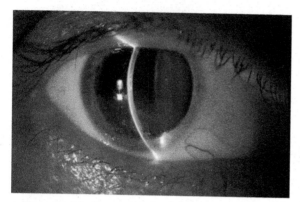

▲ **Figure 5–16.** Demonstration with fluorescein staining of punctuate epithelial erosions found in dry eye syndrome due to Sjögren syndrome, with greater distribution of epithelial lesions inferiorly. (Used with permission from University of California, Davis, Cornea and External Diseases.)

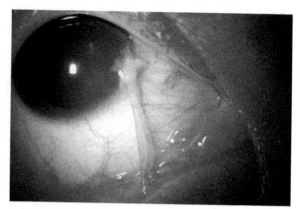

▲ **Figure 5–17.** Symblepharon formation in mucous membrane pemphigoid.

rheumatoid arthritis, it is known as secondary rather than primary Sjögren syndrome. The syndrome is overwhelmingly more common in women at or beyond menopause than in other groups, although men and younger women may also be affected. The lacrimal gland is infiltrated with lymphocytes and occasionally with plasma cells, leading to atrophy and destruction of the glandular structures.

Dry eye syndrome is characterized by bulbar conjunctival hyperemia (especially in the palpebral aperture) and symptoms of irritation that are out of proportion to the mild inflammatory sign, with pain increasing by the afternoon and evening but being absent or only slight in the morning. It often begins as a mild conjunctivitis with a mucoid discharge. Blotchy epithelial lesions appear on the cornea, more prominently in its lower half (Figure 5–16), and filaments may be seen. Rose bengal or lissamine green staining of the cornea and conjunctiva in the palpebral aperture is a helpful diagnostic test. The tear film is diminished and often contains shreds of mucus. Results of the Schirmer test are abnormal.

Conjunctival scrapings may show increased numbers of goblet cells. Lacrimal gland enlargement occurs uncommonly in patients with Sjögren syndrome. The principal diagnostic investigations in Sjögren syndrome are detection of antibodies against Ro (SSA) and La (SSB) and lymphocytic and plasma cell infiltration of the accessory salivary glands in a labial biopsy obtained by means of a simple surgical procedure.

Treatment is directed toward preserving and improving the quality of the tear film with artificial tears, obliteration of the puncta, and side shields, moisture chambers, and Buller shields. Topical corticosteroid or calcineurin inhibitor may be required in some cases.

(Dry eye syndrome [keratoconjunctivitis sicca] is discussed further in the subsequent section on Tears.)

MUCOUS MEMBRANE (OCULAR CICATRICIAL) PEMPHIGOID

Mucous membrane pemphigoid usually begins as a nonspecific chronic conjunctivitis that is resistant to therapy. The conjunctiva may be affected alone or, as indicated by its name, in combination with the mouth, nose, esophagus, vulva, and skin. The conjunctivitis leads to progressive scarring, obliteration of the fornices (especially the lower fornix), symblepharon formation (Figure 5–17), and entropion with trichiasis. The patient complains of pain, irritation, and blurring of vision. The cornea is affected only secondarily as a result of trichiasis and lack of the precorneal tear film. The disease is often more severe in women than in men and typically occurs in middle life, very rarely before age 45. In women, it may progress to blindness in a year or less; in men, progress is slower, and spontaneous remission sometimes occurs.

Conjunctival biopsies may contain eosinophils, and the basement membrane will stain positively with certain immunofluorescent stains (IgG, IgM, IgA complement). Active inflammatory disease may respond to dapsone or conventional immunosuppressants but newer agents, such as tumor necrosis factor (TNF) antagonist, increasingly are being used. The secondary consequences, such as tear deficiency, trichiais, and ocular toxicity need to be recognized and treated appropriately. Generally, the course is long and the prognosis poor, with blindness due to complete symblepharon and corneal desiccation.

CHEMICAL OR IRRITATIVE CONJUNCTIVITIS

IATROGENIC CONJUNCTIVITIS FROM TOPICALLY APPLIED DRUGS

A toxic follicular conjunctivitis or an infiltrative, nonspecific conjunctivitis, followed by scarring, is often produced by the prolonged administration of topical medications such as idoxuridine, brimonidine, apraclonidine, and dipivefrin, or by preservatives in eye drops. Silver nitrate instilled into the conjunctival sac at birth (Credé prophylaxis) is a frequent cause of mild chemical conjunctivitis. If tear production is reduced by continual irritation, the conjunctiva can be further damaged by the lack of dilution of the noxious agent as it is instilled into the conjunctival sac.

Conjunctival scrapings often contain keratinized epithelial cells, a few polymorphonuclear neutrophils, and an occasional oddly shaped cell. Treatment consists of stopping the offending agent and using bland drops or none at all. Often the conjunctival reaction persists for weeks or months after its cause has been eliminated.

OCCUPATIONAL CONJUNCTIVITIS FROM CHEMICALS & IRRITANTS

Acids, alkalies, smoke, wind, and almost any irritating substance that enters the conjunctival sac may cause conjunctivitis. Some common irritants are fertilizers, soaps, deodorants, hair sprays, tobacco, makeup preparations (mascara, etc), and various acids and alkalies. In certain areas, smog has become the most common cause of mild chemical conjunctivitis. The specific irritant in smog has not been positively identified, and treatment is nonspecific. There are no permanent ocular effects, but affected eyes are frequently chronically red and irritated.

In acid burns, the acids denature the tissue proteins and the effect is immediate. Alkalies do not denature the proteins, but tend to penetrate the tissues deeply and rapidly and to linger in the conjunctival tissue. Once in contact with the ocular surface, alkalies saponify fatty acids and continue to inflict damage for hours or days, depending on the molar concentration of the alkali and the amount introduced. Adhesions between the bulbar and palpebral conjunctiva (symblepharon) and corneal scarring are more likely to occur if the offending agent is an alkali. In either event, pain, injection, photophobia, and blepharospasm are the principal symptoms of caustic burns. A careful history will usually identify the precipitating event.

Immediate and profuse irrigation of the conjunctival sac with water or saline solution is of great importance, and any solid material should be removed mechanically. Do not use chemical antidotes. Further treatment may involve intensive topical steroids, ascorbate and citrate eye drops, cycloplegics, antiglaucoma treatment as necessary, cold compresses, and systemic analgesics (see Chapter 19). Bacterial conjunctivitis is treated with an appropriate antibacterial agent. Corneal involvement may require amniotic membrane graft, limbal stem cell transplantation, or corneal transplantation. Symblepharon may require reconstruction of the conjunctiva. Severe conjunctival and corneal burns have a poor prognosis even with surgery, but if proper treatment is started immediately, scarring may be minimized and the prognosis improved.

CATERPILLAR HAIR CONJUNCTIVITIS (OPHTHALMIA NODOSUM)

On rare occasions, caterpillar hairs are introduced into the conjunctival sac, where they produce one or many granulomas (ophthalmia nodosum). Under magnification, each granuloma is seen to contain a small foreign body.

Treatment by removal of each hair individually is effective. If a hair is retained, invasion of the sclera and uveal tract may occur.

CONJUNCTIVITIS OF UNKNOWN CAUSE

FOLLICULOSIS

Folliculosis is a widespread benign, bilateral, noninflammatory conjunctival condition characterized by follicular hypertrophy. It is more common in children than in adults, and the symptoms are minimal. The follicles are more numerous in the lower than in the upper cul-de-sac and palpebral conjunctiva. There is no associated inflammation or papillary hypertrophy, and complications do not occur.

There is no treatment for folliculosis, which disappears spontaneously after a course of 2–3 years. The cause is unknown, but folliculosis may be only a manifestation of a generalized adenoidal hypertrophy.

CHRONIC FOLLICULAR CONJUNCTIVITIS (AXENFELD'S CONJUNCTIVITIS)

Chronic follicular conjunctivitis is a bilateral transmissible disease of children characterized by numerous follicles in the upper and lower palpebral conjunctiva. There are minimal conjunctival exudates and minimal inflammation but no complications. Treatment is ineffective, but the disease is self-limited within 2 years.

OCULAR ROSACEA

Ocular rosacea is a common complication of acne rosacea and probably occurs more often in light-skinned people, especially those of northern European ancestry. It is usually a blepharoconjunctivitis, but in severe cases, corneal ulceration and scarring may also occur. The patient generally complains of mild injection and irritation, but discomfort increases if there is acute corneal involvement.

There is dilation of the blood vessels of the eyelid margin (Figure 5–18) and frequently an accompanying staphylococcal blepharitis. The conjunctiva is hyperemic, especially in the exposed interpalpebral region. Less often, there may be a nodular conjunctivitis with small gray nodules on the bulbar conjunctiva, especially near the limbus, which may ulcerate superficially. The lesions can be

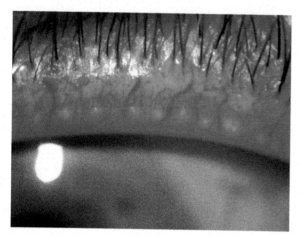

▲ **Figure 5–18.** Dilation of the blood vessels of the eyelid margin in the blepharitis of ocular rosacea.

differentiated from phlyctenules by the fact that even after they subside, large dilated vessels persist. Microscopic examination of the nodules shows lymphocytes and epithelial cells.

The peripheral cornea may ulcerate, characteristically with a narrow base at the limbus and a wider infiltrate centrally; vascularize, with the resulting pannus often being wedge- or spade-shaped and situated predominantly inferiorly; and scar (Figure 5–19).

Treatment of ocular rosacea consists of the elimination of hot, spicy foods and of alcoholic beverages, which are responsible for dilation of the facial vessels (Figure 5–20). Any secondary staphylococcal infection, which may also result in conjunctival concretions (Figure 5–21), should be treated. A course of oral tetracycline, standard doxycycline, or sustained-release doxycycline may be used, with a maintenance dose often being needed to control more severe disease.

Ocular rosacea is a chronic, recurrent disease and may respond poorly to treatment. If the cornea is not affected, the visual prognosis is good, but corneal lesions tend to recur and progress, and the vision grows steadily worse over a period of years.

PSORIASIS

Psoriasis vulgaris usually affects the areas of the skin not exposed to the sun, but in about 10% of cases, lesions appear on the skin of the eyelids, and the plaques may extend to the conjunctiva, where they cause irritation, a foreign-body sensation, and tearing. Psoriasis also causes nonspecific chronic conjunctivitis with considerable mucoid discharge. Rarely, the cornea may show marginal ulceration or a deep, vascularized opacity.

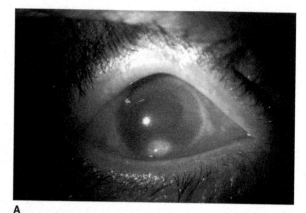

A

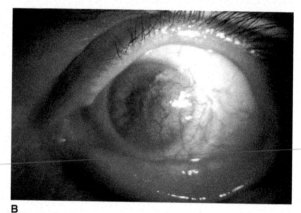

B

▲ **Figure 5–19.** Keratitis in ocular rosacea. **A:** Acute corneal ulceration with base at the limbus and wider infiltrate centrally. **B:** Chronic keratitis with pannus and scarring. (Used with permission from University of California, Davis, Cornea and External Diseases.)

The conjunctival and corneal lesions wax and wane with the skin lesions and are not affected by specific treatment. In rare cases, conjunctival scarring (symblepharon, trichiasis), corneal scarring, and occlusion of the nasolacrimal duct have occurred.

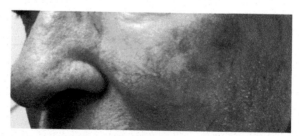

▲ **Figure 5–20.** Skin lesions in acne rosacea.

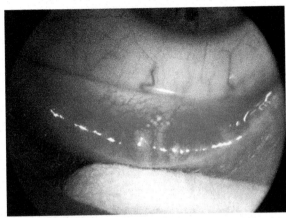

▲ **Figure 5–21.** Multiple concretions on the inferior tarsus. These are often associated with chronic lid disease caused by staphylococcal species.

STEVENS-JOHNSON SYNDROME, TOXIC EPIDERMAL NECROLYSIS, AND ERYTHEMA MULTIFORME

Stevens-Johnson syndrome and **toxic epidermal necrolysis,** the more extensive variant of the same disease, as well as **erythema multiforme,** cause skin and mucous membrane lesions, the latter possibly leading to cicatrizing conjunctivitis with the potential for severe corneal dryness and scarring (see Chapter 16). The skin lesion is an erythematous, urticarial bullous eruption that appears suddenly and is often distributed symmetrically. Bilateral conjunctivitis, often membranous, is a common manifestation. The patient complains of pain, irritation, discharge, and photophobia. The cornea becomes affected secondarily, and vascularization and scarring may seriously reduce vision.

Cultures are negative for bacteria, and conjunctival scrapings show a preponderance of polymorphonuclear cells. Systemic steroids are thought to shorten the course of the systemic disease but have little or no effect on the eye lesions. Careful cleansing of the conjunctiva to remove the accumulated secretion is helpful, however, and tear replacement may be indicated. If trichiasis and entropion supervene, they should be corrected. Topical steroids probably have no beneficial effect, and their protracted use can cause corneal melting and perforation.

The acute episode usually lasts about 6 weeks, but the conjunctival scarring, loss of tears, and complications from entropion and trichiasis may result in prolonged morbidity and progressive corneal cicatrization.

DERMATITIS HERPETIFORMIS

Dermatitis herpetiformis is a rare skin disorder characterized by symmetrically grouped erythematous papulovesicular, vesicular, or bullous lesions. The disease has a predilection for the posterior axillary fold, the sacral region, the buttocks, and the forearms. Itching is often severe. Rarely, a pseudomembranous conjunctivitis occurs and may result in cicatrization resembling that seen in mucous membrane pemphigoid. The skin eruption and conjunctivitis usually respond readily to systemic sulfones or sulfapyridine.

EPIDERMOLYSIS BULLOSA

This is a rare hereditary disease characterized by vesicles, bullae, and epidermal cysts. The lesions occur chiefly on the extensor surfaces of the joints and other areas exposed to trauma. The severe dystrophic type that leads to scarring may also produce conjunctival scars similar to those seen in dermatitis herpetiformis and mucous membrane pemphigoid. No known treatment is satisfactory.

SUPERIOR LIMBIC KERATOCONJUNCTIVITIS

Superior limbic keratoconjunctivitis is usually bilateral and limited to the upper tarsus and upper limbus. The principal complaints are irritation and hyperemia. The signs are papillary hypertrophy of the upper tarsus, redness of the superior bulbar conjunctiva, thickening and keratinization of the superior limbus, epithelial keratitis, recurrent superior filaments, and superior micropannus. Rose bengal staining is a helpful diagnostic test (Figure 5–22). The keratinized epithelial cells and mucous debris pick up the stain. Scrapings from the upper limbus show keratinizing epithelial cells.

In about 50% of cases, the condition has been associated with abnormal function of the thyroid gland. Applying 0.5% or 1% silver nitrate to the upper palpebral conjunctiva and allowing the tarsus to drop back onto the upper limbus usually result in shedding of the keratinizing cells and relief of symptoms for 4–6 weeks. This treatment can be repeated. There are no complications, and the disease usually runs a course of 2–4 years.

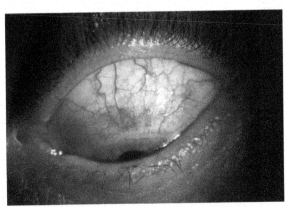

▲ **Figure 5–22.** Superior limbic keratoconjunctivitis after staining with rose bengal.

In severe cases, one may consider 5-mm resection of the perilimbal superior conjunctiva.

LIGNEOUS CONJUNCTIVITIS

This is a rare bilateral, chronic or recurrent, pseudomembranous or membranous conjunctivitis that arises early in life, predominantly in young girls, and often persists for many years. Granulomas are often associated with it, and the lids may feel very hard. Recent studies have shown an underlying type 1 plasminogen deficiency in patients suffering from ligneous conjunctivitis. Cyclosporine has been an effective treatment. Future therapies will focus on topical delivery of plasminogen.

REITER SYNDROME

A triad of disease manifestations—nonspecific urethritis, arthritis, and conjunctivitis—constitutes Reiter syndrome. Iritis can also occur, but tends to be a late complication. The syndrome occurs much more often in men than in women and has been found in association with HLA-B27 antigen. The conjunctivitis is papillary in type and usually bilateral. Conjunctival scrapings contain polymorphonuclear cells. No bacteria grow in cultures. The arthritis usually affects the large weight-bearing joints. There is no satisfactory treatment, although nonsteroidal anti-inflammatory agents may be effective. Corticosteroids usually help in resolution of iridocyclitis if present.

MUCOCUTANEOUS LYMPH NODE SYNDROME (KAWASAKI DISEASE)

This is a childhood vasculitis that can cause potentially fatal cardiac disease. As well as bilateral nonpurulent conjunctivitis, the clinical manifestations include fever, oropharyngeal abnormalities, erythema of the palms or soles, edema of the hands or feet, rash on the trunk, and cervical lymphadenopathy.

CONJUNCTIVITIS ASSOCIATED WITH SYSTEMIC DISEASE

CONJUNCTIVITIS IN GRAVES OPHTHALMOPATHY

In Graves ophthalmopathy, the conjunctiva may be red and chemotic, and the patient may complain of copious tearing. As the disease progresses, the chemosis increases, and in advanced cases, the chemotic conjunctiva may extrude between the lids (Figure 5–23), leading to corneal exposure that is exacerbated by any proptosis.

Treatment is directed toward control of the thyroid disease, and every effort must be made to protect the conjunctiva and cornea by bland ointment, surgical lid adhesions (tarsorrhaphy) if necessary, or even orbital decompression

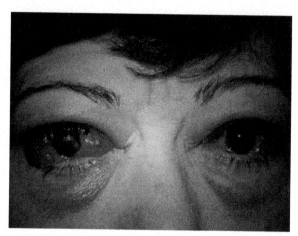

▲ **Figure 5–23.** Graves ophthalmopathy with marked chemosis leading to conjunctival prolapse, keratinization, and injection and inadequate corneal wetting. (Used with permission from Jed Rabinovitch, MD and Wills Eye Hospital Cornea Service.)

if the lids do not close enough to cover the cornea and conjunctiva.

GOUTY CONJUNCTIVITIS

Patients with gout often complain of a "hot eye" during attacks. On examination, a mild conjunctivitis is found that is less severe than suggested by the symptoms. Gout may also be associated with episcleritis or scleritis, iridocyclitis, keratitis, vitreous opacities, and retinopathy. Treatment is aimed at controlling the gouty attack with colchicine and allopurinol.

CARCINOID CONJUNCTIVITIS

In carcinoid, the conjunctiva is sometimes congested and cyanotic as a result of the secretion of serotonin by the chromaffin cells of the gastrointestinal tract. The patient may complain of a "hot eye" during such attacks.

CONJUNCTIVITIS SECONDARY TO DACRYOCYSTITIS OR CANALICULITIS

CONJUNCTIVITIS SECONDARY TO DACRYOCYSTITIS

Both pneumococcal conjunctivitis (often unilateral and unresponsive to treatment) and beta-hemolytic streptococcal conjunctivitis (often hyperacute and purulent) may be secondary to chronic dacryocystitis (see Chapter 4). The nature and source of the conjunctivitis in both instances are often missed until the lacrimal system is investigated.

CONJUNCTIVITIS SECONDARY TO CANALICULITIS

Canaliculitis due to canalicular infection with *Actinomyces israelii* or *Candida* species (or, very rarely, *Aspergillus* species) may cause unilateral mucopurulent conjunctivitis, often chronic (see Chapter 4). The source of the condition is often missed unless the characteristic hyperemic, pouting punctum is noted. Expression of the canaliculus (upper or lower, whichever is involved) is curative provided the entire concretion is removed.

Conjunctival scrapings show a predominance of polymorphonuclear cells. Cultures (unless anaerobic) are usually negative. *Candida* grows readily on ordinary culture media, but almost all of the infections are caused by *A israelii*, which requires an anaerobic medium.

II. DEGENERATIVE DISEASES OF THE CONJUNCTIVA

PINGUECULA

Pingueculae are extremely common in adults. They appear as yellow nodules on both sides of the cornea (more commonly on the nasal side) in the area of the palpebral aperture (Figure 5–24). The nodules, consisting of hyaline and yellow elastic tissue, rarely increase in size, but inflammation is common. In general, no treatment is required, but in certain cases of pingueculitis, weak topical steroids (eg, prednisolone 0.12%) or topical nonsteroidal anti-inflammatory agents may be given.

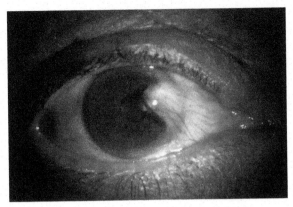

▲ **Figure 5–25.** Pterygium encroaching on the cornea and invading the visual axis.

PTERYGIUM

A pterygium is a fleshy, triangular encroachment of a pinguecula onto the cornea, usually on the nasal side bilaterally (Figure 5–25). It is thought to be an irritative phenomenon due to ultraviolet light, drying, and windy environments, since it is common in persons who spend much of their lives out of doors in sunny, dusty, or sandy, windblown surroundings. The pathologic findings in the conjunctiva are the same as those of pinguecula. In the cornea, there is replacement of Bowman's layer by hyaline and elastic tissue.

If the pterygium is enlarging and encroaches on the pupillary area, it should be removed surgically along with a small portion of superficial clear cornea beyond the area of encroachment. Conjunctival autograft at the time of surgical excision has been shown to reduce the risk of recurrent disease.

III. MISCELLANEOUS DISORDERS OF THE CONJUNCTIVA

LYMPHANGIECTASIS

Lymphangiectasis is characterized by localized small, clear, tortuous dilations in the conjunctiva (Figure 5–26). They are merely dilated lymph vessels, and no treatment is indicated unless they are irritating or cosmetically objectionable. They can then be cauterized or excised.

CONGENITAL CONJUNCTIVAL LYMPHEDEMA

This is a rare entity, unilateral or bilateral, and characterized by pinkish, fleshy edema of the bulbar conjunctiva. Usually observed as an isolated entity at birth, the condition is thought to be due to a congenital defect in the lymphatic

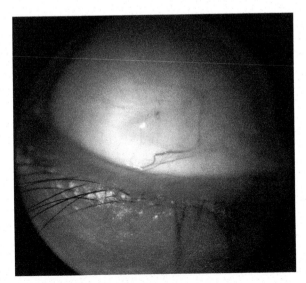

▲ **Figure 5–24.** Pingueculum.

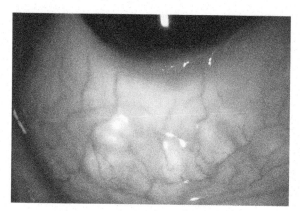

▲ **Figure 5–26.** Conjunctival lymphangiectasis. Note the clear tortuous dilations in the conjunctiva.

drainage of the conjunctiva. It has been observed in chronic hereditary lymphedema of the lower extremities (Milroy's disease) and is thought to be an ocular manifestation of this disease rather than an associated anomaly.

CYSTINOSIS

Cystinosis is a rare congenital disorder of amino acid metabolism characterized by widespread intracellular deposition of cystine crystals in various body tissues, including the conjunctiva and cornea. Three types are recognized: childhood, adolescent, and adult. Life expectancy is reduced in the first two types.

SUBCONJUNCTIVAL HEMORRHAGE

This common disorder may occur spontaneously, usually in only one eye, in any age group. Its sudden onset and bright-red appearance usually alarm the patient (Figure 5–27). The hemorrhage is caused by rupture of a small conjunctival vessel, sometimes preceded by a bout of severe coughing or sneezing.

The best treatment is reassurance. The hemorrhage usually absorbs in 2–3 weeks.

In rare instances, if the hemorrhages are bilateral or recurrent, the possibility of blood dyscrasias should then be ruled out.

OPHTHALMIA NEONATORUM

Ophthalmia neonatorum in its broad sense refers to any infection of the newborn conjunctiva. In its narrow and commonly used sense, however, it refers to a conjunctival infection, chiefly gonococcal, that follows contamination of the baby's eyes during its passage through the mother's cervix and vagina or during the postpartum period. Because gonococcal conjunctivitis can rapidly cause blindness, the cause of all cases of ophthalmia neonatorum should be verified by examination of smears of exudate, epithelial scrapings, cultures, and rapid tests for gonococci.

Gonococcal neonatal conjunctivitis causes corneal ulceration and blindness if not treated immediately. Chlamydial neonatal conjunctivitis (inclusion blennorrhea) is less destructive but can last months if untreated and may be followed by pneumonia. Other causes include infections with staphylococci, pneumococci, *Haemophilus*, and HSV and silver nitrate prophylaxis.

The time of onset is important but not entirely reliable in clinical diagnosis since the two principal types, gonorrheal ophthalmia and inclusion blennorrhea, have widely differing incubation periods: gonococcal disease, 2–3 days; and chlamydial disease, 5–12 days. The third important birth canal infection (HSV-2 keratoconjunctivitis) has a 2- to 3-day incubation period and is potentially quite serious because of the possibility of systemic dissemination.

Treatment for neonatal gonococcal conjunctivitis is with ceftriaxone, 125 mg as a single intramuscular dose; a second choice is kanamycin, 75 mg intramuscularly. To treat chlamydial conjunctivitis in newborns, erythromycin oral suspension is effective at a dosage of 50 mg/kg/d in four divided doses for 2 weeks. In both gonococcal and chlamydial conjunctivitis, the parents need to be treated. Herpes simplex keratoconjunctivitis is treated with acyclovir, 30 mg/kg/d in three divided doses for 14 days. Neonatal disease from HSV requires hospitalization because of the potential neurologic or systemic manifestations. Other types of neonatal conjunctivitis are treated with erythromycin, gentamicin, or tobramycin ophthalmic ointment four times daily.

Credé 1% silver nitrate prophylaxis is effective for the prevention of gonorrheal ophthalmia but not inclusion blennorrhea or herpetic infection. The slight chemical conjunctivitis induced by silver nitrate is minor and of short duration. Accidents with concentrated solutions can be avoided by using wax ampules specially prepared for

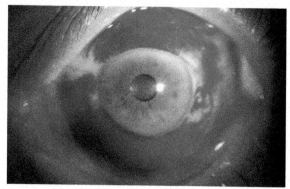

▲ **Figure 5–27.** Spontaneous subconjunctival hemorrhage while on warfarin. (Used with permission from University of California, Davis, Cornea and External Diseases.)

Credé prophylaxis. Tetracycline and erythromycin ointment are effective substitutes.

OCULOGLANDULAR DISEASE (PARINAUD OCULOGLANDULAR SYNDROME)

This is a group of conjunctival diseases, usually unilateral, characterized by low-grade fever, grossly visible preauricular adenopathy, and one or more conjunctival granulomas. The most common cause is cat-scratch disease, but there are many other causes, including *Mycobacterium tuberculosis, Treponema pallidum, Francisella tularensis, Pasteurella (Yersinia) pseudo-tuberculosis, C trachomatis* serovars L1, L2, and L3, and *C immitis.*

Conjunctival Cat-Scratch Disease

This protracted but benign granulomatous conjunctivitis is found most commonly in children who have been in intimate contact with cats. The child often runs a low-grade fever and develops a reasonably enlarged preauricular node and one or more conjunctival granulomas. These may show focal necrosis and may sometimes ulcerate. The regional adenopathy does not suppurate. The clinical diagnosis is supported by serology.

The disease appears to be caused by a slender pleomorphic gram-negative bacillus (*Bartonella* [formerly *Rochalimaea*] *henselae*), which grows in the walls of blood vessels. With special stains, this organism can be seen in biopsies of conjunctival tissue. The organism closely resembles *Leptotrichia buccalis,* and the disease was previously known as leptotrichosis conjunctivae (Parinaud conjunctivitis). The organism is commonly found in the mouth in humans and always in the mouth in cats. The eye may be contaminated by saliva on the child's fingers or by cat saliva on the child's pillow. *Afipia felis* has been incriminated also and may still play a role.

The disease is self-limited (without corneal or other complications) and resolves in 2–3 months. The conjunctival nodule can be excised; in the case of a solitary granuloma, this may be curative. Systemic tetracyclines may shorten the course but should not be given to children under 7 years of age.

Conjunctivitis Secondary to Neoplasms (Masquerade Syndrome)

When examined superficially, a neoplasm of the conjunctiva or lid margin is often misdiagnosed as a chronic infectious conjunctivitis or keratoconjunctivitis. Since the underlying lesion is often not recognized, the condition has been referred to as masquerade syndrome. The masquerading neoplasms on record are conjunctival capillary carcinoma, conjunctival carcinoma in situ, infectious papilloma of the conjunctiva, sebaceous gland carcinoma, and verrucae. Verrucae and molluscum tumors of the lid margin may desquamate toxic tumor material that produces a chronic conjunctivitis, keratoconjunctivitis, or (rarely) keratitis alone.

5.2. Conjunctival Tumors
James J. Augsburger, MD, and Zélia M. Corrêa, MD, PhD

This section presents an overview of the most common and most important neoplasms, hamartomas, and choristomas of the conjunctiva. Readers are referred to other sections of this chapter for information about inflammatory and degenerative lesions of the conjunctiva (eg, pingueculum and pterygium) that can simulate conjunctival neoplasms.

BENIGN TUMORS OF CONJUNCTIVA

Benign neoplasms are acquired tumors composed of atypical but not malignant cells. They may enlarge slowly but have little or no invasive potential and no metastatic capability. **Hamartomas** are congenital tumors composed of normal or near normal cells and tissues that occur normally at that anatomic site but are present in abnormally excessive amounts.

Choristomas are congenital cellular tumors consisting of normal cells and tissue elements that do not occur normally at that anatomic site.

Conjunctival Nevus

Conjunctival nevus is a benign neoplasm that arises from melanocytes, which exist normally within the basal layers of the conjunctival stratified squamous epithelium. It appears to be the most commonly encountered conjunctival neoplasm, but its exact incidence has never been calculated. It affects males and females equally, but it is almost exclusively a unilateral unifocal lesion. It is usually first noted during the first decade of life, but occasional lesions of this type do not become apparent until the teenage years or even later. Clinically conjunctival nevus appears as a dark brown to

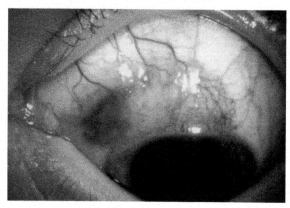

▲ **Figure 5–28.** Conjunctival nevus of superior limbal and bulbar conjunctiva with variable intensity of melanotic pigmentation and microcysts visible in the less pigmented areas.

tan lesion, which is most characteristically located adjacent to the limbus in the interpalpebral fissure (Figure 5–28). Less frequently, it involves the semilunar fold or caruncle. Slitlamp biomicroscopy frequently reveals tiny intralesional cysts and fine blood vessels. The lesion can grow to over 5 mm in diameter and over 1 mm in thickness in some individuals, especially if it contains multiple microcysts. Treatment consists of surgical excision of the entire lesion.

▶ Limbal Dermoid

Limbal dermoid is the most common conjunctival choristoma. It consists of a variety of cells and tissues of mesenchymal (mesodermal) origin, including fat cells, fibroblasts, and hair follicles. The typical lesion appears as a slightly elevated dome-shaped white mass straddling the limbus (Figure 5–29). On slitlamp biomicroscopy, fine hair shafts are frequently evident on the lesion's surface. Unilateral unifocal lesions of this type frequently occur as isolated abnormalities, but bilateral limbal dermoids are usually a sign of Goldenhar syndrome. Small lesions of this type can usually be left alone, but larger ones that extend to or near the visual axis or cause pronounced irregular astigmatism are usually managed by penetrating or lamellar keratoplasty.

▶ Conjunctival Hemangioma

Conjunctival hemangioma is a hamartoma composed of conjunctival blood vessels. It is present at birth but may not become apparent until it enlarges and becomes more evident cosmetically. It is virtually always a unilateral lesion. It appears clinically as a prominent collection of large caliber blood vessels thickening the conjunctiva (Figure 5–30). Some of the deeper blood vessels of the lesion may extend into the sclera. Unlike capillary hemangiomas of the eyelids and orbit, conjunctival hemangiomas rarely regress spontaneously. The principal indication for treatment is bothersome cosmetic appearance of the hemangioma, but no treatment has been shown to be both safe and effective. Attempted surgical excision can be complicated by difficult to control bleeding and incomplete removal that fails to improve or worsens the cosmetic abnormality. Cryotherapy is sometimes effective in inducing at least partial regression.

▶ Conjunctival Lymphangioma

Conjunctival lymphangioma is a hamartoma composed of dilated lymphatic channels lined by endothelial cells. Although congenital in nature, such lesions frequently do not appear until older childhood. They often enlarge abruptly during episodes of upper respiratory infection and may even fill with blood. Like conjunctival hemangiomas, these lesions are notoriously difficult if not impossible to eradicate by attempted surgical excision.

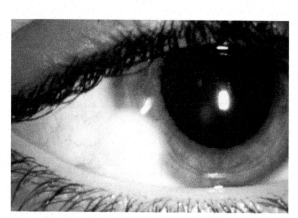

▲ **Figure 5–29.** Limbal dermoid exhibiting typical off-white color and inferotemporal location.

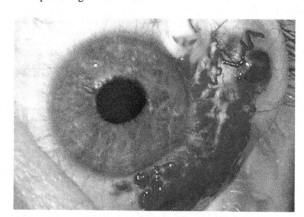

▲ **Figure 5–30.** Cavernous hemangioma of conjunctiva, composed of large-caliber blood vessels, some of which appear to extend into the underlying sclera.

CONJUNCTIVAL TUMORS INTERMEDIATE BETWEEN BENIGN AND MALIGNANT

The tumors described in the following paragraphs are categorized as neoplasms of borderline malignancy. If biopsy is performed, pathologic study may reveal benign cells, malignant cells, or cells that are judged to be borderline even by cytologic criteria. Tumors that cannot be classified unequivocally as either completely benign or definitely malignant are frequently referred to as premalignant or precancerous lesions.

Primary Acquired Melanosis of Conjunctiva

Primary acquired melanosis (PAM) of the conjunctiva is an acquired melanocytic hyperplasia of conjunctival melanocytes. It is almost exclusively a unilateral unifocal lesion. It affects males and females with equal frequency. It rarely develops before middle age and becomes evident most often in older individuals. It can arise from the limbal, bulbar, forniceal, or even palpebral conjunctiva. Clinically, it appears as a flat to minimally elevated dark brown patch of conjunctiva in an area that was normal in appearance previously (Figure 5–31). If it involves the limbal conjunctiva, it may extend into the corneal epithelium. The lesion usually enlarges slowly for several years. Prominent patches of PAM occasionally give rise to conjunctival melanomas (see later section on Conjunctival Melanoma), so they are appropriately regarded as premalignant lesions. Larger lesions should be excised or biopsied for histopathologic study. The crucial pathologic features are the degree of atypia of the melanocytic cells and the extent of conjunctival epithelial replacement by such cells. High-risk PAM that cannot be excised completely can be eliminated by cryotherapy or topical drug therapy using mitomycin C, 5-fluorouracil, or interferon alpha-2b.

Conjunctival Dysplasia

Dysplasia of the conjunctival stratified squamous epithelium is a disordered growth and maturation of the epithelium that can be a precursor to squamous cell carcinoma (see later in this chapter). Lesions of this type are almost always unilateral and unifocal and appear at the limbus in the interpalpebral fissure. It almost always occurs in middle-aged to older persons. The typical lesion appears as an irregular off-white thickening of the limbal conjunctiva. Accumulation of keratin within the disordered cells sometimes results in focal leukoplakia (white patch of hyperkeratotic epithelium). Because such lesions cannot be distinguished clinically from squamous cell carcinoma, surgical excision is usually recommended.

Intraepithelial Neoplasia of Conjunctiva and Cornea

Intraepithelial neoplasia of the conjunctiva and cornea (CIN) is a premalignant to in situ malignant disorder affecting the conjunctival and/or corneal stratified squamous epithelium. It occurs in middle-aged to older adults and is most evident in the corneal epithelium. On slitlamp biomicroscopy, CIN appears as a translucent area of mild corneal epithelial thickening without vascularization or hyperkeratosis (Figure 5–32). It may be limited to the peripheral cornea or extend through the visual axis. It is frequently associated with one or more foci of conjunctival squamous cell carcinoma (see later in this chapter). It is usually managed by surgical removal of the visibly abnormal epithelial cells or topical therapy using mitomycin C, 5-fluorouracil, or interferon alpha-2b.

Lymphoid Hyperplasia of Conjunctiva

Lymphoid hyperplasia of the conjunctiva is an infiltrative disorder of the conjunctival substantia propria in which the

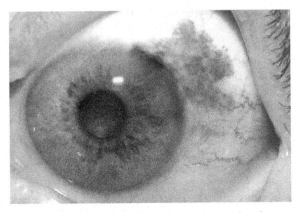

▲ **Figure 5–31.** Conjunctival primary acquired melanosis (PAM).

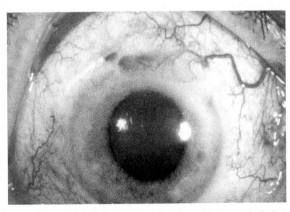

▲ **Figure 5–32.** Corneal and conjunctival intraepithelial neoplasia (CIN) predominantly manifesting as mild translucency of the upper two-thirds of the corneal epithelium.

infiltrates are composed of mildly to moderately atypical lymphocytic cells. This lesion is generally regarded as borderline between benign inflammatory lymphoid infiltrates and malignant lymphoma (see later in this chapter). It usually does not develop until middle age. It affects both males and females, and it can be unifocal, multifocal, or diffuse in one or both eyes. The typical lesion is a pink mass within the bulbar or forniceal conjunctiva. If the lesion is prominent, incisional biopsy or excision is indicated to exclude malignant lymphoma. Some patients with lesions classified pathologically as lymphoid hyperplasia eventually develop extraophthalmic foci of systemic lymphoma, so patients with this type of conjunctival lesion are usually treated with relatively low-dose external beam radiation therapy to the affected eye or eyes and monitored periodically over the ensuing years for signs of systemic lymphoma.

MALIGNANT CONJUNCTIVAL TUMORS

Malignant conjunctival tumors are composed of morphologically abnormal cells that frequently exhibit anaplastic features. Invasive clinical and pathologic features are generally evident, and regional and distant metastases are potential sequelae.

▶ Squamous Cell Carcinoma of Conjunctiva

Squamous cell carcinoma of the conjunctiva is an acquired malignant neoplasm composed of very atypical neoplastic cells arising from the stratified squamous epithelium. It usually affects middle-aged to elderly persons except in xeroderma pigmentosum, in which it tends to develop early in life. It is almost exclusively unilateral and unifocal. It occurs more commonly in males than in females. It usually develops at the limbus in the interpalpebral fissure.

The typical lesion appears as (1) a focal leukoplakic lesion (Figure 5–33), (2) a gelatinous conjunctival mass (Figure 5–34),

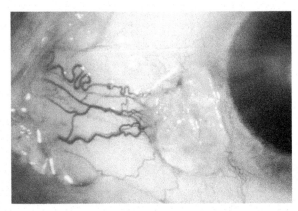

▲ **Figure 5–34.** Gelatinous type of squamous cell carcinoma of the limbal conjunctiva with prominent conjunctival blood vessels extending to the tumor.

or (3) a papillary tumor (Figure 5–35). If neglected or particularly aggressive, conjunctival squamous cell carcinoma can invade the sclera and extend intraocularly, or invade the orbit. Excision of the lesion is generally regarded to be the treatment of choice. At the time of surgery, cryotherapy to the conjunctiva surrounding and the sclera underlying the excisional defect is frequently performed to reduce the chance of local tumor recurrence. If clinical examination or pathologic study of the excised specimen suggests residual neoplasia, supplemental topical therapy with mitomycin C, 5-fluorouracil, or interferon alpha-2b is frequently provided.

▶ Mucoepidermoid Carcinoma of Conjunctiva

Mucoepidermoid carcinoma of the conjunctiva is a particularly aggressive variant of conjunctival squamous cell carcinoma. The tumor tends to be ill-defined and lumpy and frequently exhibits

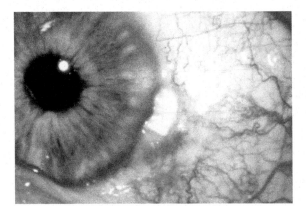

▲ **Figure 5–33.** Leukoplakic type of squamous cell carcinoma of the limbal conjunctiva; the surface white plaque (leukoplakia) is a result of focal hyperkeratosis.

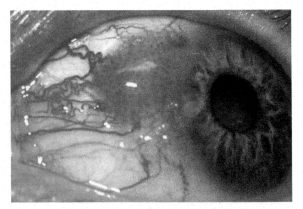

▲ **Figure 5–35.** Papillary type of squamous cell carcinoma of the limbal conjunctiva with prominent conjunctival blood vessels extending to the tumor.

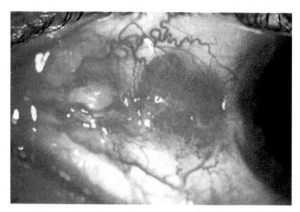

▲ **Figure 5–36.** Mucoepidermoid carcinoma of conjunctiva, manifesting as papillary type anteriorly and subepithelial nodule posteriorly.

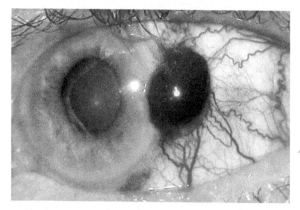

▲ **Figure 5–37.** Nodular conjunctival melanoma at the limbus, with prominent conjunctival blood vessels extending to the tumor and a small patch of primary acquired melanosis inferiorly.

a yellowish color (Figure 5–36). It tends to be highly invasive and frequently extends into the orbit by the time it is diagnosed. In most cases, orbital exenteration is performed to eliminate it.

Conjunctival Melanoma

Conjunctival melanoma is an acquired malignant neoplasm that arises from the intraepithelial melanocytes of the conjunctiva. It is almost exclusively unilateral but may be multifocal in some patients if it arises from pre-existing primary acquired melanosis (see earlier in this chapter). It usually affects middle-aged or older individuals. It affects both males and females with equal frequency, but it is much more common in Caucasians than in non-Caucasians. It can arise from any region of the conjunctiva (limbal, bulbar, forniceal, palpebral, or caruncular), but it is most common near the limbus in the interpalpebral area. The typical tumor appears as a dark brown nodular mass that is densely vascularized by conjunctival blood vessels (Figure 5–37). It frequently attains a thickness of 1 to 3 mm before it is recognized. It has the capability of invading the conjunctival stromal, extending into the conjunctival lymphatics, and metastasizing to regional lymph nodes in the head and neck and then to distant organs. Unfavorable prognostic factors for metastasis and metastatic death include larger tumor size, involvement of the fornix or caruncle, and local recurrence following attempted surgical excision. Treatment usually consists of wide surgical excision followed by conjunctival closure using sliding or transposition flaps or a mucous membrane graft. Supplemental cryotherapy to the retained conjunctiva adjacent to the excisional defect at the time of surgical excision or subsequent topical therapy using mitomycin C, 5-fluorouracil, or interferon alpha-2b is frequently performed to reduce the likelihood of local tumor relapse. Regional lymph node dissection at the time of initial treatment should be considered in cases with high-risk features.

A substantial proportion of patients with larger conjunctival melanomas that involved the fornix or caruncle at the time of treatment will eventually develop metastasis and die of that metastasis despite aggressive local therapy.

Conjunctival Lymphoma

Malignant lymphoma of the conjunctiva is an infiltrative neoplasm of the conjunctival substantia propria in which the infiltrates are composed of atypical lymphocytic cells. It usually occurs in middle-aged and older persons. It affects both males and females, and it can be unifocal, multifocal, or diffuse in one or both eyes. The typical lesion is a pink mass within the bulbar or forniceal conjunctiva (Figure 5–38). If the lesion is prominent clinically, incisional or excisional

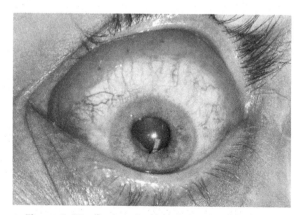

▲ **Figure 5–38.** Conjunctival lymphoma involving 180° of the superior forniceal conjunctiva, found to be malignant by histopathologic and immunohistochemical analysis.

biopsy is indicated for pathologic studies of the tissue to establish the diagnosis. Approximately 20% of patients with lesions classified pathologically as malignant lymphoma eventually develop extraophthalmic foci of systemic lymphoma, so patients with this type of conjunctival tumor are usually treated by fractionated external beam radiation therapy to the affected eye or eyes and monitored periodically over the ensuing years for signs of systemic lymphoma.

▶ Kaposi's Sarcoma of Conjunctiva

Kaposi's sarcoma of the conjunctiva is an acquired neoplasm composed of pleomorphic, malignant cells that become densely vascularized. It develops most commonly in individuals with AIDS. It is most common in middle-aged and older men. It is usually unilateral and unifocal but can be bilateral and multifocal. The typical lesion is a nodular red mass that is frequently hemorrhagic. Excision, cryotherapy, and focal radiation therapy can be employed to treat individual lesions, but whole-body therapy is generally indicated because lesions of the same type eventually develop in many bodily sites in individuals with AIDS.

5.3. Tears

Francisco J. Garcia-Ferrer, MD

Tears form a thin layer approximately 7–10 μm thick that covers the corneal and conjunctival epithelium. The functions of this ultrathin layer are (1) to make the cornea a smooth optical surface by abolishing minute surface epithelial irregularities; (2) to wet and protect the delicate surface of the corneal and conjunctival epithelium; (3) to inhibit the growth of microorganisms by mechanical flushing and antimicrobial action; and (4) to provide the cornea with necessary nutrient substances.

LAYERS OF THE TEAR FILM

The tear film is composed of three primary layers (Figure 5–39).

1. The superficial lipid layer is a monomolecular film derived from meibomian glands. It is thought to retard evaporation and form a watertight seal when the lids are closed.

2. The middle aqueous layer is elaborated by the major and minor lacrimal glands and contains water-soluble substances (salts and proteins).

3. The deep mucinous layer is composed of glycoprotein and overlies the corneal and conjunctival epithelial cells. The epithelial cell membranes are composed mainly of lipoproteins and are therefore relatively hydrophobic. Mucin is partly adsorbed onto the corneal epithelial cell membranes and is anchored by the microvilli of the surface epithelial cells. This provides a new hydrophilic surface for the aqueous tears to spread over, which is wetted by a lowering of surface tension.

COMPOSITION OF TEARS

The normal tear volume is estimated to be 7 ± 2 μL in each eye. Albumin accounts for 60% of the total protein in tear fluid. Immunoglobulins IgA, IgG, and IgE as well as lysozymes make up the remaining 40% of total protein. IgA

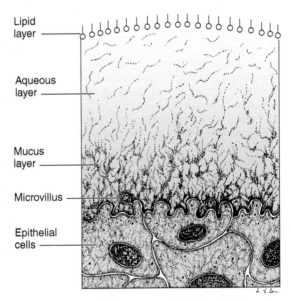

▲ **Figure 5–39.** The three primary layers of the tear film covering the superficial epithelial layer of the cornea.

predominates and differs from serum IgA in that it is not only transudated from serum but is produced by plasma cells located in the lacrimal gland. In certain allergic conditions such as vernal conjunctivitis, the IgE concentration of tear fluid increases. Tear lysozymes form 21–25% of the total protein and—acting synergistically with gamma globulins and other nonlysozyme antibacterial factors—represent an important defense mechanism against infection. Other tear enzymes may also play a role in diagnosis of certain clinical entities, for example, hexosaminidase assay for diagnosis of Tay-Sachs disease.

K$^+$, Na$^+$, and Cl$^-$ also occur in higher concentrations in tears than in plasma. Tears contain a small amount of glucose (5 mg/dL) and urea (0.04 mg/dL), and changes in blood concentration parallel changes in tear glucose and urea levels. The average pH of tears is 7.35, although there is a wide normal variation (5.20–8.35). Under normal conditions, tear fluid is isotonic. Tear film osmolarity ranges from 295 to 309 mosm/L.

DRY EYE SYNDROME (KERATOCONJUNCTIVITIS SICCA)

Dryness of the eye may result from any disease associated with deficiency of the tear film components (aqueous, mucin, or lipid), lid surface abnormalities, or epithelial abnormalities. Hence, there are many causes of dry eye syndrome (keratoconjunctivitis sicca) (Table 5–3). Primary Sjögren syndrome, an immune-mediated disorder of the lacrimal and salivary glands, characteristically manifesting as dry mouth as well as dry eyes, is the most important specific disease entity (see previous section on Conjunctiva).

▶ Etiology

Many of the causes of dry eye syndrome affect more than one component of the tear film or lead to ocular surface alterations that secondarily cause tear film instability. Histopathologic features include loss of conjunctival goblet

---

Table 5–3. Etiology and Diagnosis of Dry Eye Syndrome

I. Etiology
  A. Conditions characterized by hypofunction of the lacrimal gland:
    1. Congenital
      a. Familial dysautonomia (Riley-Day syndrome)
      b. Aplasia of the lacrimal gland (congenital alacrima)
      c. Ectodermal dysplasia
    2. Acquired
      a. Systemic diseases
        (1) Primary and secondary Sjögren syndrome
        (2) Progressive systemic sclerosis
        (3) Sarcoidosis
        (4) Leukemia, lymphoma
        (5) Amyloidosis
        (6) Hemochromatosis
      b. Infection
        (1) Mumps
      c. Injury
        (1) Surgical removal of, or damage to, lacrimal gland
        (2) Irradiation
        (3) Chemical burn
      d. Medications
        (1) Antihistamines
        (2) Antimuscarinics: atropine, scopolamine
        (3) Beta-adrenergic blockers: timolol
      e. Neurogenic (eg, facial nerve palsy)
  B. Conditions characterized by mucin deficiency:
    1. Avitaminosis A
    2. Stevens-Johnson syndrome, toxic epidermal necrolysis, and erythema multiforme
    3. Mucous membrane pemphigoid
    4. Chronic conjunctivitis, eg, trachoma
    5. Chemical burns
    6. Medications, including eye drop preservatives
    7. Folk remedies, eg, kermes

  C. Conditions characterized by lipid deficiency:
    1. Lid margin scarring
    2. Blepharitis
  D. Defective spreading of the tear film:
    1. Eyelid abnormalities
      a. Defects, coloboma
      b. Ectropion or entropion
      c. Keratinization of lid margin
      d. Decreased or absent blinking
        (1) Neurologic disorders (eg, facial nerve palsy)
        (2) Hyperthyroidism
        (3) Contact lens
        (4) Drugs
        (5) Herpes simplex keratitis
        (6) Leprosy
      e. Lagophthalmos
        (1) Nocturnal lagophthalmos
        (2) Hyperthyroidism
        (3) Leprosy
    2. Conjunctival abnormalities
      a. Pterygium
      b. Symblepharon
    3. Proptosis

II. Diagnostic Tests:
  A. Schirmer test without anesthesia
  B. Tear break-up time
  C. Ocular ferning test
  D. Impression cytology
  E. Fluorescein staining
  F. Rose bengal and lissamine green staining
  G. Tear lysozyme
  H. Tear film osmolality
  I. Tear lactoferrin

cells, abnormal enlargement of nongoblet epithelial cells, increased cellular stratification, and increased keratinization.

▶ Clinical Findings

Patients with dry eyes complain most frequently of a scratchy or sandy (foreign-body) sensation. Other common symptoms are itching, excessive mucus secretion, inability to produce tears, a burning sensation, photosensitivity, redness, pain, and difficulty in moving the lids. On gross examination, the eyes may appear normal, but on careful slitlamp examination, subtle indications of the presence of chronic dryness and irritation are found. The most characteristic feature is interruption or absence of the tear meniscus at the lower lid margin. Tenacious yellowish mucus strands are sometimes seen in the lower conjunctival fornix. The bulbar conjunctiva loses its normal luster and may be thickened, edematous, and hyperemic.

The corneal epithelium shows varying degrees of fine punctate stippling in the interpalpebral fissure. The damaged corneal and conjunctival epithelial cells stain with 1% rose bengal, and defects in the corneal epithelium stain with fluorescein (Figure 5–16). In the late stages of keratoconjunctivitis sicca, filaments may be seen—one end of each filament attached to the corneal epithelium and the other end moving freely (Figure 5–40).

Accurate diagnosis and grading of dry eye syndrome can be achieved using various diagnostic tests (Table 5–3).

A. Schirmer Test

Schirmer strips (Whatman filter paper No. 41) are inserted into the lower conjunctival cul-de-sac at the junction of the mid and temporal thirds of the lower lid (see Figure 2–26). The moistened exposed portion is measured 5 minutes after insertion. When performed without anesthesia, the test measures the function of the main lacrimal gland, whose secretory activity is stimulated by the irritating nature of the filter paper. Less than 10 mm of wetting without anesthesia is considered abnormal.

Schirmer tests can be performed after topical anesthesia (0.5% tetracaine) to measure the function of the accessory lacrimal glands, but the test is considered unreliable. Less than 5 mm in 5 minutes is abnormal.

The Schirmer test is a screening test for assessment of tear production. False-positive and false-negative results occur. Low readings are sporadically found in normal eyes, and normal tests may occur in dry eyes—especially those secondary to mucin deficiency.

B. Tear Film Break-Up Time

Measurement of the tear film break-up time may sometimes be useful to estimate the mucin content of tear fluid. Deficiency in mucin may not affect the Schirmer test, which quantifies tear production, but may lead to instability of the tear film, resulting in its rapid break-up. "Dry spots" (Figure 5–41) are formed in the tear film, followed by exposure of the corneal or conjunctival epithelium. This process ultimately damages the epithelial cells, which can then be stained with rose bengal. Damaged epithelial cells may be shed from the cornea, leaving areas susceptible to punctate staining when the corneal surface is flooded with fluorescein.

The tear film break-up time is measured by applying a slightly moistened fluorescein strip to the bulbar conjunctiva and asking the patient to blink. The tear film is then scanned with the aid of the cobalt filter on the slitlamp while the patient refrains from blinking. The time that elapses before the first dry spot appears in the corneal fluorescein layer is

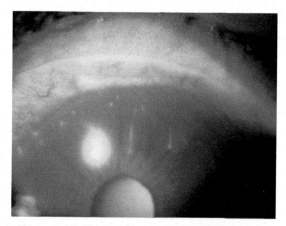

▲ **Figure 5–40.** Corneal filaments highlighted by fluorescein stain. (Used with permission from Jed Rabinovitch, MD and Wills Eye Hospital Cornea Service.)

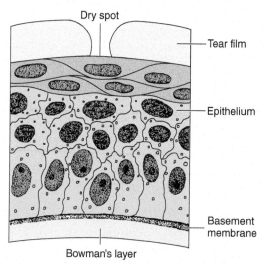

▲ **Figure 5–41.** Baring of the corneal epithelium following formation of a dry spot in the tear film.

the tear film break-up time. Normally it is over 15 seconds, but it will be reduced appreciably by the use of local anesthetics, by manipulating the eye, or by holding the lids open. Tear film break-up time is reduced in eyes with aqueous tear deficiency and is always shorter than normal in eyes with mucin deficiency.

C. Ocular Ferning Test

A simple and inexpensive qualitative test for the study of conjunctival mucus is performed by drying conjunctival scrapings on a clean glass slide. Microscopic arborization (ferning) is observed in normal eyes. In patients with cicatrizing conjunctivitis (mucous membrane pemphigoid, Stevens-Johnson syndrome, toxic epidermal necrolysis, erythema multiforme, diffuse conjunctival cicatrization), ferning of the mucus is reduced or absent.

D. Impression Cytology

Impression cytology is a method by which goblet cell densities on the conjunctival surface can be counted. In normal persons, the goblet cell population is highest in the infranasal quadrant. Loss of goblet cells has been documented in trachoma, mucous membrane pemphigoid, Stevens-Johnson syndrome, and avitaminosis A.

E. Fluorescein Staining

Touching the conjunctiva with a dry strip of fluorescein is a good indicator of wetness, and the tear meniscus can be seen easily. Fluorescein will stain the eroded and denuded areas as well as microscopic defects of the corneal epithelium (Figure 5–16).

F. Rose Bengal and Lissamine Green Staining

Rose bengal (Figure 5–22) and lissamine green are equally sensitive for staining the conjunctiva. Both dyes will stain all desiccated nonvital epithelial cells of the conjunctiva and to a lesser extent the cornea. Unlike rose bengal, lissamine green does not cause significant irritation.

G. Tear Lysozyme Assay

Reduction in tear lysozyme concentration usually occurs early in the course of Sjögren syndrome and is helpful in diagnosis. Tears can be collected on Schirmer strips and assayed, usually by spectrophotometric methods.

H. Tear Osmolality

Hyperosmolality of tears has been documented in dry eye syndrome and in contact lens wearers and is thought to be a consequence of decreased corneal sensitivity. Reports claim that hyperosmolality is the most specific test for dry eye syndrome. Hyperosmolality may be found even when Schirmer test and staining with rose bengal and lissamine green are normal.

I. Lactoferrin

Tear lactoferrin is low in patients with hyposecretion of the lacrimal gland. Testing kits are commercially available.

► Complications

Early in the course of dry eye syndrome, vision is slightly impaired. As the condition worsens, discomfort can become disabling. In advanced cases, corneal ulceration, corneal thinning, and perforation may develop. Secondary bacterial infection occasionally occurs, and corneal scarring and vascularization may result in marked reduction in vision. Early treatment may prevent these complications.

► Treatment

The patient should understand that dry eye syndrome is a chronic condition and complete relief is unlikely except in mild cases when the corneal and conjunctival epithelial changes are reversible. Artificial tears, particularly preservative-free tears in more advanced cases, are the mainstay of symptomatic treatment. Aqueous deficiency can be treated with various preparations. The simplest are physiologic (0.9%) or hypoosmotic (0.45%) solutions of sodium chloride, which can be used as frequently as every half-hour, but in most cases are needed only three or four times a day. More prolonged duration of action can be achieved with drop preparations containing a mucomimetic such as methylcellulose, polyvinyl alcohol, or polyacrylic acid (carbomers), by using petrolatum ointment during the day and particularly during sleep, or with a hydroxypropyl cellulose (Lacrisert) insert. Mucomimetics, which also include sodium hyaluronate and autologous serum, are particularly indicated when there is mucin deficiency. If there is tenacious mucus, mucolytic agents (eg, acetylcysteine, 10% or 20% one drop six times daily) may be helpful. Additional relief can be achieved by using humidifiers, moisture-chamber spectacles, or swim goggles.

Disease modification can be achieved with topical anti-inflammatory agents such as corticosteroids, of which loteprednol is favored because of its low risk of intraocular adverse effects, or calcineurin inhibitors, of which cyclosporine 0.05% ophthalmic emulsion (Restasis) twice a day has been used most widely. Diquafosol eye drops promote water transfer and mucin secretion in ocular tissues.

Patients with excessive tear lipids may require specific instructions for removal of lipid strands from the eyelid margin. Antibiotics topically or systemically may be necessary. Dietary supplementation with omega-3 fatty acids or flax seed oil has been advocated to modulate favorably meibomian gland secretion. Topical vitamin A may be useful in reversing ocular surface metaplasia.

All chemical preservatives in artificial tears induce a certain amount of corneal toxicity. Benzalkonium chloride is the most damaging of the commonly used preparations. Patients who require frequent drops fare better with nonpreserved solutions. Preservatives can also cause idiosyncratic reactions. This is most common with thimerosal.

Patients with dry eyes from any cause are more likely to have concurrent infections. Chronic blepharitis is common and should be treated with appropriate lid hygiene and topical antibiotics as needed. If there is acne rosacea, treatment with systemic doxycycline may be helpful.

Surgical treatment for dry eyes includes insertion of temporary (collagen) or extended (silicone) punctal plugs to retain lacrimal secretions. Permanent closure of the puncta and canaliculi can be achieved by thermal, electrocautery, or laser treatment. Injection of botulinum toxin into the medial lower eyelid is reported to improve discomfort by reducing tear drainage.

REFERENCES

Conjunctiva

Abelson MB et al: Advances in pharmacotherapy for allergic conjunctivitis. Expert Opin Pharmacother 2015;16:1219. [PMID: 25943976]

Adebayo A et al: Shifting trends in in vitro antibiotic susceptibilities for common bacterial conjunctival isolates in the last decade at the New York Eye and Ear Infirmary. Graefes Arch Clin Exp Ophthalmol 2011;249:111. [PMID: 20532549]

Al-Amri AM: Long-term follow-up of tacrolimus ointment for treatment of atopic keratoconjunctivitis. Am J Ophthalmol 2014;157:280. [PMID: 24439439]

Azari AA et al: Conjunctivitis: A systematic review of diagnosis and treatment. JAMA 2013;310:1721. [PMID: 24150468]

Brémond-Gignac D et al: Atopic keratoconjunctivitis in children: Clinical features and diagnosis. Ophthalmology 2016;123:435. [PMID: 26278858]

Brunner M et al: Control of ocular disease in mucous membrane pemphigoid. Klin Monbl Augenheilkd 2014;231:331. [PMID: 24771161]

Castillo M et al: Topical antihistamines and mast cell stabilisers for treating seasonal and perennial allergic conjunctivitis. Cochrane Database Syst Rev 2015;6:CD009566. [PMID: 26028608]

Chansaenroj J et al: Epidemic outbreak of acute haemorrhagic conjunctivitis caused by coxsackievirus A24 in Thailand, 2014. Epidemiol Infect 2015;143:3087. [PMID: 25824006]

Chhipa SA et al: Ocular manifestation, complications and aetiological factors in Stevens-Johnson syndrome/toxic epidermal necrolysis. J Pak Med Assoc 2015;65:62. [PMID: 25831677]

Chigbu DI et al: Update and clinical utility of alcaftadine ophthalmic solution 0.25% in the treatment of allergic conjunctivitis. Clin Ophthalmol 2015;9:1215. [PMID: 26185412]

Çoban-Karataş M et al: Efficacy of topical 0.05% cyclosporine treatment in children with severe vernal keratoconjunctivitis. Turk J Pediatr 2014;56:410. [PMID: 25818961]

Ejere HO et al: Face washing promotion for preventing active trachoma. Cochrane Database Syst Rev 2015;2:CD003659. [PMID: 25697765]

Erdinest N et al: Topical immunomodulators in the management of allergic eye diseases. Curr Opin Allergy Clin Immunol 2014;14:457. [PMID: 25054831]

Fukushima A et al: Therapeutic effects of 0.1% tacrolimus eye drops for refractory allergic ocular diseases with proliferative lesion or corneal involvement. Br J Ophthalmol 2014;98:1023. [PMID: 24695688]

González-López JJ et al: Topical cyclosporine for atopic keratoconjunctivitis. Cochrane Database Syst Rev 2012;9:CD009078. [PMID: 22972132]

Guglielmetti S et al: Atopic keratoconjunctivitis and atopic dermatitis. Curr Opin Allergy Clin Immunol 2010;10:478. [PMID: 20720488]

Gupta S et al: Steroid-induced glaucoma and childhood blindness. Br J Ophthalmol 2015;99:1454. [PMID: 26002945]

Habtamu E et al: Epilation for minor trachomatous trichiasis: Four-year results of a randomised controlled trial. PLoS Negl Trop Dis 2015;9:e0003558. [PMID: 25768796]

Han Y et al: Corticosteroids for preventing postherpetic neuralgia. Cochrane Database Syst Rev 2013;3:CD005582. [PMID: 23543541]

Ihler F et al: Ragweed-induced allergic rhinoconjunctivitis: Current and emerging treatment options. J Asthma Allergy 2015;8:15. [PMID: 25733916]

Jain R et al: Stevens-Johnson syndrome: The role of an ophthalmologist. Surv Ophthalmol 2016;61:369. [PMID: 26829569]

Jalbert I et al: Environmental aeroallergens and allergic rhinoconjunctivitis. Curr Opin Allergy Clin Immunol 2015;15:476. [PMID: 26258925]

Jhanji V et al: Adenoviral keratoconjunctivitis. Surv Ophthalmol 2015;60:435. [PMID: 26077630]

Kaniwa N et al: Drugs causing severe ocular surface involvements in Japanese patients with Stevens-Johnson syndrome/toxic epidermal necrolysis. Allergol Int 2015;64:379. [PMID: 26433536]

Keklikci U et al: Topical cyclosporine a 0.05% eyedrops in the treatment of vernal keratoconjunctivitis: Randomized placebo-controlled trial. Adv Clin Exp Med 2014;23:455. [PMID: 24979519]

Kiiski V et al: Long-term safety of topical pimecrolimus and topical tacrolimus in atopic blepharoconjunctivitis. JAMA Dermatol 2014;150:571. [PMID: 24500107]

Kim DH et al: The role of systemic immunomodulatory treatment and prognostic factors on chronic ocular complications in Stevens-Johnson syndrome. Ophthalmology 2015;122:254. [PMID: 25262319]

Lee YC et al: Human adenovirus type 8 epidemic keratoconjunctivitis with large corneal epithelial full-layer detachment: An endemic outbreak with uncommon manifestations. Clin Ophthalmol 2015;9:953. [PMID: 26060391]

Leonardi A et al: Epidemiology of allergic conjunctivitis: Clinical appearance and treatment patterns in a population-based study. Curr Opin Allergy Clin Immunol 2015;15:482. [PMID: 26258920]

Leonardi A et al: Allergic conjunctivitis: A cross-sectional study. Clin Exp Allergy 2015;45:1118. [PMID: 25809830]

Li Z et al: Topical fluorometholone versus diclofenac sodium in cases with perennial allergic conjunctivitis. Eye Contact Lens 2015;41:310. [PMID: 26322818]

Martins TG et al: Corneal complication caused by gonococcal conjunctivitis. Einstein (Sao Paulo) 2015;13:474. [PMID: 26018149]

McAnena L et al: Prevalence of gonococcal conjunctivitis in adults and neonates. Eye 2015;29:875. [PMID: 25907207]

McLaurin E et al: Phase 3 randomized double-masked study of efficacy and safety of once-daily 0.77% olopatadine hydrochloride ophthalmic solution in subjects with allergic conjunctivitis using the conjunctival allergen challenge model. Cornea 2015;34:1245. [PMID: 26266427]

Medina NH et al: Acute hemorrhagic conjunctivitis epidemic in São Paulo State, Brazil, 2011. Rev Panam Salud Publica 2016;39:137. [PMID: 27754516]

Moore D et al: Preventing ophthalmia neonatorum. Can J Infect Dis Med Microbiol. 2015;26:122. [PMID: 26236350]

Mpyet C et al: Global elimination of trachoma by 2020: A work in progress. Ophthalmic Epidemiol 2015;22:148. [PMID: 26158572]

Pucci N et al: Tacrolimus vs. cyclosporine eyedrops in severe cyclosporine-resistant vernal keratoconjunctivitis: A randomized, comparative, double-blind, crossover study. Pediatr Allergy Immunol 2015;26:256. [PMID: 25712437]

Qiu W et al: Punctal plugs versus artificial tears for treating primary Sjögren's syndrome with keratoconjunctivitis SICCA: A comparative observation of their effects on visual function. Rheumatol Int 2013;33:2543. [PMID: 23649850]

Ram J et al: Images in clinical medicine. Giant papillae in vernal keratoconjunctivitis. N Engl J Med 2014;370:1636. [PMID: 24758619]

Shattock AJ et al: Control of trachoma in Australia: A model-based evaluation of current interventions. PLoS Negl Trop Dis 2015;9:e0003474. [PMID: 25860143]

Solomon A: Corneal complications of vernal keratoconjunctivitis. Curr Opin Allergy Clin Immunol 2015;15:489. [PMID: 26258926]

Sotozono C et al: Predictive factors associated with acute ocular involvement in Stevens-Johnson syndrome and toxic epidermal necrolysis. Am J Ophthalmol 2015;160:228. [PMID: 25979679]

Suzuki T et al: Conjunctivitis caused by Neisseria gonorrhoeae isolates with reduced cephalosporin susceptibility and multidrug resistance. J Clin Microbiol 2013;51:4246. [PMID: 24025911]

Szeto SK et al: Prevalence of ocular manifestations and visual outcomes in patients with herpes zoster ophthalmicus. Cornea 2017;36:338. [PMID: 27741018]

US Preventive Services Task Force: Ocular prophylaxis for gonococcal ophthalmia neonatorum: Reaffirmation recommendation statement. Am Fam Physician 2012;85:195. [PMID: 22335221]

Van Zyl L et al: Prevalence of chronic ocular complications in Stevens-Johnson syndrome and toxic epidermal necrolysis. Middle East Afr J Ophthalmol 2014;21:332. [PMID: 25371640]

West SK et al: Trachoma control: 14 years later. Ophthalmic Epidemiol 2015;22:145. [PMID: 26158571]

Wilson DJ et al: Comparing the efficacy of ophthalmic NSAIDs in common indications: A literature review to support cost-effective prescribing. Ann Pharmacother 2015;49:727. [PMID: 25725037]

Conjunctival Tumors

Ballalai PL et al: Long-term results of topical mitomycin C 0.02% for primary and recurrent conjunctival-corneal intraepithelial neoplasia. Ophthal Plast Reconstr Surg 2009;25:296. [PMID: 19617789]

Baum TD et al: Primary acquired melanosis of the conjunctiva. Int Ophthalmol Clin 1997;37:61. [PMID: 9429932]

Brownstein S: Malignant melanoma of the conjunctiva. Cancer Control 2004;11:310. [PMID: 15377990]

Carrau RL et al: Mucoepidermoid carcinoma of the conjunctiva. Ophthal Plast Reconstr Surg 1994;10:163. [PMID: 7947443]

Chalasani R et al: Role of topical chemotherapy for primary acquired melanosis and malignant melanoma of the conjunctiva and cornea: Review of the evidence and recommendations for treatment. Clin Experiment Ophthalmol 2006;34:708. [PMID: 16970772]

Damato B et al: Conjunctival melanoma and melanosis: A reappraisal of terminology, classification and staging. Clin Experiment Ophthalmol 2008;36:786. [PMID: 19128387]

Damato B et al: Management of conjunctival melanoma. Expert Rev Anticancer Ther 2009;9:1227. [PMID: 19761427]

Doganay S et al: Surgical excision, cryotherapy, autolimbal transplantation and mitomycin-C in treatment of conjunctival-corneal intraepithelial neoplasia. Int Ophthalmol 2005;26:53. [PMID: 16779567]

Dugel PU et al: Treatment of ocular adnexal Kaposi's sarcoma in acquired immune deficiency syndrome. Ophthalmology 1992;99:1127. [PMID: 1495793]

Gichuhi S et al: Risk factors for ocular surface squamous neoplasia in Kenya: A case-control study. Trop Med Int Health 2016;21:1522. [PMID: 27714903]

Hamam R et al: Conjunctival/corneal intraepithelial neoplasia. Int Ophthalmol Clin 2009;49:63. [PMID: 19125065]

Heffler KF: Tumors of the cornea and conjunctiva. Curr Opin Ophthalmol 1995;6:32. [PMID: 10172412]

Kao A et al: Management of primary acquired melanosis, nevus, and conjunctival melanoma. Cancer Control 2016;23:117. [PMID: 27218788]

Kim JW et al: Topical treatment options for conjunctival neoplasms. Clin Ophthalmol 2008;2:503. [PMID: 19668748]

Kirkegaard MM et al: Conjunctival lymphoma: An international multicenter retrospective study. JAMA Ophthalmol 2016;134:406. [PMID: 26891973]

Lee GA et al: Ocular surface squamous neoplasia. Surv Ophthalmol 1995;39:429. [PMID: 7660300]

Lommatzsch PK et al: Malignant conjunctival melanoma. Clinical review with recommendations for diagnosis, therapy and follow-up. Klin Monbl Augenheilkd 2002;219:710. [German] [PMID: 12447715]

Pe'er J: Ocular surface squamous neoplasia. Ophthalmol Clin North Am 2005;18:1. [PMID: 15763187]

Poothullil AM et al: Topical medical therapies for ocular surface tumors. Semin Ophthalmol 2006;21:161. [PMID: 16912014]

Ringeisen AL et al: Bulbar conjunctival molluscum contagiosum. Ophthalmology 2016;123:294. [PMID: 26802706]

Rodriguez-Sains RS: Pigmented conjunctival neoplasms. Orbit 2002;21:231. [PMID: 12187419]

Shields CL et al: Conjunctival nevi: Clinical features and natural course in 410 consecutive patients. Arch Ophthalmol 2004;122:167. [PMID: 14769591]

Shields CL et al: Conjunctival tumors in children. Curr Opin Ophthalmol 2007;18:351. [PMID: 17700226]

Shields CL et al: Conjunctival lymphoid tumors: Clinical analysis of 117 cases and relationship to systemic lymphoma. Ophthalmology 2001;108:979. [PMID: 11320031]

Shields CL et al: Conjunctival tumors in 5002 cases. Comparative analysis of benign versus malignant counterparts. The 2016 James D. Allen Lecture. Am J Ophthalmol 2017;173:106. [PMID: 27725148]

Suarez MJ: Clinicopathological features of ophthalmic neoplasms arising in the setting of xeroderma pigmentosum. Ocul Oncol Pathol 2015;2:112. [PMID: 27172099]

Tsai PS et al: Treatment of conjunctival lymphomas. Semin Ophthalmol 2005;20:239. [PMID: 16352495]

Yoon YD et al: Tumors of the cornea and conjunctiva. Curr Opin Ophthalmol 1997;8:55. [PMID: 10170445]

Tears

Ames P et al: Cyclosporine ophthalmic emulsions for the treatment of dry eye: A review of the clinical evidence. Clin Investig (Lond) 2015;5:267. [PMID: 25960865]

Bron AJ et al: Rethinking dry eye disease: A perspective on clinical implications. Ocul Surf 2014;12:S1. [PMID: 24725379]

Bukhari AA: Botulinum neurotoxin type A versus punctal plug insertion in the management of dry eye disease. Oman J Ophthalmol. 2014;7:61. [PMID: 25136228]

Dogru M et al: Changing trends in the treatment of dry-eye disease. Expert Opin Investig Drugs 2013;22:1581. [PMID: 24088227]

Foulks GN et al: Clinical guidelines for management of dry eye associated with Sjögren disease. Ocul Surf 2015;13:118. [PMID: 25881996]

Keating GM: Diquafosol ophthalmic solution 3%: A review of its use in dry eye. Drugs 2015;75:911. [PMID: 25968930]

Koh S: Clinical utility of 3% diquafosol ophthalmic solution in the treatment of dry eyes. Clin Ophthalmol 2015;9:865. [PMID: 26028958]

Lee HS et al: Efficacy of hypotonic 0.18% sodium hyaluronate eye drops in patients with dry eye disease. Cornea 2014;33:946. [PMID: 24915018]

Marcet MM et al: Safety and efficacy of lacrimal drainage system plugs for dry eye syndrome: A report by the American Academy of Ophthalmology. Ophthalmology 2015;122:1681. [PMID: 26038339]

Mohammadpour M et al: Trachoma: Past, present and future. J Curr Ophthalmol 2016;28:165. [PMID: 27830198]

Moscovici BK et al: Treatment of Sjögren's syndrome dry eye using 0.03% tacrolimus eye drop: Prospective double-blind randomized study. Cont Lens Anterior Eye 2015;38:373. [PMID: 25956572]

Sacchetti M et al: Systematic review of randomised clinical trials on topical ciclosporin A for the treatment of dry eye disease. Br J Ophthalmol 2014;98:1016. [PMID: 24344232]

Wan KH et al: Efficacy and safety of topical 0.05% cyclosporine eye drops in the treatment of dry eye syndrome: A systematic review and meta-analysis. Ocul Surf 2015;13:213. [PMID: 26045239]

Wu D et al: Efficacy and safety of topical diquafosol ophthalmic solution for treatment of dry eye: A systematic review of randomized clinical trials. Cornea 2015;34:644. [PMID: 25909234]

Cornea

Ahmed Al-Maskari, FRCOphth, and
Daniel F. P. Larkin, MD, FRCOphth

CLINICAL ASSESSMENT OF CORNEAL DISEASE: SYMPTOMS & SIGNS

Thorough clinical assessment is crucial in corneal disease as diagnosis is feasible in most cases on the basis of history and clinical examination. A history of trauma or contact lens wear can often be elicited, with foreign bodies and abrasions being the two most common acute corneal abnormalities. Identifying any past or family history of corneal disease can be critical. Herpes simplex infection and corneal erosion are often recurrent, but since recurrent erosion is extremely painful and herpetic keratitis is not, they can be differentiated by the history. Use of topical medications, including nonprescription preparations, should be elicited. Topical corticosteroids predispose to bacterial, fungal, and viral disease, especially herpes simplex keratitis. Many medications and preservatives can cause contact dermatitis or corneal toxicity. Toxicity is an important cause of corneal and conjunctival disease. The keys to examination of the cornea are adequate illumination and magnification, making the slitlamp essential. Examining the reflection as light is moved carefully over the entire cornea identifies rough areas indicative of epithelial defects. Fluorescein staining highlights superficial epithelial lesions that might otherwise not be apparent. Examination, particularly after trauma, is facilitated by instillation of a local anesthetic. Further methods of imaging in corneal disease are listed in Table 6–1.

MICROBIAL KERATITIS

Microbial keratitis is a major cause of visual loss throughout the world. Prevention, early diagnosis, and prompt management are essential to avoid long-term visual impairment. Table 6–2 outlines the most common risk factors for microbial keratitis. Examination of corneal scrapings, using Gram and Giemsa stains, may allow identification of the organism, particularly bacteria. Cultures for bacteria, fungi, *Acanthamoeba*, or viruses should be undertaken

at presentation if indicated clinically or later if there is lack of response to treatment. Polymerase chain reaction (PCR) provides rapid identification of herpes viruses, *Acanthamoeba*, and fungi. Appropriate therapy is instituted as soon as the necessary specimens have been obtained. It is important that laboratory results are interpreted in conjunction with the clinical picture.

1. BACTERIAL KERATITIS

Many types of bacterial corneal ulcers look alike and vary only in severity. This is especially true of ulcers caused by opportunistic bacteria (eg, alpha-hemolytic streptococci, *Staphylococcus aureus*, *Staphylococcus epidermidis*, *Nocardia*, and *Mycobacterium chelonae*), which often cause indolent corneal ulcers that tend to spread slowly and superficially.

▶ *Streptococcus pneumoniae* (Pneumococcal) Keratitis (Figure 6–1)

Pneumococcal corneal ulcer usually manifests 24–48 hours after inoculation of an abraded cornea. It typically produces a well-circumscribed ulcer that spreads from the original site of infection toward the center of the cornea. The advancing border shows active ulceration and infiltration as the trailing border begins to heal. The superficial corneal layers become involved first and then the deep layers. The cornea surrounding the ulcer is often clear. Hypopyon is common. Scrapings from the leading edge of a pneumococcal corneal ulcer usually contain gram-positive lancet-shaped diplococci. See Table 6–3 for recommended antibiotic treatment. Any concurrent dacryocystitis and nasolacrimal duct obstruction should be treated.

▶ *Pseudomonas aeruginosa* Keratitis

Pseudomonas corneal ulcer begins as a gray infiltrate at the site of a break in the corneal epithelium (Figure 6–2). Severe

Table 6–1. Methods of Corneal Imaging

Method	Description	Applications
Corneal topography (see Chapter 2)	Computer analysis of keratoscopy images to produce three-dimensional corneal profile displayed as refractive power, elevation, and thickness maps. Wavefront aberrometry to analyze the quality of the optical image may be incorporated.	Diagnosis and monitoring of corneal ectasia
Specular microscopy	High-magnification image of corneal endothelium.	Diagnosis of endothelial disorders; quantification of endothelial cell density
Anterior segment optical coherence tomography (OCT)	Cross-sectional image of cornea and anterior chamber.	Measure depth of corneal scars; assessment of position of endothelial grafts
Confocal microscopy	Imaging of cellular structure of the cornea and corneal nerves.	Diagnosis of *Acanthamoeba* and filamentary fungal keratitis

pain is common. The lesion tends to spread rapidly in all directions because of proteolytic enzymes produced by the organisms. Although superficial at first, the ulcer may quickly affect the entire cornea with devastating consequences, including extensive stromal loss, corneal perforation, and intraocular infection. There is often a large hypopyon that tends to increase in size as the ulcer progresses.

Pseudomonas corneal infection is usually associated with soft contact lenses, especially overnight wear. The organism has been shown to adhere to the surface of soft contact lenses. Scrapings from the ulcer may contain long, thin, gram-negative rods that are often scanty. See Table 6–3 for recommended antibiotic treatment.

▷ *Moraxella liquefaciens* Keratitis

M liquefaciens (diplobacillus of Petit) causes an indolent oval ulcer that usually affects the inferior cornea and progresses into the deep stroma over a period of days. There is usually little or no hypopyon, and the surrounding cornea is usually clear. *M liquefaciens* ulcer often occurs in a patient with alcoholism, diabetes mellitus, or other causes of immunosuppression. Scrapings may contain large, square-ended gram-negative diplobacilli. See Table 6–3 for recommended antibiotic treatment. Treatment can be difficult and prolonged.

Table 6–2. Main Risk Factors for Microbial Keratitis

Contact lens wear
Ocular surface disease
Trauma
Ocular surgery

▷ Group A *Streptococcus* Keratitis

Central corneal ulcers caused by beta-hemolytic streptococci have no identifying features. The surrounding corneal stroma is often infiltrated and edematous, and there is usually a moderately large hypopyon. Scrapings often contain gram-positive cocci in chains. See Table 6–3 for recommended antibiotic treatment.

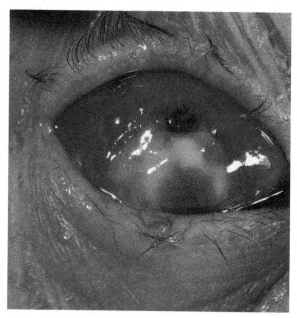

▲ **Figure 6–1.** Pneumococcal corneal ulcer with iris prolapsing through superior peripheral corneal perforation.

Table 6–3. Treatment of Microbial Keratitis

Type	First-Line Treatment	Regimen	Second-Line Treatment	Comments
Bacterial	Topical fluoroquinolone (eg, ofloxacin, moxifloxacin)	Hourly day and night for 48 hours, then hourly during the day for 3 days, then 4 times daily until resolution	Topical cefuroxime (fortified 5%) and gentamicin (fortified 1.5%)	
Chlamydial	Oral azithromycin, doxycycline, erythromycin, or tetracycline (see Chapter 5)		Topical sulfonamide, tetracycline, erythromycin, or rifampicin (see Chapter 5)	
Mycobacterial	Topical amikacin 2.5% and levofloxacin	Hourly day and night for 48 hours then taper down	Topical azithromycin	
Fungal	Filamentary: Topical natamycin Yeasts: Topical amphotericin (0.15%)	Hourly day and night for 24 hours, then hourly during the day until signs of healing, then 4 times daily until resolution	Topical voriconazole (1%)	For severe cases, add topical chlorhexidine (0.2%) and oral voriconazole
Viral	Topical acyclovir or ganciclovir	5 times daily for 1 week then 3 times daily for 1 week	Topical trifluorothymidine	
Acanthamoeba	Biguanide (eg, polyhexamethylene biguanide 0.02%) and/or diamidine (eg, hexamidine 0.1%)	Hourly day and night for 48 hours, then hourly during the day for 3 days, then every 2 hours for 3–4 weeks, then 4 times daily		

▶ *Staphylococcus aureus, Staphylococcus epidermidis,* & Alpha-Hemolytic *Streptococcus* Keratitis

Central corneal ulcers caused by these organisms have become more common, many of them in corneas compromised by topical corticosteroid use. The ulcers are often indolent but may be associated with hypopyon and some surrounding corneal infiltration. They are often superficial, and the ulcer bed feels firm when scraped. Scrapings may contain gram-positive cocci singly, in pairs, or in chains. Infectious crystalline keratopathy (in which the corneal infiltrate has

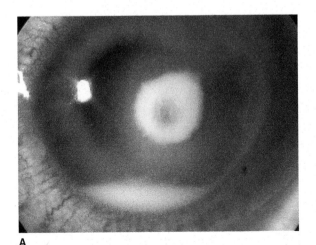

A

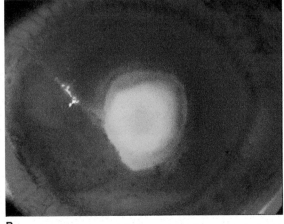

B

▲ **Figure 6–2. A:** *Pseudomonas* ulcer related to 24-hour contact lens wear. **B:** Fluorescein highlighting the epithelial defect.

a branching appearance) is typically associated with long-term therapy with topical corticosteroid; the disease is often caused by alpha-hemolytic streptococci as well as nutritionally deficient streptococci. See Table 6–3 for recommended antibiotic treatment.

Chlamydial Keratitis

All five principal types of chlamydial conjunctivitis (trachoma, inclusion conjunctivitis, primary ocular lymphogranuloma venereum, parakeet or psittacosis conjunctivitis, and feline pneumonitis conjunctivitis) may be accompanied by corneal lesions. Only in trachoma and lymphogranuloma venereum, however, are they blinding or visually damaging. The corneal lesions of trachoma have been extensively studied and are of great diagnostic importance. In order of appearance, they consist of (1) epithelial microerosions affecting the upper third of the cornea; (2) micropannus; (3) subepithelial round opacities, commonly called trachoma pustules; (4) limbal follicles and their cicatricial remains, known as Herbert's peripheral pits; (5) gross pannus; and (6) extensive, diffuse, subepithelial cicatrization. Mild cases of trachoma may have only epithelial keratitis and micropannus and may heal without impairing vision.

The rare cases of lymphogranuloma venereum have far fewer characteristic changes but are known to have developed blindness secondary to diffuse corneal scarring and total pannus. The remaining types of chlamydial infection cause only micropannus, epithelial keratitis, and, rarely, subepithelial opacities that are not visually significant. Several methods of identifying chlamydia are available through any competent laboratory.

Chlamydial keratoconjunctivitis responds to systemic azithromycin, doxycycline, erythromycin, or tetracycline (see Table 6–3 and Chapter 5). Topical sulfonamides, tetracyclines, erythromycin, and rifampin are also effective.

Mycobacterium chelonae & Nocardia Keratitis

Ulcers due to *M chelonae* and *Nocardia* are rare. They often follow trauma and are often associated with contact with soil. The ulcers are indolent, and the bed of the ulcer often has radiating lines that make it look like a cracked windshield. Hypopyon may or may not be present. Scrapings may contain acid-fast slender rods (*M chelonae*) or gram-positive filamentous, often branching organisms (*Nocardia*). See Table 6–3 for recommended antibiotic treatment.

2. FUNGAL KERATITIS

Fungal corneal ulcers once were seen only in agricultural settings, but with the advent of contact lenses, immunosuppressive disease, and corticosteroid use, these infections are seen in a variety of populations. The use of corticosteroids

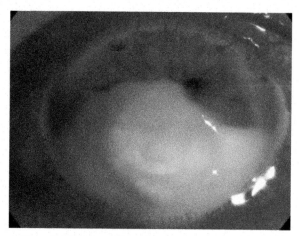

▲ Figure 6–3. Fungal keratitis.

is contraindicated in fungal disease; by altering the natural immune response and enhancing collagenase activity, these drugs are counterproductive.

Fungal ulcers are indolent and typified by an infiltrate with irregular edges, often a hypopyon, marked inflammation of the globe, superficial ulceration, and satellite lesions (usually infiltrates at sites distant from the main area of ulceration) (Figure 6–3). Underlying the principal lesion, and the satellite lesions as well, there is often an endothelial plaque associated with a severe anterior chamber reaction. Corneal abscesses frequently occur.

Most fungal ulcers are caused by opportunists such as *Candida*, *Fusarium*, *Aspergillus*, *Penicillium*, *Cephalosporium*, and others. There are no identifying features that help to differentiate one type of fungal ulcer from another, although the hyphae typical of filamentous fungi are characteristic on in vivo confocal microscopy.

Scrapings from fungal corneal ulcers, except those caused by *Candida*, contain hyphal elements; scrapings from *Candida* ulcers usually contain pseudohyphae or yeast forms that show characteristic budding. See Table 6–3 for recommended antifungal treatment.

3. VIRAL KERATITIS

Herpes Simplex Virus Keratitis

Herpes simplex virus (HSV) keratitis occurs in two forms: primary and recurrent. It is a common cause of corneal scarring and loss of vision. The epithelial form is the ocular counterpart of labial herpes, with which it shares immunologic and pathologic features as well as having a similar time course. The only difference is that the clinical course of the keratitis may be prolonged because of the avascularity of the corneal stroma, which retards the migration of lymphocytes and macrophages to the lesion. HSV ocular infection in the immunocompetent host is often self-limited, but in the immunologically compromised host, including patients treated with topical corticosteroids, its course can be chronic and damaging. Stromal and endothelial disease has previously been thought to be a purely immunologic response to virus particles or virally induced cellular changes. However, there is increasing evidence that active viral infection can occur within stromal and possibly endothelial cells as well as in other tissues within the anterior segment, such as the iris and trabecular endothelium. This highlights the need to assess the relative role of viral replication and host immune responses prior to and during therapy for HSV disease. Topical corticosteroids may control damaging inflammatory responses but at the expense of facilitation of viral replication. Thus, whenever topical corticosteroids are to be used, antivirals are likely to be necessary. Any patient undergoing topical corticosteroid therapy for HSV eye disease must be under the supervision of an ophthalmologist.

Serologic studies suggest that most adults have been exposed to the virus, although many do not recollect any episodes of clinical disease. Following primary infection, the virus establishes latency in the trigeminal ganglion. The factors influencing the development of recurrent disease, including its site, have yet to be unraveled. There is increasing evidence that the severity of disease is at least partly determined by the strain of virus involved. Most HSV infections of the cornea are still caused by HSV type 1, which causes labial herpes, but in both infants and adults, a few cases caused by HSV type 2, which causes genital herpes, have been reported. The corneal lesions caused by the two types are indistinguishable.

In most cases, diagnosis is made clinically on the basis of characteristic dendritic or geographic ulcers and greatly reduced or absent corneal sensation. Culture and PCR for viral DNA are used for accurate identification of HSV from tissue and fluid as well as from corneal epithelial cells.

A. Clinical Findings

Primary ocular herpes simplex is infrequently seen, but manifests as a vesicular blepharoconjunctivitis, occasionally with corneal involvement, and usually occurs in young children. It is generally self-limited, without causing significant ocular damage. Topical antiviral therapy may be used as prophylaxis against corneal involvement and as therapy for corneal disease.

Attacks of the common recurrent type of HSV keratitis are triggered by fever, overexposure to ultraviolet light, trauma, the onset of menstruation, or some other local or systemic source of immunosuppression. Unilaterality is the rule, but bilateral lesions develop in 4–6% of cases and are seen most often in atopic patients.

1. The first symptoms of HSV keratitis are usually irritation, photophobia, and tearing. There is often a history of nonocular herpetic infection. When the central cornea is affected, there is also some reduction in vision.

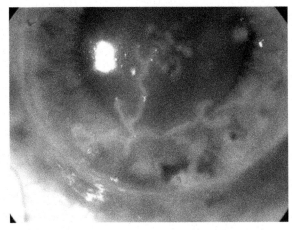

▲ **Figure 6–4.** Dendritic ulcer of herpes simplex epithelial keratitis.

2. HSV keratitis is classified clinically as epithelial, stromal, or endothelial.

1. Epithelial HSV Keratitis—The most characteristic lesion is the **dendritic ulcer**, which occurs in the corneal epithelium, has a branching, linear pattern with feathery edges, and has terminal bulbs at its ends (Figure 6–4). Fluorescein staining makes the dendrite easy to identify. HSV keratitis can also resemble many corneal diseases and must be considered in the differential diagnosis. A typical feature of HSV keratitis is reduced corneal sensation.

Geographic ulceration is a form of chronic dendritic disease in which the delicate dendritic lesion takes a broader form and the edges of the ulcer lose their feathery quality. HSV also may cause a blotchy epithelial keratitis and stellate epithelial keratitis, but these are usually transitory and often become typical dendrites within 1–2 days.

Subepithelial opacities can be caused by HSV infection. A ghost-like image, corresponding in shape to the original epithelial defect but slightly larger, can be seen in the area immediately underlying the epithelial lesion. As a rule, these subepithelial lesions do not persist for more than a few months.

Peripheral lesions of the cornea can also be caused by HSV. They are usually linear and show a loss of epithelium before the underlying corneal stroma becomes infiltrated. This is in contrast to the marginal ulcer associated with bacterial hypersensitivity, for example, to S aureus in staphylococcal blepharitis, in which the infiltration precedes the loss of the overlying epithelium. Distinguishing the two disorders is important because treatment of marginal immune ulcers can include use of topical corticosteroid, which is contraindicated in active HSV infection. Testing for corneal sensation is unreliable in peripheral herpetic disease. The patient is apt to be far less photophobic than a patient with nonherpetic corneal disease.

2. Stromal HSV Keratitis—Focal areas of stromal infiltration and edema, often accompanied by vascularization, are likely to be predominantly due to viral replication. Corneal thinning, necrosis, and perforation may develop rapidly, particularly if topical corticosteroids are being used without antiviral cover. If there is stromal disease in the presence of epithelial ulceration, it may be difficult to differentiate bacterial or fungal superinfection from herpetic disease. The features of the epithelial disease need to be carefully scrutinized for herpetic characteristics, but a bacterial or fungal component may be present, and the patient must be managed accordingly. Stromal necrosis also may be caused by an acute immune reaction, again complicating the diagnosis with regard to active viral disease. Hypopyon may be seen with necrosis as well as secondary bacterial or fungal infection.

Disciform keratitis is the most common form of HSV stromal keratitis. The stroma is edematous in a central, disk-shaped area, without significant infiltration and usually without vascularization. The edema may be sufficient to produce folds in Descemet membrane. Keratic precipitates may lie directly under the disciform lesion but may also involve the entire endothelium because of the frequently associated anterior uveitis. The pathogenesis of disciform keratitis is generally regarded as an immunologic reaction to viral antigens in the stroma or endothelium, but active viral disease cannot be ruled out. Like most herpetic lesions in immunocompetent individuals, disciform keratitis is normally self-limited, lasting weeks to months. Edema is the most prominent sign, and healing can occur with minimal scarring and vascularization.

3. Endothelial HSV Keratitis—A similar clinical appearance to disciform keratitis is seen with **primary endothelial HSV keratitis (endotheliitis)**, which can be associated with anterior uveitis, raised intraocular pressure, and focal inflammation of the iris. Viral replication within the various anterior chamber structures is thought to be responsible.

B. Treatment

The treatment of HSV keratitis should be directed at eliminating viral replication within the cornea while minimizing the damaging effects of the inflammatory response.

1. Debridement—An effective way to treat dendritic keratitis is epithelial debridement since the virus is located in the epithelium, and debridement will also reduce the viral antigenic load to the corneal stroma. Healthy epithelium adheres tightly to the cornea, but infected epithelium is easy to remove. Debridement is accomplished with a tightly wound cotton-tipped applicator. Adjunctive therapy with a topical antiviral accelerates epithelial healing.

2. Drug Therapy—The topical antiviral agents used in herpetic keratitis are trifluridine, ganciclovir, and acyclovir. (Topical acyclovir for ophthalmic use is not approved in the United States.) Ganciclovir and acyclovir are more effective in stromal disease than the others. Oral antivirals like acyclovir are valuable, particularly in atopic individuals who are susceptible to aggressive ocular and dermal (eczema herpeticum) herpetic disease. They may be used instead of topical antivirals to avoid corneal toxicity. Dose of oral acyclovir for active disease is 400 mg five times daily in immunocompetent patients and 800 mg five times daily in immunocompromised and atopic patients. Prophylactic dose in recurrent disease is 400 mg twice daily. Famciclovir or valacyclovir may also be used.

Viral replication in the immunocompetent patient, particularly when confined to the corneal epithelium, usually is self-limited and scarring is minimal. If it becomes necessary to use topical corticosteroids because of the severity of the inflammatory response in the stroma, appropriate antiviral therapy is essential to control viral replication. Problems in the management of HSV keratitis are often due to inappropriate use of multiple topical treatments, including antivirals, antibiotics, and corticosteroids, resulting in adverse effects including epithelial toxicity. Frequently, using oral or topical antivirals and tapering the corticosteroids will result in marked improvement. Long-term antiviral therapy may predispose to antiviral resistance.

3. Surgical Treatment—Keratoplasty (especially anterior lamellar keratoplasty, if feasible, because it has the advantage over penetrating keratoplasty of reduced potential for corneal graft rejection) may be indicated for visual rehabilitation in patients with severe corneal scarring, but it should not be undertaken until the herpetic disease has been inactive for many months. Postoperatively, recurrent herpetic infection may occur as a result of the surgical trauma and the topical corticosteroids necessary to prevent corneal graft rejection. It may also be difficult to distinguish corneal graft rejection from recurrent stromal disease. Oral antiviral agents should be used for several months after keratoplasty to cover the use of topical corticosteroids.

Corneal perforation due to progressive herpetic stromal disease or superinfection with bacteria or fungi may necessitate emergency penetrating keratoplasty. Cyanoacrylate glue can be used to seal a small perforation (Figure 6–5), and lamellar "patch" grafts have been successful in selected cases. Therapeutic soft contact lens, tarsorrhaphy, or amniotic membrane transplant may be required to heal persistent epithelial defects in HSV keratitis.

▶ Varicella-Zoster Virus Keratitis

Varicella-zoster virus (VZV) infection occurs in two forms: primary (varicella) and recurrent (herpes zoster). Ocular manifestations are uncommon in varicella but common in ophthalmic zoster. In varicella (chickenpox), the usual eye lesions are pocks on the lids and lid margins. Rarely, keratitis occurs (typically a peripheral stromal lesion with

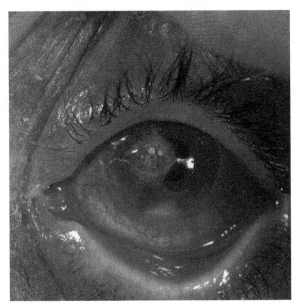

▲ **Figure 6–5.** Medical-grade cyanoacrylate glue sealing small paracentral corneal perforation.

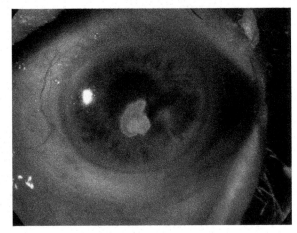

▲ **Figure 6–6.** Secondary bacterial infection of anesthetic cornea following herpes zoster keratitis.

vascularization), and still more rarely, epithelial keratitis occurs with or without pseudodendrites. Disciform keratitis, with uveitis of varying duration, has been reported.

In contrast to the rare and benign corneal lesions of varicella, the relatively frequent ophthalmic herpes zoster is often accompanied by keratouveitis that varies in severity according to the immune status of the patient. Thus, although children with zoster keratouveitis usually have benign disease, the aged have severe and sometimes blinding disease. Corneal complications in ophthalmic zoster often occur if there is a skin eruption in areas supplied by the nasociliary branch of the ophthalmic division of the fifth cranial nerve.

Unlike recurrent HSV keratitis that usually affects only the epithelium, herpes zoster keratitis affects the stroma and anterior uvea at onset. The epithelial lesions are blotchy and amorphous except for an occasional linear pseudodendrite that only vaguely resembles the true dendrites of HSV keratitis. Stromal opacities consist of edema and mild cellular infiltration and initially are subepithelial. Deep stromal disease can follow with necrosis and vascularization. A disciform keratitis sometimes develops and resembles HSV disciform keratitis. Loss of corneal sensation, with the risk of neurotrophic keratitis, is always a prominent feature and often persists for months after the corneal lesion appears to have healed (Figure 6–6). The associated uveitis tends to persist for weeks or months, but with time, it eventually heals. Scleritis (sclerokeratitis) can be a serious feature of VZV ocular disease.

Intravenous and oral antivirals have been used successfully in herpes zoster ophthalmicus, particularly in

immunocompromised patients. The dose for oral acyclovir is 800 mg five times daily for 10–14 days; for oral valacyclovir, 1 g three times daily for 7–10 days; and for oral famciclovir, 500 mg every 8 hours for 7–10 days. Therapy needs to be started within 72 hours after appearance of the rash. The role of topical antivirals is less certain. Topical corticosteroids may be necessary to treat severe keratitis, uveitis, and secondary glaucoma. The use of systemic corticosteroids is controversial. They may be indicated to reduce the incidence and severity of postherpetic neuralgia, but the risk of steroid complications is significant. Systemic acyclovir has little influence on the development of postherpetic neuralgia. Patients with facial and scalp lesions should be seen for several months after the onset of the skin lesions because the keratitis can be delayed.

▶ **Adenovirus Keratitis**

Keratitis usually accompanies all types of adenovirus conjunctivitis, reaching its peak 5–7 days after onset of the conjunctivitis. It is a fine epithelial keratitis best seen with the slitlamp after instillation of fluorescein. The minute lesions may group together to make up larger ones.

The epithelial keratitis is often followed by subepithelial opacities. In epidemic keratoconjunctivitis (EKC), which is due to adenovirus types 8 and 19, the subepithelial lesions are round and grossly visible (Figure 5–5). They appear 8–15 days after onset of the conjunctivitis and may persist for months or even (rarely) for several years. Similar lesions occur exceptionally in other adenoviral infections (eg, those caused by types 3, 4, and 7) but tend to be transitory and mild, lasting a few weeks at most. Subepithelial opacities usually resolve with topical corticosteroid but often recur, so such treatment with its risk of adverse effects is best avoided. Topical cyclosporine and tacrolimus also are effective.

Other Viral Keratitis

A fine epithelial keratitis may be seen in other viral infections, such as measles (in which the central cornea is affected predominantly), rubella, mumps, infectious mononucleosis, acute hemorrhagic conjunctivitis, Newcastle disease conjunctivitis, and verruca of the lid margin. A superior epithelial keratitis and pannus often accompany molluscum contagiosum nodules on the lid margin, which is a feature of human immunodeficiency virus (HIV) infection.

Acanthamoeba Keratitis

Acanthamoeba is a free-living protozoan that thrives in polluted water containing bacteria and organic material. Corneal infection with *Acanthamoeba* is usually associated with soft contact lens wear, including silicone hydrogel lenses, or overnight wear of rigid (gas-permeable) contact lenses to correct refractive errors (orthokeratology). There have been cases associated with a particular contact lens solution, probably related to insufficient anti-*Acanthamoeba* efficacy. It may also occur in non–contact lens wearers after exposure to contaminated water or soil.

The initial symptoms are pain out of proportion to the clinical findings, redness, and photophobia. The characteristic clinical signs are indolent corneal ulceration, stromal ring, and perineural infiltrates (Figure 6–7), but patients often present with changes confined to the corneal epithelium.

The diagnosis is established by culturing on nonnutrient agar with an overlay of *Escherichia coli*. Better results are obtained by corneal biopsy than corneal scraping, since histopathologic examination for amebic forms (trophozoites or cysts) can also be undertaken. In vivo confocal microscopy is a newer diagnostic technique by which cysts can be directly identified. Often the amebic forms can be identified in or cultured from solutions from contact lens storage cases.

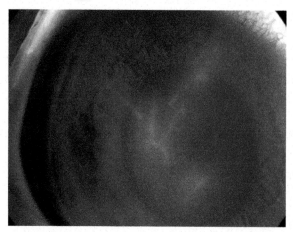

▲ **Figure 6-7.** *Acanthamoeba* keratitis with perineural infiltrates.

The differential diagnosis includes herpetic keratitis, with which it is frequently confused, and fungal, mycobacterial, or *Nocardia* keratitis.

In the early stages of the disease, epithelial debridement may be beneficial. Medical treatment is usually started with intensive topical biguanide (usually polyhexamethylene biguanide) and/or diamidine (such as propamidine isethionate) (Table 6–3). *Acanthamoeba* species may have variable drug sensitivities and may acquire drug resistance. An important principle is that drugs must be cysticidal. Effectiveness of treatment is hampered by the organisms' ability to encyst within the corneal stroma, necessitating prolonged treatment. Corticosteroids are not indicated in the treatment of *Acanthamoeba* keratitis unless required to control severe inflammation.

Keratoplasty may be necessary in advanced disease to arrest progression of the infection or after resolution and scarring to restore vision. If the organism reaches the sclera, medical and surgical treatments have high failure rates.

STERILE KERATITIS

Marginal Keratitis

The majority of marginal corneal ulcers are benign but extremely painful. They are secondary to acute or chronic bacterial conjunctivitis, particularly staphylococcal blepharoconjunctivitis and less often *Haemophilus* conjunctivitis. They are not an infectious process, however, and scrapings do not contain the causal bacteria. They are the result of sensitization to bacterial products; antibody from the limbal vessels reacts with antigen that has diffused through the corneal epithelium.

Marginal infiltrates and ulcers start as oval or linear infiltrates, separated from the limbus by a lucid interval, and only later may ulcerate and vascularize. They are self-limited, usually lasting from 7 to 10 days, but those associated with staphylococcal blepharoconjunctivitis usually recur. Treatment for blepharitis (shampoo scrubs, antimicrobials) usually will clear the problem; topical corticosteroids may be needed for severe cases. Topical corticosteroid preparations shorten their course and relieve symptoms, which are often severe, but treatment of the underlying blepharoconjunctivitis is essential if recurrences are to be prevented. Before starting corticosteroid therapy, great care must be taken to distinguish this entity from marginal herpetic keratitis. Marginal herpetic keratitis is usually almost symptomless because of corneal anesthesia, whereas hypersensitivity-type marginal ulcer is painful.

Mooren Ulcer (Figure 6–8)

The cause of Mooren ulcer is still unknown, but an autoimmune origin is suspected. It is a marginal ulcer, unilateral in 60–80% of cases, and characterized by painful, progressive excavation of the limbus and peripheral

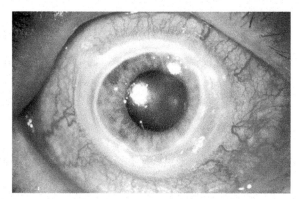

▲ **Figure 6–9.** Three hundred sixty degrees of peripheral ulcerative keratitis in a patient with rheumatoid arthritis.

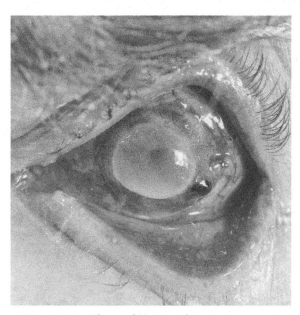

▲ **Figure 6–8.** Advanced Mooren ulcer.

cornea that often leads to loss of the eye. It occurs most commonly in old age but does not seem to be related to any of the systemic diseases that most often afflict the aged. It is unresponsive to both antibiotics and topical corticosteroids. Surgical excision of the limbal conjunctiva in an effort to remove sensitizing substances has recently been advocated. Lamellar tectonic keratoplasty has been used with success in selected cases. Systemic immunosuppressive therapy often is necessary to control moderate or advanced disease.

Phlyctenular Keratoconjunctivitis

Phlyctenules are localized accumulations of lymphocytes, monocytes, macrophages, and neutrophils. They appear first at the limbus, but in recurrent attacks, they may involve the bulbar conjunctiva and cornea. Corneal phlyctenules, often bilateral, cicatrize and vascularize, but conjunctival phlyctenules leave no trace.

Phlyctenular keratoconjunctivitis is a delayed hypersensitivity response, in most cases in developed countries to *S aureus* or other bacteria that proliferate on the lid margin in association with blepharitis. It may also occur in response to *Mycobacterium tuberculosis*, which was formerly a major cause of visual loss.

Untreated phlyctenules spontaneously regress after 10–14 days. Topical corticosteroid therapy shortens their duration and decreases scarring and vascularization. In the staphylococcal type, the acute staphylococcal infection and chronic blepharitis need to be treated.

Peripheral Ulcerative Keratitis (Marginal Keratitis in Autoimmune Disease) (Figure 6–9)

The peripheral cornea receives its nourishment from the aqueous humor, the limbal capillaries, and the tear film. It is contiguous with the subconjunctival lymphoid tissue and the lymphatic arcades at the limbus. The perilimbal conjunctiva appears to play an important role in the pathogenesis of corneal lesions that arise both from local ocular disease and from systemic disorders, particularly those of autoimmune origin. There is a striking similarity between the limbal capillary network and the renal glomerular capillary network. On the endothelial basement membranes of the capillaries of both networks, immune complexes are deposited and immunologic disease results. Thus, the peripheral cornea often participates in such autoimmune diseases as rheumatoid arthritis, polyarteritis nodosa, systemic lupus erythematosus, scleroderma, granulomatosis with polyangiitis (Wegener's granulomatosis), ulcerative colitis, Crohn's disease, and relapsing polychondritis. The corneal changes are secondary to scleral inflammation, with or without scleral vascular closure (see Chapter 7). The clinical signs include vascularization, infiltration and opacification, and peripheral guttering that may progress to perforation. Mooren ulcer may be an example of advanced peripheral ulcerative keratitis (PUK). Treatment is directed toward control of the associated systemic disease; topical therapy usually is ineffective, and systemic use of potent immunosuppressants often is required. Corneal perforation may require cyanoacrylate glue (Figure 6–5), lamellar patch grafting, or full-thickness keratoplasty.

Vitamin a Deficiency

The typical corneal ulcer associated with avitaminosis A is centrally located and bilateral, gray, and indolent, with a definite lack of corneal luster in the surrounding area. The cornea becomes soft and necrotic (keratomalacia), and perforation is common. The epithelium of the conjunctiva is keratinized, as evidenced by the presence of a Bitot's spot. This is a foamy, wedge-shaped area in the conjunctiva, usually on the temporal side, with the base of the wedge at the limbus and the apex extending toward the lateral canthus. Within the triangle, the conjunctiva is furrowed concentrically with the limbus, and dry flaky material can be seen falling from the area into the inferior cul-de-sac. A stained conjunctival scraping from a Bitot's spot will show keratinized epithelial cells.

Avitaminosis A corneal ulceration usually results from dietary lack of vitamin A or impaired absorption from the gastrointestinal tract. It may develop in an infant who has a feeding problem; in an adult who is on a restricted or generally inadequate diet; or in any person with biliary obstruction, since bile in the gastrointestinal tract is necessary for the absorption of vitamin A, or other causes of malabsorption. Lack of vitamin A causes a generalized keratinization of the epithelium throughout the body. The conjunctival and corneal changes together are known as **xerophthalmia.** Since the epithelium of the air passages is affected, many patients, if not treated, will die of pneumonia. Avitaminosis A also causes a generalized retardation of osseous growth. This is extremely important in infants; for example, if the skull bones do not grow and the brain continues to grow, increased intracranial pressure and papilledema can result.

Mild vitamin A deficiency should be treated in adults with a dose of 30,000 U/d for 1 week. Advanced cases will require much higher doses initially (20,000 U/kg/d). The average daily requirement of vitamin A is 1500–5000 IU for children, according to age, and 5000 IU for adults. Highly pigmented vegetables are the best source of dietary vitamin A.

Neurotrophic Keratitis

Trigeminal nerve dysfunction, due to trauma, surgery, tumor, inflammation, or any other cause, may result in corneal anesthesia with loss of the blink reflex, one of the cornea's defense mechanisms, as well as lack of trophic factors important for epithelial function. In the early stages of neurotrophic keratitis, there is diffuse blotchy epithelial edema. Subsequently there is loss of the epithelium (neurotrophic ulcer), which may extend over a large area of the cornea.

In the absence of corneal sensation, even a severe keratitis may produce little discomfort. Patients must be warned to look out for redness of the eye, reduced vision, corneal abnormality, or increased conjunctival discharge and to seek ophthalmic care as soon as any of these develop. Keeping the cornea moist with artificial tears and lubricant ointments may help to protect it. Swim goggles may be useful at night.

Once neurotrophic keratitis develops, it must be treated promptly. The most effective management is to keep the eye closed by careful horizontal taping of the eyelids, by tarsorrhaphy, or by means of ptosis induced with botulinum toxin. Secondary corneal infection must be treated promptly. Topical nerve growth factor drops can be used to promote the healing of epithelial defects, and autologous serum drops may be beneficial in long-term surface maintenance.

Exposure Keratitis

Exposure keratitis may develop in any situation in which the cornea is not properly moistened and covered by the eyelids. Examples include proptosis from any cause, ectropion, floppy lid syndrome, the absence of part of an eyelid as a result of trauma, and inability to close the lids, as in Bell's palsy. The two factors at work are the drying of the cornea and its exposure to minor trauma. The uncovered cornea is particularly subject to drying during sleeping hours, and swim goggles may be useful at night. If an ulcer develops, it usually follows minor trauma and occurs in the inferior third of the cornea. Exposure keratitis is sterile but can become secondarily infected.

The therapeutic objective is to provide protection and moisture for the entire corneal surface. The treatment method depends on the underlying condition: eyelid surgery, correction of exophthalmos, eye shield, or the options mentioned earlier in the discussion of neurotrophic keratitis. The combination of corneal anesthesia and exposure is particularly likely to result in severe keratitis.

Drug-Induced Epithelial Keratitis

Epithelial keratitis is commonly seen in patients using antiviral medications, particularly trifluridine, and several of the broad-spectrum and medium-spectrum antibiotics, such as neomycin, gentamicin, and tobramycin. It is usually a coarse superficial keratitis affecting predominantly the lower half of the cornea and interpalpebral fissure. It may cause permanent scarring. The preservatives in eye drops, particularly benzalkonium chloride (BAK) and thimerosal, are common causes of toxic keratitis.

Keratoconjunctivitis Sicca (Including Sjögren Syndrome)

Epithelial filaments in the lower half of the cornea are the cardinal signs of this autoimmune disease, in which secretion of the lacrimal and accessory lacrimal glands is diminished or eliminated. There is also a blotchy epithelial keratitis that affects mainly the lower half. Severe cases develop mucous pseudofilaments that stick to the corneal epithelium.

This pattern of keratitis also occurs in cicatrizing conjunctival diseases such as ocular mucous membrane pemphigoid, in which destruction of goblet cells of the conjunctiva results in mucus deficiency, such that any tears fail to wet the corneal epithelium effectively.

Treatment of keratoconjunctivitis sicca is frequent use of tear substitutes and lubricating ointments, of which there are many commercial preparations. Preservative-free preparations are preferable. Mucus deficiency requires treatment with mucus substitutes in addition to artificial tears. Topical cyclosporine 0.1%, a T-cell inhibitor, occasionally can reestablish goblet cell (mucin) density. Topical vitamin A may help to reverse epithelial keratinization. Autologous or allogeneic serum drops can be helpful in severe cases. Moisture chambers or swim goggles may be required. Lacrimal punctal plugs and punctal occlusion are important in the management of advanced cases, as are room humidifiers.

CORNEAL ECTASIA

▶ Keratoconus

Keratoconus is a stromal shape disorder that is relatively prevalent in all ethnic groups and may be inherited as an autosomal recessive or autosomal dominant trait. It is usually bilateral and asymmetric but may be unilateral. Symptoms caused by the refractive consequences typically commence in the second decade of life. Keratoconus has been associated with a number of diseases, including Down's syndrome, atopic dermatitis, retinitis pigmentosa, Marfan's syndrome and Ehlers-Danlos syndrome. Pathologically, there are disruptive changes in Bowman layer, stromal thinning, and ruptures in Descemet membrane.

Blurred vision is the only symptom. Many patients present with rapidly increasing myopic astigmatism. Signs include cone-shaped cornea; linear narrow folds centrally in Descemet membrane (Vogt's lines), which are pathognomonic; an iron ring around the base of the cone (Fleischer's ring); and, in extreme cases, indentation of the lower lid by the cornea when the patient looks down (Munson's sign). There is an irregular or scissor reflex on retinoscopy and a distorted corneal reflection with Placido disk or keratoscope even early in the disease. Color-coded topography provides earliest and more qualitative information on the degree of corneal distortion and irregular steepening (Figure 2–25). Early topographic signs of keratoconus (forme fruste) suggest possible progressive stromal thinning and refractive change and an unsuitable candidate for laser refractive surgery.

Acute hydrops of the cornea may occur, manifested by sudden diminution of vision associated with central corneal edema (Figure 6–10). This arises as a consequence of rupture of Descemet membrane. Usually it clears gradually without treatment but often leaves apical and Descemet membrane scarring.

Keratoconus is often slowly progressive and usually stabilizes in the fourth decade of life. Corneal collagen cross-linking has been shown to be effective in arresting the progression of keratoconus. It is therefore essential that

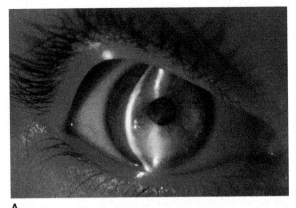

A

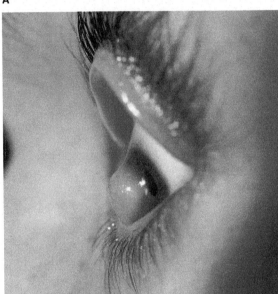

B

▲ **Figure 6–10.** Acute corneal hydrops due to keratoconus. **A:** Slitlamp view of milder case. **B:** Lateral view of more severe case.

newly diagnosed patients are reviewed every 6–12 months with serial corneal topography scans to monitor progression. Corneal collagen cross-linking involves diffusing riboflavin into the corneal stroma then shining ultraviolet A light to trigger a chemical reaction, which is thought to strengthen intercollagen bonds in the corneal stroma. Rigid contact lenses will markedly improve vision in the early stages by correcting irregular astigmatism. Keratoconus is one of the most common indications for corneal transplantation, either anterior lamellar or penetrating. Surgery is indicated when a contact lens can no longer be effectively worn or to restore stromal transparency following hydrops.

If a corneal transplant is done before extreme corneal thinning occurs, the prognosis is excellent; good best-corrected vision is achieved in over 85% of eyes after 4 years and in over 70% of eyes after 14 years. Best vision after deep lamellar or penetrating keratoplasty may require a rigid contact lens. Insertion of corneal intrastromal ring segments may improve best corrected vision and contact lens tolerance.

CORNEAL DEGENERATION

The corneal degenerations are a rare group of slowly progressive, bilateral, degenerative disorders that usually appear in the second or third decades of life. Some are hereditary. Other cases follow ocular inflammatory disease, and some are of unknown cause.

▶ Terrien Disease

Terrien disease is a rare bilateral symmetric degeneration characterized by marginal thinning of the upper nasal quadrants of the cornea. Men are more commonly affected than women, and the condition occurs more frequently in the third and fourth decades. There are no symptoms except for mild irritation during occasional inflammatory episodes, and the condition is slowly progressive. The clinical picture consists of marginal thinning and peripheral vascularization with lipid deposition. Perforation is a complication, especially from trauma. Tectonic (structural) keratoplasty may be required. Histopathologic studies of affected corneas have revealed vascularized connective tissue with fibrillary degeneration and fatty infiltration of collagen fibers. Because the course of progression is slow and the central cornea is spared, the prognosis is reasonably good.

▶ Band (Calcific) Keratopathy

Band keratopathy is characterized by the deposition of calcium salts in a band-like pattern in the anterior layers of the cornea. The keratopathy is usually limited to the interpalpebral area. The calcium deposits are noted in the basement membrane, Bowman layer, and anterior stromal lamellas. A clear margin separates the calcific band from the limbus, and clear holes may be seen in the band. Symptoms include irritation, injection, and blurring of vision.

Calcific band keratopathy has been described in a number of inflammatory, metabolic, and degenerative conditions. It is characteristically associated with juvenile idiopathic arthritis. It has been described in long-standing inflammatory conditions of the eye, glaucoma, and failed retinal detachment surgery. Band keratopathy may also be associated with hyperparathyroidism. The standard method of removing band keratopathy consists of removal of the corneal epithelium by curettage under topical anesthesia followed by irrigation of the cornea with a sterile 0.01 molar solution of ethylenediaminetetraacetic acid (EDTA) (edetate

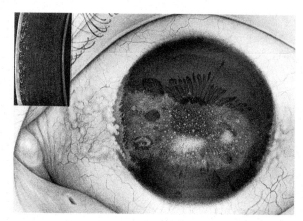

▲ **Figure 6–11.** Diagram of climatic droplet (Labrador) keratopathy including cross-sectional view (*inset*). (Used with permission from A. Ahmad.)

calcium) or application of EDTA with a cotton-tip applicator. The rigid sheets of calcium deposits can be lifted and dissected away with a sharp blade. Final smoothing of the area is accomplished best with the excimer laser (phototherapeutic keratectomy).

▶ Climatic Droplet Keratopathy (Spheroid Degeneration of the Cornea) (Figure 6–11)

Climatic droplet keratopathy affects mainly people who work out of doors. The corneal degeneration is thought to be caused by exposure to ultraviolet light and is characterized in the early stages by fine subepithelial yellow droplets in the peripheral cornea. As the disease advances, the droplets become central, with subsequent corneal clouding causing blurred vision. Treatment in advanced cases is corneal transplantation.

▶ Salzmann Nodular Degeneration

This disorder is usually preceded by corneal inflammation, particularly phlyctenular keratoconjunctivitis or trachoma. Symptoms include redness, irritation, and blurring of vision. There is degeneration of the superficial cornea that involves the stroma, Bowman layer, and epithelium, with superficial whitish-gray elevated nodules sometimes occurring in chains. Rigid contact lenses will significantly improve visual acuity in most cases. Corneal transplantation is rarely required, but superficial lamellar keratectomy or phototherapeutic (excimer laser) keratectomy may be necessary.

▶ Arcus Senilis

Arcus senilis is an extremely common, bilateral, benign peripheral corneal degeneration. Its prevalence is strongly associated with age. It is also associated with hypercholesterolemia and

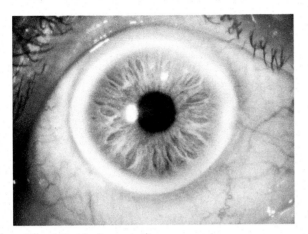

▲ **Figure 6–12.** Arcus senilis.

hypertriglyceridemia. Blood lipid studies should be performed in affected individuals under age 50.

Pathologically, lipid droplets involve the entire corneal thickness but are more concentrated in the superficial and deep layers, being relatively sparse in the corneal stroma.

There are no symptoms. Clinically, arcus senilis appears as a hazy gray ring about 2 mm in width and with a clear space between it and the limbus (Figure 6–12). No treatment is necessary, and there are no complications.

INHERITED CORNEAL DYSTROPHIES

This group of disorders of the cornea of unknown cause is characterized by bilateral and symmetrical abnormal deposits and associated alteration in the normal corneal architecture that may or may not interfere with vision. These corneal dystrophies usually manifest themselves by age 20 but sometimes later. They may be stationary or slowly progressive throughout life. Corneal transplantation, when indicated, improves vision in most patients with hereditary corneal dystrophy.

Corneal dystrophies are classified anatomically as epithelial and subepithelial, epithelial-stromal, stromal, or endothelial (Table 6–4). The more common dystrophies are described in the following sections.

▶ Epithelial & Subepithelial

A. Epithelial Basement Membrane Dystrophy

Microcysts, dots, or map or fingerprint patterns are seen at the level of the epithelial basement membrane, hence the older names Cogan's microcystic dystrophy and map-dot-fingerprint dystrophy. Confocal microscopy demonstrates abnormal epithelial basement membrane protruding into the epithelium, as well as epithelial cell abnormalities and

microcysts. Recurrent erosion is common. Vision usually is not significantly affected.

B. Meesmann Corneal Dystrophy

This slowly progressive disorder is characterized by microcystic areas in the epithelium. The onset is in early childhood. The main symptom is slight irritation, and vision is slightly affected. The inheritance is autosomal dominant.

▶ Epithelial-Stromal

These are due to mutations of the transforming growth factor beta-induced 1 (*TGFB1*) gene.

A. Reis-Bücklers Dystrophy

This is dominantly inherited and initially affects the Bowman layer. It manifests in childhood as recurrent erosion. Opacification of the Bowman layer gradually occurs, and the epithelium is irregular. No vascularization is usually noted. Vision may be markedly reduced.

B. Lattice Dystrophy

This starts as fine, branching linear opacities in the Bowman layer in the central area and spreads to the periphery. The deep stroma may become involved, but the process does not reach the Descemet membrane. Recurrent erosion often occurs. Histologic examination reveals amyloid deposits in the collagen fibers. Corneal transplantation, usually penetrating keratoplasty but possibly deep lamellar keratoplasty, is common, as is recurrence of the dystrophy in the graft. The hereditary pattern for lattice dystrophy is autosomal dominant.

C. Granular Dystrophy

This usually asymptomatic, slowly progressive corneal dystrophy most often begins in early childhood. The lesions consist of central, fine, whitish "granular" lesions in the stroma of the cornea. The epithelium and Bowman layer may be affected late in the disease. Visual acuity is slightly reduced. Histologically, the cornea shows uniform deposition of hyaline material. Corneal transplantation is not needed except in very severe and late cases. The inheritance is autosomal dominant.

▶ Stromal

A. Macular Dystrophy

This type of stromal corneal dystrophy is manifested by a dense gray central opacity that starts in the Bowman layer. The opacity tends to spread toward the periphery and later involves all depths of the stroma. Recurrent corneal erosion may occur, and vision can be severely impaired. Histologic examination shows deposition of acid mucopolysaccharide

Table 6–4. International Anatomic Classification of Corneal Dystrophies (IC3D)

Location	Name	Inheritance	Genetic Locus	Gene	Age of Onset
Epithelial and subepithelial	Epithelial basement membrane dystrophy (EBMD)	Most cases have no family history	5q31	TGFBI (2 families)	Adulthood; rarely in childhood
	Epithelial recurrent erosion dystrophies (EREDs)	AD	Unknown	Unknown	Early childhood
	Subepithelial mucinous corneal dystrophy (SMCD)	AD (possibly X-linked)	Unknown	Unknown	0–10
	Meesmann corneal dystrophy (MECD)	AD	12q13 17q12 (Stocker-Holt variant)	KRT3 KRT12 (Stocker-Holt variant)	Early childhood
	Lisch epithelial corneal dystrophy (LECD)	X-linked dominant	Xp22.3	Unknown	Childhood
	Gelatinous drop-like corneal dystrophy (GDLD)	AR	1p32	TACSTD2	0–20
Epithelial-stromal TGFBI	Reis-Bücklers corneal dystrophy (RBCD)	AD	5q31	TGFBI	Childhood
	Thiel-Behnke corneal dystrophy (TBCD)	AD	5q31	TGFBI	Early childhood
	Lattice corneal dystrophy type 1 (classic) (LCD1) and variants	AD	5q31	TGFBI	0–20
	Granular corneal dystrophy, type 1 (classic) (GCD1) and type 2 (GCD2)	AD	5q31	TGFBI	Childhood
Stromal	Macular corneal dystrophy (MCD)	AR	16q22	CHST6	Childhood
	Schnyder corneal dystrophy (SCD)	AD	1p36	UBIAD1	0–30
	Congenital stromal corneal dystrophy (CSCD)	AD	12q21.33	DCN	Congenital
	Fleck corneal dystrophy (FCD)	AD	2q34	PIKFYVE	Congenital or early childhood
	Posterior amorphous corneal dystrophy (PACD)	AD	12q21.33	Deletion of KERA, LUM, DCN, and EPYC	0–10
	Central cloudy dystrophy of François (CCDF)	Unknown	Unknown	Unknown	0–10
	Pre-Descemet corneal dystrophy (PDCD)	Unknown	Unknown	Unknown (Xp22.31 if associated with X-linked ichthyosis)	Usually after 30
Endothelial	Fuchs endothelial corneal dystrophy (FECD)	Mostly unknown but some AD	Early onset: 1p34.3-p32 Late onset: Multiple loci	Early onset: COL8A2	Mostly after age 30
	Posterior polymorphous corneal dystrophy (PPCD)	AD	PPCD1: 20p11.2-q11.2 PPCD2: 1p34.3-p32.3 PPCD3: 10p11.22	PPCD1: unknown PPCD2: COL8A2 PPCD3: ZEB1	Early childhood

(continued)

Table 6–4. International Anatomic Classification of Corneal Dystrophies (IC3D) (*Continued*)

Location	Name	Inheritance	Genetic Locus	Gene	Age of Onset
	Congenital hereditary endothelial dystrophy (CHED)	AR	20p13	*SLC4A11*	Congenital
	X-linked endothelial corneal dystrophy (XECD)	X-linked dominant	Xq25	Unknown	Congenital

Abbreviations: AD, autosomal dominant; AR, autosomal recessive; CHST6, carbohydrate sulfotransferase 6; COL8A2, collage, type VIII, alpha-2; DCN, decorin; EPYC, epiphycan; KERA, keratocan; KRT3, keratin K3; KRT12, keratin K12; LUM, lumican; PIKFYE, phosphoinositide kinase, FYVE finger containing; SLC4A11, solute carrier family 4, sodium borate transporter, member 11; TACSTD2, tumor-associated calcium signal transducer 2; TGFBI, transforming growth factor beta-induced; UBIAD1, UbiA prenyltransferase domain containing 1; ZEB1, zinc finger E box-binding homeobox 1.
Source: Data from Weiss JS et al. IC3D classification of corneal dystrophies - Edition 2. Cornea 2015;34(2):117-159. (Available at: http://www .corneasociety.org/.)

in the stroma and degeneration of the Bowman layer. Penetrating or deep keratoplasty is often required. The inheritance is autosomal recessive.

▶ **Endothelial**

A. Fuchs' Dystrophy

This disorder begins in the third or fourth decade and is slowly progressive. It is familial in some patients, in whom symptom onset is much earlier. Initial symptoms are glare and misting of vision in the morning. Women are more commonly affected than men. There are central wart-like deposits (guttata) on Descemet membrane, thickening of Descemet membrane, and defects of size and shape of the endothelial cells. Decompensation of the endothelium may occur, particularly after cataract surgery, and leads to edema of the corneal stroma and epithelium, causing blurring of vision. Corneal haze is slowly progressive. Histologic examination of the cornea reveals the wart-like excrescences on Descemet membrane. Thinning and pigmentation of the endothelium and thickening of Descemet membrane are characteristics. Endothelial keratoplasty, generally combined with cataract surgery if this has not been performed previously, is indicated once symptoms become troublesome.

B. Posterior Polymorphous Dystrophy

This is a common disorder with onset in early childhood. Polymorphous plaques of calcium crystals are observed in the deep stromal layers. Vesicular lesions may be seen in the endothelium. Edema occurs in the deep stroma. The condition is asymptomatic in most cases, but in severe cases, epithelial and total stromal edema may occur. The inheritance is autosomal dominant.

THYGESON SUPERFICIAL PUNCTATE KERATITIS

Superficial punctate keratitis is an uncommon chronic and recurrent bilateral disorder more common in females. It is characterized by discrete and elevated oval epithelial opacities that show punctate staining with fluorescein, mainly in the pupillary area. The opacities are not visible grossly but can be easily seen with the slitlamp or loupe. Subepithelial opacities underlying the epithelial lesions are often observed as the epithelial disease resolves. No causative organism has been identified, but a virus is suspected. Blurring of vision and photophobia are the symptoms. The conjunctiva is not involved.

Epithelial keratitis secondary to staphylococcal blepharoconjunctivitis is differentiated from superficial punctate keratitis by its involvement of the lower third of the cornea and lack of subepithelial opacities. Epithelial keratitis in trachoma is ruled out by its location in the upper third of the cornea and the presence of pannus. Many other forms of keratitis involving the superficial cornea are unilateral or are eliminated by the history.

Short-term instillation of weak corticosteroid drops will often cause disappearance of the opacities and subjective improvement, but recurrences are the rule. The ultimate prognosis is good since there is no scarring or vascularization of the cornea. Untreated, the disease runs a protracted course of 1–3 years. Long-term treatment with topical corticosteroids may prolong the course of the disease for many years and lead to steroid-induced cataract and glaucoma. Therapeutic soft contact lenses have been used to control symptoms in especially bothersome cases. Cyclosporine drops, 1% or 2%, can be an effective substitute for corticosteroids.

RECURRENT CORNEAL EROSION

This is a fairly common and serious mechanical corneal disorder that presents some classic signs and symptoms but may be easily missed if it is not looked for specifically. The patient is usually awakened during the early morning hours by a pain in the affected eye. The pain is continuous, and the eye becomes red, irritated, and photophobic. When the patient attempts to open the eyes in the morning, the lid pulls off the loose epithelium, resulting in pain and redness.

There are three types of recurrent corneal erosions:

1. **Acquired recurrent erosion (traumatic):** The patient usually gives a history of previous corneal injury. It is unilateral, it occurs with equal frequency in men and women, and the family history is negative. The recurrent erosion occurs most frequently in the center below the pupil regardless of the location of the previous injury.

2. **Recurrent erosion associated with corneal disease:** After corneal ulceration heals, the epithelium may break down in a recurrent fashion (as in HSV "metaherpetic" ulcer).

3. **Recurrent erosion associated with corneal dystrophies:** Recurrent erosions of the cornea may be observed in patients with epithelial basement membrane dystrophy, lattice dystrophy, and Reis-Bücklers corneal dystrophy.

Recurrent corneal erosion is due to a defect in anchoring of the corneal epithelium between the epithelial basement membrane and Bowman layer, due to faulty hemidesmosome connections. The epithelium is loose and vulnerable to separation.

Instillation of a local anesthetic relieves the symptoms immediately, and fluorescein staining will show the eroded area, typically a small area in the lower central cornea. Healed erosions often exhibit subepithelial debris.

Treatment consists of a pressure bandage on the eye to promote healing. The cornea usually heals in 2–3 days. To reduce the risk of recurrence and promote continued healing, a bland ophthalmic ointment at bedtime is used for several months. In more severe cases, artificial tears are instilled during the day. Hypertonic ointment (sodium chloride 5%) drops are often helpful. Therapeutic soft contact lens, needle micropuncture of the Bowman layer, and phototherapeutic keratectomy are useful in cases that do not respond to more conservative management.

LIMBAL EPITHELIAL STEM CELL DEFICIENCY

Corneal epithelial cells are essential in maintaining the integrity and transparency of the anterior corneal surface. These cells are derived from a population of stem cells based at the limbus. The causes of limbal stem cell deficiency are listed in Table 6–5. Careful slitlamp examination is required to detect signs of early stem cell deficiency. These include loss of epithelial cell transparency, abnormal corneal staining, and superficial vascularization. Advanced stem cell deficiency may cause epithelial

Table 6–5. Causes of Limbal Epithelial Stem Cell Deficiency

Trauma	Chemical injury Thermal injury
Autoimmune/inflammatory	Mucous membrane pemphigoid Stevens-Johnson syndrome Graft-versus-host disease
Iatrogenic	Limbal surgery Drop toxicity
Congenital	Aniridia Ectodermal dysplasia
Advanced pterygium	
Ocular surface neoplasia	
Long-term contact lens wear	

irregularity with recurrent persistent epithelial defects. This can in turn lead to stromal inflammation and corneal melting. The diagnosis can be confirmed by impression cytology, which involves taking samples of epithelial cells by placing filter paper on the cornea. Immunohistochemical staining and microscopy can then identify the cytokeratin expressed in harvested cells and check for the presence of goblet cells. The presence of cytokeratin 3 and 12 indicates normal corneal epithelial phenotype, whereas the presence of cytokeratin 19 along with goblet cells confirms the presence of conjunctival phenotype epithelial cells on the corneal surface. Management of limbal stem cell deficiency includes various techniques of stem-cell transplantation, either as a block of autologous limbus from the contralateral eye or allogeneic limbus from a relative or cadaveric donor, or ex vivo expanded stem cell populations generated from small biopsies from these sites.

CORNEAL DEPOSITION

Vortex dystrophy, or cornea verticillata, due to deposits in basal epithelium manifests as pigmented lines or whorls spreading over the entire corneal surface. Visual acuity is not markedly affected. Usually due to drugs (amiodarone, chloroquine and hydroxychloroquine, indomethacin, or phenothiazines), it also occurs in Fabry's disease.

CORNEAL TRANSPLANTATION

Corneal transplantation (keratoplasty) is indicated for a number of serious corneal conditions, for example, scarring, edema, thinning, and distortion. Table 6–6 lists the different types of keratoplasty and their indications.

Younger donors are preferred for penetrating and deep lamellar endothelial keratoplasties because there is a direct relationship between age and the health and number of the endothelial cells, but older corneas (50–65 years) are entirely

Table 6–6. Types of Keratoplasty (Corneal Graft)

Types of Keratoplasty	Abbreviations	Description	Indications
Penetrating keratoplasty	PK	Full-thickness corneal transplant	Full-thickness stromal scar Combined stromal and endothelial pathology
Deep anterior lamellar keratoplasty	DALK	Replacement of all corneal layers except DM and endothelium	Any corneal disorder with healthy endothelium (eg, keratoconus, corneal dystrophies, postinfection scars)
Endothelial keratoplasty	DSEK/DSAEK (Descemet stripping automated endothelial keratoplasty)	Replacement of endothelium and DM with donor endothelium, DM, and thin layer of posterior stroma	Endothelial failure (eg, Fuchs' endothelial disease, pseudophakic bullous keratopathy, corneal transplant endothelial failure)
	DMEK (Descemet membrane endothelial keratoplasty)	Replacement of endothelium and DM with donor endothelium and DM (no stroma)	
Tectonic keratoplasty		Full-thickness graft to repair a corneal perforation	Impending or actual corneal perforation
Rotational keratoplasty		Patient's own cornea trephined and rotated to move a scar out of the visual axis	Full-thickness corneal scar that can be rotated out of the visual axis

Abbreviation: DM, Descemet membrane.

satisfactory if the endothelial cell count is adequate. Because of the rapid endothelial cell death rate, the eyes should be enucleated soon after death and refrigerated immediately. Corneoscleral disks stored in nutrient media at 4°C may be used up to 10 days after donor death, and preservation in tissue culture media allows storage at 34°C for as long as 6 weeks.

For lamellar and deep lamellar keratoplasty, corneas can be frozen, dehydrated, or refrigerated for several weeks; the endothelial cells are not important in these partial-thickness procedures involving the anterior cornea.

Diseases, like chemical injuries (see Chapter 19), in which loss of limbal stem cells leads to failure of corneal epithelialization, may benefit from limbal stem cell transplants, from the fellow eye or a donor eye, or amniotic membrane transplants, particularly in preparation for corneal transplantation. For severe corneal disease unsuitable for corneal transplantation, various artificial corneas (keratoprostheses) have been attempted with increasing success.

Techniques

For penetrating or lamellar keratoplasty, the recipient eye is prepared by a partial-thickness cutting of a circle of diseased cornea, such as with a suction trephine, and full-thickness removal with scissors or partial-thickness removal with dissection. For endothelial keratoplasty, the recipient endothelium is removed using instruments inserted into the anterior chamber.

For penetrating keratoplasty, the donor corneoscleral cap is placed endothelium up on a suction Teflon block;

the trephine is pressed down into the cornea, and a full-thickness button is punched out. For lamellar, deep lamellar, and endothelial keratoplasty, the process is adapted, using a microkeratome or femtosecond laser to remove the required portion of cornea from a corneoscleral cap or whole globe. Precut tissue for endothelial keratoplasty is now available from eye banks in developed countries.

Developments in sutures (Figure 6–13), instruments, and microscopes, as well as changes in surgical techniques,

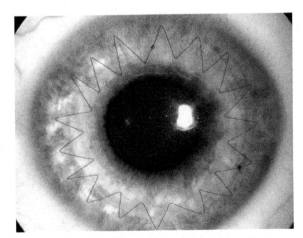

▲ **Figure 6–13.** Penetrating keratoplasty with 10–0 nylon running suture.

have significantly improved the prognosis in all patients requiring corneal transplants. Reducing and managing postoperative astigmatism and corneal graft rejection continue to be major problems, particularly after penetrating keratoplasty (see Chapter 16). Early suture removal guided by topographical mapping can be useful to minimize post-graft astigmatism.

REFRACTIVE CORNEAL SURGERY

The inconvenience of spectacles to many wearers and the complications associated with contact lenses have resulted in increasing popularity of refractive surgery.

Lasers

Refractive laser surgery involves modifying the curvature of the cornea to achieve a desired refractive outcome (see Chapter 23). In **LASIK (laser in situ keratomileusis)**, a femtosecond laser or microkeratome is used to cut a thin anterior lamellar corneal flap, which is folded back (Table 6–7). Excimer laser ablation of the stromal bed produces programmed reshaping of the cornea, and then the flap is repositioned. In the surface ablation techniques, such as **photorefractive keratectomy (PRK)**, the cornea is laser ablated after manual removal of only the epithelium. Excimer laser delivery in all these techniques can be further refined by wavefront-guided technology to take account of the optical aberrations of individual eyes.

Laser refractive surgery is mostly used for myopia but can also treat astigmatism or hyperopia. Long-term visual results are about the same for the various techniques, but each has its advantages and disadvantages. In large ablations, especially with LASIK, the possibility of ectasia must be considered. LASIK produces the most rapid recovery, both visually and in terms of discomfort. The surface ablation techniques are particularly indicated for thin corneas and patients at risk of corneal trauma such as in contact sport. Complications of laser refractive corneal surgery include unexpected refractive outcome, fluctuating refraction, irregular astigmatism, regression, flap or interface problems, stromal haze, corneal ectasia, and infection. Previous laser refractive corneal surgery results in particular difficulties when determining intraocular lens power for cataract surgery.

Procedures to Correct Astigmatism

Astigmatism continues to be a problem following penetrating and anterior lamellar keratoplasty and after cataract surgery. Astigmatism after keratoplasty may be improved by various surgical procedures, including relaxing incisions and wedge resections. PRK or topography-guided excimer laser surface ablation may be helpful. Refinements of incision, including adjustment of location according to preoperative corneal astigmatism, are useful in preventing postoperative astigmatism after cataract surgery.

Intrastromal Corneal Implants

PMMA (polymethyl methacrylate) ring segments can be placed in the corneal stroma to adjust the corneal shape and thus reduce astigmatism. An intrastromal pocket is created with a femtosecond laser at 80% corneal depth. One or two ring segments are then implanted through a 1.2-mm vertical incision into the stromal pocket. The size and location of the ring segments are decided based on the corneal topography. The refractive outcome of ring implants in keratoconus can be unpredictable, but they can be useful in moderate keratoconus patients who are intolerant to contact lenses.

Table 6–7. Corneal Refractive Procedures

	Procedure	Technique	Indication
LASIK (laser in situ keratomileusis)	Excimer laser	Cutting and lifting anterior corneal flap, then ablation of the stromal bed with excimer laser	Refractive error
PRK (photorefractive keratectomy)		Surface ablation of the corneal surface and stroma	
Corneal intrastromal ring implant	KeraRing/Intacs	PMMA (polymethyl methacrylate segment) implanted in corneal stromal pocket	Keratoconus
Arcuate keratotomy	Manual or femtosecond laser	Subtotal corneal stromal incisions, steep axis to reduce astigmatism	Natural or postkeratoplasty astigmatism

REFERENCES

Ang M et al: Five-year graft survival comparing Descemet stripping automated endothelial keratoplasty and penetrating keratoplasty. Ophthalmology 2016;123:1646. [PMID: 27262764]

Aristeidou A et al: The evolution of corneal and refractive surgery with the femtosecond laser. Eye Vis (Lond) 2015;2:12. [PMID: 26605365]

Arnalich-Montiel F et al: Corneal surgery in keratoconus: Which type, which technique, which outcomes? Eye Vis (Lond) 2016;3:2. [PMID: 26783544]

Atallah MR et al: Limbal stem cell transplantation: Current perspectives. Clin Ophthalmol 2016;10:593. [PMID: 27099468]

Avadhanam VS et al: A brief review of Boston type-1 and osteoodonto keratoprostheses. Br J Ophthalmol 2015;99:878. [PMID: 25349081]

Avni Zauberman N et al: Anterior stromal puncture for the treatment of recurrent corneal erosion syndrome: Patient clinical features and outcomes. Am J Ophthalmol 2014;157:273. [PMID: 24439438]

Bajracharya L et al: Outcome of therapeutic penetrating keratoplasty in a tertiary eye care center in Nepal. Clin Ophthalmol 2015;9:2299. [PMID: 26673279]

Barsam A et al: Case-control study of risk factors for acute corneal hydrops in keratoconus. Br J Ophthalmol. 2016 Jul 7. [Epub ahead of print] [PMID: 27388247]

Bhadange Y et al: Comparison of culture-negative and culture-positive microbial keratitis: Cause of culture negativity, clinical features and final outcome. Br J Ophthalmol 2015;99:1498. [PMID: 25911069]

Carnt N et al: The impact of topical corticosteroids used in conjunction with antiamoebic therapy on the outcome of *Acanthamoeba* keratitis. Ophthalmology 2016;123:984. [PMID: 26952591]

Carnt N et al: Strategies for the prevention of contact lens-related *Acanthamoeba* keratitis: A review. Ophthalmic Physiol Opt 2016;36:77. [PMID: 26691018]

Carrijo-Carvalho LC et al: Therapeutic agents and biocides for ocular infections by free-living amoebae of *Acanthamoeba* genus. Surv Ophthalmol 2016 Nov 8. [Epub ahead of print] [PMID: 27836717]

Centers for Disease Control and Prevention (CDC). Adenovirus-associated epidemic keratoconjunctivitis outbreaks—four states, 2008-2010. MMWR Morb Mortal Wkly Rep 2013;62:637. [PMID: 23945769]

Cheung N et al: Emerging trends in contact lens-related infections. Curr Opin Ophthalmol 2016;27:327. [PMID: 27176217]

Cope JR et al: *Acanthamoeba* keratitis among rigid gas permeable contact lens wearers in the United States, 2005 through 2011. Ophthalmology 2016;123:1435. [PMID: 27117780]

Diez-Feijóo E et al: Clinical presentation and causes of recurrent corneal erosion syndrome: Review of 100 patients. Cornea 2014;33:571. [PMID: 24699561]

Diez-Feijóo E et al: Optical coherence tomography findings in recurrent corneal erosion syndrome. Cornea 2015;34:290. [PMID: 25532997]

Edell AR et al: Herpes simplex and herpes zoster eye disease: Presentation and management at a city hospital for the underserved in the United States. Eye Contact Lens 2013;39:311. [PMID: 23771014]

Estopinal CB et al: Geographic disparities in the etiology of bacterial and fungal keratitis in the United States of America. Semin Ophthalmol 2016;31:345. [PMID: 27101474]

Ghanem RC et al: Tacrolimus for the treatment of subepithelial infiltrates resistant to topical steroids after adenoviral keratoconjunctivitis. Cornea 2014;33:1210. [PMID: 25188789]

Godefrooij DA et al: Nationwide reduction in the number of corneal transplantations for keratoconus following the implementation of cross-linking. Acta Ophthalmol 2016;94:675. [PMID: 27213687]

Gospe SM 3rd et al: Keratomalacia in a patient with psychogenic vitamin A deficiency. Cornea 2016;35:405. [PMID: 26785304]

Gupta N et al: Prevalence of corneal diseases in the rural Indian population: The Corneal Opacity Rural Epidemiological (CORE) study. Br J Ophthalmol 2015;99:147. [PMID: 25395684]

Handor H et al: Ophthalmologists beware of adenoviruses. Pan Afr Med J 2014;17:205. [PMID: 25161749]

Ho JW et al: Microbiological profiles of fungal keratitis: A 10-year study at a tertiary referral center. J Ophthalmic Inflamm Infect 2016;6:5. [PMID: 26897131]

Hoddenbach JG et al: Clinical presentation and morbidity of contact lens-associated microbial keratitis: A retrospective study. Graefes Arch Clin Exp Ophthalmol 2014;252:299. [PMID: 24281783]

Inoue Y. Review of clinical and basic approaches to corneal endotheliitis. Cornea 2014;33:S3. [PMID: 25170583]

Iovieno A et al: *Acanthamoeba* sclerokeratitis: Epidemiology, clinical features, and treatment outcomes. Ophthalmology 2014;121:2340. [PMID: 25097155]

James SH et al: A possible pitfall in acyclovir prophylaxis for recurrent herpetic keratitis. J Infect Dis 2013;208:1353. [PMID: 23901076]

Kwon JW et al: Analyses of factors affecting endothelial cell density in an eye bank corneal donor database. Cornea 2016;35:1206. [PMID: 27310882]

Lalitha P et al: Trends in bacterial and fungal keratitis in South India, 2002-2012. Br J Ophthalmol 2015;99:192. [PMID: 25143391]

Li SM et al: Laser-assisted subepithelial keratectomy (LASEK) versus photorefractive keratectomy (PRK) for correction of myopia. Cochrane Database Syst Rev 2016;2:CD009799. [PMID: 26899152]

Li X et al: Age distribution of various corneal diseases in China by histopathological examination of 3112 surgical specimens. Invest Ophthalmol Vis Sci 2014;55:3022. [PMID: 24722694]

Lin BR et al: Identification of the first de novo UBIAD1 gene mutation associated with Schnyder corneal dystrophy. J Ophthalmol. 2016;2016:1968493. [PMID: 27382485]

Lin YB et al: Fingernail-induced corneal abrasions: Case series from an ophthalmology emergency department. Cornea 2014;33:691. [PMID: 24831196]

Lin ZN et al: Characteristics of corneal dystrophies: A review from clinical, histological and genetic perspectives. Int J Ophthalmol 2016;9:904. [PMID: 27366696]

Maharana PK et al: Recent advances in diagnosis and management of mycotic keratitis. Indian J Ophthalmol 2016;64:346. [PMID: 27380973]

Mandathara PS et al: Outcome of keratoconus management: Review of the past 20 years' contemporary treatment modalities. Eye Contact Lens 2016 May 11. [Epub ahead of print] [PMID: 27171132]

Mastropasqua L et al: Understanding the pathogenesis of neurotrophic keratitis: The role of corneal nerves. J Cell Physiol 2017;232:717. [PMID: 27683068]

Matthaei M et al: Changing indications in penetrating keratoplasty: A systematic review of 34 years of global reporting. Transplantation 2016 Jun 22. [Epub ahead of print] [PMID: 27336399]

Maycock NJ et al: Update on *Acanthamoeba* keratitis: Diagnosis, treatment, and outcomes. Cornea 2016;35:713. [PMID: 26989955]

McClintic SM et al: Visual outcomes in treated bacterial keratitis: Four years of prospective follow-up. Invest Ophthalmol Vis Sci 2014;55:2935. [PMID: 24618327]

McDonald EM et al: Topical antibiotics for the management of bacterial keratitis: An evidence-based review of high quality randomised controlled trials. Br J Ophthalmol 2014;98:1470. [PMID: 24729078]

McDonald EM et al: A prospective study of the clinical characteristics of patients with herpes simplex and varicella zoster keratitis, presenting to a New Zealand emergency eye clinic. Cornea 2015;34:279. [PMID: 25532996]

McGrath LA et al: Techniques, indications and complications of corneal debridement. Surv Ophthalmol 2014;59:47. [PMID: 24239444]

Mencucci R et al: Management of recurrent corneal erosions: Are we getting better? Br J Ophthalmol 2014;98:150. [PMID: 24421300]

Mundey K et al: Unexplained anterior uveitis: Viral causes. J Clin Diagn Res 2015;9:NL01. [PMID: 26435979]

Ni N et al: Use of adjunctive topical corticosteroids in bacterial keratitis. Curr Opin Ophthalmol 2016;27:353. [PMID: 27096374]

Njoya JM et al: Herpetic epithelial keratitis. QJM 2015;108:595. [PMID: 25524905]

Oliver VF et al: The genetics and pathophysiology of IC3D category 1 corneal dystrophies: A review. Asia Pac J Ophthalmol (Phila) 2016;5:272. [PMID: 27213768]

Park PJ et al: Corneal lymphangiogenesis in herpetic stromal keratitis. Surv Ophthalmol 2015;60:60. [PMID: 25444520]

Prajna NV et al: Effect of oral voriconazole on fungal keratitis in the Mycotic Ulcer Treatment Trial II (MUTT II): A randomized clinical trial. JAMA Ophthalmol 2016;134:1365. [PMID: 27787540]

Prakash G et al: The three faces of herpes simplex epithelial keratitis: A steroid-induced situation. BMJ Case Rep 2015;2:2015. [PMID: 25837655]

Punia RS et al: Spectrum of fungal keratitis: Clinicopathologic study of 44 cases. Int J Ophthalmol 2014;7:114. [PMID: 24634875]

Ramamurthy S et al: Outcomes of repeat keratoplasty for failed therapeutic keratoplasty. Am J Ophthalmol 2016;162:83. [PMID: 26558523]

Reddy JC et al: Risk factors and clinical outcomes of bacterial and fungal scleritis at a tertiary eye care hospital. Middle East Afr J Ophthalmol 2015;22:203. [PMID: 25949079]

Robaei D et al: The impact of topical corticosteroid use before diagnosis on the outcome of *Acanthamoeba* keratitis. Ophthalmology 2014;121:1383. [PMID: 24630688]

Rolinski J et al: Immunological aspects of acute and recurrent herpes simplex keratitis. J Immunol Res 2014;2014:513560. [PMID: 25276842]

Rubino P et al: Anterior segment findings in vitamin A deficiency: A case series. Case Rep Ophthalmol Med 2015;2015:181267. [PMID: 26509090]

Sacchetti M et al: Diagnosis and management of neurotrophic keratitis. Clin Ophthalmol 2014;8:571. [PMID: 24672223]

Santhiago MR et al: Ectasia risk factors in refractive surgery. Clin Ophthalmol 2016;10:713. [PMID: 27143849]

Schaftenaar E et al: Early- and late-stage ocular complications of herpes zoster ophthalmicus in rural South Africa. Trop Med Int Health 2016;21:334. [PMID: 26663773]

Schein OD. Evidence-based treatment of fungal keratitis. JAMA Ophthalmol 2016;134:1372. [Epub ahead of print] [PMID: 27787542]

Serna-Ojeda JC et al: Herpes simplex virus disease of the anterior segment in children. Cornea 2015;34(Suppl 10):S68. [PMID: 26266435]

Sharma N et al: Demographic profile, clinical features and outcome of peripheral ulcerative keratitis: A prospective study. Br J Ophthalmol 2015;99:1503. [PMID: 25935428]

Sharma N et al: Gatifloxacin 0.3% versus fortified tobramycin-cefazolin in treating nonperforated bacterial corneal ulcers: Randomized, controlled trial. Cornea 2016;35:56. [PMID: 26509763]

Sharma S et al: Re-appraisal of topical 1% voriconazole and 5% natamycin in the treatment of fungal keratitis in a randomised trial. Br J Ophthalmol 2015;99:1190. [PMID: 25740805]

Song X et al: A multi-center, cross-sectional study on the burden of infectious keratitis in China. PLoS One 2014;9:e113843. [PMID: 25438169]

Srinivasan M et al: Visual recovery in treated bacterial keratitis. Ophthalmology 2014;121:1310. [PMID: 24612976]

Steger B et al: Femtosecond laser-assisted lamellar keratectomy for corneal opacities secondary to anterior corneal dystrophies: An interventional case series. Cornea 2016;35:6. [PMID: 26509759]

Szeto SK et al: Prevalence of ocular manifestations and visual outcomes in patients with herpes zoster ophthalmicus. Cornea 2016 Oct 12. [Epub ahead of print] [PMID: 27741018]

Tallab RT et al: Corticosteroids as a therapy for bacterial keratitis: An evidence-based review of "who, when and why." Br J Ophthalmol 2016;100:731. [PMID: 26743622]

Tsatsos M et al: Herpes simplex virus keratitis: an update of the pathogenesis and current treatment with oral and topical antiviral agents. Clin Exp Ophthalmol 2016;44:824. [Epub ahead of print] [PMID: 27273328]

Vazirani J et al: Autologous simple limbal epithelial transplantation for unilateral limbal stem cell deficiency: Multicentre results. Br J Ophthalmol 2016;100:1416. [PMID: 26817481]

Weiss JS. The Oskar Fehr Lecture. Klin Monbl Augenheilkd 2016;233:708. [PMID: 27315290]

Weiss JS et al: IC3D classification of corneal dystrophies—edition 2. Cornea 2015;34:117. [PMID: 25564336]

Uveal Tract & Sclera

7

Emmett T. Cunningham, Jr., MD, PhD, MPH,
James J. Augsburger, MD, Zélia M. Corrêa, MD, PhD, and
Carlos Pavesio, MD, FRCOphth

7.1. Uveitis

Emmett T. Cunningham, Jr., MD, PhD, MPH

UVEITIS

The uveal tract consists of the choroid, ciliary body, and iris (Figure 7–1). The term "uveitis" denotes inflammation of the iris (iritis, iridocyclitis), ciliary body (intermediate uveitis, cyclitis, peripheral uveitis, or pars planitis), or choroid (choroiditis). Common usage, however, includes inflammation of the retina (retinitis), retinal vasculature (retinal vasculitis), and intraocular portion of the optic nerve (papillitis). Uveitis may also occur secondary to inflammation of the cornea (keratitis), sclera (scleritis), or both (sclerokeratitis). Uveitis usually affects people 20–50 years of age and accounts for 10–20% of cases of legal blindness in developed countries. Uveitis is more common in the developing world than in the developed countries, due in large part to the greater prevalence of infections that can affect the eye, such as toxoplasmosis and tuberculosis.

▶ Clinical Findings

A. Symptoms and Signs (Table 7–1)

Inflammation of the uveal tract has many causes and may involve one or more regions of the eye simultaneously. Anatomically, intraocular inflammation can be classified as anterior uveitis, intermediate uveitis, posterior uveitis, or diffuse or panuveitis (Figure 7–2).

    Anterior uveitis is most common and is usually unilateral and acute in onset. Typical symptoms include pain, photophobia, and blurred vision. Examination usually reveals circumcorneal redness with minimal injection of the palpebral conjunctiva or discharge. The pupil may be small (miosis) or irregular due to the formation of posterior synechiae. Inflammation limited to the anterior chamber is called "iritis," whereas inflammation involving both the anterior chamber and the anterior vitreous is often referred to as "iridocyclitis." Corneal sensation and intraocular pressure should be checked in every patient with uveitis. Decreased sensation occurs in patients with herpetic uveitis due to simplex or varicella-zoster virus infection or leprosy (see Chapter 15), whereas increased intraocular pressure can occur with herpes simplex virus, varicella-zoster virus, cytomegalovirus, toxoplasmosis, syphilis, sarcoidosis, or an uncommon form of iridocyclitis called glaucomatocyclitic crisis, also known as the Posner-Schlossman syndrome. Clumps of white cells and inflammatory debris termed keratic precipitates are usually evident on the corneal endothelium in patients with active inflammation. Keratic precipitates may be large and so-called "mutton fat" or "granulomatous" (Figure 7–3), small and nongranulomatous, or stellate. Granulomatous or nongranulomatous keratic precipitates are usually located inferiorly in a wedge-shaped region known as Arlt's triangle. Stellate keratic precipitates, in contrast, are usually distributed evenly over the entire corneal endothelium and may be seen in uveitis due to herpes simplex virus, varicella-zoster virus, cytomegalovirus, toxoplasmosis, Fuchs heterochromic iridocyclitis, and sarcoidosis. Keratic precipitates may also be localized to an area of prior or active keratitis, most frequently in herpetic keratouveitis. Iris nodules may be present at the iris margin (Koeppe nodules), within the iris

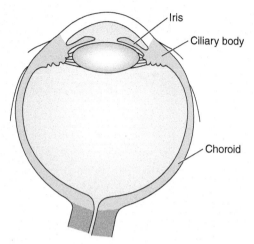

▲ **Figure 7–1.** The uveal tract consists of the iris, ciliary body, and choroid.

Table 7–1. Common Points of Differentiation of Granulomatous and Nongranulomatous Uveitis

	Nongranulomatous	Granulomatous
Onset	Acute	Insidious
Pain	Marked	None or minimal
Photophobia	Marked	Slight
Blurred vision	Moderate	Marked
Circumcorneal flush	Marked	Slight
Keratic precipitates	Small white	Large gray ("mutton fat")
Pupil	Small and irregular	Small and irregular (variable)
Posterior synechiae	Sometimes	Sometimes
Iris nodules	None	Sometimes
Site	Anterior	Anterior, posterior, or panuveitis
Course	Acute	Chronic
Recurrence	Common	Sometimes

stroma (Busacca nodules), or in the anterior chamber angle (Berlin nodules). Evidence for granulomatous disease, such as mutton fat keratic precipitates or iris nodules, may indicate an infectious cause of uveitis or one of a relatively limited number of noninfectious causes, including sarcoidosis, Vogt-Koyanagi-Harada disease, sympathetic ophthalmia, endophthalmitis, lens-induced uveitis, or multiple sclerosis. Particularly severe anterior chamber inflammation may result in layering of inflammatory cells in the inferior angle (hypopyon). The most common cause of hypopyon uveitis in North America and Europe is HLA-B27–associated uveitis, whereas the most common cause of hypopyon uveitis in Asia is Behçet disease. The iris should be examined carefully for evidence of atrophy or transillumination, which can occur in a sectoral or patchy pattern in the setting of herpetic uveitis, or diffusely with Fuchs heterochromic iridocyclitis, also known as Fuchs uveitis syndrome. The presence of anterior (Figure 7–4) or posterior (Figures 7–5 and 7–6) synechiae should also be noted, as this can predispose the patient to ocular hypertension or glaucoma.

Intermediate uveitis, also called cyclitis, peripheral uveitis, or pars planitis, is the second most common type of intraocular inflammation. The hallmark of intermediate uveitis is vitreous inflammation. Intermediate uveitis is typically bilateral and tends to affect patients in their late teens or early adult years. Men and women are affected equally. Typical symptoms include floaters and blurred vision. Pain, photophobia, and redness are usually absent or minimal, although these symptoms may be more prominent at onset.

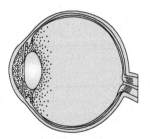
Anterior uveitis
(Iritis, iridocyclitis)

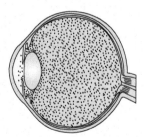
Intermediate uveitis
(Pars planitis, cyclitis)

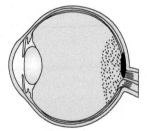
Posterior uveitis
(Retinitis, choroiditis, papillitis)

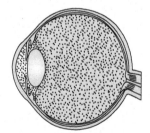
Panuveitis
(Diffuse uveitis)

▲ **Figure 7–2.** Anatomic classification of uveitis, including anterior uveitis, intermediate uveitis, posterior uveitis, and panuveitis. [Modified after Cunningham ET Jr. Diagnosis and management of acute anterior uveitis. American Academy of Ophthalmology, Focal Points 2002, Volume XX, Number 1 (Section 1 of 3).]

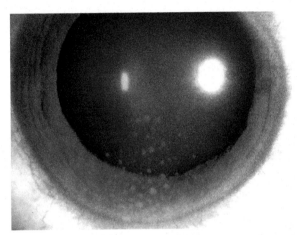

▲ **Figure 7–3.** Granulomatous keratic precipitates located on the inferior corneal endothelium in Arlt's triangle.

The most striking finding on examination is vitritis, often accompanied by vitreous condensates, either free-floating as "snowballs" or layered over the pars plana and ciliary body as "snowbanking." Mild anterior chamber inflammation may be present, but if significant, the inflammation is more appropriately termed diffuse uveitis or panuveitis (see later in the chapter). The cause of intermediate uveitis is unknown in the vast majority of patients, although sarcoidosis and multiple sclerosis account for 10–20% of cases. Syphilis and tuberculosis, although uncommon, should be excluded in all patients. The most common complications of intermediate uveitis include cystoid macular edema, retinal vasculitis, and neovascularization of the optic disk and retina.

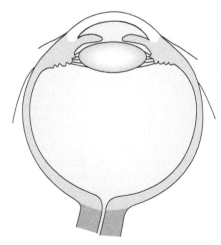

▲ **Figure 7–4.** Anterior synechiae (adhesions). The peripheral iris adheres to the cornea. Ocular hypertension or glaucoma may result.

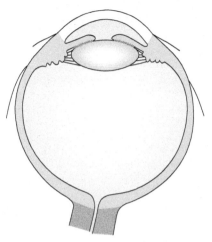

▲ **Figure 7–5.** Posterior synechiae. The iris adheres to the lens. Iris seclusion, iris bombé, ocular hypertension, and glaucoma may result.

Posterior uveitis includes retinitis, choroiditis, retinal vasculitis, and papillitis, which may occur alone or in combination. Symptoms typically include floaters, loss of visual field or scotomas, or decreased vision, which can be severe. Retinal detachment, although infrequent, occurs most commonly in posterior uveitis and may be tractional, rhegmatogenous, or exudative in nature.

B. Laboratory Testing

Laboratory testing is usually not required for patients with mild uveitis and a recent history of trauma or surgery—or with clear evidence of herpes simplex or herpes zoster virus infection, such as a concurrent vesicular dermatitis,

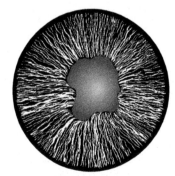

▲ **Figure 7–6.** Posterior synechiae (anterior view). The iris is adherent to the lens in several places as a result of previous inflammation, causing an irregular, fixed pupil. Appropriate treatment with corticosteroids and cycloplegic/mydriatic agents can often prevent such synechiae.

dendritic or disciform keratitis, or sectoral iris atrophy. Laboratory testing is often deferred for otherwise healthy and asymptomatic young to middle-aged patients with a first episode of mild to moderately severe acute, unilateral, non-granulomatous iritis or iridocyclitis that responds promptly to treatment with topical corticosteroids and cycloplegic/mydriatic agents. Patients with recurrent, severe, bilateral, granulomatous, intermediate, posterior, or panuveitis should be tested, however, as should any patient whose uveitis fails to respond promptly to standard therapy. Testing for syphilis should include both a Venereal Disease Research Laboratory (VDRL) or rapid plasma reagin (RPR) test and a more specific test for anti–*Treponema pallidum* antibodies, such as the FTA-ABS or MHA-TP assays. Sarcoidosis should be excluded by chest x-ray and serum angiotensin-converting enzyme (ACE) or lysozyme level testing. Tuberculosis should be excluded by the same chest x-ray and by either skin testing using both purified protein derivative (PPD) or by an interferon-γ release assay (IGRA), such as the QuantiF-ERON-TB Gold or T-SPOT.TB tests. Although the IGRAs provide markedly increased specificity for patients with prior bacillus Calmette-Guérin (BCG) vaccination, a remote history of BCG vaccination should not preclude PPD skin testing in areas where IGRAs are not available, since the PPD test should become negative (< 5 mm induration) within 5 years following BCG vaccination. Testing other than for syphilis, tuberculosis, and sarcoidosis should be tailored to findings elicited on history or identified on physical examination. Examples might include an antinuclear antibody (ANA) titer for a young child with chronic iridocyclitis and arthritis suspected of having juvenile idiopathic arthritis (JIA); an HLA-B27 histocompatibility antigen test for patients with arthritis, psoriasis, urethritis, or symptoms consistent with inflammatory bowel disease; or toxoplasmosis immunoglobulin (Ig) G and IgM titers for a patient with unilateral panuveitis and focal retinochoroiditis.

▶ Differential Diagnosis

The differential diagnosis for eye redness and decreased vision is extensive and somewhat beyond the scope of this brief overview. However, entities commonly confused with uveitis include conjunctivitis, distinguished by the presence of discharge and redness involving both the palpebral and bulbar conjunctiva; keratitis, distinguished by the presence of epithelial staining or defects or by stromal thickening or infiltrate; and acute angle-closure glaucoma, associated with markedly raised intraocular pressure, corneal haziness and edema, and a narrow anterior chamber angle, often best visualized in the uninvolved fellow eye. (See Inside Front Cover.)

▶ Complications & Sequelae

Anterior uveitis can produce both anterior (Figure 7–4) and posterior synechiae (Figures 7–5 and 7–6). Anterior synechiae can impede aqueous outflow at the chamber angle and cause ocular hypertension or glaucoma. Posterior synechiae, when extensive, can cause secondary angle-closure glaucoma by producing pupillary seclusion and forward bulging of the iris (iris bombé). Early and aggressive use of corticosteroids and cycloplegic/mydriatic agents lessens the likelihood of these complications.

Both anterior and posterior chamber inflammation promote lens thickening and opacification. Early in the course, this can cause a simple shift in refractive error, usually toward myopia. With time, however, cataract progression often limits best-corrected vision. Treatment involves removal of the cataract, but should be done only when the intraocular inflammation is well controlled for at least 6 months, since the risk of intraoperative and postoperative complications is greater in patients with active uveitis. Aggressive use of local and systemic corticosteroids is usually necessary before, during, and after cataract surgery in these patients.

Cystoid macular edema is a common cause of visual loss in patients with uveitis and may be observed in the setting of severe anterior or intermediate uveitis. Longstanding or recurrent macular edema can cause permanent loss of vision due to cystoid degeneration. Both fluorescein angiography and optical coherence tomography can be used to diagnose cystoid macular edema and to monitor its response to therapy.

Retinal detachments, including tractional, rhegmatogenous, and exudative forms, occur infrequently in patients with posterior, intermediate, or panuveitis. Exudative retinal detachment suggests significant choroidal inflammation and occurs most commonly in association with Vogt-Koyanagi-Harada disease, sympathetic ophthalmia, and posterior scleritis or in association with severe retinitis or retinal vasculitis.

▶ Treatment

Corticosteroids and cycloplegic/mydriatic agents are the mainstays of therapy for uveitis. Care should be taken to rule out an epithelial defect and ruptured globe when a history of trauma is elicited and to check corneal sensation and intraocular pressure to rule out herpes virus infection. Aggressive topical therapy with a potent corticosteroid, such as 1% prednisolone acetate, one or two drops in the affected eye every 1 or 2 hours while awake, usually provides good control of anterior inflammation. Prednisolone acetate is a suspension and needs to be shaken vigorously prior to each use. A cycloplegic/mydriatic agent, such as homatropine 2% or 5%, used two to four times daily, helps prevent synechia formation and reduces discomfort from ciliary spasm.

Noninfectious intermediate, posterior, and panuveitis respond best to sub-Tenon injections of triamcinolone acetonide, usually 1 mL (40 mg) given superotemporally. Intraocular triamcinolone acetonide, 0.05–0.1 mL (2–4 mg), or oral prednisone, 0.5–1.5 mg/kg/d, can also be effective. Corticosteroid-sparing agents such as methotrexate, azathioprine, mycophenolate mofetil, cyclosporine, tacrolimus, cyclophosphamide, chlorambucil, or the tumor necrosis factor (TNF)-α inhibitors can be required to treat severe or chronic forms of noninfectious inflammation, particularly when there is systemic involvement. Therapy for selected granulomatous forms of uveitis is outlined in Table 7–2.

▶ Complications of Treatment

Cataract and glaucoma are the most common complications of corticosteroid therapy. Cycloplegic/mydriatic agents weaken accommodation and can be particularly bothersome to patients under 45 years of age. Because oral corticosteroids or noncorticosteroid immunosuppressants can cause numerous systemic complications, dosing and monitoring are best done in close collaboration with an internist, rheumatologist, or oncologist experienced with the use of such agents.

▶ Course & Prognosis

The course and prognosis of uveitis depend to a large extent on the severity, location, and cause of the inflammation. In general, severe inflammation takes longer to treat and is more likely to cause intraocular damage and loss of vision than mild or moderate inflammation. Moreover, anterior uveitis tends to respond more promptly than intermediate, posterior, or panuveitis. Retinal, choroidal, or optic nerve involvement tends to be associated with a poorer prognosis.

ANTERIOR UVEITIS (TABLE 7–3)

1. UVEITIS ASSOCIATED WITH JOINT DISEASE

About 20% of children with the pauciarticular form of juvenile idiopathic arthritis (JIA) (formerly known as juvenile rheumatoid arthritis [JRA] in the United States and juvenile chronic arthritis [JCA] in the United Kingdom) develop a chronic bilateral nongranulomatous iridocyclitis. Girls are affected four to five times more commonly than boys. JIA-associated uveitis is usually detected at 5–6 years of age following the insidious onset of cataract (leukocoria), a difference in color of the two eyes (heterochromia), a difference in the size or shape of the pupil (anisocoria), or ocular misalignment (strabismus). Often these findings are first noted at a screening vision test performed at school. There is no correlation between the onset of the arthritis and that of the uveitis, which may precede the onset of arthritis by up to 10 years. The knee is the most commonly involved joint. The cardinal signs of the disease are cells and flare in the anterior chamber, small- to medium-sized white keratic precipitates with or without flecks of fibrin on the endothelium, posterior

Table 7–2. Treatment of Granulomatous Uveitis

	Anti-Infective Chemotherapy	Use of Corticosteroids
Toxoplasmosis	If central vision is threatened, give pyrimethamine, 75 mg by mouth as a loading dose for 2 days followed by 25–50 mg once daily for 4 weeks, in combination with trisulfapyrimidines (sulfadiazine, sulfamerazine, and sulfamethazine, 0.167 g of each per tablet), 2 g by mouth as loading dose followed by 0.5–1 g 4 times daily for 4 weeks. If a fall in the white blood cell or platelet count occurs during therapy, give folinic acid (leucovorin), 1 mL IM twice weekly or 3 mg orally twice weekly. Alternative chemotherapeutic approach for ocular toxoplasmosis: 800 mg sulfamethoxazole with 160 mg trimethoprim by mouth twice daily, or clindamycin 300 mg by mouth 4 times a day with sulfonamides (as above), or spiramycin 1 g by mouth 3 times daily, or minocycline 100 mg by mouth daily for 3–4 weeks.	If the response is not favorable after 2 weeks, continue the anti-infective therapy and give systemic corticosteroids, eg, prednisone, 0.5 mg/kg/d with tapering over 3–4 weeks. Do not stop anti-infective therapy prior to stopping corticosteroids.
Tuberculosis	Isoniazid, 300 mg by mouth daily, rifampicin, 450–600 mg by mouth daily, and pyridoxine, 50 mg by mouth daily, for 6–9 months; with ethambutol, 15 mg/kg by mouth daily, and pyrazinamide, 1.5–2 g by mouth daily, for initial 2 months.	If a favorable response does not occur in 6 weeks, continue antimycobacterial therapy and give systemic corticosteroids, eg, prednisone, 0.5–1 mg/kg/d, with tapering as allowed by response.
Sarcoidosis	Treat with local corticosteroids, cycloplegic/mydriatic agents, and, as needed, with systemic corticosteroids such as prednisone, 0.5–1 mg/kg/d, with tapering as allowed by response. The usual contraindications to systemic corticosteroid therapy apply. A corticosteroid-sparing agent is occasionally required.	
Sympathetic ophthalmia	Treat with local corticosteroids, cycloplegic/mydriatic agents, and systemic corticosteroids in high doses, eg, prednisone, 1–1.5 mg/kg/d. The usual contradictions to systemic corticosteroid therapy apply, and a corticosteroid-sparing agent is often required.	

Table 7–3. Causes of Anterior Uveitis

Autoimmune
Juvenile idiopathic arthritis
Sarcoidosis
Tubulointerstitial nephritis with uveitis (TINU)
Ankylosing spondylitis
Reiter's syndrome (reactive arthritis)
Inflammatory bowel disease (ulcerative colitis, Crohn's disease)
Psoriatic arthritis
Lens-induced uveitis

Infections
Syphilis
Tuberculosis
Leprosy (Hansen's disease)
Herpes simplex virus
Varicella-zoster virus
Cytomegalovirus
Onchocerciasis
Leptospirosis

Malignancy
Retinoblastoma
Leukemia
Lymphoma
Malignant melanoma
Metastasis

Other
Idiopathic
Trauma, including penetrating injury
Retinal detachment
Fuchs heterochromic iridocyclitis (Fuchs uveitis syndrome)
Glaucomatocyclitic crisis (Posner-Schlossman syndrome)

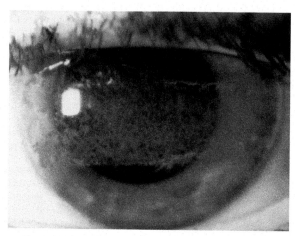

▲ **Figure 7–7.** Extensive band keratopathy in a young girl with juvenile idiopathic arthritis (JIA).

synechiae formation, often progressing to seclusion of the pupil, and cataract. Band keratopathy (Figure 7–7), secondary ocular hypertension or glaucoma, and cystoid macular edema can also be present and cause loss of vision. Patients suspected of having JIA should be evaluated by a rheumatologist and tested for a positive ANA titer.

Treatment of JIA-associated uveitis is challenging. Topical corticosteroids, nonsteroidal anti-inflammatory agents, and cycloplegic/mydriatic agents are all of value. In resistant cases, systemic immunosuppression with noncorticosteroid immunosuppressants such as methotrexate, mycophenolate mofetil, or TNF-α inhibitors may be required to control the disease. Cataract surgery is associated with a relatively high risk of postoperative exacerbations, and intraocular lens implantation is usually contraindicated.

Up to 50% of patients with **ankylosing spondylitis** develop anterior uveitis. There is a marked preponderance for men. The uveitis can vary in severity from mild to severe and often produces pain, photophobia, and blurred vision. Limbal injection is usually present. Keratic precipitates, though usually present, are rarely granulomatous, and iris

nodules do not occur. Posterior synechiae, peripheral anterior synechiae, cataracts, and glaucoma are common complications following severe, recurrent, or poorly controlled bouts of inflammation. Macular edema is uncommon, but can occur when the inflammation is severe and spills over to involve the vitreous. Recurrence is the rule and may involve either eye, although bilateral simultaneous involvement is atypical. The HLA-B27 histocompatibility antigen is present in approximately 50% of patients with acute nongranulomatous iritis or iridocyclitis seen in tertiary referral centers, but may be as high as 90% in community practice. Of those patients with anterior uveitis who are HLA-B27 positive, roughly half will experience a nonocular complication of their disease—most commonly ankylosing spondylitis, but Reiter's syndrome (reactive arthritis), inflammatory bowel disease, and psoriatic arthritis may also occur. Imaging and colonoscopy can occasionally confirm diagnoses suspected on clinical grounds.

2. FUCHS HETEROCHROMIC IRIDOCYCLITIS (FUCHS UVEITIS SYNDROME)

Fuchs heterochromic iridocyclitis is uncommon, accounting for less than 5% of all cases of uveitis. The onset is typically insidious during the third or fourth decade of life. Redness, pain, and photophobia tend to be minimal. Patients usually complain of blurred vision due to cataract. Iris heterochromia, best appreciated with natural lighting, can be subtle and is often most obvious over the iris sphincter muscle. Keratic precipitates are often small and stellate and scattered over the entire endothelium. Abnormal blood vessels may be seen in the chamber angle on gonioscopy. Posterior synechiae are uncommon, although they may occur in some patients following cataract surgery. A vitreous reaction may be present in 10% of patients. While loss of stromal pigment tends to make heavily pigmented eyes look hypochromic, stromal atrophy affecting lightly colored irides can actually reveal underlying pigment epithelium on the posterior surface of the iris, causing paradoxic hyperchromia. Pathologically, the iris and ciliary body show moderate atrophy with patchy depigmentation and diffuse infiltration of lymphocytes and plasma cells.

Cataract eventually develops in most patients, whereas glaucoma occurs in 10–15% of cases. The prognosis is generally good. Cataract surgery can usually be performed without complication, and most patients with glaucoma can be managed with topical medications alone. Bleeding of abnormal angle vessels at the time of anterior segment surgery is known as Amsler's sign.

3. LENS-INDUCED UVEITIS

Lens-induced (phacogenic) uveitis is an autoimmune disease directed against lens antigens. There are no data at present to substantiate the suggestion that lens material per se is toxic, so the term "phacotoxic uveitis" should be avoided. The classic case occurs when the lens develops a hypermature cataract and the lens capsule leaks lens material into the posterior and anterior chambers. This material elicits an inflammatory reaction characterized by accumulation of plasma cells, mononuclear phagocytes, and a few polymorphonuclear cells. Typical anterior uveitis symptoms of pain, photophobia, and blurred vision are common. Lens-induced uveitis may also occur following lens trauma or cataract surgery with retained lens material. Phacolytic glaucoma is a common complication. Definitive treatment requires removal of the lens material. Concurrent treatment with corticosteroids, cycloplegic/mydriatic agents, and intraocular pressure–lowering medications is often necessary.

INTERMEDIATE UVEITIS (CYCLITIS, PERIPHERAL UVEITIS, PARS PLANITIS)

Intermediate uveitis affects mainly the intermediate zone of the eye—ciliary body, principally the pars plana, peripheral retina, and vitreous. The cause is unknown in most cases, although syphilis, tuberculosis, and sarcoidosis should be ruled out with appropriate laboratory and ancillary testing. Multiple sclerosis should also be considered, particularly when supportive signs or symptoms are present. Intermediate uveitis is seen mainly among young adults, affects men and women equally, and is bilateral in up to 80% of cases. Common complaints include floaters and blurred vision. Pain, redness, and photophobia are unusual but can accompany a severe first attack. Adequate examination of the ciliary body, pars plana, and peripheral retina requires use of an indirect ophthalmoscope and scleral depression, which often reveals vitreous condensations in the form of snowballs and

snowbanking. Adjacent retinal vasculitis is common. Anterior chamber inflammation is invariably mild, and posterior synechiae are uncommon. Posterior subcapsular cataract and cystoid macular edema are the most common causes of decreased vision. In severe cases, cyclitic membranes and retinal detachments may occur. Secondary glaucoma is rare. Corticosteroids are used mainly to treat cystoid macular edema or retinal neovascularization. Topical corticosteroids should be tried for 3–4 weeks to identify patients predisposed to development of corticosteroid-induced ocular hypertension. If no improvement is noted and ocular hypertension does not develop, a posterior sub-Tenon or intraocular injection of triamcinolone acetonide, 40 mg/mL, may be effective. Patients with intermediate uveitis usually do well with cataract surgery.

POSTERIOR UVEITIS (TABLE 7–4)

The retina, choroid, and optic nerve are affected by a variety of infectious and noninfectious disorders, the more common of which are listed in Table 7–4.

Table 7–4. Causes of Posterior Uveitis

Infectious disorders
  Viruses
    Cytomegalovirus, herpes simplex virus, varicella-zoster virus, rubella virus, rubeola virus
  Bacteria
    Agents of tuberculosis, brucellosis, sporadic and endemic syphilis; *Borrelia* (Lyme disease); and various hematogenously spread gram-positive and gram-negative pathogens
  Fungi
    Candida, Histoplasma, Cryptococcus, Aspergillus
  Parasites
    Toxoplasma, Toxocara, Cysticercus, Onchocerca

Noninfectious disorders
  Autoimmune disorders
    Behçet disease
    Vogt-Koyanagi-Harada disease
    Systemic lupus erythematosus
    Granulomatosis with polyangiitis
    Sympathetic ophthalmia
    Retinal vasculitis
  Malignancies
    Intraocular lymphoma
    Malignant melanoma
    Leukemia
    Metastatic lesions
  Unknown etiology
    Sarcoidosis
    Serpiginous choroiditis
    Birdshot chorioretinopathy
    Acute multifocal placoid pigment epitheliopathy
    Multiple evanescent white dot syndrome

Most cases of posterior uveitis are associated with some form of systemic disease. The cause can often be established on the basis of (1) the morphology of the lesions, (2) the mode of onset and course of the disease, or (3) the association with systemic symptoms or signs. Other considerations are the age of the patient and whether involvement is unilateral or bilateral. Laboratory and ancillary tests are often helpful.

Lesions of the posterior segment of the eye can be focal, multifocal, geographic, or diffuse. Those that tend to cause clouding of the overlying vitreous should be differentiated from those that give rise to little or no vitreous cells. The type, distribution, and severity of vitreous opacities should be described. Inflammatory lesions of the posterior segment are generally insidious in onset, but some may be accompanied by abrupt and profound visual loss.

Worldwide, the most common causes of retinitis in immunocompetent patients are toxoplasmosis, syphilis, and Behçet disease, whereas the most common causes of choroiditis are sarcoidosis, tuberculosis, and Vogt-Koyanagi-Harada disease. Inflammatory papillitis or optic neuritis can be caused by any of these diseases, but multiple sclerosis should always be suspected, particularly when associated with eye pain worsened by movement (see Chapter 14). Less common causes of posterior uveitis include intraocular lymphoma, acute retinal necrosis (ARN) syndrome, sympathetic ophthalmia, and the "white dot" syndromes such as multiple evanescent white dot syndrome (MEWDS) or acute multifocal posterior placoid epitheliopathy (AMPPE).

▶ Diagnosis & Clinical Features

Diagnostic clues and clinical features of the more commonly encountered posterior uveitis syndromes are described below.

A. Age of the Patient

Posterior uveitis in patients under 3 years of age can be caused by a "masquerade syndrome" such as retinoblastoma or leukemia. Infectious causes of posterior uveitis in this age group include congenital toxoplasmosis, toxocariasis, and perinatal infections due to syphilis, cytomegalovirus, herpes simplex virus, varicella-zoster virus, or rubella virus.

In the age group from 4 to 15 years, the most common causes of posterior uveitis are toxoplasmosis and toxocariasis. Uncommon causes include syphilis, tuberculosis, sarcoidosis, Behçet syndrome, and Vogt-Koyanagi-Harada disease.

In the age group from 16 to 50 years, the differential diagnosis for posterior uveitis includes syphilis, tuberculosis, sarcoidosis, toxoplasmosis, Behçet disease, Vogt-Koyanagi-Harada disease, and ARN syndrome.

Patients over age 50 years who present with posterior uveitis may have syphilis, tuberculosis, sarcoidosis, intraocular lymphoma, birdshot chorioretinitis, ARN syndrome, toxoplasmosis, or endogenous endophthalmitis.

B. Laterality

Unilateral posterior uveitis favors a diagnosis of toxoplasmosis, toxocariasis, ARN syndrome, or endogenous bacterial or fungal infection.

C. Symptoms

1. Reduced vision—Reduced visual acuity may be present in all types of posterior uveitis but especially in the setting of a macular lesion or retinal detachment. Every patient should be examined for an afferent pupillary defect, which, when present, signifies optic nerve or widespread retinal dysfunction.

2. Ocular injection—Eye redness is uncommon in strictly intermediate or posterior uveitis, but can occur in panuveitis.

3. Pain—Pain is atypical in posterior uveitis, but can occur in endophthalmitis, posterior scleritis, or optic neuritis caused by multiple sclerosis.

D. Signs

Signs important in the diagnosis of posterior uveitis include hypopyon formation, granuloma formation, glaucoma, vitritis, morphology of the lesions, vasculitis, retinal hemorrhages, and scar formation.

1. Hypopyon—Disorders of the posterior segment that may be associated with significant anterior inflammation and hypopyon include syphilis, tuberculosis, sarcoidosis, endogenous endophthalmitis, Behçet disease, and leptospirosis. When this occurs, the uveitis is more appropriately termed diffuse or panuveitis.

2. Type of uveitis—Anterior granulomatous uveitis may be associated with conditions that affect the posterior retina and choroid, including syphilis, tuberculosis, sarcoidosis, toxoplasmosis, Vogt-Koyanagi-Harada disease, and sympathetic ophthalmia. On the other hand, nongranulomatous anterior uveitis may be associated with Behçet disease, ARN syndrome, intraocular lymphoma, or the white dot syndromes.

3. Glaucoma—Acute ocular hypertension in association with posterior uveitis can occur with toxoplasmosis, ARN syndrome due to herpes simplex virus or varicella-zoster virus, sarcoidosis, or syphilis.

4. Vitritis—Posterior uveitis is often associated with vitritis, usually due to leakage from the inflammatory foci, from retinal vessels, or from the optic nerve head. Severe vitritis tends to occur with infections involving the posterior pole, such as toxoplasmic retinochoroiditis or bacterial endophthalmitis, whereas mild to moderate inflammation usually occurs with primary outer retinal and choroidal inflammatory disorders. Serpiginous choroiditis and presumed ocular histoplasmosis are typically accompanied by little if any vitritis.

5. Morphology and location of lesions—

A. Retina—The retina is the primary target of many types of infectious agents. Toxoplasmosis is the most common cause of retinitis in immunocompetent hosts. The active lesion of toxoplasmosis is generally seen in the company of old, healed scars that may be heavily pigmented. The lesions may appear in a juxtapapillary location and often give rise to retinal vasculitis. The vitreous is generally clouded when large lesions are present. In contrast, retinal infection with herpes viruses, such as cytomegalovirus and varicella-zoster virus, is more common in immunocompromised hosts. Rubella and rubeola virus retinal infections occur primarily in infants, where they tend to produce diffuse pigmentary changes involving the outer retina referred to as "salt and pepper" retinopathy (see Chapter 15).

B. Choroid—The choroid is the primary target of granulomatous processes such as tuberculosis and sarcoidosis. Patients with tuberculosis and sarcoidosis may present with a focal, multifocal, or geographic choroiditis. Both multifocal and diffuse infiltrations of the choroid occur in Vogt-Koyanagi-Harada disease and sympathetic ophthalmia. Birdshot chorioretinopathy and presumed ocular histoplasmosis syndrome, in contrast, almost always produce multifocal choroiditis.

C. Optic nerve—Primary inflammatory papillitis can occur from syphilis, tuberculosis, sarcoidosis, toxoplasmosis, multiple sclerosis, Lyme disease, intraocular lymphoma, or systemic *Bartonella henselae* infection (cat-scratch disease). Peripapillary serous retinal detachment and/or macular star are often present in eyes with *B henselae* infection.

E. Trauma

A history of trauma in patients with uveitis raises the possibility of intraocular foreign body or sympathetic ophthalmia. Surgical trauma, including routine operations for cataract and glaucoma, may introduce micro-organisms into the eye and lead to acute or subacute endophthalmitis.

F. Mode of Onset

The onset of posterior uveitis may be acute and sudden or slow and insidious. Diseases of the posterior segment of the eye that tend to present with sudden loss of vision include toxoplasmic retinochoroiditis, ARN syndrome, and bacterial endophthalmitis. Most other causes of posterior uveitis have a more insidious onset.

1. OCULAR TOXOPLASMOSIS

Toxoplasmosis is caused by *Toxoplasma gondii*, an obligate intracellular protozoan. The ocular lesions may be acquired in utero or following systemic infection. Constitutional symptoms may be mild and easily missed. The domestic cat and other feline species serve as definitive hosts for the parasite. Susceptible women who acquire the disease during pregnancy may transmit the infection to the fetus, where it can be fatal. Sources of human infection include oocysts in soil or airborne in dust, undercooked meat containing bradyzoites (encysted forms of the parasite), and tachyzoites (proliferative form) transmitted across the placenta.

► Clinical Findings

A. Symptoms and Signs

Patients with toxoplasmic retinochoroiditis present with a history of floaters and blurred vision. In severe cases, there may also be pain and photophobia. The ocular lesions consist of fluffy-white areas of focal necrotic retinochoroiditis that may be small or large and single or multiple. Active edematous lesions are often adjacent to healed retinal scars (Figure 7–8). Retinal vasculitis and hemorrhage can be observed. Cystoid macular edema can accompany lesions in or near the macula. Iridocyclitis is frequently seen in patients with severe infections, and intraocular pressure may be raised.

B. Laboratory Findings

A positive serologic test for *T gondii* with consistent clinical signs is considered diagnostic. An increase in antibody titer is usually not detected during reactivation, but raised IgM titer provides strong evidence for recently acquired infection.

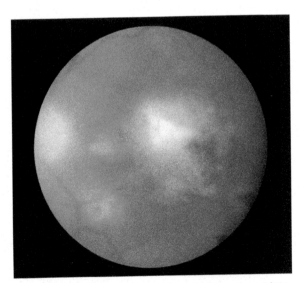

▲ **Figure 7–8.** Recurrent toxoplasmic retinochoroiditis involving the macula, with new fluffy-white lesion adjacent to healed pigmented scar. (Used with permission from S. Patel.)

Treatment

Small lesions in the retinal periphery not associated with significant vitritis require no treatment. In contrast, severe or posterior infections are usually treated for 4–6 weeks with pyrimethamine, 25–50 mg daily, and trisulfapyrimidine, 0.5–1 g four times daily. Loading doses of 75 mg of pyrimethamine daily for 2 days and 2 g of trisulfapyrimidine as a single dose should be given at the start of therapy. Patients are usually also given 3 mg of leucovorin calcium twice weekly to prevent bone marrow depression. A complete blood count should be performed weekly during therapy (Table 7–2).

An alternative approach for the treatment of ocular toxoplasmosis consists of administration of 800 mg of sulfamethoxazole with 160 mg of trimethoprim by mouth twice daily for 3–4 weeks, or clindamycin, 300 mg by mouth four times daily, with trisulfapyrimidine, 0.5–1 g four times daily. Clindamycin causes pseudomembranous colitis in 10–15% of patients. Other antibiotics effective in ocular toxoplasmosis include spiramycin and minocycline. Choroidal neovascularization can be treated with photodynamic therapy (PDT) or intravitreal anti-VEGF (vascular endothelial growth factor) injections.

Anterior uveitis associated with ocular toxoplasmosis may be treated with topical corticosteroids and cycloplegic/mydriatic agents. Long-acting periocular corticosteroid injections are contraindicated. Topical glaucoma medications are occasionally necessary. Systemic corticosteroids can be used in conjunction with antimicrobial therapy for vision-threatening inflammatory lesions but should never be used for a prolonged period in the absence of antimicrobial coverage.

2. HISTOPLASMOSIS

In some areas of the United States where histoplasmosis is endemic (the Ohio and Mississippi River Valley areas), the diagnosis of choroiditis due to presumed ocular histoplasmosis is common. Patients usually have a positive skin test to histoplasmin and demonstrate "punched-out" spots in the posterior or peripheral fundus. These spots are small, irregularly round or oval, and usually depigmented centrally with a finely pigmented border. Peripapillary atrophy and hyperpigmentation occur frequently. Macular lesions may produce choroidal neovascularization, a complication that should be suspected in every patient with presumed ocular histoplasmosis who presents with decreased vision or evidence of subretinal fluid or hemorrhage. Choroidal neovascularization is effectively treated with corticosteroids, PDT, or intravitreal anti-VEGF injections (see Chapter 10).

3. OCULAR TOXOCARIASIS

Toxocariasis results from infection with *Toxocara cati* (an intestinal parasite of cats) or *Toxocara canis* (an intestinal parasite of dogs). Visceral larva migrans is a disseminated systemic infection occurring in a young child (Table 7–5). Ocular involvement occurs less frequently in visceral larva migrans.

Ocular toxocariasis may occur without systemic manifestations. Children acquire the disease by close association with pets and by eating dirt (pica) contaminated with *Toxocara* ova. The ingested ova form larvae that penetrate the intestinal mucosa and gain access to the systemic circulation and finally to the eye. The parasite does not infect the intestinal tract of humans.

Clinical Findings

A. Symptoms and Signs

The disease is usually unilateral. *Toxocara* larvae lodge in the retina and die, leading to a marked inflammatory reaction and local production of *Toxocara* antibodies. Children are typically brought to the ophthalmologist because of a red eye, blurred vision, or a whitish pupil (leukocoria).

Three clinical presentations are recognized: (1) a localized posterior granuloma, usually near the optic nerve head or fovea; (2) a peripheral granuloma involving the pars plana, often producing an elevated mass that mimics the snowbank of intermediate uveitis; and (3) chronic endophthalmitis.

B. Laboratory Findings

Characteristic clinical findings and a positive enzyme-linked immunosorbent assay (ELISA) for anti-*Toxocara* antibodies,

Table 7–5. Comparison between Visceral and Ocular Larva Migrans

	Visceral Larva Migrans	Ocular Larva Migrans[1]
Average age at onset	2 years	7 years
Fever	+	–
Abdominal symptoms (pain, nausea, diarrhea)	+	–
Nonspecific pulmonary disease	+	–
Hepatosplenomegaly	+	–
Eosinophilia	+	–
Hypergammaglobulinemia	+	–
ELISA (serum anti-*Toxocara* antibodies)	+	±
ELISA (aqueous *Toxocara* antibodies)	–	+
Ocular finding[1]	–	+

[1]Ocular findings of ocular larva migrans; diffuse chronic panuveitis, posterior pole granuloma, or peripheral granuloma.

even at low titer, confirm the diagnosis of ocular toxocariasis. Negative ELISAs are common but do not rule out the possibility of ocular infection. Positive antibody titers of the ocular fluids from patients with suspected ocular toxocariasis have been demonstrated in the setting of a negative serum ELISA, but the test is not routinely available and, in any case, is seldom necessary.

▶ **Treatment**

Systemic or periocular injections of corticosteroids should be given when there is evidence of significant intraocular inflammation. Vitrectomy may be necessary in patients with marked vitreous opacity or with significant preretinal traction. Systemic anthelmintic therapy is not indicated for limited ocular disease and, in fact, may worsen the inflammation by producing more rapid killing of the intraocular parasite.

4. ACQUIRED IMMUNODEFICIENCY SYNDROME

Uveitis is common in patients infected with the human immunodeficiency virus (HIV), particularly in advanced stages of the illness when acquired immunodeficiency syndrome (AIDS) develops (see Chapter 15). CD4 T lymphocyte counts are a good predictor of the risk of opportunistic infections, with the majority occurring at counts of less than 100 cells/μL. Uveitis occurs most commonly in the setting of posterior segment infection. Cytomegalovirus retinitis, a geographic retinitis often accompanied by hemorrhage (Figure 7–9), occurred in 30–40% of HIV-positive patients at some point in the course of their illness prior to the advent of combination antiretroviral therapy. Other herpesviruses,

such as varicella-zoster and herpes simplex, can produce a similar retinitis but are usually distinguished by a very rapid progression. Infections caused by other organisms, such as *T gondii, Treponema pallidum, Cryptococcus neoformans, Mycobacterium tuberculosis,* and *Mycobacterium avium-intracellulare,* occur in less than 5% of HIV-positive patients but should be considered, particularly when there is a history of infection or exposure, when choroiditis is present, or when the retinitis is atypical in appearance or fails to respond to antiviral therapy. Intraocular lymphoma occurs in less than 1% of HIV-positive patients but should be considered when the retinitis is atypical or is unresponsive to antiviral treatment, especially when neurologic symptoms are present. Diagnosis usually requires vitreous biopsy.

PANUVEITIS (TABLE 7–6)

The term "panuveitis" is used to denote a more or less uniform cellular infiltration of both the anterior and posterior segments, together with involvement of the retina, choroid, and/or optic disk. Associated findings, such as retinitis, vasculitis, or choroiditis, can occur and often prompt further diagnostic testing. Tuberculosis, sarcoidosis, and syphilis should always be considered in patients with diffuse uveitis. Less common causes include sympathetic ophthalmia, Vogt-Koyanagi-Harada disease, Behçet syndrome, birdshot chorioretinopathy, and intraocular lymphoma.

1. TUBERCULOUS UVEITIS

Tuberculosis can cause any type of uveitis but deserves special consideration when granulomatous keratic precipitates or iris or choroidal granulomas are present. Such granulomas, or tubercles, consist of giant and epithelioid cells.

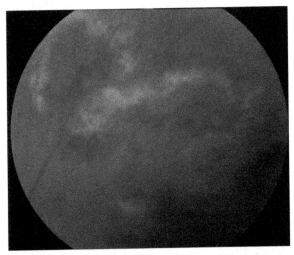

▲ **Figure 7–9.** Cytomegalovirus retinitis with perivascular geographic hemorrhagic retinitis.

Table 7–6. Causes of Panuveitis

Sarcoidosis
Tuberculosis
Syphilis
Onchocerciasis
Leptospirosis
Brucellosis
Sympathetic ophthalmia
Behçet disease
Multiple sclerosis
Cysticercosis
Vogt-Koyanagi-Harada disease
Masquerade syndromes:
   Retinoblastoma
   Leukemia
   Lymphoma
   Retinitis pigmentosa
Retinal intraocular foreign body

Caseating necrosis is characteristic on histopathologic examination. Although the infection is said to be transmitted from a primary focus elsewhere in the body, uveal tuberculosis is uncommon in patients with active pulmonary tuberculosis (see Chapter 15). Evaluation should include a chest x-ray and either skin testing with a PPD or an IGRA. Treatment should involve three or more antituberculous medicines for 6–9 months (Table 7–2).

2. SARCOIDOSIS

Sarcoidosis is a chronic granulomatous disease of unknown cause, usually presenting in the fourth or fifth decade of life. Pulmonary involvement occurs in most patients. Virtually every organ system can be involved, including the skin, bones, liver, spleen, central nervous system, and eyes. The tissue reaction is much less severe than in tuberculous uveitis, and caseation can rarely occur. Anergy on skin testing supports the diagnosis. When the parotid glands are involved, the disease is called uveoparotid fever, or Heerfordt's disease. When the lacrimal glands are involved, the disease is called Mikulicz's syndrome.

Uveitis occurs in approximately 25% of patients with systemic sarcoidosis. As with tuberculosis, any form of uveitis can occur, but sarcoid deserves special consideration when the uveitis is granulomatous or when retinal phlebitis is present, particularly in black patients.

The diagnosis can be supported by an abnormal chest x-ray, especially when hilar adenopathy is present, or by raised serum ACE, lysozyme, or calcium levels. The strongest evidence comes from histopathologic demonstration of noncaseating granulomas in affected tissues such as lung or conjunctiva. However, biopsies should only be taken when suspicious lesions are clearly evident. A gallium scan of the head, neck, and thorax can provide evidence for subclinical inflammation of the lacrimal, parotid, or salivary glands or of paratracheal or pulmonary lymph nodes.

Corticosteroid therapy given early in the disease may be effective, but recurrences are common. Long-term therapy may require the use of corticosteroid-sparing agents such as methotrexate, azathioprine, or mycophenolate mofetil (Table 7–2).

3. SYPHILIS

Syphilis is an uncommon but treatable cause of uveitis. Intraocular inflammation occurs almost exclusively during the secondary and tertiary stages of infection. All types of uveitis occur. Associated retinitis (Figure 7–10) and papillitis are common. Widespread atrophy and hyperplasia of the retinal pigment epithelium can occur late if untreated. Testing should include one of the commonly used (and less expensive) tests for the production of *T pallidum*–induced anticardiolipin antibodies, such as the VDRL or RPR test, as well

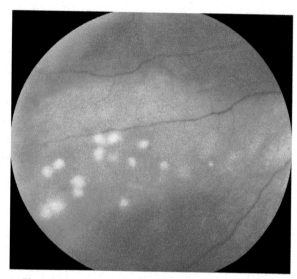

▲ **Figure 7–10.** Characteristic "ground glass" appearance and overlying superficial retinal precipitates in a patient with syphilitic retinitis. (Used with permission from J. M. Jumper.)

as a test for the more specific anti–*T pallidum* antibodies, such as the FTA-ABS or MHA-TP. While the FTA-ABS and MHA-TP tests display high sensitivity and specificity during both secondary and tertiary stages of infection, the VDRL and RPR can be falsely negative in up to 30% of patients with late or latent disease. Falsely positive results can occur in the setting of other spirochetal infections, biliary cirrhosis, or collagen-vascular disease, whereas falsely negative results can occur in severely immunocompromised patients. Patients with uveitis and a positive serologic test for syphilis should undergo examination of the cerebrospinal fluid to rule out neurosyphilis. Treatment consists of aqueous crystalline penicillin G, 4 million units, given intravenously every 4 hours for 14 days.

4. SYMPATHETIC OPHTHALMIA

Sympathetic ophthalmia is a rare but devastating bilateral granulomatous uveitis that comes on 10 days to many years following a perforating eye injury. The vast majority of cases occur within 1 year after injury. The cause is not known, but the disease is probably related to hypersensitivity to some element of the pigment-bearing cells in the uvea. It very rarely occurs following uncomplicated intraocular surgery for cataract or glaucoma and even less commonly following endophthalmitis.

The injured, or exciting, eye becomes inflamed first, and the fellow, or sympathizing, eye secondarily. Patients usually complain of photophobia, redness, and blurred vision, although the presence of floaters may be the primary

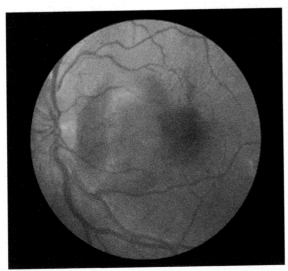

Figure 7–11. Sympathetic ophthalmia with exudative retinal detachment. (Used with permission from H. R. McDonald.)

complaint. The uveitis is usually diffuse. Soft yellow-white exudates in the deep layer of the retina (Dalen-Fuchs nodules) are sometimes seen in the posterior segment. Serous retinal detachments can also occur (Figure 7–11).

The recommended treatment of a severely injured sightless eye is enucleation, or possibly evisceration, within 10 days after injury. The sympathizing eye should be treated aggressively with local or systemic corticosteroids. Long-term corticosteroid-sparing immunosuppressant therapy is often required (Table 7–2). Without treatment, the disease progresses relentlessly to complete bilateral blindness.

UVEITIS IN DEVELOPING COUNTRIES

All forms of uveitis mentioned above also occur in developing countries, and some, such as toxoplasmosis and tuberculosis, are relatively common. In addition, more than 95% of all HIV-positive patients live in developing countries, particularly in sub-Saharan Africa and Southeast Asia. In these regions, otherwise opportunistic infections such as cytomegalovirus retinitis are increasing at an alarming rate. A few infectious causes of uveitis deserve special mention, since they occur almost exclusively in patients who either live in or visit developing countries.

1. LEPTOSPIROSIS

Uveitis occurs in up to 10% of patients infected with the spirochete *Leptospira*. Humans are accidental hosts, infected most commonly by contact with or ingestion of infected water supplies. Wild and domestic animals, including rodents, dogs, pigs, and cattle, are the natural hosts and shed large quantities of infectious organisms in their urine. Farmers, veterinarians, and those who work or swim in waters fed by agricultural runoff are at particularly high risk.

Clinical Findings

A. Symptoms and Signs

Fever, malaise, and headache are common constitutional symptoms. Renal failure and death can occur in up to 30% of untreated patients. The uveitis may be of any type but is typically diffuse and often associated with hypopyon and retinal vasculitis.

B. Laboratory Findings

Culture of live organisms is only possible early in the infection. Sensitive and specific anti-*Leptospira* antibody tests are available for use on blood or cerebrospinal fluid. A fourfold rise in antibody titer is strong evidence for recent infection.

Treatment

Treatment of severe infections includes penicillin, 1.5 million units intravenously every 6 hours for 10 days. Less severe infections can be treated with doxycycline, 100 mg given orally twice daily for 7 days. Topical corticosteroids and cycloplegic/mydriatic agents should be used in conjunction with antibiotic therapy to minimize the complications of anterior uveitis. Posterior sub-Tenon injection of corticosteroids may be necessary for severe intermediate, posterior, or diffuse forms of inflammation.

2. ONCHOCERCIASIS

Onchocerciasis is caused by *Onchocerca volvulus*. The disease afflicts about 15 million people in Africa and Central America and is a major cause of blindness. It is transmitted by *Simulium damnosum*, a black fly that breeds in areas of rapidly flowing streams—thus the term "river blindness." Microfilariae picked up from the skin by the fly mature into larvae that become adult worms in 1 year. The adult parasite produces cutaneous nodules 5–25 mm in diameter on the trunk, thighs, arms, head, and shoulders. Microfilariae cause itching, and healing of skin lesions may lead to loss of skin elasticity and areas of depigmentation.

Clinical Findings

A. Symptoms and Signs

Skin nodules may be seen. The cornea reveals nummular keratitis and sclerosing keratitis. Microfilariae swimming actively in the anterior chamber look like silver threads.

Death of the microfilariae causes an intense inflammatory reaction and severe uveitis, vitritis, and retinitis. Focal retinochoroiditis may be seen. Optic atrophy may develop secondary to glaucoma.

B. Laboratory Findings

The diagnosis of onchocerciasis is made by skin biopsy and microscopic examination looking for live microfilariae.

▶ Treatment

The preferred treatment for onchocerciasis is with nodulectomy and ivermectin. Diethylcarbamazine and suramin have significant toxicity and should be used only when ivermectin is not available.

The great advantage of ivermectin over diethylcarbamazine is that a single oral dose of 100 or 200 µg/kg reduces the worm burden in the skin and anterior chamber more slowly and therefore with a significant reduction in systemic and ocular reactions. The reduction also persists longer.

The minimum effective dose remains to be determined. A dose of 100 µg/kg may be as effective as 200 µg/kg and is associated with fewer of the mild and transient side effects, such as fever and headache. Treatment is repeated at 6 or 12 months.

Topical therapy with corticosteroids and cycloplegic/mydriatic agents is helpful for uveitis.

3. CYSTICERCOSIS

Cysticercosis is an uncommon cause of serious ocular morbidity. The disease is endemic in Mexico, Central and South America, and parts of Africa and Asia, with ocular involvement occurring in about one-third of affected patients. Ocular cysticercosis is caused either by the ingestion of eggs of *Taenia solium* or by reverse peristalsis in cases of intestinal obstruction caused by adult tapeworms. Eggs mature and embryos penetrate intestinal mucosa, thus gaining access to the circulation. The larvae (*Cysticercus cellulosae*) is the most common tapeworm that invades the human eye.

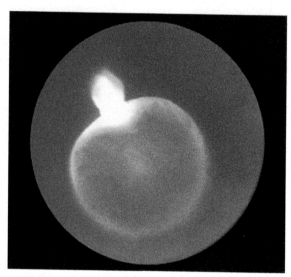

▲ **Figure 7–12.** Cysticercosis with intravitreal cyst. (Used with permission from G. R. O'Connor.)

▶ Clinical Findings

The larvae may reach the subretinal space, producing acute retinitis with retinal edema and subretinal exudates, or the vitreous cavity (Figure 7–12), where a translucent cyst with a dense white spot formed by the invaginated scolex develops. Larvae may live in the eye for as long as 2 years. Death of the larvae inside the eye leads to a severe inflammatory reaction. Movements of larvae within the ocular tissue may stimulate a chronic inflammatory reaction and fibrosis. In rare instances, the larva may be seen in the anterior chamber. Involvement of the brain can cause seizures. Focal calcification may be seen in the subcutaneous tissues by x-ray.

▶ Treatment

Treatment of intraocular cysticercosis is by surgical removal, usually by pars plana vitrectomy.

7.2. Uveal Tumors

James J. Augsburger, MD, and Zélia M. Corrêa, MD, PhD

This section presents an overview of the most common and most important neoplasms, hamartomas, and choristomas of the uvea. Neoplastic tumors of the ciliary body epithelium (Chapter 10) and nonneoplastic lesions and disorders of the fundus that can simulate uveal melanoma and other uveal neoplasms (eg, subretinal and suprachoroidal hematomas, nodular posterior scleritis, disciform fibrovascular lesion associated with neovascular age-related macular degeneration, and inflammatory chorioretinal granulomas) are discussed in other parts of this book.

BENIGN UVEAL TUMORS

Benign neoplasms are acquired tumors composed of cells that are atypical but not abnormal enough to be classified as malignant. They may enlarge slowly, but have little or no invasive potential and no metastatic capability. **Hamartomas** are congenital tumors composed of normal or near-normal cells that exist normally in that anatomic site but are present in abnormally excessive amount. **Choristomas** are congenital cellular tumors consisting of normal cells and tissue elements that do not occur normally in that anatomic site.

▶ Uveal Nevus

Uveal nevus is a benign acquired neoplasm composed of mildly atypical uveal melanocytes. It can develop within any portion of the uvea (iris, ciliary body, or choroid), but the choroid is involved most frequently. Epidemiologic studies have shown uveal nevi to be rare in infants and children, uncommon in teenagers and young adults, but relatively frequent in older individuals. Cross-sectional clinical and autopsy studies have identified such lesions in about 2% to 10% of eyes of Caucasians over the age of 50 years. These lesions are believed to occur with similar frequency in non-Caucasians, but they are much more likely to be overlooked clinically because of the more pronounced melanotic pigmentation of the normal choroid that obscures the lesion in such individuals.

The typical uveal nevus is a dark brown to tan lesion regardless of where in the uvea it develops. Most uveal nevi are small (less than 3 mm maximal basal diameter and less than 0.5 mm maximal thickness) when first identified, and only about 5% ever achieve a size greater than 5 mm in diameter and/or greater than 1 mm in thickness. Lesions of the iris are likely to be noted by the patient as a cosmetic lesion but may be detected on routine eye examination. Because of their readily visible nature, iris nevi are usually detected when they are quite small (Figure 7–13). In contrast, choroidal nevi (Figure 7–14) are usually detected incidentally during routine examination or examination for coincidental visual symptoms. Iris nevi generally appear bland without prominent intrinsic vascularity on slitlamp biomicroscopy; however, they can be associated with peaking of the pupil toward the lesion and localized eversion of the pupil margin (ectropion iridis). Choroidal nevi typically appear as thin gray to brown choroidal lesions with feathered margins that blend imperceptibly into the surrounding normal choroid. Drusen are frequently present on the surface of such lesions. Some larger choroidal nevi have small clumps of orange pigment (lipofuscin) on their surface and limited overlying and surrounding exudative subretinal fluid. Rarely, choroidal neovascularization with subretinal bleeding and/or exudation develops over a choroidal nevus.

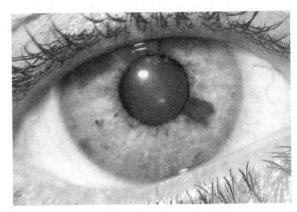

▲ **Figure 7–13.** Typical iris nevus involving pupillary margin. Note also the multiple tiny iris freckles.

Unequivocally typical uveal nevi require no treatment. However, choroidal nevi that are associated with exudative subretinal fluid involving the macula and causing visual blurring and distortion may be treated by focal laser therapy to sites of leakage identified on fluorescein angiography, and choroidal neovascularization associated with a choroidal nevus may be treated by intravitreal anti-VEGF therapy, photodynamic therapy, laser hyperthermia to the entire melanocytic choroidal tumor, or focal photocoagulation depending on its location and extent.

Melanocytoma of the optic disk is a variant of uveal nevus. Typically it is a dark brown to almost black intrapapillary mass (Figure 7–15). Fundus biomicroscopy frequently

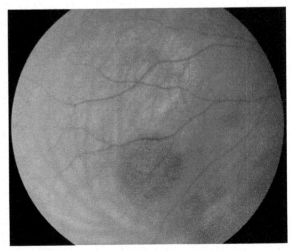

▲ **Figure 7–14.** Typical melanocytic choroidal nevus underlying retinal blood vessels and only about 0.25 mm thick by ultrasonography.

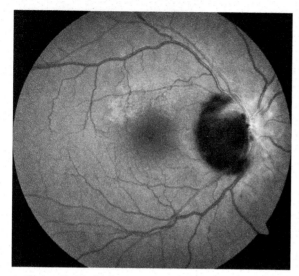

▲ **Figure 7–15.** Melanocytoma of the optic disk, with typical black color of lesion and replacement of retinal nerve fibers by tumor tissue.

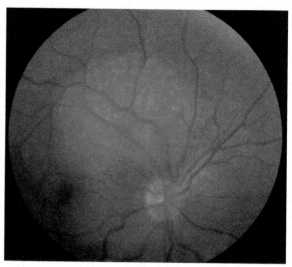

▲ **Figure 7–16.** Circumscribed choroidal hemangioma just superior to optic disk and fovea, with shallow exudative subretinal fluid involving the central macula.

shows darkly melanotic tumor cells invading the retinal nerve fiber layer at the disk, and there can be progressive reduction of visual field.

Many uveal nevi exhibit limited long-term growth, so this is not compelling evidence that a nevus is malignant or has transformed into a malignant melanoma. However, large lesion size and substantial or rapid growth should always prompt reconsideration of the diagnosis (see later section on Nevus versus Melanoma Category).

▶ Circumscribed Choroidal Hemangioma

Circumscribed choroidal hemangioma is sometimes classified as a hamartoma even though it is rarely, if ever, detected at birth or identified in the neonatal period. It is a localized overgrowth of choroidal blood vessels and almost exclusively unilateral and unifocal. There is no recognized familial tendency. The average age at detection is late 30s to early 40s. Clinically, there is a localized, round to oval, dome-shaped, reddish-orange mass that is centered posterior to the ocular equator (Figure 7–16). The posterior margin is almost always within 2 optic disk diameters of the optic disk and/or foveola. At detection, diameter is usually less than 10 mm and thickness is usually less than 3.5 mm, although diameter greater than 15 mm and thickness greater than 5 mm are encountered occasionally. If the circumscribed choroidal hemangioma develops in the macula, it frequently causes progressive cystic degeneration of the overlying retina with permanently reduced vision. Juxtapapillary extramacular location is frequently associated with progressive accumulation of exudative subretinal fluid, resulting in blurring and distortion of vision if there is involvement of the central macula. Circumscribed choroidal hemangioma tends to enlarge slowly.

Fluorescein angiography of circumscribed choroidal hemangioma typically shows early hyperfluorescence of the relatively large-caliber choroidal blood vessels and late diffuse hyperfluorescence of the entire lesion, but there may be less definition than anticipated. Indocyanine green angiography (ICGA) is generally considered to be more useful. Typically it shows well-defined diffuse early hyperfluorescence of the entire lesion and late washout of its central portion that is not evident until 20 to 30 minutes after dye injection. B-scan ocular ultrasonography shows a fusiform to dome-like cross-sectional shape, characteristically with relatively strong internal sonoreflectivity similar to orbital fat.

The most commonly employed initial treatment for small to medium visually symptomatic circumscribed choroidal hemangioma is photodynamic laser therapy, which generally results in pronounced flattening of the hemangioma and prompt, sustained resolution of associated exudative subretinal fluid. Large circumscribed choroidal hemangiomas associated with bullous exudative retinal detachment and/or prominent fibrous metaplasia of the overlying retinal pigment epithelium may require plaque radiation therapy or some method of relatively low-dose external beam radiation therapy to stabilize and/or shrink the tumor and eliminate retinal detachment. Factors adversely influencing the visual outcome include larger size or subfoveal location of the hemangioma, extensive retinal detachment, and worse visual acuity prior to treatment.

Diffuse Choroidal Hemangioma

Diffuse choroidal hemangioma is a diffuse congenital overgrowth (malformation) of relatively normal-appearing choroidal blood vessels with no recognized familial inheritance pattern. It is usually unilateral, but bilateral involvement has been reported. It typically occurs in conjunction with an ipsilateral congenital cutaneous facial nevus flammeus affecting the eyelids and periorbital region, which is a characteristic lesion of Sturge-Weber syndrome.

Diffuse choroidal hemangioma appears as reddish-orange thickening of the choroid that tends to be most pronounced around the optic disk and in the macula (Figure 7–17). The optic disk cup of the affected eye frequently appears large and deep because of the circumpapillary choroidal thickening. Visual loss is caused by progressive cystic retinal degeneration of the macula, chronic secondary exudative retinal detachment, and/or associated secondary glaucoma.

Photodynamic therapy or plaque radiotherapy (brachytherapy) to accentuated areas of choroidal vascular thickening may eliminate secondary subretinal fluid in the macula, but low-dose external beam radiation therapy to the posterior ocular segment is sometimes necessary to stabilize the hemangioma and eliminate associated subretinal fluid.

Choroidal Osteoma

Choroidal osteoma is a benign uveal neoplasm composed of mature bone tissue. Because bone does not normally occur in the uvea, choroidal osteoma is sometimes classified as a choristoma even though it has not been detected at birth or

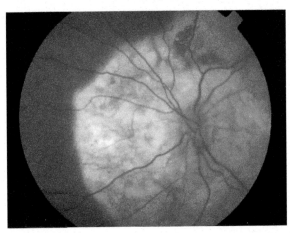

▲ **Figure 7–18.** Choroidal osteoma in typical circumpapillary location. The tumor has a pale color with well-defined smooth margins. There are small-caliber blood vessels on its surface and localized subretinal blood superiorly.

in a neonate. It predominantly affects women (9:1 female-to-male ratio) and is bilateral in approximately 20% of cases. It is always unifocal in affected eyes. There is no generally recognized familial tendency.

Choroidal osteoma is usually first detected during the second or third decade of life. The characteristic appearance is a rather well-defined golden to off-white juxtapapillary or circumpapillary choroidal plate-like lesion with smoothly curved margins (Figure 7–18). In most cases, it enlarges slowly, but retains a plate-like cross section. The retinal pigment epithelium is frequently disrupted and clumped over the tumor, and the overlying sensory retina may be thinned or cystic. Choroidal neovascularization frequently develops from the surface of the osteoma and leads to further visual loss due to accumulation of exudative and/or hemorrhagic subretinal fluid and exudates and eventual subretinal fibrosis. If the osteoma involves the central macula, usually there is profound permanent visual loss. Choroidal neovascularization due to extramacular choroidal osteoma with visual symptoms can be treated by intravitreal anti-VEGF agents, photodynamic laser therapy, or laser photocoagulation. Spontaneous and laser-induced regression, or at least decalcification, of choroidal osteomas has been reported, but this is not usually associated with improvement of visual acuity. Because the tumor has no recognized malignant potential, no destructive treatment for the tumor is indicated.

UVEAL TUMORS INTERMEDIATE BETWEEN BENIGN AND MALIGNANT

Some uveal tumors are categorized as intermediate between benign and malignant because they cannot be categorized reliably as either benign or malignant by clinical examination.

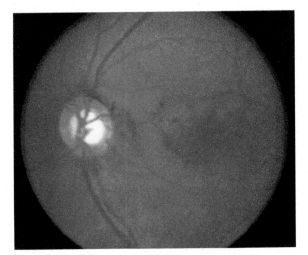

▲ **Figure 7–17.** Diffuse choroidal hemangioma surrounding the optic disk, with its cup appearing large and deep because of the pronounced circumpapillary choroidal vascular thickening. There is clumping of the retinal pigment epithelium in the central macula.

Biopsy may reveal benign cells, malignant cells, or borderline malignant cells according to cytologic or histologic criteria.

Nevus versus Melanoma Category

Approximately 95% of uveal nevi never exceed 5 mm in maximal basal diameter and 1 mm in thickness, but the remaining 5% can achieve substantially larger dimensions. Uveal nevi are substantially more common than uveal melanomas, so there is considerable overlap between nevi and melanomas among lesions with a 5- to 10-mm basal diameter and/or 1- to 3.5-mm thickness, of which those without clearly invasive clinical features are sometimes referred to as "suspicious nevi," "nevomas," or "indeterminate pigmented uveal tumors." An iris lesion that might be categorized in this way would be larger (especially in thickness) than the typical iris nevus and associated with peaking of the pupil toward the lesion, eversion of the pupil margin (ectropion iridis), and possibly abnormally prominent intralesional blood vessels (Figure 7–19) but would not exhibit seeding onto the adjacent iris, implantation tumors on the trabecular meshwork, or full-thickness iris replacement (demonstrable by ultrasound biomicroscopy). A choroidal or ciliary body tumor that might be categorized in this way would also be larger (especially in thickness) than the typical choroidal nevus, but would exhibit clinical features of dormancy, such as prominent clumps of black retinal pigment epithelial pigment and prominent drusen on its surface, and limited if any indication of growth activity, such as small clumps of orange pigment (lipofuscin) on its surface and limited overlying or surrounding exudative subretinal fluid (Figure 7–20). In the absence of a tumor specimen that can be evaluated

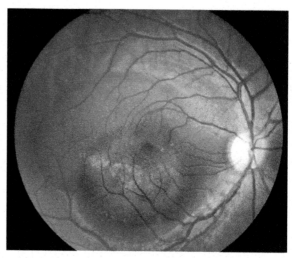

▲ **Figure 7–20.** Melanocytic subfoveal choroidal tumor in nevus versus melanoma category (choroidal nevoma). This visually symptomatic tumor was 2 mm thick. It exhibits a prominent ring of subretinal orange pigment (lipofuscin) on its surface and an associated blister of overlying and surrounding exudative subretinal fluid. It was left untreated, spontaneously flattening slightly with disappearance of the orange pigment and subretinal fluid. Follow-up for over 25 years has shown no reactivation.

pathologically, one can never be certain which of these tumors is benign (nevus) and which is malignant (melanoma). Because of this diagnostic uncertainty, some ocular tumor experts recommend diagnostic biopsy, usually by fine-needle aspiration, for any small lesions in this category prior to any treatment.

Atypical Lymphoid Hyperplasia of the Uvea

Atypical lymphoid hyperplasia of the uvea (previously termed benign reactive lymphoid hyperplasia) is focal or diffuse infiltration of the uvea by activated but benign-appearing lymphoid cells. Pathologically, the lymphoid cells are frequently organized into germinal centers that are evident on low- to high-power microscopy. Immunohistochemically, the lymphoid cells comprising the infiltrates are usually of B-cell lineage but frequently exhibit polyclonal features. Clinically, these lesions appear as tan to creamy focal to diffuse infiltrates in the iris or choroid. B-scan ultrasonography shows generalized choroidal thickening (sometimes with locally accentuated prominence) in diffuse cases, and ultrasound biomicroscopy confirms the solid soft tissue character of iris and iridociliary infiltrates. The retina usually remains attached or shows limited shallow detachment over the choroidal infiltration, but progressive disruption of the retinal

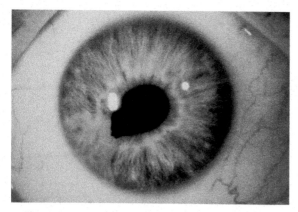

▲ **Figure 7–19.** Amelanotic melanocytic iris neoplasm in nevus versus melanoma category (iris nevoma). Note peaking of the pupil, limited ectropion iridis, and intralesional blood vessels. Histopathologic study of the excised tumor showed it to be a spindle A melanocytic tumor (ie, a nevus).

pigment epithelium develops in many cases. There may be focal or diffuse pink anterior epibulbar masses reminiscent of primary conjunctival lymphoma, or posterior peribulbar extraocular soft tissue masses that may only be evident on B-scan ultrasonography, computed tomography scanning, or magnetic resonance imaging. Biopsy, usually transcleral incisional biopsy, is required to establish the diagnosis and rule out malignant uveal lymphoma. Treatment usually consists of relatively low-dose fractionated external beam radiation therapy that usually results in prompt and sustained clinical regression. If vision is poor prior to treatment, it may not recover even if all of the uveal infiltrates completely regress. Occasional patients with atypical lymphoid hyperplasia of the uvea develop systemic lymphoma, so all affected patients should probably be monitored for systemic disease.

MALIGNANT UVEAL TUMORS

The component cells of malignant uveal tumor are clearly abnormal morphologically. Invasive clinical and pathologic features are generally evident, and metastasis may occur.

▶ Primary Uveal Melanoma

Primary uveal melanoma is an acquired malignant neoplasm that arises from uveal melanocytes. It is almost always unilateral and unifocal. Although characteristic chromosomal abnormalities are present within individual tumor cells, primary uveal melanoma does not usually exhibit any familial hereditary pattern. Uveal melanomas are rare in persons under the age of 20 years but become progressively more frequent with advancing age. The average age at diagnosis is 40 to 45 years for iris melanoma and 55 to 60 years for choroidal and ciliary body melanoma. Primary uveal melanoma affects both men and women. The cumulative lifetime incidence in whites is 1 in 2000–2500 persons. In the United States, the overall mean age-adjusted incidence is approximately 5 per million persons per year. Risk factors include ocular melanocytosis, cutaneous dysplastic nevus syndrome (familial atypical multiple mole—melanoma [FAMM] syndrome), lighter iris color, white race (98% of cases), and increasing age. In Europe a correlation has been identified between increasing incidence and increasing latitude, consistent with a protective effect of ocular pigmentation.

Iris melanomas are frequently detected by the patient or family member as a newly appearing or changing spot on the iris, whereas choroidal melanomas and most ciliary body melanomas are not evident cosmetically and are detected on fundus examination prompted by visual symptoms or on routine examination. Typically, iris melanoma is a dark brown to tan nodular iris mass that replaces the normal iris stroma (Figure 7–21). It frequently attracts prominent intralesional blood vessels and routinely causes peaking and/or splinting of the pupil and ectropion iridis. Loss of cohesiveness of the tumor cells frequently results in satellite tumors

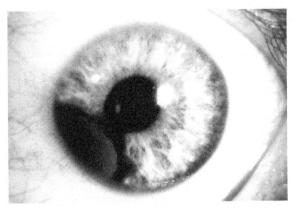

▲ **Figure 7–21.** Darkly melanotic iris melanoma, filling the anterior chamber angle inferonasally and approximately 3 mm thick. Histopathologic study of the excised tumor confirmed it to be a melanoma.

on the adjacent iris and in the angle on the trabecular meshwork, commonly leading to secondary glaucoma.

Typically ciliary body or ciliochoroidal melanoma is a dark nodular peripheral fundus mass (Figure 7–22) associated with prominent localized dilation of blood vessels in the overlying sclera (sentinel blood vessels). The tumor sometimes extends into the peripheral iris, where it may be evident on slitlamp biomicroscopy and gonioscopy. If thick enough, it may indent and even displace the crystalline lens and cause progressive astigmatism. The tumor occasionally

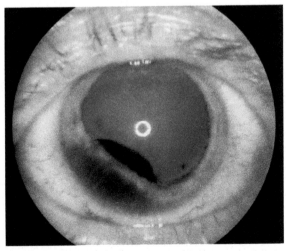

▲ **Figure 7–22.** Darkly melanotic ciliary body melanoma, which has invaded the peripheral iris, with the main portion of the melanoma lying posterior to the iris and indenting the lens.

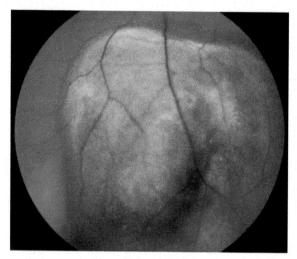

▲ **Figure 7–23.** Primary nonuniformly melanotic choroidal melanoma with dome-shaped configuration.

invades the overlying sclera and extends to the external surface of the eye, where it appears as a dark brown flat to nodular vascularized episcleral mass.

Typically choroidal melanoma is a dark brown to pale golden subretinal mass (Figure 7–23) that, at detection, has a largest basal diameter of at least 7 mm and/or thickness of more than 3 mm. Average largest basal diameter is 12–13 mm, and average thickness is 6–6.5 mm. The most common tumor shape is a dome with round or oval base. The most distinctive shape is a mushroom-like nodule with nodular apical eruption through Bruch's membrane. Occasional choroidal melanomas have a geographic multinodular or diffuse shape.

Ultrasound biomicroscopy (UBM) is useful for determining the size, shape, and precise location of the margins of iris and iridociliary body melanomas prior to planned treatment and for following them after treatment to monitor for regression or local relapse. B-scan ultrasonography is appropriate for determining the size, shape, and intraocular location of choroidal and ciliary body melanomas; identifying scleral invasion and transscleral extension to the orbit; and showing (on dynamic imaging) vascular pulsations within the tumor. It is also useful for monitoring after eye-preserving treatment, such as plaque radiotherapy (brachytherapy) and proton beam irradiation, for regression or relapse.

Patients with primary uveal melanoma are at risk of metastasis, especially to the liver, regardless of how the primary intraocular tumor is managed. Prognostic factors for metastasis and metastatic death include tumor size (larger size unfavorable), location (ciliary body least favorable, iris most favorable), melanocytic cell type (epithelioid least favorable, spindle most favorable), vasculogenic mimicry pattern (complex loops and networks unfavorable), and chromosome 3 status (monosomy unfavorable, disomy favorable) and gene expression profile (Class 2 unfavorable, Class 1 favorable) of tumor cells.

Several different treatment options are available for primary uveal melanomas of different sizes, intraocular locations, and associated clinical features. Enucleation is appropriate for extremely large intraocular tumor, tumor surrounding or invading the optic disk, or an eye that is blind and painful due to the tumor. Iodine-125 (I-125; United States) or ruthenium-106 (Europe) plaque radiotherapy and proton beam irradiation are the most commonly employed treatments for small to relatively large choroidal and ciliary body melanomas. In some centers, they are also being used with increasing frequency instead of iridectomy and iridocyclectomy for many iris and iridociliary melanomas. All three types of radiation therapy usually induce tumor shrinkage, which is sustained long term, but are frequently associated with delayed-onset radiation-induced cataract, retinopathy, and optic neuropathy, and may possibly result in iris neovascularization, neovascular glaucoma, and profound or even total visual loss. Transscleral tumor resection is employed in a few centers for selected ciliary body and choroidal melanomas, almost always in conjunction with preoperative proton beam irradiation or postoperative plaque radiotherapy. Transvitreal endoresection of selected postequatorial choroidal melanomas is undertaken in a few centers, almost always in conjunction with preoperative plaque or proton beam radiation therapy. No prospective comparative clinical trials of surgical resection versus enucleation or plaque radiotherapy have been reported. Transpupillary infrared laser hyperthermia (transpupillary thermotherapy [TTT]) has been used extensively in some centers to treat selected small posterior melanocytic choroidal tumors believed to be melanomas, but as sole therapy, it has largely been abandoned, as was laser photocoagulation before it, because of unacceptably high rates of local tumor relapse and even transscleral tumor extension into the orbit. TTT and laser photocoagulation are still used to supplement plaque radiotherapy in some centers, mainly for juxtapapillary and macular choroidal melanomas. Most iris and iridociliary melanomas are treated by surgical excision (iridectomy, iridocyclectomy) or plaque radiotherapy.

There is no compelling evidence that any method of treatment of primary uveal melanomas improves survival. There are no natural history data of survival in uveal melanoma that encompass the entire spectrum from extremely small asymptomatic lesions of uncertain pathologic nature to frankly malignant tumors filling much or all of the eye. In the absence of such information, there is no valid standard against which to judge effectiveness of any treatment. It has been suggested that the longer survival of patients with smaller tumors at the time of treatment demonstrates that treatment is effective if provided early enough, but there are no comparative clinical trials comparing survival in treated versus untreated primary uveal melanomas of any defined size category.

The Collaborative Ocular Melanoma Study (COMS) in the United States and a number of retrospective but statistically adjusted comparative survival studies have shown that enucleation and I-125 plaque radiotherapy of medium to relatively large choroidal melanomas provide equivalent posttreatment rates of metastasis and mortality. COMS also showed that low-dose fractionated external beam radiation therapy prior to enucleation of large choroidal melanoma did not improve survival compared with enucleation alone.

Metastasis from uveal melanoma is associated with extremely poor survival. Although mean survival is longer if limited metastasis is detected by presymptomatic surveillance than if there is symptomatic, advanced metastasis at detection, there is no evidence that aggressive treatments, such as surgical metastasectomy or hepatic artery infusion chemotherapy, at any stage provide clinically significant improvement in survival. Furthermore, no adjuvant therapy has been shown to prevent or delay metastasis.

▶ Uveal Metastasis of Nonophthalmic Primary Cancer

Nonophthalmic primary cancers can metastasize hematogenously to the uvea. Clinically apparent uveal metastasis typically is off-white to pink to gold (most carcinomas) or to dark brown (skin melanomas). Iris metastasis typically is a progressively enlarging discohesive mass (Figure 7–24) that may be associated with variable blurred vision, ocular pain, signs of intraocular inflammation, and raised intraocular pressure. Choroid metastasis typically is a round to oval dome-shaped mass (Figure 7–25) that is frequently associated with overlying and surrounding exudative subretinal fluid out of proportion to the size of the tumor. Although the most frequent situation is a solitary metastatic tumor in one eye (80% of cases), about 20% of patients will have two or more discrete metastatic tumors in one or both eyes. If left untreated, most uveal metastases enlarge measurably within days to a few weeks.

The nonophthalmic primary cancers that most commonly give rise to clinically detected uveal metastases are breast cancer in women, lung cancer in men, and colon cancer in both groups.

Uveal metastasis from nonophthalmic primary cancer is the most common malignant intraocular neoplasm. In the United States, approximately 25% of all deaths are attributable to cancer. Of these deaths, about 50% are attributable to the effects of metastatic disease. At autopsy, approximately 90% of patients dying of metastatic disease have at least microscopically evident metastatic cells within ocular blood vessels and/or other intraocular tissues, but only about 10% of such patients have uveal tumors that an ophthalmologist might be expected to detect by clinical examination. Many of these patients are likely to have developed their clinically detectable uveal metastatic disease during the final phase of their illness. Only about 50% experience symptoms that prompt clinical evaluation resulting in detection of the uveal metastatic disease.

Because the eye embryologically is an outgrowth of the brain, metastatic tumor to the eye should be regarded as metastasis to the brain. About 20% of patients with a metastatic tumor in one or both eyes will have a concurrent intracranial metastasis detectable by computed tomography or magnetic resonance imaging scan. Uveal metastasis is

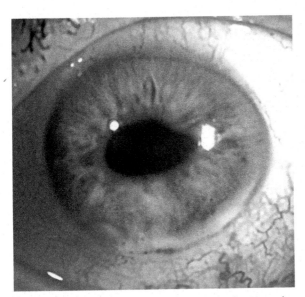

▲ **Figure 7–24.** Multinodular metastasis to the iris and inferior anterior chamber angle from primary lung cancer, causing distortion of the pupil.

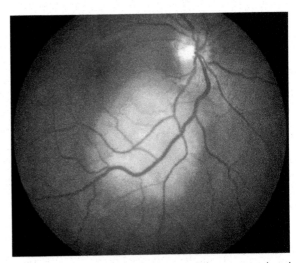

▲ **Figure 7–25.** Unifocal homogeneously creamy colored metastasis to the choroid from primary breast cancer.

associated with very poor survival. The median survival following detection of uveal metastasis is approximately 6 months, ranging from 12 months in breast cancer to 3 months in skin melanoma. Treatment for symptomatic uveal metastasis usually consists of palliative external beam radiation therapy, chemotherapy appropriate to the type of cancer, or both.

Primary Uveal Lymphoma

Primary uveal lymphoma is a relatively uncommon but important subcategory of **primary intraocular lymphoma**. Most cases of primary intraocular lymphoma are characterized by accumulation of malignant lymphoid cells in the vitreous (usually bilaterally), beneath the retinal pigment epithelium, and sometimes within the sensory retina, and are associated with antecedent, concurrent, or subsequent lymphoma in the brain and cerebrospinal fluid (see Primary Vitreoretinal Lymphoma in Chapter 10). Conversely, primary uveal lymphoma is characterized by focal or diffuse infiltration of the uvea, almost always unilaterally, by malignant lymphocytes and occasionally subsequent development of systemic (non–central nervous system) lymphoma. This form of lymphoma bears more similarity to primary conjunctival lymphoma (see Chapter 5) than to primary vitreoretinal lymphoma. Rarely, predominantly vitreoretinal disease can be caused by systemic B-cell lymphoma.

The lymphoid cells infiltrating the uvea in primary uveal lymphoma tend to be more abnormal in morphologic appearance on microscopy than those associated with atypical lymphoid hyperplasia (see above). Germinal centers within the uvea are unlikely, and immunohistochemical staining and flow cytometry tend to show a more monoclonal character to the cells. As in primary vitreoretinal lymphoma, the lymphoid cells are usually of B-cell lineage. Clinically, the uveal infiltrates of primary uveal lymphoma appear as tan to creamy, focal to diffuse infiltrates in the iris or choroid (Figure 7–26). B-scan ultrasonography shows generalized choroidal thickening (sometimes with locally accentuated prominence) in diffuse cases, and ultrasound biomicroscopy confirms the solid soft tissue character of iris and iridociliary infiltrates. The retina usually remains

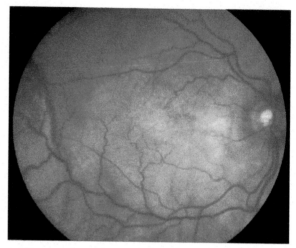

▲ **Figure 7–26.** Diffuse uveal lymphoid infiltration of primary uveal lymphoma, with focal accentuation temporally.

attached or shows limited shallow detachment in areas of choroidal infiltration, but progressive disruption of retinal pigment epithelium overlying the infiltrates develops in many cases. There may be focal or diffuse pink anterior epibulbar masses reminiscent of primary conjunctival lymphoma and/or posterior peribulbar extraocular soft tissue masses that may only be evident on B-scan ultrasonography, but epibulbar lesions are more common in atypical lymphoid hyperplasia (see above).

Treatment of primary uveal lymphoma usually consists of fractionated external beam radiation therapy, typically resulting in prompt, sustained clinical regression. If vision is poor prior to treatment, it may not recover even if all of the uveal infiltrates regress completely. In aggressive, neglected, or misdiagnosed cases, the eye can become blind and painful with congestive features and diffuse intraocular bleeding that can necessitate enucleation. About 20% of patients with primary uveal lymphoma develop systemic lymphoma, so all affected patients should be monitored for systemic disease.

7.3. Sclera
Carlos Pavesio, MD, FRCOphth

The human sclera consists almost entirely of collagen and comprises five-sixths of the outer tunic of the eye, extending from the cornea anteriorly to the optic foramen posteriorly.

The shape is, in part, maintained by the presence of the intraocular contents and the intraocular pressure. However, the sclera must be rigid enough to provide relatively constant conditions for the intraocular pressure so that, when the eyeball is moved, the intraocular pressure does not fluctuate. In addition, the opacity of the sclera ensures that internal light scattering does not affect the retinal image and the sclera must protect the intraocular contents from injury. Conditions that lead to alterations of these properties may result in changes to vision and eventually, in very severe cases, destruction of the globe with significant or total loss of vision.

Apart from potentially being affected by local factors, the sclera may also be involved in systemic conditions and may be the first manifestation of such problems. This makes the role of the ophthalmologist very important in their recognition.

INFLAMMATORY CONDITIONS

1. EPISCLERITIS

The inflammation is localized to the episclera and tends to affect young people, typically in the third and fourth decades of life, and is more prevalent in women. The condition is benign, tends to be recurrent, and is typically self-limiting. It is unilateral in about two-thirds of cases. Although usually lasting for 1–2 weeks, the duration of episcleritis varies widely between individuals.

The onset is almost always sudden, with the eye becoming red and uncomfortable within an hour of the start of the attack. Patients may also report heat, ocular surface discomfort and irritation, and tenderness. In nodular cases, one or more nodules can develop, and the redness tends to progress over a few days, but is always confined to the nodules, which may also become quite tender.

On examination, the inflammation will be limited to the episclera and may be diffuse, involving one or more quadrants as in simple episcleritis (Figure 7–27), or it may be localized in to a small area, which is swollen producing a nodular episcleritis (Figure 7–28). There is no involvement of the underlying sclera, and keratitis and uveitis are uncommon.

In most cases the cause is unknown, but an association with a local or systemic disorder, such as gout, ocular rosacea, atopy, infection, or collagen-vascular disease can be found in up to one-third of the patients.

Even though episcleritis can cause great distress and is unsightly and uncomfortable, there are no long-term complications in simple disease, and in nodular disease, complications are rare and confined to changes in the adjacent cornea and sclera after multiple attacks at the same location.

Many patients become aware of warning symptoms prior to the onset of disease, and in such cases, the frequent use of topical corticosteroids may be beneficial. In the absence of a known etiology, treatment can include the use of chilled artificial tears and eventually topical corticosteroids in more

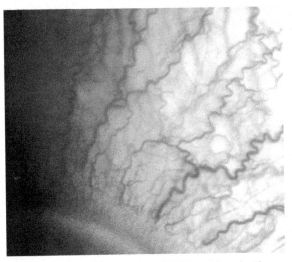

▲ **Figure 7–27. Diffuse episcleritis.** (Reproduced with permission from Watson PG et al, eds. *The Sclera and Systemic Disorders.* 2nd ed. London, England: Butterworth–Heinemann; 2004. Copyright © Elsevier.)

intense cases. Topical nonsteroidal anti-inflammatory drugs (NSAIDs) tend not to be effective. In the presence of a local or systemic disorder, the treatment becomes specific and directed to the underlying condition. In some more resistant cases, the use of oral NSAIDs may be beneficial. The use of systemic corticosteroids is usually restricted to cases associated with an underlying collagen-vascular disease.

2. SCLERITIS

In contrast to episcleritis, scleritis is a much more severe condition, not only because of the intense symptoms, especially pain, but also because it may result in structural damage to

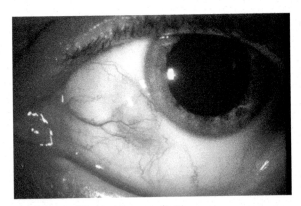

▲ **Figure 7–28. Nodular episcleritis.**

the globe and carries a much stronger association with an underlying condition.

Scleritis is uncommon, accounting for less than a quarter of all scleral disease. The average age of onset is 48 years, with a range of 11–87 years. Patients over the age of 60 years have a greater likelihood of more severe disease and of developing complications including visual loss.

Most often, the inflammatory process is driven primarily by an immunologic response, and less commonly, it can be precipitated by local factors such as trauma or infections (Table 7–7). There is associated systemic disease in up to two-thirds of patients.

Scleritis is one of the very few severely painful eye diseases. However, it is important to remember that even though pain is usually a predominant feature, it may be absent in patients with posterior scleritis and in patients with a unique form of scleral thinning without overt inflammatory features, known as scleromalacia perforans, which usually occurs in association with rheumatoid arthritis. The pain of scleritis is described typically as a deep, boring pain, affecting the periocular bones and often referred to the face, cheek, and jaw as a consequence of involvement of the fifth cranial nerve. The pain typically worsens at night, often waking the patient in the early morning hours, and common

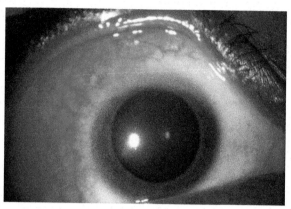

▲ **Figure 7–29.** Anterior diffuse scleritis. (Reproduced with permission from Pavesio C. Scleritis. In: Gupta A, Gupta V, Herbort CP, Khairallah M, eds. *Uveitis Text and Imaging*. New Delhi, India: Jaypee Brothers Medical Publishers Ltd; 2009.) See color insert.

analgesics typically offer little symptomatic relief. Other symptoms can include photophobia and reduction of vision.

Anterior scleritis may show different degrees of severity. A key clinical sign is deep violaceous discoloration of the globe due to dilation of the deep episcleral plexus, which can be diffuse or nodular. Diffuse (Figure 7–29) and nodular (Figure 7–30) diseases are less severe in terms of response to therapy and complications and also tend to occur in younger individuals. Necrotizing disease is much more aggressive. It tends to occur in older patients and may present with typical inflammatory features, when it is known as

Table 7–7. Causes of Scleritis

Autoimmune diseases
Rheumatoid arthritis
Granulomatosis with polyangiitis
Relapsing polychondritis
Polyarteritis nodosa
Systemic lupus erythematosus
Ulcerative colitis
Psoriatic arthritis
IgA nephropathy

Infections
Tuberculosis
Atypical *Mycobacterium*
Syphilis
Leprosy
Herpes simplex
Herpes zoster
Pseudomonas
Staphylococcus
Streptococcus

Others
Sarcoidosis
Physical agents (irradiation, thermal burns)
Chemical agents (alkali or acid burns)
Mechanical causes (trauma, surgery)
Lymphoma
Rosacea
Gout

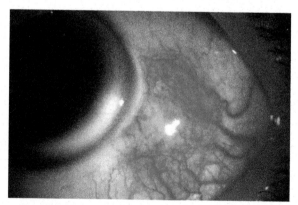

▲ **Figure 7–30.** Anterior nodular scleritis. (Reproduced with permission from Pavesio C. Scleritis. In: Gupta A, Gupta V, Herbort CP, Khairallah M, eds. *Uveitis Text and Imaging*. New Delhi, India: Jaypee Brothers Medical Publishers (P) Ltd; 2009.)

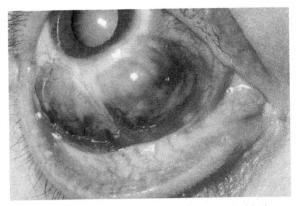

▲ **Figure 7–31.** Scleromalacia perforans in an elderly woman with rheumatoid arthritis.

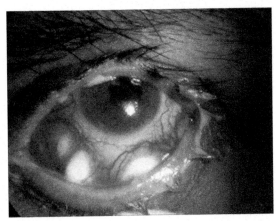

▲ **Figure 7–33.** Necrotizing scleritis following pars plana vitrectomy.

necrotizing scleritis, or without any overt clinical features of inflammation (scleromalacia perforans) (Figure 7–31). Up to two-thirds of patients with the necrotizing scleritis have an underlying systemic disease, and either form may result in staphyloma formation (Figure 7–32). Surgically induced necrotizing scleritis (SINS) is a type of necrotizing scleritis triggered by surgical procedures, especially those involving scleral intervention or the local use of antimetabolites (Figure 7–33).

Complications of anterior scleritis include increased transparency of the sclera, staphyloma formation, corneal thinning and vascularization, uveitis, and elevation of intraocular pressure. All are more common in the necrotizing forms of the disease. Visual loss may occur as a consequence of direct corneal involvement, astigmatism due to the loss of scleral support, cataract, uveitis, or glaucoma.

Posterior scleritis, which involves the nonvisible portion of the sclera, is a serious, potentially blinding condition that tends to be underdiagnosed and is often treated late. The manifestations include pain, which is not always present; visual disturbance in the form of blurring or distortion, sometimes due to induced myopia; and hypertropia and/or diplopia due to involvement of extraocular muscles. There may be severe visual loss due to macular or optic nerve involvement, but it is not possible to predict in which cases such progression will occur.

Possible other more obvious manifestations include proptosis, choroidal folds (Figure 7–34), fundus mass, exudative

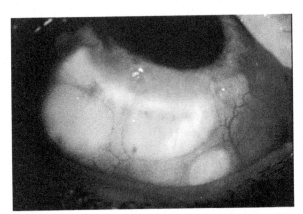

▲ **Figure 7–32.** Necrotizing scleritis resulting in staphyloma. (Reproduced with permission from Pavesio C. Scleritis. In: Gupta A, Gupta V, Herbort CP, Khairallah M, eds. *Uveitis Text and Imaging.* New Delhi, India: Jaypee Brothers Medical Publishers (P) Ltd; 2009.)

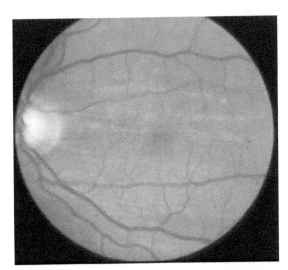

▲ **Figure 7–34.** Posterior scleritis with choroidal folds and optic disk swelling. (Reproduced with permission from Watson PG et al, eds. *The Sclera and Systemic Disorders.* 2nd ed. London, England: Butterworth-Heinemann; 2004. Copyright © Elsevier.)

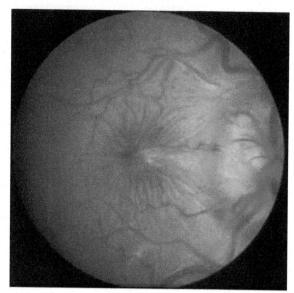

△ **Figure 7–35.** Posterior scleritis with optic disk swelling and retinal folds involving the macula. (Reproduced with permission from Watson PG et al, eds. *The Sclera and Systemic Disorders.* 2nd ed. London, England: Butterworth Heinemann; 2004. Copyright © Elsevier.)

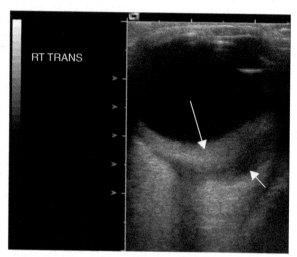

△ **Figure 7–36.** B-scan ultrasonography demonstrating scleral thickening **(arrow)** and fluid in the posterior sub-Tenon's space **(arrowhead).**

retinal detachment, and optic disk swelling (Figure 7–35). Posterior scleritis can be very difficult to diagnose clinically, and the diagnosis can be confirmed or, in some cases, first suggested by the detection of thickening of the posterior coats of the eye by ultrasonography or computed tomography. Posterior scleritis needs to be differentiated from other causes of choroidal thickening. The presence of fluid in sub-Tenon's space is usually quite helpful (Figure 7–36).

The most frequent causes of scleritis are listed in Table 7–7. Infectious causes of scleritis are much less common, and most cases are associated with trauma or surgical procedures, especially retinal detachment surgery with scleral buckle placement, or occur in patients with an active systemic infection. Investigations are usually guided by the medical history.

Management decisions depend on the type of presentation and risk of complications. Anterior diffuse and nodular scleritis tend to respond well to a systemic NSAID, and options include indomethacin, 75 mg daily; ibuprofen, 600 mg daily; or flurbiprofen, 300 mg daily. In most cases, pain will respond quite quickly, which is a good indication that the treatment is effective. In cases where there is no response after 2 weeks of therapy, treatment can be increased to include the use of systemic corticosteroids. Topical corticosteroids can be used mainly to improve control of symptoms or to treat associated anterior uveitis, but they have little effect on the course of the scleral inflammation.

In cases of necrotizing disease, initial treatment should be oral corticosteroids, usually prednisolone 1 mg/kg/d. Frequently, an additional immunosuppressant becomes necessary. Intravenous methylprednisolone, 1 g per day for 3 consecutive days, is occasionally needed in severe cases. Cyclophosphamide is a useful agent in necrotizing disease, especially cases associated with granulomatosis with polyangiitis, and may induce disease remission. Other useful agents include azathioprine, mycophenolate mofetil, and, less frequently, cyclosporine A. The treatment of posterior scleritis follows the same principles of treatment as for severe anterior scleritis. The use of biologics, especially anti-TNF agents, is also becoming an option in cases of refractory scleritis.

Surgical intervention should be reserved for cases of scleral or corneal perforation to preserve integrity of the globe.

Infectious scleritis is rare. It is classified as exogenous, which is the more common type and includes posttraumatic and postsurgical infections as well as extension of infections arising in adjacent structures, particularly the cornea, or endogenously, such as syphilis and tuberculosis. The infection may be bacterial, fungal, viral, or parasitic. The clinical presentation may be similar to noninfectious scleritis, leading to delayed recognition. Specimens obtained by scrapings are stained with Gram and Giemsa stains and cultured on blood, chocolate, and Sabouraud agars and in brain-heart and thioglycolate broths. However, scleral biopsy is frequently necessary to establish the correct diagnosis. Molecular methods such as polymerase chain reaction are also useful.

Empirical aggressive topical, subconjunctival, and systemic antimicrobial therapy is commenced immediately and adjusted according to the results of stains and cultures. Prolonged therapy is usually required. Steroid therapy may be helpful but needs to be avoided in *Pseudomonas* and fungal infections.

OTHER AFFECTIONS OF THE SCLERA

1. NONINFLAMMATORY THINNING OF THE SCLERA

The sclera may be thinned as a result of dysgenesis or disease. Ectasia is when the sclera alone becomes stretched, whereas involvement of both the sclera and the underlying uveal tissue is more properly termed a staphyloma.

A. Congenital Anomalies

Colobomas of the sclera are rare, but occasionally, the sclera fuses incompletely during development, leaving a large ectatic area inferior to the disk, invariably accompanied by uveal tract and retinal colobomas. In peripapillary ectasia, the entire area around the disk bulges outward. Ectasia of the anterior sclera is rare.

B. Acquired Ectasia

Prolonged elevation of intraocular pressure early in infancy, as may occur with congenital glaucoma, can lead to stretching and thinning of the sclera. Buphthalmos is the term used to describe these very large eyes.

C. Staphyloma

This is the term used for ectatic sclera that has become attached to the underlying uvea. Staphylomas may occur following severe scleritis or uveitis (Figure 7–37) and may be anterior, equatorial, or posterior. Anterior staphylomas, located anterior to the equator, are termed calary when they are over the ciliary body and intercalary when they are between the ciliary body and the limbus. They most probably result from a combination of inflammation and high intraocular pressure. They can also develop following surgery, such as trabeculectomy. The majority of posterior staphyloma develop as a result of pathological myopia, but they can also result from congenital, infective, and inflammatory disorders.

3. NONINFLAMMATORY THICKENING OF THE SCLERA

A. Nanophthalmos

This happens when the eye develops normally until the embryonic fissure has closed, but then grows very slowly in all dimensions, resulting in a very small eye and consequently high hyperopia. With age, these individuals are prone to develop acute angle closure, because the crystalline lens has a normal size and continues to grow normally. There is also a risk of uveal effusion syndrome.

B. Idiopathic

Abnormal thickening of the posterior coats of the eye can be demonstrated by ultrasonography in some patients without any evidence of inflammation and without resulting in visual loss.

REFERENCES

Uveitis

Abbouda A et al: Psoriasis and psoriatic arthritis-related uveitis: Different ophthalmological manifestations and ocular inflammation features. Semin Ophthalmol 2016 Jul 15:1. [Epub ahead of print] [PMID: 27419848]

Abusamra K et al: Intraocular lymphoma: Descriptive data of 26 patients including clinico-pathologic features, vitreous findings, and treatment outcomes. Ocul Immunol Inflamm 2016 Jul 20:1. [Epub ahead of print] [PMID: 27438792]

Accorinti M et al: Cytomegalovirus anterior uveitis: Long-term follow-up of immunocompetent patients. Graefes Arch Clin Exp Ophthalmol 2014;252:1817. [PMID: 25138606]

Arantes TE et al: Ocular involvement following postnatally acquired *Toxoplasma gondii* infection in Southern Brazil: A 28-year experience. Am J Ophthalmol 2015;159:1002. [PMID: 25743338]

Azad S et al: Pars plana vitrectomy with in vivo cyst lysis for intraocular cysticercosis. Ophthalmic Surg Lasers Imaging Retina 2016;47:665. [PMID: 27434899]

Aziz HA et al: Sympathetic ophthalmia: Clinicopathologic correlation in a consecutive case series. Retina 2015;35:1696. [PMID: 25719985]

Breazzano MP et al: Features of cutaneous malignant melanoma metastatic to the retina and vitreous. Ocul Oncol Pathol 2015;2:80. [PMID: 27172390]

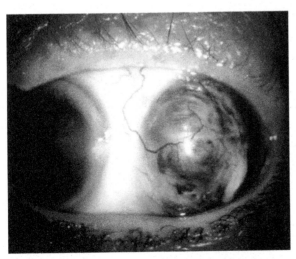

▲ **Figure 7–37.** Large temporal staphyloma following scleritis.

Bustillo JL et al: Cuban Ocular Toxoplasmosis Epidemiology Study (COTES): Incidence and prevalence of ocular toxoplasmosis in Central Cuba. Br J Ophthalmol 2015;99:382. [PMID: 25253767]

Chen SC et al: Patterns and etiologies of uveitis at a tertiary referral center in Taiwan. Ocul Immunol Inflamm 2016 Jul 27:1. [Epub ahead of print] [PMID: 27463023]

Ching Wen Ho D et al: A review of the role of intravitreal corticosteroids as an adjuvant to antibiotics in infectious endophthalmitis. Ocul Immunol Inflamm 2016 Nov 16:1. [Epub ahead of print] [PMID: 27849402]

Cho H et al: Endogenous endophthalmitis in the American and Korean population: An 8-year retrospective study. Ocul Immunol Inflamm 2016 Jul 26:1-8. [Epub ahead of print] [PMID: 27459423]

Chocron IM et al: Ophthalmic manifestations of relapsing acute childhood leukemia. J AAPOS 2015;19:284. [PMID: 25890837]

Cimino L et al: Vitreoretinal lymphomas misdiagnosed as uveitis: Lessons learned from a case series. Indian J Ophthalmol 2016;64:369. [PMID: 27380976]

Clarke SLN et al: Juvenile idiopathic arthritis-associated uveitis. Pediatr Rheumatol Online J 2016;14:27. [PMID: 27121190]

Couto C et al: Chronic anterior uveitis in children. Ocul Immunol Inflamm 2016;24:392. [PMID: 27191963]

Crawford CM et al: A review of the inflammatory chorioretinopathies: The white dot syndromes. ISRN Inflamm 2013;2013:783190. [PMID: 24294536]

Cunningham ET Jr et al: Necrotizing herpetic retinitis. Ocul Immunol Inflamm 2014;22:167. [PMID: 24856278]

Cunningham ET Jr et al: Uveitis in children and adolescents. Ocul Immunol Inflamm 2016;24:365. [PMID: 27471956]

D'Ambrosio EM et al: Clinical features and complications of the HLA-B27-associated acute anterior uveitis: A metanalysis. Semin Ophthalmol. 2016 Jul 12:1. [Epub ahead of print] [PMID: 27404944]

Despreaux R et al: Ocular toxocariasis: Clinical features and long-term visual outcomes in adult patients. Am J Ophthalmol 2016;166:162. [PMID: 27066722]

Diaz RI et al: Ocular histoplasmosis syndrome. Surv Ophthalmol 2015;60:279. [PMID: 25841248]

Dick AD et al: Risk of ocular complications in patients with noninfectious intermediate uveitis, posterior uveitis, or panuveitis. Ophthalmology 2016;123:655. [PMID: 26712559]

Durand ML: Endophthalmitis. Clin Microbiol Infect 2013;19:227. [PMID: 23438028]

Fend F et al: How we diagnose and treat vitreoretinal lymphoma. Br J Haematol 2016;173:680. [PMID: 27133587]

Gao F et al: Clinical patterns of uveitis in a tertiary center in North China. Ocul Immunol Inflamm. 2016 Apr 12:1. [Epub ahead of print] [PMID: 27070829]

Gupta A et al: Microbiology and visual outcomes of culture-positive bacterial endophthalmitis in Oxford, UK. Graefes Arch Clin Exp Ophthalmol 2014;252:1825. [PMID: 25028312]

Haake DA et al: Leptospirosis in humans. Curr Top Microbiol Immunol 2015;387:65. [PMID: 25388133]

Harrell M et al: Current treatment of toxoplasma retinochoroiditis: An evidence-based review. J Ophthalmol 2014;2014:273506. [PMID: 25197557]

Horneff G et al: Comparison of treatment response, remission rate and drug adherence in polyarticular juvenile idiopathic arthritis patients treated with etanercept, adalimumab or tocilizumab. Arthritis Res Ther 2016;18:272. [PMID: 27881144]

Jackson TL et al: Systematic review of 342 cases of endogenous bacterial endophthalmitis. Surv Ophthalmol 2014;59:627. [PMID: 25113611]

Jijelava KP et al: Diffuse anterior retinoblastoma: A review. Saudi J Ophthalmol 2013;27:135. [PMID: 24227977]

Johnson JS et al: A 25-year-old man with exudative retinal detachments and infiltrates without hematological or neurological findings found to have relapsed precursor T-cell acute lymphoblastic leukemia. Case Rep Ophthalmol 2015;6:321. [PMID: 26483676]

Jones JL et al: Follow-up of the 1977 Georgia outbreak of toxoplasmosis. Am J Trop Med Hyg 2016;94:1299. [PMID: 27044565]

Kashani AH et al: The emergence of Klebsiella pneumoniae endogenous endophthalmitis in the USA: Basic and clinical advances. J Ophthalmic Inflamm Infect 2013;3:28. [PMID: 23514342]

Keino H et al: Clinical features of uveitis in children and adolescents at a tertiary referral centre in Tokyo. Br J Ophthalmol 2016 Jun 22. [Epub ahead of print] [PMID: 27335142]

Kempen JH et al: Remission of intermediate uveitis: Incidence and predictive factors. Am J Ophthalmol 2016;164:110. [PMID: 26772874]

Khan S et al: Pediatric infectious endophthalmitis: A review. J Pediatr Ophthalmol Strabismus 2014;51:140. [PMID: 24877526]

Kim DY et al: Recent clinical manifestation and prognosis of fungal endophthalmitis: A 7-year experience at a tertiary referral center in Korea. J Korean Med Sci 2015;30:960. [PMID: 26130961]

Kim M et al: Anti-TNFα treatment for HLA-B27 positive ankylosing spondylitis-related uveitis. Am J Ophthalmol 2016;170:32. [PMID: 27470062]

Kitazawa K et al: Diffuse anterior retinoblastoma with sarcoidosis-like nodule. Case Rep Ophthalmol 2015;6:443. [PMID: 26955346]

Knickelbein JE et al: Multimodal imaging of the white dot syndromes and related diseases. J Clin Exp Ophthalmol 2016;7:570. [PMID: 27482471]

Kopplin LJ et al: Review for disease of the year: Epidemiology of HLA-B27 associated ocular disorders. Ocul Immunol Inflamm 2016;24:470. [PMID: 27232197]

Legendre M et al: Clinicopathologic characteristics, treatment, and outcomes of tubulointerstitial nephritis and uveitis syndrome in adults: A national retrospective strobe-compliant study. Medicine (Baltimore) 2016;95:e3964. [PMID: 27367994]

Lim HW et al: Endogenous endophthalmitis in the Korean population: A six-year retrospective study. Retina 2014;34:592. [PMID: 24056527]

Mahajan S et al: Clinical characteristics of primary vitreoretinal lymphoma in an Indian population. Ocul Immunol Inflamm 2016 Mar 22:1. [Epub ahead of print] [PMID: 27003620]

Mehta S et al: Outcomes of cataract surgery in patients with uveitis: A systematic review and meta-analysis. Am J Ophthalmol 2014;158:676. [PMID: 24983790]

Minos E et al: Birdshot chorioretinopathy: Current knowledge and new concepts in pathophysiology, diagnosis, monitoring and treatment. Orphanet J Rare Dis 2016;11:61. [PMID: 27175923]

Mohammadi Z et al: Ocular manifestations in a child with systemic brucellosis. J Res Med Sci 2014;19:677. [PMID: 25364370]

Moradi A et al: Risk of hypotony in juvenile idiopathic arthritis (JIA)-associated uveitis. Am J Ophthalmol 2016;169:113. [PMID: 27345732]

Mustafa OM et al: Hypopyon and Klebsiella sepsis. N Engl J Med 2016;374:e33. [PMID: 27355556]

Nagashima T et al: Three cases of tubulointerstitial nephritis and uveitis syndrome with different clinical manifestations. Int Ophthalmol 2016 Aug 10. [Epub ahead of print] [PMID: 27511057]

Northey LC et al: Syphilitic uveitis and optic neuritis in Sydney, Australia. Br J Ophthalmol 2015;99:1215. [PMID: 25788666]

O'Keefe GA et al: Vogt-Koyanagi-Harada disease. Surv Ophthalmol 2017;62:1. [PMID: 27241814]

Olsen TG et al: The association between multiple sclerosis and uveitis. Surv Ophthalmol 2017;62:89. [PMID: 27491475]

Oray M et al: Fulminant ocular toxoplasmosis: The hazards of corticosteroid monotherapy. Ocul Immunol Inflamm 2016;24:637. [PMID: 26647176]

Oray M et al: Ocular morbidities of juvenile idiopathic arthritis-associated uveitis in adulthood: Results from a tertiary center study. Graefes Arch Clin Exp Ophthalmol 2016;254:1841. [PMID: 27084082]

Ozdal PC et al: Pars planitis: Epidemiology, clinical characteristics, management and visual prognosis. J Ophthalmic Vis Res 2015;10:469. [PMID: 27051493]

Patel AK et al: Risk of retinal neovascularization in cases of uveitis. Ophthalmology 2016;123:646. [PMID: 26686964]

Patel AV et al: Unilateral eye findings: A rare herald of acute leukemia. Ocul Oncol Pathol 2016;2:166. [PMID: 27239459]

Patel SN et al: Endogenous endophthalmitis associated with intravenous drug abuse. Retina 2014;34:1460. [PMID: 24418848]

Pathanapitoon K et al: Clinical spectrum of HLA-B27-associated ocular inflammation. Ocul Immunol Inflamm 2016 Jul 18:1. [Epub ahead of print] [PMID: 27428361]

Pathanapitoon K et al: Looking for ocular tuberculosis: Prevalence and clinical manifestations of patients with uveitis and positive QuantiFERON/TB Gold Test. Ocul Immunol Inflamm. 2016 Nov 16:1. [Epub ahead of print] [PMID: 27849401]

Paulus YM et al: Prospective trial of endogenous fungal endophthalmitis and chorioretinitis rates, clinical course, and outcomes in patients with fungemia. Retina 2016;36:1357. [PMID: 26655621]

Phatak S et al: Controversies in intraocular lens implantation in pediatric uveitis. J Ophthalmic Inflamm Infect 2016;6:12. [PMID: 27009616]

Pradhan E et al: Antibiotics versus no treatment for toxoplasma retinochoroiditis. Cochrane Database Syst Rev 2016;5:CD002218. [PMID: 27198629]

Raja H et al: Ocular manifestations of tick-borne diseases. Surv Ophthalmol 2016;61:726. [PMID: 27060746]

Ratra D et al: Endogenous endophthalmitis: A 10-year retrospective study at a tertiary hospital in South India. Asia Pac J Ophthalmol (Phila) 2015;4:286. [PMID: 26181589]

Reich M et al: Influence of drug therapy on the risk of recurrence of ocular toxoplasmosis. Br J Ophthalmol 2016;100:195. [PMID: 26163541]

Reichstein D. Primary vitreoretinal lymphoma: An update on pathogenesis, diagnosis and treatment. Curr Opin Ophthalmol 2016;27:177. [PMID: 26859131]

Rishi E et al: Syphilitic uveitis as the presenting feature of HIV. Indian J Ophthalmol 2016;64:149. [PMID: 27050352]

Sadiq MA et al: Endogenous endophthalmitis: diagnosis, management, and prognosis. J Ophthalmic Inflamm Infect 2015;5:32. [PMID: 26525563]

Schaftenaar E et al: Uveitis is predominantly of infectious origin in a high HIV and TB prevalence setting in rural South Africa. Br J Ophthalmol 2016;100:1312. [PMID: 27307174]

Schwartzman S: Advancements in the management of uveitis. Best Pract Res Clin Rheumatol 2016;30:304. [PMID: 27886802]

Shah JS et al: Tubercular uveitis with ocular manifestation as the first presentation of tuberculosis: A case series. J Clin Diagn Res 2016;10:NR01. [PMID: 27134908]

Shah M et al: Endophthalmitis caused by nontuberculous mycobacterium: Clinical features, antimicrobial susceptibilities, and treatment outcomes. Am J Ophthalmol 2016;168:150. [PMID: 27048999]

Sharma S et al: Endophthalmitis patients seen in a tertiary eye care centre in Odisha: A clinico-microbiological analysis. Indian J Med Res 2014;139:91. [PMID: 24604043]

Siak J et al: The pattern of uveitis among Chinese, Malays, and Indians in Singapore. Ocul Immunol Inflamm 2016 Jul 15:1. [Epub ahead of print] [PMID: 27419535]

Silpa-Archa S et al: Birdshot retinochoroidopathy: Differences in clinical characteristics between patients with early and late age of onset. Ocul Immunol Inflamm 2016 Apr 12:1. [Epub ahead of print] [PMID: 27070723]

Silpa-Archa S et al: Vogt-Koyanagi-Harada syndrome: Perspectives for immunogenetics, multimodal imaging, and therapeutic options. Autoimmun Rev 2016;15:809. [PMID: 27060382]

Silveira C et al: Ocular involvement following an epidemic of Toxoplasma gondii infection in Santa Isabel do Ivaí, Brazil. Am J Ophthalmol 2015;159:1013. [PMID: 25743340]

Steeples LR et al: Staphylococcal endogenous endophthalmitis in association with pyogenic vertebral osteomyelitis. Eye (Lond) 2016;30:152. [PMID: 26449198]

Suelves AM et al: Nuclear cataract as an early predictive factor for recalcitrant juvenile idiopathic arthritis-associated uveitis. J AAPOS 2016;20:232. [PMID: 27164426]

Sun L et al: Risk factors of uveitis in ankylosing spondylitis: An observational study. Medicine (Baltimore) 2016;95:e4233. [PMID: 27428230]

Teussink MM et al: Multimodal imaging of the disease progression of birdshot chorioretinopathy. Acta Ophthalmol 2016;94:815. [PMID: 27230297]

Tranos P et al: Current perspectives of prophylaxis and management of acute infective endophthalmitis. Adv Ther 2016;33:7276. [PMID: 26935830]

Tsirouki T et al: A focus on the epidemiology of uveitis. Ocul Immunol Inflamm 2016 Jul 28:1. [Epub ahead of print] [PMID: 27467180]

Tsuboi M et al: Prognosis of ocular syphilis in patients infected with HIV in the antiretroviral therapy era. Sex Transm Infect 2016;92:605. [PMID: 27044266]

Vaziri K et al: Endophthalmitis: State of the art. Clin Ophthalmol 2015;9:95. [PMID: 25609911]

Vilela RC et al: Etiological agents of fungal endophthalmitis: Diagnosis and management. Int Ophthalmol 2014;34:707. [PMID: 24081913]

Woo JH et al: Characteristics of cytomegalovirus uveitis in immunocompetent patients. Ocul Immunol Inflamm 2015;23:378. [PMID: 25207970]

Yalçındağ FN et al: Demographic and clinical characteristics of uveitis in Turkey: The first National Registry report. Ocul Immunol Inflamm 2016 Jul 28:1. [Epub ahead of print] [PMID: 27467500]

Zagora SL et al: Etiology and clinical features of ocular inflammatory diseases in a tertiary referral centre in Sydney, Australia. Ocul Immunol Inflamm 2016 Nov 30:1. [Epub ahead of print] [PMID: 27901620]

Zhang R et al: Clinical manifestations and treatment outcomes of syphilitic uveitis in a Chinese population. J Ophthalmol 2016;2016:2797028. [PMID: 27144014]

Uveal Tumors

Afshar AR et al: Uveal melanoma: Evidence for efficacy of therapy. Int Ophthalmol Clin 2015;55:23. [PMID: 25436491]

Alameddine RM et al: Review of choroidal osteomas. Middle East Afr J Ophthalmol 2014;21:244. [PMID: 25100910]

Al-Jamal RT et al: The Pediatric Choroidal and Ciliary Body Melanoma Study: A survey by the European Ophthalmic Oncology Group. Ophthalmology 2016;123:898. [PMID: 26854035]

Andreoli MT et al: Epidemiological trends in uveal melanoma. Br J Ophthalmol 2015;99:1550. [PMID: 25904122]

Arepalli S et al: Choroidal metastases: Origin, features, and therapy. Indian J Ophthalmol 2015;63:122. [PMID: 25827542]

Aronow ME et al: Uveal lymphoma: clinical features, diagnostic studies, treatment selection, and outcomes. Ophthalmology 2014;121:334. [PMID: 24144449]

Aziz HA et al: Vision loss following episcleral brachytherapy for uveal melanoma: Development of a vision prognostication tool. JAMA Ophthalmol 2016;134:615. [PMID: 27101414]

Ben-Shabat I et al: Long-term follow-up evaluation of 68 patients with uveal melanoma liver metastases treated with isolated hepatic perfusion. Ann Surg Oncol 2016;23:1327. [PMID: 26628434]

Biewald E et al: Endoresection of large uveal melanomas: Clinical results in a consecutive series of 200 cases. Br J Ophthalmol 2016 Apr 27. [Epub ahead of print] [PMID: 27121095]

Chattopadhyay C et al: Uveal melanoma: From diagnosis to treatment and the science in between. Cancer 2016;122:2299. [PMID: 26991400]

Choudhary MM et al: Uveal melanoma: Evidence for adjuvant therapy. Int Ophthalmol Clin 2015;55:45. [PMID: 25436492]

Correa ZM. Assessing prognosis in uveal melanoma. Cancer Control 2016;23:93. [PMID: 27218785]

Gokhale R et al: Diagnostic fine-needle aspiration biopsy for iris melanoma. Asia Pac J Ophthalmol (Phila) 2015;4:89. [PMID: 26065351]

Hau SC et al: Evaluation of iris and iridociliary body lesions with anterior segment optical coherence tomography versus ultrasound B-scan. Br J Ophthalmol 2015;99:81. [PMID: 25091953]

Kaliki S et al: Uveal melanoma: Estimating prognosis. Indian J Ophthalmol 2015;63:93. [PMID: 25827538]

Kamran SC et al: Outcomes of proton therapy for the treatment of uveal metastases. Int J Radiat Oncol Biol Phys 2014;90:1044. [PMID: 25442038]

Kivelä T. Diagnosis of uveal melanoma. Dev Ophthalmol 2012;49:1. [PMID: 22042009]

Klingenstein A et al: Quality of life in the follow-up of uveal melanoma patients after enucleation in comparison to CyberKnife treatment. Graefes Arch Clin Exp Ophthalmol 2016;254:1005. [PMID: 26573389]

Lee E et al: Optic disc melanocytoma report of 5 patients from Singapore with a review of the literature. Asia Pac J Ophthalmol (Phila) 2015;4:273. [PMID: 26181587]

Moser JC et al: The Mayo Clinic experience with the use of kinase inhibitors, ipilimumab, bevacizumab, and local therapies in the treatment of metastatic uveal melanoma. Melanoma Res 2015;25:59. [PMID: 25396683]

Nathan P et al: Uveal melanoma UK national guidelines. Eur J Cancer 2015;51:2404. [PMID: 26278648]

Nichols EE et al: Disparities in uveal melanoma: Patient characteristics. Semin Ophthalmol 2016;31:296. [PMID: 27128153]

Rishi P et al: Using risk factors for detection and prognostication of uveal melanoma. Indian J Ophthalmol 2015;63:110. [PMID: 25827540]

Rishi P et al: Biopsy techniques for intraocular tumors. Indian J Ophthalmol 2016;64:415. [PMID: 27488148]

Salomão DR et al: Vitreoretinal presentation of secondary large B-cell lymphoma in patients with systemic lymphoma. JAMA Ophthalmol 2013;131:1151. [PMID: 23744124]

Schuermeyer I et al: Depression, anxiety, and regret before and after testing to estimate uveal melanoma prognosis. JAMA Ophthalmol 2016;134:51. [PMID: 26539659]

Schwab C et al: New insights into oculodermal nevogenesis and proposal for a new iris nevus classification. Br J Ophthalmol 2015;99:644. [PMID: 25359901]

Seibel I et al: Predictive risk factors for radiation retinopathy and optic neuropathy after proton beam therapy for uveal melanoma. Graefes Arch Clin Exp Ophthalmol 2016;254:1787. [PMID: 27376824]

Sellam A et al: Fine needle aspiration biopsy in uveal melanoma: Technique, complications, and outcomes. Am J Ophthalmol 2016;162:28. [PMID: 26556006]

Shields CL et al: Iris nevus growth into melanoma: Analysis of 1611 consecutive eyes: The ABCDEF guide. Ophthalmology 2013;120:766. [PMID: 23290981]

Shields CL et al: Choroidal melanoma: Clinical features, classification, and top 10 pseudomelanomas. Curr Opin Ophthalmol 2014;25:177. [PMID: 24614143]

Shields CL et al: Prognosis of uveal melanoma based on race in 8100 patients: The 2015 Doyne Lecture. Eye (Lond) 2015;29:1027. [PMID: 26248525]

Shields JA et al: Management of posterior uveal melanoma: Past, present, and future: The 2014 Charles L. Schepens lecture. Ophthalmology 2015;122:414. [PMID: 25439690]

Shields CL et al: American Joint Committee on Cancer classification of uveal melanoma (anatomic stage) predicts prognosis in 7,731 patients: The 2013 Zimmerman Lecture. Ophthalmology 2015;122:1180. [PMID: 25813452]

Shields CL et al: Melanoma of the eye: Revealing hidden secrets, one at a time. Clin Dermatol 2015;33:183. [PMID: 25704938]

Sikuade MJ et al: Outcomes of treatment with stereotactic radiosurgery or proton beam therapy for choroidal melanoma. Eye (Lond) 2015;29:1194. [PMID: 26160531]

Singh AD. Prognostication of uveal melanoma: A work in progress. JAMA Ophthalmol 2016;134:740. [PMID: 27124594]

Singh AD et al: Fine-needle aspiration biopsy of uveal melanoma: Outcomes and complications. Br J Ophthalmol 2016;100:456. [PMID: 26231747]

Takiar V et al: A choice of radionuclide: Comparative outcomes and toxicity of ruthenium-106 and iodine-125 in the definitive treatment of uveal melanoma. Pract Radiat Oncol 2015;5:e169. [PMID: 25423888]

Tarmann L et al: Ruthenium-106 plaque brachytherapy for uveal melanoma. Br J Ophthalmol 2015;99:1644. [PMID: 25979763]

Triozzi PL et al: Adjuvant therapy of uveal melanoma: Current status. Ocul Oncol Pathol 2014;1:54. [PMID: 27175362]

Turcotte S et al: Primary transpupillary thermotherapy for choroidal indeterminate melanocytic lesions. Can J Ophthalmol 2014;49:464. [PMID: 25284104]

Verma V et al: Clinical outcomes of proton radiotherapy for uveal melanoma. Clin Oncol (R Coll Radiol) 2016;28:e17. [PMID: 26915706]

Weis E et al: Management of uveal melanoma: A consensus-based provincial clinical practice guideline. Curr Oncol 2016;23:e57. [PMID: 26966414]

Sclera

Al Barqi M et al: Clinical features and visual outcomes of scleritis patients presented to tertiary care eye centers in Saudi Arabia. Int J Ophthalmol 2015;8:1215. [PMID: 26682176]

Bernauer W et al: Five-year outcome in immune-mediated scleritis. Graefes Arch Clin Exp Ophthalmol 2014;252:1477. [PMID: 25007956]

Cao JH et al: Rituximab in the treatment of refractory noninfectious scleritis. Am J Ophthalmol 2016;164:22. [PMID: 26766304]

Das S et al: Postoperative necrotizing scleritis: A report of four cases. Middle East Afr J Ophthalmol. 2014;21:350. [PMID: 25371644]

Diaz JD et al: Treatment and management of scleral disorders. Surv Ophthalmol 2016 Jun 15. [Epub ahead of print] [PMID: 27318032]

Diogo MC et al: CT and MR imaging in the diagnosis of scleritis. AJNR Am J Neuroradiol 2016;37:2334. [PMID: 27444937]

Doshi RR et al: The spectrum of postoperative scleral necrosis. Surv Ophthalmol 2013;58:620. [PMID: 23410842]

Fénolland JR et al: Syphilitic scleritis. Ocul Immunol Inflamm 2016;24:93. [PMID: 24833404]

Gonzalez-Gonzalez LA et al: Clinical features and presentation of infectious scleritis from herpes viruses: A report of 35 cases. Ophthalmology 2012;119:1460. [PMID: 22463821]

González-López JJ et al: Bilateral posterior scleritis: Analysis of 18 cases from a large cohort of posterior scleritis. Ocul Immunol Inflamm 2016;24:16. [PMID: 26471249]

Ho YF et al: Infectious scleritis in Taiwan: A 10-year review in a tertiary-care hospital. Cornea 2014;33:838. [PMID: 24977990]

Hodson KL et al: Epidemiology and visual outcomes in patients with infectious scleritis. Cornea 2013;32:466. [PMID: 22902495]

Lavric A et al: Posterior scleritis: Analysis of epidemiology, clinical factors, and risk of recurrence in a cohort of 114 patients. Ocul Immunol Inflamm 2016;24:6. [PMID: 26134101]

Oray M et al: Diagnosis and management of non-infectious immune-mediated scleritis: Current status and future prospects. Expert Rev Clin Immunol 2016;12:827. [PMID: 27055583]

Pradhan ZS et al: Infectious scleritis: Clinical spectrum and management outcomes in India. Indian J Ophthalmol 2013;61:590. [PMID: 24212312]

Ramenaden ER et al: Clinical characteristics and visual outcomes in infectious scleritis: A review. Clin Ophthalmol 2013;7:2113. [PMID: 24235809]

Reddy JC et al: Risk factors and clinical outcomes of bacterial and fungal scleritis at a tertiary eye care hospital. Middle East Afr J Ophthalmol 2015;22:203. [PMID: 25949079]

Sainz-de-la-Maza M et al: Scleritis associated with relapsing polychondritis. Br J Ophthalmol 2016;100:1290. [PMID: 26888976]

Shoughy SS et al: Clinical manifestations and outcome of tuberculous sclerokeratitis. Br J Ophthalmol 2016;100:1301. [PMID: 26701691]

Suhler EB et al: Rituximab therapy for refractory scleritis: Results of a phase I/II dose-ranging, randomized, clinical trial. Ophthalmology 2014;121:1885. [PMID: 24953794]

Wakefield D et al: Scleritis: Immunopathogenesis and molecular basis for therapy. Prog Retin Eye Res 2013;35:44. [PMID: 23454614]

Watson PG et al, eds: *The Sclera and Systemic Disorders*, 3rd ed. London, England: J P Medical Ltd; 2012.

Lens

Richard A. Harper, MD

The (crystalline) lens contributes to focusing of images on the retina. It is positioned just posterior to the iris and is supported by **zonular fibers** arising from the ciliary body and inserting onto the equatorial region of the lens capsule (see Figure 1–12). The lens capsule is a basement membrane that surrounds the lens substance. Epithelial cells near the lens equator divide throughout life and continually differentiate into new lens fibers, so that older lens fibers are compressed into a central **nucleus;** younger, less-compact fibers around the nucleus make up the **cortex.** Because the lens is avascular and has no innervation, it must derive nutrients from the aqueous humor. Lens metabolism is primarily anaerobic owing to the low level of oxygen dissolved in the aqueous.

Accommodation is the eye's ability to adjust its focus from distance to near due to changes of the shape of the lens. Its inherent elasticity allows the lens to become more or less spherical depending on the amount of tension exerted by the zonular fibers on the lens capsule. Zonular tension is controlled by the action of the ciliary muscle that, when contracted, relaxes zonular tension. The lens then assumes a more spherical shape, resulting in increased dioptric power to bring near objects into focus. Ciliary muscle relaxation reverses this sequence of events, causing the lens to flatten and bringing distant objects into view. As the lens ages, accommodation gradually reduces as lens elasticity decreases.

PHYSIOLOGY OF SYMPTOMS

Symptoms associated with lens disorders are primarily visual. **Presbyopia** is the reduced ability with age to perform near tasks due to decreased accommodation. Loss of lens transparency (cataract) results in blurred vision for near and distance. Surgical removal of the lens or its complete dislocation from the visual axis results in an **aphakic refractive state;** severely blurred vision results from loss of over one-third of the eye's refractive power, the majority still being provided by the curvature of the cornea.

The lens is best examined with the pupil dilated. A magnified view of the lens can be obtained with a slitlamp or by using the direct ophthalmoscope with a high plus (+10) setting.

CATARACT

The term cataract refers to any opacity in the lens. Aging is the most common cause, but many other factors can be involved, including trauma, toxins, systemic disease (such as diabetes), smoking, and heredity. Age-related cataract is a common cause of visual impairment. The prevalence of cataracts is around 50% in individuals age 65–74, increasing to about 70% for those over 75.

The pathogenesis of cataracts is incompletely understood. They are characterized by protein aggregates that scatter light and reduce transparency and other protein alterations that result in yellow or brown discoloration. Factors that contribute to cataract formation include oxidative damage (from free radical reactions), ultraviolet light damage, and malnutrition. No medical treatment has been established to retard or reverse the underlying chemical changes. At present, evidence for a protective effect from B vitamins, multivitamins, or carotenoids is inconclusive.

Most cataracts are not visible to the casual observer until they become dense enough to cause severe vision loss. On ophthalmoscopy, the ocular fundus becomes increasingly more difficult to visualize as the lens opacity becomes denser until the fundus reflection is completely absent. A **mature cataract** is one in which all of the lens substance is opaque; the **immature cataract** has some transparent regions. If the lens takes up water, it may become **intumescent.** In the **hypermature cataract,** cortical proteins have become liquid. This liquid may escape through the intact capsule, leaving a shrunken lens with a wrinkled capsule. A hypermature cataract in which the lens nucleus floats freely in the capsular bag is called a **morgagnian cataract** (Figure 8–1).

The severity of cataract, assuming that no other eye disease is present, is judged primarily by the patient's symptoms and the visual acuity. Generally speaking, the decrease in visual

acuity is directly proportionate to the density of the cataract. However, some individuals who have clinically significant cataracts when examined with the ophthalmoscope or slitlamp see well enough to carry on with normal activities. Others have a decrease in visual acuity out of proportion to the observed degree of lens opacification. This is due to distortion of the image by the partially opaque lens or the cataract being located in the posterior visual axis. The Cataract Management Guideline Panel recommends reliance on clinical judgment combined with visual acuity as the best guide to the appropriateness of surgery but recognizes the need for flexibility, with due regard to a patient's particular functional and visual needs, the environment, and other risks, all of which may vary widely.

AGE-RELATED CATARACT (FIGURES 8–1 AND 8–2)

Loss of clarity in the lens nucleus results in **nuclear sclerosis**. The earliest symptom may be improved near vision without glasses ("second sight") due to increased refractive power of the central lens, creating a myopic (nearsighted) shift in refraction. Other symptoms may include poor hue discrimination, a need for increased light, and monocular diplopia. Most nuclear cataracts are bilateral but may be asymmetric.

Cortical cataracts are caused by changes in hydration of lens fibers creating clefts in a radial pattern around the equatorial region. They also tend to be bilateral, but they are often asymmetric. Visual function is variably affected, depending on how near the opacities are to the visual axis.

Posterior subcapsular cataracts are located in the cortex adjacent to the posterior capsule. They tend to cause visual symptoms earlier in their development owing to involvement of the visual axis. Common symptoms include glare and reduced vision under bright lighting conditions. This lens opacity can also result from trauma, corticosteroid use (topical or systemic), inflammation, or exposure to ionizing radiation.

Age-related cataract is usually slowly progressive. If surgery is indicated, lens extraction improves visual acuity in over 90% of cases. The remainder of patients either has preexisting retinal damage or, in rare cases, develops complications that prevent significant visual improvement, for example, intraocular hemorrhage perioperatively, or infection, retinal detachment, or glaucoma postoperatively.

CHILDHOOD CATARACT (FIGURES 8–3 AND 8–4)

Childhood cataracts are divided into two groups: **congenital (infantile) cataracts**, which are present at birth or appear shortly thereafter, and **acquired cataracts**, which occur later and are usually related to a specific cause. Either type may be unilateral or bilateral.

About one-third of childhood cataracts are hereditary, while another third are secondary to metabolic or infectious diseases or associated with a variety of syndromes. The final one-third result from undetermined causes. Acquired cataracts arise most commonly from trauma, either blunt or penetrating. Other causes include uveitis, acquired ocular infections, diabetes, and drugs.

▶ Clinical Findings

A. Congenital Cataract

Congenital lens opacities are common and often visually insignificant (see also Chapter 17). Opacity that is out of the visual axis or not dense enough to interfere significantly with light transmission requires no treatment other than observation. Dense central congenital cataracts require surgery.

Congenital cataracts that cause significant visual loss must be detected early, preferably in the newborn nursery by the pediatrician or family physician. Large, dense, white cataracts may present as leukocoria (white pupil), noticeable by the parents, but many dense cataracts cannot be seen by the parents. Unilateral infantile cataracts that are dense, central, and larger than 2 mm in diameter will cause permanent deprivation amblyopia if not treated within the first 2 months of life and thus require surgical management on an urgent basis. Even then, there must be careful attention to avoidance of amblyopia (see also Chapter 17) related to postoperative anisometropia (difference in focus power between the two eyes). Equally dense bilateral cataracts may require less-urgent management, although bilateral deprivation amblyopia can result. When surgery is undertaken, there must be as short an interval as is reasonably possible between treatment of the two eyes.

B. Acquired Cataract

Acquired cataracts often do not require the same urgent care (aimed at preventing amblyopia) as infantile cataracts because the children are usually older and the visual system more mature. Surgical assessment is based on the location, size, and density of the cataract, but a period of observation along with subjective visual acuity testing is helpful. Because unilateral cataract in children will not produce any symptoms or signs that parents would routinely notice, screening programs are important for case finding.

TRAUMATIC CATARACT

Traumatic cataract (Figures 8–5 to 8–7) is most commonly due to a foreign body injury to the lens or blunt trauma to the eyeball. Air rifle pellets and fireworks are a frequent cause; less-frequent causes include arrows, rocks, contusions, and ionizing radiation. Most traumatic cataracts are preventable. In industry, the best safety measure is a good pair of safety goggles.

The lens usually becomes white soon after the entry of a foreign body, since interruption of the lens capsule allows

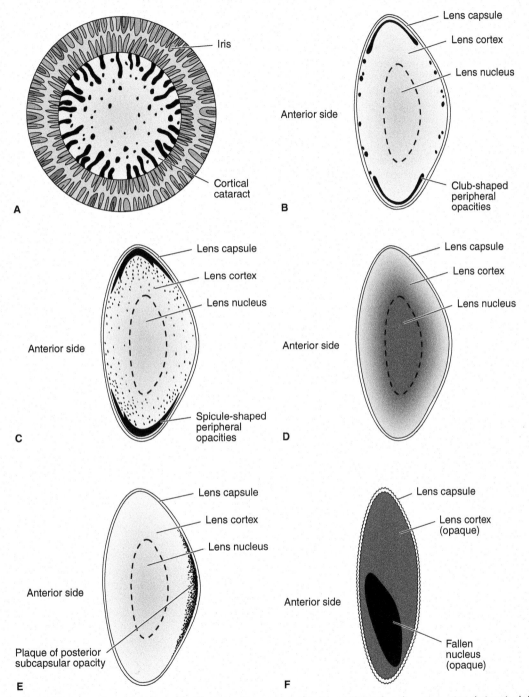

▲ **Figure 8–1.** Age-related cataract. **A** and **B:** "Coronary" type cortical cataract (frontal and cross-sectional views): club-shaped peripheral opacities with clear central lens; slowly progressive. **C:** "Cuneiform" type cortical cataract: peripheral spicules and central clear lens; slowly progressive. **D:** Nuclear sclerotic cataract: diffuse opacity principally affecting nucleus; slowly progressive. **E:** Posterior subcapsular cataract: plaque of granular opacity on posterior capsule; may be rapidly progressive. **F:** "Morgagnian" type (hypermature lens): the entire lens is opaque, and the lens nucleus has fallen inferiorly.

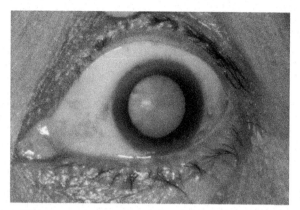

▲ **Figure 8-2.** Mature age-related cataract viewed through a dilated pupil.

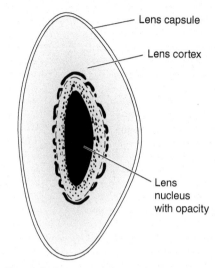

▲ **Figure 8-4.** Congenital cataract, zonular type. One zone of lens involved. The cortex is relatively clear.

fluid to penetrate into the lens structure. The patient often gives a history of striking metal upon metal. For example, a minute fragment of a steel hammer may pass through the cornea and lens and lodge in the vitreous or retina.

CATARACT SECONDARY TO INTRAOCULAR DISEASE ("COMPLICATED CATARACT")

Cataract may develop as a direct effect of intraocular disease upon the physiology of the lens (eg, severe recurrent uveitis). The cataract usually begins in the posterior subcapsular area and may eventually involve the entire lens structure. Intraocular diseases commonly associated with the development of cataracts are chronic or recurrent uveitis, glaucoma, retinitis pigmentosa, and retinal detachment. The visual prognosis is not as good as in ordinary age-related cataract due to the underlying ocular disease.

CATARACT ASSOCIATED WITH SYSTEMIC DISEASE

Bilateral cataracts occur in many systemic disorders including diabetes mellitus (Figure 8-8), hypocalcemia (of any cause), myotonic dystrophy, atopic dermatitis, galactosemia, and Down, Lowe (oculo-cerebro-renal), and Werner syndromes (see Chapters 15 and 18).

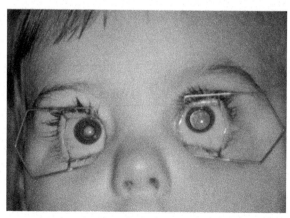

▲ **Figure 8-3.** Congenital cataract (right eye) with dilated pupils.

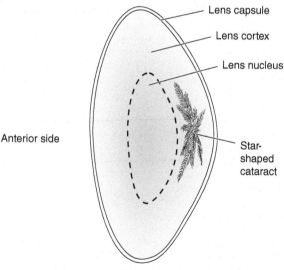

▲ **Figure 8-5.** Traumatic "star-shaped" cataract in the posterior lens. This is usually due to ocular contusion and is only detectable through a well-dilated pupil.

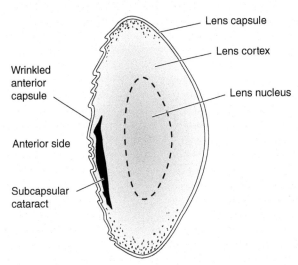

▲ **Figure 8–6.** Traumatic cataract with wrinkled anterior capsule.

DRUG-INDUCED CATARACT

Corticosteroids administered over a long period of time, either systemically (oral or inhaled) or in drop form, can cause lens opacities. Other drugs associated with cataract include phenothiazines and amiodarone (see Chapter 22).

CATARACT SURGERY

Cataract surgery is the most commonly performed surgical procedure worldwide. The generally preferred method in **adults and older children** preserves the posterior portion of

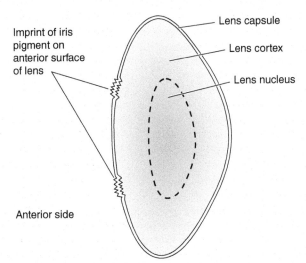

▲ **Figure 8–7.** Imprint of iris pigment on anterior surface of lens.

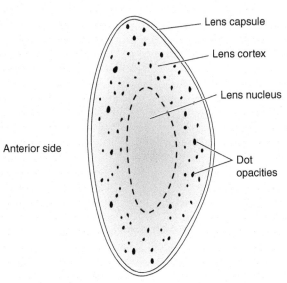

▲ **Figure 8–8.** Punctate dot cataract. This type of cataract is sometimes seen as an ocular complication of diabetes mellitus. It may also be congenital.

the lens capsule and thus is known as **extracapsular cataract extraction**. An incision is made at the limbus or in the peripheral cornea, either superiorly or temporally. An opening is created in the anterior capsule (anterior capsulorhexis), and the nucleus and cortex of the lens are removed. (The femtosecond laser can be used for the initial incision, capsulorhexis, and other parts of the procedure, but its value for routine use is uncertain.) An intraocular lens is placed in the empty "capsular bag," thus supported by the intact posterior capsule.

The technique of **phacoemulsification** is now the most common form of extracapsular cataract extraction in developed countries. It uses a handheld ultrasonic vibrator to disintegrate the hard nucleus such that the nuclear material and cortex can be aspirated through a small incision of approximately 2.5 to 3 mm. This same incision size is then adequate for insertion of foldable intraocular lenses. If a rigid intraocular lens is used, the wound needs to be extended to approximately 5 mm. In developing countries, particularly rural areas, the instruments for phacoemulsification are often not available. **Manual sutureless small incision cataract surgery** (MSICS) is based on the traditional nuclear expression form of extracapsular cataract extraction, in which the nucleus is removed intact, but using a small incision. The cortex is removed by manual aspiration. MSICS may be indicated for dense cataracts unsuitable for phacoemulsification.

The main intraoperative complication of extracapsular surgery is posterior capsular tear, for which the main predisposing factors include previous trauma, dense cataract, unstable lens, and small pupil, possibly leading to displacement of nuclear material into the vitreous ("dropped nucleus") that generally necessitates complex vitreoretinal surgery. Postoperatively,

there may be secondary opacification of the posterior capsule that requires discission using the neodymium:YAG laser (see Posterior Capsule Opacification later in the chapter).

Intraocular Lenses

There are many styles of intraocular lenses, but most designs consist of a central optic and two legs (or **haptics**) to maintain the optic in position. The optimal intraocular lens position is within the capsular bag following an extracapsular procedure. This is associated with the lowest incidence of postoperative complications, such as pseudophakic bullous keratopathy, glaucoma, iris damage, hyphema, and lens decentration. The newest posterior chamber lenses are made of flexible materials such as silicone and acrylic polymers, allowing the lens implant to be folded and thus decreasing the required incision size. Lenses with **multifocal optics** can provide good vision for both near and distance without glasses. If there is inadvertent damage to the posterior capsule during extracapsular surgery, an intraocular lens can be placed in the anterior chamber or sutured to lie in the ciliary sulcus. Methods of calculating the correct dioptric power of an intraocular lens are discussed in Chapter 21. If an intraocular lens cannot be safely placed or is contraindicated, postoperative refractive correction generally requires a contact lens or aphakic spectacles.

Postoperative Care

The patient is usually ambulatory on the day of surgery but is advised to move cautiously and avoid straining or heavy lifting for about a month. The eye may be patched on the day of surgery. Protection at night by a metal shield is often suggested for several days after surgery. Topical postoperative antibiotics and anti-inflammatory drops are used for 4–6 weeks after surgery.

Complications of Adult Cataract Surgery

Cataract surgery in adults has a very low rate (2–5%) of complications that result in permanent impairment of vision. The most serious but rare complications are perioperative intraocular hemorrhage (< 0.5%) and postoperative intraocular infection (endophthalmitis, 0.1%), either of which can result in severe visual loss or removal of the eye. Suspicion of endophthalmitis requires vitreous tap for microscopy and culture and intravitreal injection of antibiotics (see Table 22–1). Vitrectomy is sometimes indicated (see Chapter 9). Other complications include retinal detachment, cystoid macular edema, glaucoma, corneal edema, and ptosis.

Posterior Capsule Opacification

About 10% of eyes require treatment for posterior capsule opacification following uncomplicated phacoemulsification surgery (Figure 8–9).

Persistent lens epithelium on the capsule favors regeneration of lens fibers, giving the posterior capsule a "fish egg"

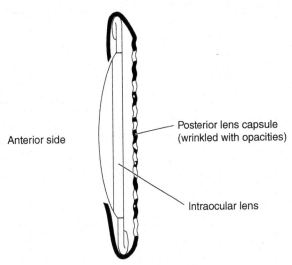

▲ **Figure 8–9.** Posterior capsule opacification ("after-cataract").

appearance (Elschnig's pearls). The proliferating epithelium may produce multiple layers, leading to opacification. These cells may also undergo myofibroblastic differentiation. Their contraction produces numerous tiny wrinkles in the posterior capsule, resulting in visual distortion.

The neodymium:YAG laser provides a noninvasive method of creating an optical window in the posterior capsule (see Chapter 23). Complications include a transient rise in intraocular pressure, damage to the intraocular lens, and rupture of the anterior hyaloid face with forward displacement of vitreous into the anterior chamber, potentially leading to rhegmatogenous retinal detachment or cystoid macular edema. The rise in intraocular pressure is usually detectable within 3 hours after treatment and resolves within a few days with treatment. Small pits or cracks may occur on the intraocular lens but usually have no effect on visual acuity.

Childhood Cataract Surgery

Cataract surgery in young children is often hindered by more difficult anterior capsulorhexis, as well as the frequent need to make an opening in the posterior capsule (posterior capsulorhexis) and to remove part of the vitreous (anterior vitrectomy) to reduce the incidence of posterior capsule opacification, which is much higher than after adult cataract surgery. The cataracts are less dense than in adults and can usually be removed by an irrigation–aspiration technique, without the need for phacoemulsification.

Optical correction can consist of spectacles in older bilaterally aphakic children, but most childhood cataract operations are followed by contact lens correction, with adjustment of power as the refractive status of the eye changes with growth. Intraocular lenses are also used in some cases. They avoid the difficulties associated with contact lens wear, but there are difficulties calculating the appropriate power.

Prognosis

The visual prognosis for childhood cataract patients requiring surgery is not as good as that for patients with age-related cataract. The associated amblyopia and occasional anomalies of the optic nerve or retina limit the degree of useful vision that can be achieved in this group of patients. The prognosis for improvement of visual acuity is worst following surgery for unilateral congenital cataracts and best for incomplete bilateral congenital cataracts that are slowly progressive. Glaucoma is a common long-term complication.

DISLOCATED LENS (ECTOPIA LENTIS)

Partial or complete lens dislocation (subluxation) (Figure 8–10) may be hereditary or due to trauma.

Hereditary Lens Dislocation

Hereditary lens dislocation is usually bilateral and may be an isolated familial anomaly or due to inherited connective tissue disorder such as homocystinuria, Marfan syndrome, or Weill-Marchesani syndrome (see Chapter 15). The vision is blurred, particularly if the lens is dislocated out of the line of vision. If dislocation is partial, the edge of the lens and the zonular fibers holding it in place can be seen in the pupil. If the lens is completely dislocated into the vitreous, it may be visible with an ophthalmoscope.

A partially dislocated lens may be complicated by cataract formation. If that is the case, the cataract may have to be removed, but there is a significant risk of vitreous loss, predisposing to retinal detachment. If the lens is free in the vitreous, it may lead in later life to the development of glaucoma of a type that responds poorly to treatment. If dislocation is partial and the lens is clear, the visual prognosis is good.

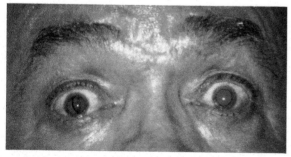

▲ **Figure 8–10.** Partially dislocated (subluxed) lens (right eye) with dilated pupils.

Traumatic Lens Dislocation

Partial or complete traumatic lens dislocation may occur following a contusion injury such as a blow to the eye with a fist. If the dislocation is partial, there may be no visual symptoms; but if the lens is floating in the vitreous, the patient will have significantly blurred vision. Iridodonesis, a quivering of the iris when the patient moves the eye, is a common sign of lens dislocation and is due to the lack of lens support. This is present both in partially and in completely dislocated lenses but is more marked in the latter.

Uveitis and glaucoma are common complications of dislocated lens, particularly if dislocation is complete. If there are no complications, dislocated lenses are best left untreated. If uveitis or uncontrollable glaucoma occurs, lens extraction may need to be done despite the poor results possible from this operation. For completely dislocated lenses, the technique of choice is pars plana lensectomy or phacofragmentation, depending on the density of cataract. Some partially dislocated (subluxed) lenses are amenable to phacoemulsification with various adaptations, such as capsular tension rings or support hooks.

REFERENCES

Agarkar S et al: Incidence, management, and visual outcomes in pediatric endophthalmitis following cataract surgery by a single surgeon. J AAPOS 2016;20:415. [PMID: 27343836]

American Academy of Ophthalmology Cataract and Anterior Segment Panel: Preferred Practice Pattern Guidelines. Cataract in the adult eye. American Academy of Ophthalmology, 2011. Available at: http://www.aaojournal.org/content/preferred-practice-pattern

Ang GS et al: Manual small incision cataract surgery in a United Kingdom university teaching hospital setting. Int Ophthalmol 2010;30:23. [PMID: 19129974]

Behndig A et al: One million cataract surgeries: Swedish National Cataract Register 1992-2009. J Cataract Refract Surg 2011;37:1539. [PMID: 21782099]

Braga-Mele R et al: Multifocal intraocular lenses: Relative indications and contraindications for implantation. J Cataract Refract Surg 2014;40:313. [PMID: 24461503]

Celano M et al: Motor skills of children with unilateral visual impairment in the Infant Aphakia Treatment Study. Dev Med Child Neurol 2016;58:154. [PMID: 26084944]

Chang JR et al: Risk factors associated with incident cataracts and cataract surgery in the Age-related Eye Disease Study (AREDS): AREDS report number 32. Ophthalmology 2011;1180:2113. [PMID: 21684602]

Chu CJ et al: Risk factors and incidence of macular edema after cataract surgery: A database study of 81984 Eyes. Ophthalmology 2016;123:316. [PMID: 26681390]

Coleman AL. How big data informs us about cataract surgery: The LXXII Edward Jackson Memorial Lecture. Am J Ophthalmol 2015;160:1091. [PMID: 26432566]

Cooper K et al: The cost-effectiveness of second-eye cataract surgery in the UK. Age Ageing 2015;44:1026. [PMID: 26410365]

de Silva SR et al: Phacoemulsification with posterior chamber intraocular lens versus extracapsular cataract extraction (ECCE) with posterior chamber intraocular lens for age-related cataract. Cochrane Database Syst Rev 2014;1:CD008812. [PMID: 24474622]

Findl O et al: Interventions for preventing posterior capsule opacification. Cochrane Database Syst Rev 2010;2:CD003738. [PMID: 20166069]

Freedman SF et al: Glaucoma-related adverse events in the first 5 years after unilateral cataract removal in the Infant Aphakia Treatment Study. JAMA Ophthalmol 2015;133:907. [PMID: 25996491]

Garcia-Gutierrez S et al: Impact of clinical and patient-reported outcomes on patient satisfaction with cataract extraction. Health Expect 2014;17:765. [PMID: 22784407]

Glaser TS et al: The association of dietary lutein plus zeaxanthin and B vitamins with cataracts in the Age-Related Eye Disease Study: AREDS Report No. 37. Ophthalmology 2015;122:1471. [PMID: 25972257]

González N et al: Factors affecting cataract surgery complications and their effect on the postoperative outcome. Can J Ophthalmol 2014;49:72. [PMID: 24513361]

Grewal DS et al: Femtosecond laser-assisted cataract surgery-current status and future directions. Surv Ophthalmol 2016;61:103. [PMID: 26409902]

Hartmann EE et al: Stereopsis results at 4.5 years of age in the Infant Aphakia Treatment Study. Am J Ophthalmol 2015;159:64. [PMID: 25261241]

Herrinton LJ et al: Comparative effectiveness of antibiotic prophylaxis in cataract surgery. Ophthalmology 2016;123:287. [PMID: 26459998]

Hoffman RS et al: Management of the subluxated crystalline lens. J Cataract Refract Surg 2013;39:1904. [PMID: 24286841]

Hoffman RS et al: Cataract surgery in the small eye. J Cataract Refract Surg 2015;41:2565. [PMID: 26703508]

Infant Aphakia Treatment Study Group: The infant aphakia treatment study: Design and clinical measures at enrolment. Arch Ophthalmol 2010;128:21. [PMID: 20065212]

Jabbarvand M et al: Endophthalmitis occurring after cataract surgery: Outcomes of more than 480,000 cataract surgeries, epidemiologic features, and risk factors. Ophthalmology 2016;123:295. [PMID: 26704882]

Javitt JC: Intracameral antibiotics reduce the risk of endophthalmitis after cataract surgery: Does the preponderance of the evidence mandate a global change in practice? Ophthalmology 2016;123:226. [PMID: 26802702]

Kruger SJ et al: Cost of intraocular lens versus contact lens treatment after unilateral congenital cataract surgery in the Infant Aphakia Treatment Study at age 5 years. Ophthalmology 2015;122:288. [PMID: 25439604]

Lee CM et al: The global state of cataract blindness. Curr Opin Ophthalmol 2017;28:98. [PMID: 27820750]

Lim JC et al: Tools to fight the cataract epidemic: A review of experimental animal models that mimic age related nuclear cataract. Exp Eye Res 2016;145:432. [PMID: 26391448]

Lin AA et al: Update on pediatric cataract surgery and intraocular lens implantation. Curr Opin Ophthalmol 2010;21:55. [PMID: 19855277]

Lundström M et al: Decreasing rate of capsule complications in cataract surgery: Eight-year study of incidence, risk factors, and data validity by the Swedish National Cataract Register. J Cataract Refract Surg 2011;37:1762. [PMID: 21820852]

Lundström M et al: Risk factors for endophthalmitis after cataract surgery: Predictors for causative organisms and visual outcomes. J Cataract Refract Surg 2015;41:2410. [PMID: 26703490]

Malik A et al: Local anesthesia for cataract surgery. J Cataract Refract Surg 2010;36:133. [PMID: 20117717]

Mesnard C et al: Endophthalmitis after cataract surgery despite intracameral antibiotic prophylaxis with licensed cefuroxime. J Cataract Refract Surg 2016;42:1318. [PMID: 27697250]

Morrison DG et al: Corneal changes in children after unilateral cataract surgery in the Infant Aphakia Treatment Study. Ophthalmology 2015;122:2186. [PMID: 26271843]

Nagy ZZ et al: Femtosecond laser cataract surgery. Eye Vis (Lond) 2015;2:11. [PMID: 26605364]

Palagyi A et al: While we waited: Incidence and predictors of falls in older adults with cataract. Invest Ophthalmol Vis Sci 2016;57:6003. [PMID: 27820872]

Plager DA et al: Complications in the first 5 years following cataract surgery in infants with and without intraocular lens implantation in the Infant Aphakia Treatment Study. Am J Ophthalmol 2014;158:892. [PMID: 25077835]

Reilly MA: A quantitative geometric mechanics lens model: Insights into the mechanisms of accommodation and presbyopia. Vision Res 2014;103:20. [PMID: 25130408]

Repka MX et al: Cataract surgery in children from birth to less than 13 years of age: Baseline characteristics of the cohort. Ophthalmology 2016;123:2462. [PMID: 27769584]

Riaz Y et al: Manual small incision cataract surgery (MSICS) with posterior chamber intraocular lens versus phacoemulsification with posterior chamber intraocular lens for age-related cataract. Cochrane Database Syst Rev 2013;10:CD008813. [PMID: 24114262]

Sachdeva V et al: Validation of guidelines for undercorrection of intra-ocular lens (IOL) power in children. Am J Ophthalmol 2017;174:17. [PMID: 27818207]

Sadiq MA et al: Genetics of ectopia lentis. Semin Ophthalmol 2013;28:313. [PMID: 24138040]

Schmier JK et al: An updated estimate of costs of endophthalmitis following cataract surgery among Medicare patients: 2010-2014. Clin Ophthalmol 2016;10:21217. [PMID: 27822008]

Shah M et al: Controversies in traumatic cataract classification and management: A review. Can J Ophthalmol 2013;48:251. [PMID: 23931462]

Sheppard JD. Topical bromfenac for prevention and treatment of cystoid macular edema following cataract surgery: A review. Clin Ophthalmol 2016;10:2099. [PMID: 27822006]

Strenk SA et al: Magnetic resonance imaging of the anteroposterior position and thickness of the aging, accommodating, phakic, and pseudophakic ciliary muscle. J Cataract Refract Surg 2010;36:235. [PMID: 20152603]

Struck MC. Long-term results of pediatric cataract surgery and primary intraocular lens implantation from 7 to 22 months of life. JAMA Ophthalmol 2015;133:1180. [PMID: 26111188]

Thompson J et al: Cataracts. Prim Care 2015;42:409. [PMID: 26319346]

Venkatesh R et al: Carbon footprint and cost-effectiveness of cataract surgery. Curr Opin Ophthalmol 2016;27:82. [PMID: 26569528]

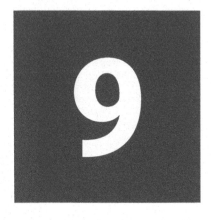

Vitreous

9

Steve Charles, MD

INTRODUCTION

During the past four decades, there has been an explosion of interest in the vitreous due to the development of vitreoretinal surgery. Previously large numbers of patients were blinded by vitreoretinal diseases. One goal of this chapter is to help the medical student, intern, resident, general ophthalmologist, and optometrist become aware of the indications for vitreoretinal surgery, many of which are time sensitive. Many vitreoretinal conditions have implications for the family medical practitioner, internist, and emergency physician.

VITREOUS ANATOMY AND ITS RELEVANCE TO PATHOLOGY

The vitreous fills the space between the lens and the retina and consists of a three-dimensional collagen fiber matrix and a hyaluronan gel (Figure 9–1). The outer surface of the vitreous, known as the cortex, is in contact with the lens (anterior vitreous cortex) and adherent in varying degrees to the surface of the retina (posterior vitreous cortex) (Figure 9–2).

Aging, hemorrhage, inflammation, trauma, myopia, and other processes often cause hypocellular contraction of the vitreous collagen matrix. The posterior vitreous cortex then separates from areas of low adherence to the retina and may produce traction on areas of greater adherence. The vitreous base extends from the equator anteriorly and is a zone of permanent and strong adherence. The vitreous never detaches from the vitreous base. The vitreous is also more adherent to the optic nerve and, to a lesser extent, the macula and retinal vessels. Adherence to the macular region is a significant factor in the pathogenesis of epimacular membrane, macular hole, vitreomacular schisis, and vitreomacular traction syndrome.

Previously it was taught that the vitreous developed cavities from a process known as syneresis, ultimately resulting in "collapse" of the vitreous. It is now believed that collagen cross-linking and selective loss of retinal adherence rather than cavity formation are the primary events. Even though the vitreous may migrate inferiorly when separated from the retina, this process causes less force at the zones of vitreoretinal adherence than the traction caused by saccadic eye motion. Saccadically induced, dynamic forces play a significant role in the development of retinal breaks (tears), damage to the retinal surface, and bleeding from torn vessels (Figure 9–3). Further contraction of the vitreous caused by invasion of retinal pigment epithelial, glial, or inflammatory cells may result in sufficient static traction to detach the retina without retinal tears.

Prior to vitreoretinal surgery, vitreous "bands" were thought to cause traction on the retina, and largely unsuccessful attempts were made to cut them with scissors. The visualization provided by vitreoretinal endoillumination systems has contributed to our knowledge of anatomy and demonstrated that these bands are contiguous with the transparent posterior vitreous cortex, which is also responsible for substantial traction. Traction bands virtually only exist when penetrating trauma creates a path through the vitreous or from severe necrosis, usually from *Toxocara canis* infection. Even these bands are usually contiguous with the posterior vitreous cortex.

EXAMINATION OF THE VITREOUS AND VITREORETINAL INTERFACE

Normal vitreous is essentially transparent but is capable of exerting substantial force on the retina. Vitreoretinal traction can often be inferred by the configuration of the retinal surface (Figure 9–4). Transparent vitreous is best seen with a narrow, off-axis slitbeam using a three-mirror contact lens and stereo biomicroscopy (Figure 9–5). Visualization is significantly enhanced by dark adaptation of the observer. A biomicroscope with a broad, on-axis slitbeam or a direct ophthalmoscope is not suitable for observing the vitreous.

Indirect ophthalmoscopes provide a large field of view, are capable of looking "around" some lenticular and vitreous

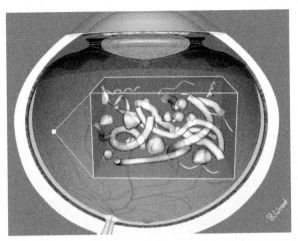

▲ **Figure 9–1.** The vitreous consists of a three-dimensional matrix of collagen fibers and a hyaluronan gel.

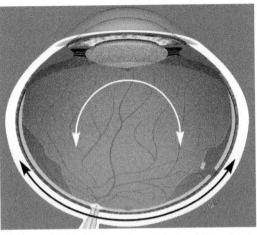

▲ **Figure 9–3.** Motion of partially detached vitreous **(white arrow)**, induced by saccades **(black arrow)** and resulting in a retinal break **(arrowhead)**.

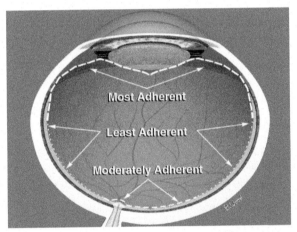

Most Adherent

Least Adherent

Moderately Adherent

▲ **Figure 9–2.** The vitreous cortex is adherent to the lens and especially to the retinal surface to varying degrees.

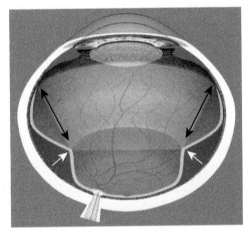

▲ **Figure 9–4.** Abnormal retinal configuration **(white arrows)** indicating vitreoretinal traction **(black arrows)**.

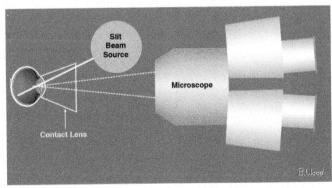

Slit Beam Source

Microscope

Contact Lens

▲ **Figure 9–5.** Narrow, off-axis slitbeam, contact lens, and biomicroscope offer the best view of transparent vitreous.

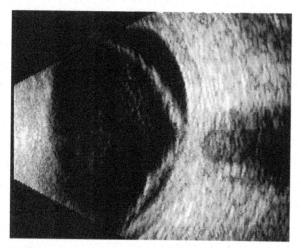

▲ **Figure 9–6.** B-scan ultrasonogram.

opacities, and provide a stereoscopic view. Many observers only attempt to look "through" the vitreous, ignoring the opportunity to look "at" the vitreous, especially if it is abnormal. Visualization of vitreoretinal traction is enhanced rather than adversely affected by eye motion. In addition, mobility of the vitreous is an excellent gauge of the extent of vitreoretinal traction. It is often possible to see some portion of the retina in eyes with substantial vitreous hemorrhages by looking at the periphery first to establish a plane of focus, known as the visual horopter. The viewing path length through semi-opaque vitreous is much less in the periphery than when attempting to visualize the optic nerve. The vitreous is often clearer superiorly. Sitting the patient up for a period of time may cause blood to migrate inferiorly, enabling a better view of the retina.

If the vitreous is too opaque to visualize the retina, B-scan ultrasonography should be used to determine if the retina is attached or a tumor, foreign body, dislocated lens, dislocated intraocular lens, or choroidal detachment is present (Figure 9–6).

Optical coherence tomography (OCT) uses light to construct a three-dimensional (3D) model of the macula and posterior retina. The 3D model is constructed from a series of optical B-scan images (see Chapter 2). Spectral domain OCT with tracking produces much better resolution and has

much shorter acquisition times than the initial time domain OCT (Figure 9–7). The resolution is approximately 5 μm. OCT is ideal for visualization of vitreomacular traction, epimacular membranes, macular holes, macular cysts, macular edema, vitreomacular schisis, subretinal fluid, pigment epithelial detachments, and choroidal neovascular membranes.

▼ SYMPTOMS OF VITREORETINAL DISEASE

FLOATERS

Most people experience "floaters" at some point during their life. These may be described as strings, spider webs, small saucer-like objects, or a transparent ring. Posterior vitreous detachment occurs in at least 70% of the population and causes the majority of floater complaints. Most floaters prove to be clinically insignificant after examination of the retina fails to reveal any retinal breaks or other pathology. Careful, timely, peripheral retina examination using an indirect ophthalmoscope through a widely dilated pupil is essential any time a patient complains of the onset of floaters. Any change in the nature of floaters is also an indication for peripheral retinal examination within a few days. Floaters secondary to posterior vitreous separation are better termed vitreous "condensations" to emphasize their origin from preexisting vitreous collagen fibers and surfaces. Erythrocytes and, on occasion, inflammatory cells can result in the patient seeing floaters, often described as saucer-like. A ring-like floater is usually a result of visualizing the zone of posterior vitreous cortex previously adherent to the optic nerve. Vitreous hemorrhage (Figure 9–8) requires careful examination to determine if an avulsed vessel or vascular disease such as diabetic retinopathy, venous occlusive disease, hemoglobinopathy, or leukemia is present. The presence of inflammatory cells demands a workup for lymphoma, sarcoidosis, candidal infection, and other systemic disorders. Although floaters are common, it is crucial that careful retinal examination be done before a patient is reassured that only posterior vitreous separation has occurred.

Small, uniform, spherical, golden objects known as asteroid hyalosis frequently occur in the vitreous (Figure 9–9). Although they have an impressive appearance, they almost never interfere with vision and need no treatment. It was

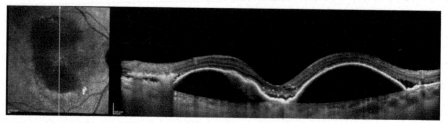

▲ **Figure 9–7.** Spectral domain optical coherence tomography.

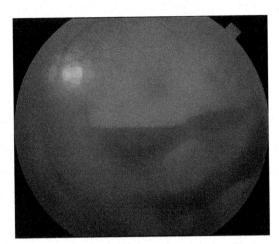

▲ **Figure 9–8.** Vitreous hemorrhage.

once taught that asteroid hyalosis is associated with diabetes, but this was subsequently disproved.

Vitrectomy is very rarely indicated for floaters. Many patients overreact to floaters and need counseling rather than surgery with its risk of retinal detachment and cataract. Although some ophthalmologists perform YAG laser vitreolysis for floaters, this is rarely effective and also has risk of retinal detachment and cataract.

LIGHT FLASHES (PHOTOPSIA)

Light flashes, better termed "photopsia," are caused by mechanical stimulation of the retina, usually secondary to the vitreous separating from the retina. Jagged, lightning-like, bilateral scintillating scotomas secondary to migraine (50% are not accompanied by a headache) are often mistakenly confused with photopsia. The majority of patients experiencing posterior vitreous separation will experience

light flashes, especially during saccades, until separation has stabilized. Posterior vitreous separation is never "complete" as the vitreous always remains attached to the peripheral vitreous base. Any patient with the recent onset of photopsia must have a timely, careful examination of the retinal periphery with a dilated pupil and indirect ophthalmoscope.

VITREORETINAL DISEASES

VITREOMACULAR DISEASE

In many vitreomacular diseases, OCT is superior to clinical examination and essential to diagnosis and treatment decisions.

Epimacular membranes (EMM) are usually caused by posterior vitreous separation. It is thought that excessive adherence of the posterior vitreous cortex to the retinal surface results in a partial-thickness retinal defect during the process of separation. Glial cells migrate through the defect onto the retinal surface and cause hypocellular contraction. EMM is treated by vitrectomy and membrane peeling, best performed with end-opening forceps, although pics and other tools are used as well. Peeling the internal limiting membrane (ILM) after peeling the EMM hastens visual recovery and eliminates striae. Patients with EMM complain of metamorphopsia and reduced vision. Usually they experience dramatic improvement after the EMM and ILM are removed.

Vitreomacular traction syndrome (VMT) was thought to be rare until the availability of OCT. It is thought that excessive adherence of the posterior vitreous cortex to the retinal surface, coupled with hypocellular vitreous contraction, results in VMT. In some cases, a layer of posterior vitreous cortex separates from the vitreous body, remaining attached to the retina and then contracting. More typically, the taut posterior vitreous cortex adherent to the macula creates macular elevation, distortion, and reduced vision. Vitrectomy usually with ILM peeling is extremely effective in managing these cases.

Macular hole development is related to posterior vitreous separation, but the exact mechanism is unknown. The Gass classification adds nothing to management decisions. The core issue is to determine by OCT if the hole is partial or full thickness. Partial-thickness holes require vitrectomy, ILM peeling, and SF6 gas if they are symptomatic or if macular cysts or schisis is present, but otherwise, they can be observed. Full-thickness holes require vitrectomy, ILM peeling, and SF6 gas, which results in at least 90% chance of significant visual improvement.

RETINAL BREAKS & RHEGMATOGENOUS RETINAL DETACHMENT

As described earlier, posterior vitreous separation in eyes with abnormal vitreoretinal adherence can result in retinal tears (breaks). Retinal breaks occur more commonly in

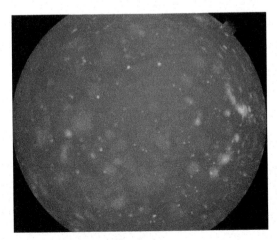

▲ **Figure 9–9.** Asteroid hyalosis.

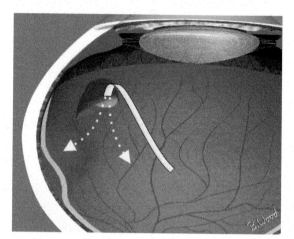

▲ **Figure 9–10.** Passage of liquid vitreous through horseshoe retinal tear leading to retinal detachment.

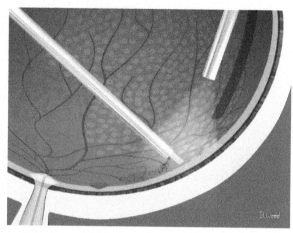

▲ **Figure 9–11.** Endolaser retinal photocoagulation.

patients with myopia as they may have lattice degeneration, which is genetically linked to myopia. Symptomatic retinal breaks are said to be more significant than asymptomatic, although patients vary widely in their reporting of symptoms. Large tears are more significant than small tears, although very small flap tears often cause retinal detachment. Small round holes, especially those inside lattice degeneration, seldom cause retinal detachment. Operculated holes or round atrophic holes are less likely to cause retinal detachment than flap (horseshoe) tears (Figure 9–10).

DIABETIC RETINOPATHY

Patients with proliferative diabetic retinopathy may bleed into the vitreous from retinal neovascularization. These patients must be managed aggressively with eye-saving panretinal photocoagulation, often combined with anti-VEGF (vascular endothelial growth factor) therapy with intravitreal injections of ranibizumab (Lucentis), aflibercept (Eylea), or bevacizumab (Avastin), although such anti-VEGF therapy is not approved by the US Food and Drug Administration. If the blood prevents visualization of the retina, ultrasound examination must be performed to rule out traction retinal detachment. Vitrectomy can be done to improve vision and apply endopanretinal photocoagulation (Figure 9–11).

Diabetic traction retinal detachments are managed using vitreoretinal surgery, incorporating techniques such as scissors segmentation (Figure 9–12) and delamination (Figure 9–13) of epiretinal membranes. Coagulation of transected neovascularization preferably is accomplished using endolaser or optionally bipolar diathermy probes (Figure 9–14).

COMPLICATIONS OF CATARACT SURGERY

Approximately 0.5–1% of cataract surgery patients ultimately develop rhegmatogenous retinal detachment, presumably related to alterations in the vitreous during or after surgery. These patients present with light flashes, photopsia, loss of peripheral vision, and loss of central vision if the macula is detached. Posterior capsule rupture and vitreous loss are often said to occur after 1% of cataract surgeries, but some evidence suggests that the incidence probably is closer to 5%. Retinal detachment is more common after capsule rupture, vitreous loss, and anterior

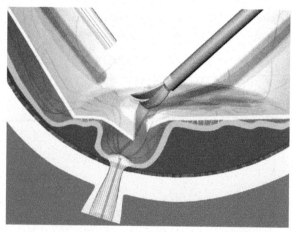

▲ **Figure 9–12.** Scissors segmentation of epiretinal membrane to release tangential traction.

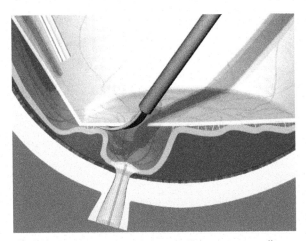

▲ **Figure 9–13.** Scissors delamination to remove adherent epiretinal membrane.

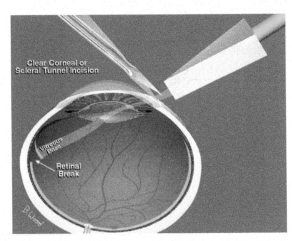

▲ **Figure 9–15.** Vitreous traction during and after cataract surgery can lead to retinal breaks and detachment.

vitrectomy, especially if cellulose sponge vitrectomy is used (Figure 9–15).

Capsule rupture during cataract surgery may result in displacement of lens material or occasionally the entire lens into the vitreous. Inflammation and phacolytic glaucoma usually develop unless only a small amount of cortex is dislocated. Vitrectomy plus lens fragmentation is very effective in removing posterior dislocated lens material (Figure 9–16).

Endophthalmitis may occur within a few days after cataract surgery and can rapidly result in loss of the eye unless recognized and treated rapidly. Most cases can be treated by performing a vitreous tap for culture and sensitivity and injecting intravitreal antibiotics. Severe cases with retained view of the retina are treated with vitrectomy as well. Even with prompt diagnosis and appropriate treatment, eyes with certain aggressive organisms often are still lost. Any patient with pain, decreased vision, or increasing inflammation soon after cataract surgery should be seen immediately to determine if endophthalmitis is present. Endophthalmitis can also result from a leaking filtering bleb, trauma, or endogenous sources such as an intravenous line or indwelling catheter, especially in immune-incompetent patients.

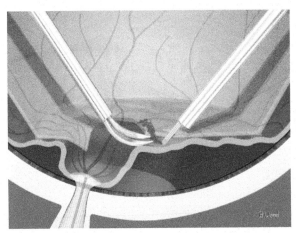

▲ **Figure 9–14.** Coagulation of transected vessels with bipolar endoilluminator during segmentation or delamination.

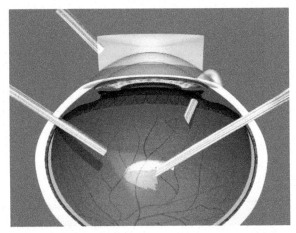

▲ **Figure 9–16.** Vitrectomy with contact lens and endoillumination to allow fragmentation and removal of posterior dislocated lens material.

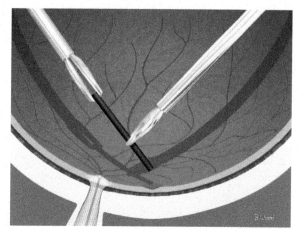

▲ **Figure 9–17.** Removal of intraocular foreign body with diamond-coated forceps.

TRAUMA

Penetrating ocular trauma often results in a vitreous hemorrhage, which may be accompanied by significant retinal damage. Vitreous mobility as judged by indirect ophthalmoscopy and ultrasonography helps determine the timing of vitrectomy after penetrating trauma without a foreign body. Mobile vitreous, even if completely opaque from hemorrhage, can be observed if ultrasound demonstrates the retina to be attached and no foreign body is present. Vitrectomy is typically performed 7–10 days after initial wound repair after posterior vitreous separation occurs, active bleeding subsides, and the cornea is clearer. If early vitreous contraction is indicated by decreased mobility, vitrectomy should be performed before fibrosis and secondary traction retinal detachment occur.

If a metallic (ferrous or copper), toxic, or potentially infectious (biologic material) intraocular foreign body is present, prompt vitrectomy and forceps removal of the foreign body are indicated (Figure 9–17) (see Chapter 19). Occasionally, a plastic or glass foreign body or a shotgun pellet can be observed without surgery or until vitreoretinal traction occurs.

SUMMARY

Study of vitreoretinal diseases is fascinating and can have a major impact on visual outcomes. New technologies and techniques are being developed at an explosive pace, producing great improvement in outcomes after vitreoretinal surgery. Many eyes formerly untreatable have had vision restored. Advances in biotechnology and OCT imaging are likely to produce phenomenal advances in the upcoming years.

REFERENCES

Binder MI et al: Endogenous endophthalmitis: An 18-year review of culture positive cases at a tertiary care center. Medicine (Baltimore) 2003;82:97. [PMID: 12640186]

Brown GC et al: Photopsias: A key to diagnosis. Ophthalmology 2015;122:2084. [PMID: 26249730]

Chalam KV et al: Concurrent removal of intravitreal lens fragments after phacoemulsification with pars plana vitrectomy prevents development of retinal detachment. Int J Ophthalmol 2015;8:89. [PMID: 25709914]

Chee YE et al: The role of vitrectomy in the management of fungal endophthalmitis. Semin Ophthalmol 2017;32:29. [PMID: 27792412]

Cho GE et al: Changing trends in surgery for retinal detachment in Korea. Korean J Ophthalmol 2014;28:451. [PMID: 25435747]

Cho H et al: Endogenous endophthalmitis in the American and Korean population: An 8-year retrospective study. Ocul Immunol Inflamm 2016 Jul 26:1. [Epub ahead of print] [PMID: 27459423]

Cohen MN et al: Management of symptomatic floaters: Current attitudes, beliefs, and practices among vitreoretinal surgeons. Ophthalmic Surg Lasers Imaging Retina 2015;46:859. [PMID: 26431302]

Dave VP et al: Endophthalmitis after pars plana vitrectomy: Clinical features, risk factors, and management outcomes. Asia Pac J Ophthalmol (Phila) 2016;5:192. [PMID: 27003734]

Fassbender JM et al: A comparison of immediate and delayed vitrectomy for the management of vitreous hemorrhage due to proliferative diabetic retinopathy. Ophthalmic Surg Lasers Imaging Retina 2016;47:35. [PMID: 26731207]

Goh YW et al: The incidence of retinal breaks in the presenting and fellow eyes in patients with acute symptomatic posterior vitreous detachment and their associated risk factors. Asia Pac J Ophthalmol (Phila) 2015;4:5. [PMID: 26068606]

Gonzalez MA et al: Outcomes of pars plana vitrectomy for patients with vitreomacular traction. Ophthalmic Surg Lasers Imaging Retina 2015;4:708. [PMID: 26247451]

Gupta B et al: Trends and emerging patterns of practice in vitreoretinal surgery. Acta Ophthalmol 2016 May 23. [Epub ahead of print] [PMID: 27213838]

Gurler B et al: Syrian civil-war-related intraocular foreign body injuries: A four-year retrospective analysis. Semin Ophthalmol. 2016 Jul 1:1. [Epub ahead of print] [PMID: 27367974]

Hurst J et al: Value of subjective visual reduction in patients with acute-onset floaters and/or flashes. Can J Ophthalmol 2015;50:265. [PMID: 26257218]

Ivanova T et al: Vitrectomy for primary symptomatic vitreous opacities: An evidence-based review. Eye (Lond) 2016;30:645. [PMID: 26939559]

Kim DY et al: Acute-onset vitreous hemorrhage of unknown origin before vitrectomy: Causes and prognosis. J Ophthalmol 2015;2015:429251. [PMID: 26504593]

Kontos A et al: Duration of intraocular gases following vitreoretinal surgery. Graefes Arch Clin Exp Ophthalmol 2017;255:231. [PMID: 27460279]

Lin H et al: Prognostic indicators of visual acuity after open globe injury and retinal detachment repair. Retina 2016;36:750. [PMID: 26469530]

Mansouri MR et al: Ocular trauma treated with pars plana vitrectomy: Early outcome report. Int J Ophthalmol 2016;9:738. [PMID: 27275432]

Melamud A et al: Early vitrectomy for spontaneous, fundus-obscuring vitreous hemorrhage. Am J Ophthalmol 2015;160:1073. [PMID: 26209230]

Midena E et al: Multimodal retinal imaging of diabetic macular edema: Toward new paradigms of pathophysiology. Graefes Arch Clin Exp Ophthalmol 2016;254:1661. [PMID: 27154296]

Milston R et al: Vitreous floaters: Etiology, diagnostics, and management. Surv Ophthalmol 2016;61:211. [PMID: 26679984]

Mitry D et al: The predisposing pathology and clinical characteristics in the Scottish retinal detachment study. Ophthalmology 2011;118:1429. [PMID: 21561662]

Mura M et al: Use of a new intra-ocular spectral domain optical coherence tomography in vitreoretinal surgery. Acta Ophthalmol 2016;94:246. [PMID: 26842922]

Oahalou A et al: Diagnostic pars plana vitrectomy and aqueous analyses in patients with uveitis of unknown cause. Retina 2014;34:108. [PMID: 23619637]

Oellers P et al: Surgery for proliferative diabetic retinopathy: New tips and tricks. J Ophthalmic Vis Res 2016;11:93. [PMID: 27195092]

Ohtomo K et al: Outcomes of late-onset bleb-related endophthalmitis treated with pars plana vitrectomy. J Ophthalmol 2015;2015:923857. [PMID: 26495137]

Palacio AC et al: Vitreomacular adhesion evolution with age in healthy human eyes. Retina 2017;37:118. [PMID: 27306115]

Reichel E et al: Prevalence of vitreomacular adhesion: an optical coherence tomography analysis in the retina clinic setting. Clin Ophthalmol 2016;10:627. [PMID: 27103782]

Schweitzer KD et al: Predicting retinal tears in posterior vitreous detachment. Can J Ophthalmol 2011;46:481. [PMID: 22153633]

Scupola A et al: 25-gauge pars plana vitrectomy for retained lens fragments in complicated cataract surgery. Ophthalmologica 2015;234:101. [PMID: 26183856]

Sharma P et al: Flashes and floaters. Prim Care 2015;42:425. [PMID: 26319347]

Sharma T et al: Surgical treatment for diabetic vitreoretinal diseases: A review. Clin Exp Ophthalmol 2016;44:340. [PMID: 27027299]

Skeie JM et al: Proteomic insight into the molecular function of the vitreous. PLoS One 2015;10:e0127567. [PMID: 26020955]

Stalmans P. A retrospective cohort study in patients with tractional diseases of the vitreomacular interface (ReCoVit). Graefes Arch Clin Exp Ophthalmol 2016;254:617. [PMID: 26899900]

Steel DH et al: The design and validation of an optical coherence tomography-based classification system for focal vitreomacular traction. Eye (Lond) 2016;30:314. [PMID: 26768921]

Sternfeld A et al: Advantages of diabetic tractional retinal detachment repair. Clin Ophthalmol 2015;9:1989. [PMID: 26604667]

Syed Z et al: Age-dependent vitreous separation from the macula in a clinic population. Clin Ophthalmol 2016;10:1237. [PMID: 27462138]

Thomas BJ et al: Pars plana vitrectomy for late vitreoretinal sequelae of infectious endophthalmitis: Surgical management and outcomes. Retina 2016 Jul 26. [Epub ahead of print] [PMID: 27465568]

Vanner EA et al: Meta-analysis comparing same-day versus delayed vitrectomy clinical outcomes for intravitreal retained lens fragments after age-related cataract surgery. Clin Ophthalmol 2014;8:2261. [PMID: 25429196]

Wu H et al: Pediatric posttraumatic endophthalmitis. Graefes Arch Clin Exp Ophthalmol 2016;254:1919. [PMID: 27067874]

Wu L et al: Anatomical and functional outcomes of symptomatic idiopathic vitreomacular traction: A natural history study from the Pan American Collaborative Retina Study Group. Retina 2016;36:1913. [PMID: 26966868]

Yonekawa Y et al: Immediate sequential bilateral pediatric vitreoretinal surgery: An international multicenter study. Ophthalmology 2016;123:1802. [PMID: 27221737]

Ziemssen F et al: Knowledge of vitreomacular traction (VMT) scenarios: Is doing nothing still a beneficial alternative and, if so, when? Graefes Arch Clin Exp Ophthalmol 2016;254:615. [PMID: 26887826]

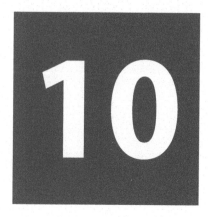

Retina

Raeba Mathew, FRCS, Sobha Sivaprasad, FRCOphth, James J. Augsburger, MD, and Zélia M. Corrêa, MD, PhD

10.1. Retina & Retinal Disorders

Raeba Mathew, FRCS, and Sobha Sivaprasad, FRCOphth

RETINA

The human retina is the most complex of the ocular tissues with a highly organized structure. It receives the visual image, produced by the optical system of the eye, and converts the light energy into an electrical signal, which undergoes initial processing and is then transmitted through the optic nerve to the visual cortex, where the structural (form, color, and contrast) and spatial (position, depth, and motion) attributes are perceived. The anatomy of the retina is described in Chapter 1, Figure 1–17 showing its layers. Function and functional disturbance in the retina often can be localized to a single layer or a single cell type.

PHYSIOLOGY

Rod and cone photoreceptors are responsible for the initial transformation, by the process of phototransduction, of light stimuli into the nerve impulses that are conducted through the visual pathways to the visual cortex. These photoreceptors are arranged such that there is an increased density of cones in the center of the macula (fovea), decreasing to the periphery, and a higher density of rods in the periphery. In the foveola, there is a nearly 1:1 relationship between each cone photoreceptor, its ganglion cell, and the emerging nerve fiber, whereas in the peripheral retina, many photoreceptors connect to the same ganglion cell. The fovea is responsible for good spatial resolution (visual acuity) and color vision, both requiring high ambient light (photopic vision) and being best at the foveola, while the remaining retina is utilized primarily for motion, contrast, and night (scotopic) vision.

The rod and cone photoreceptors are located in the avascular outermost layer of the sensory retina. Each rod photoreceptor cell contains rhodopsin, a photosensitive visual pigment embedded in the double-membrane disks of the photoreceptor outer segment. It is made up of two components, an opsin protein combined with a chromophore. The opsin in rhodopsin is scotopsin, which is formed of seven transmembrane helices. It surrounds the chromophore, retinal, which is derived from vitamin A. When rhodopsin absorbs a photon of light, 11-cis retinal is isomerized to all-trans retinal and eventually to all-trans retinol. The resulting configurational change initiates a secondary messenger cascade. Peak light absorption by rhodopsin occurs at approximately 500 nm, which is in the blue-green region of the light spectrum. Spectral sensitivity studies of cone photopigments have shown peak wavelength absorption at 430, 540, and 575 nm for blue-, green-, and red-sensitive cones, respectively. The cone photopigments are composed of 11-cis retinal bound to other opsin proteins than scotopsin.

Night (scotopic) vision is mediated entirely by rod photoreceptors. With this dark-adapted form of vision, varying shades of gray are seen but colors cannot be distinguished. As the retina becomes fully light-adapted, the spectral sensitivity of the retina shifts from a rhodopsin-dominated peak of 500 nm to approximately 560 nm, and color sensation becomes evident. An object takes on color when it selectively reflects or transmits certain wavelengths of light within the visible spectrum (400–700 nm). Daylight (photopic) vision is mediated primarily by cone photoreceptors, and twilight (mesopic) vision by a combination of cones and rods.

The photoreceptors are maintained by the retinal pigment epithelium (RPE), which plays an important role in the visual process. It is responsible for phagocytosis of the outer segments of the photoreceptors, transport of vitamins, and reduction of light scatter, as well as providing a selective barrier between the choroid and retina. The basement membrane of the RPE cells forms the inner layer of Bruch's membrane, which is otherwise composed of a specialized extracellular matrix and the basement membrane of the choriocapillaris as its outer layer. RPE cells have little capacity for regeneration.

EXAMINATION

Examination of the retina is described in Chapter 2 and depicted in Figures 2–11 to 2–17. The retina can be examined with a direct or indirect ophthalmoscope or with a slitlamp (biomicroscope) and handheld or contact biomicroscopy lens. This allows identification of the type, level, and extent of retinal disease. Retinal imaging techniques (Figures 2–28 to 2–33) are useful adjuncts to clinical examination, enabling identification of anatomical, vascular (both retinal and choroidal), and functional abnormalities. They include digital fundus photography, fundus fluorescein angiography (FFA), (cross-sectional) optical coherence tomography (OCT), indocyanine green angiography (ICGA), and fundus autofluorescence (FAF). The clinical application of visual electrophysiologic and psychophysical tests is described in Chapter 2. Recent advances in retinal imaging include wide-angle cameras, en-face OCT, and noninvasive OCT angiography. On OCT, the inner retina extends to the outer border of the inner plexiform; the outer retina extends from the external limiting membrane; and the middle retina comprises the intervening inner nuclear, outer plexiform, and outer nuclear layers.

AGE-RELATED MACULAR DEGENERATION

Age-related macular degeneration (AMD) affects the elderly and is the leading cause of irreversible blindness in the developed world. It is a complex multifactorial progressive disease. Current evidence suggests genetic susceptibility involving the complement pathway and environmental risk factors, including increasing age, white race, female gender, and smoking. Among white people over age 55 years, the 15-year incidence is 15.1% for early AMD and 4.1% for late AMD.

▶ Pathogenesis

The pathogenesis is still poorly understood. There is a switch, for which the trigger is unclear, in the outer retina–Bruch's membrane–choroid complex from age-related changes to disease that is characterized initially by accumulation of material (drusen) beneath the RPE. It is likely that multiple insults to the retinal-choroid interface result in an exaggerated degenerative process eventually causing atrophy of the RPE that is identified clinically as geographic atrophy and results in gradual decline of vision. These insults include oxidative stress, inflammation, hypoxia, and changes in extracellular matrix. As the disease progresses from the early stage of drusen accumulation to geographic atrophy, angiogenesis occurs in some eyes due to imbalance between proangiogenic and antiangiogenic cytokines in the inflammatory milieu, resulting in the growth of choroidal new vessels through single or multiple areas of weakness in Bruch's membrane into the subretinal space (neovascular AMD). The new vessels leak serous fluid and/or blood, resulting in distortion and rapid decrease of central vision.

▶ Genetic Factors

Twin studies and linkage analysis have identified multiple loci for AMD genes. The two most important are 1q25–31 (complement factor H-CFH) and 10q26 (age-related maculopathy susceptibility ARMS2/HTRA serine peptidase 1-HTRA1). Female sex and pathogenic variants at these loci (CFH-rs1061170 or ARMS2-rs10490924) are independently associated with early AMD incidence, whereas current smoking and the pathogenic variants are associated with late AMD incidence. Individuals with a pathogenic variant are more likely to develop the disease if they smoke or have a low intake of antioxidants.

▶ Classification

Various classifications have been proposed for AMD. The Beckman Initiative for Macular Research Classification Committee stages AMD according to lesions within two disk diameters of the fovea in either eye:

1. No apparent aging changes: no drusen and no pigmentary abnormalities
2. Normal aging changes: only small drusen (< 63 μm diameter) (drupelets) and no pigmentary abnormalities
3. Early AMD: medium drusen (> 63–125 μm diameter) and no pigmentary abnormalities
4. Intermediate AMD: large drusen (> 125 μm diameter) and/or any pigmentary abnormalities
5. Late AMD: neovascular AMD and/or any geographic atrophy

Drusen are identified clinically as yellow deposits that vary in size and shape and are discrete or confluent (Figure 10–1A). Histopathologically, drusen also may form diffuse subretinal deposits, either basal laminar

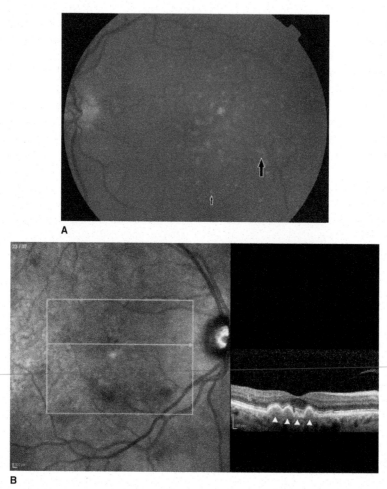

▲ **Figure 10–1.** Age-related macular degeneration (AMD). **A:** Discrete **(small arrow)** and large confluent **(large arrow)** drusen. **B:** Optical coherence tomography scan of large confluent drusen **(arrowheads)**.

deposits, formed mainly of collagen-based material and situated between the plasma and basement membranes of the RPE, or basal linear deposits, consisting of granular lipid-rich material located within Bruch's membrane. On OCT, drusen are seen as bumps between the RPE and Bruch's membrane (Figure 10–1B). On FFA during the early phase, there may be punctate hyperfluorescence corresponding to window defects due to overlying RPE atrophy, and in the late phase, the fluorescence may decrease in smaller drusen and increase in larger drusen.

Reticular pseudodrusen (subretinal drusenoid deposits) are a risk factor for the progression of AMD to advanced stages. They may be identified clinically as indistinct, interlacing, yellowish lesions occurring in the macula, typically along the superior arcades, or with autofluorescence imaging as hypofluorescent lesions against a background of mildly increased autofluorescence. They are best seen on infrared imaging as hyporeflectant lesions against a background of mild hyperreflectance. They may coexist with drusen or lie adjacent to areas of geographic atrophy or (retinal) pigment epithelial detachment (PED). They have been reported to fade with time, and choroidal new vessels may develop in these areas. (On OCT, they appear as granular hyperreflective material lying over the RPE in an undulating pattern. On FFA, they are defects in the choriocapillaris in the early phase. On ICGA, the reticular pattern may be identified as a distinctive grouping of hypofluorescent dots in the mid and late phases.)

Pigmentary abnormalities of AMD may be due to focal clumps of pigmented cells in the subretinal space and outer retina or attenuated areas of hypopigmented RPE that progress to atrophy.

Geographic atrophy is responsible for up to 20% of legal blindness attributable to AMD. It manifests as well-demarcated areas, greater than 175 μm in diameter, of atrophy of the RPE and photoreceptor cells, allowing direct visualization of the underlying choroidal vessels. Visual loss occurs once the fovea is affected. Geographic atrophy is best monitored with autofluorescence imaging, appearing as marked hypofluorescence with different patterns correlating with different rates of disease progression. Early-phase FFA shows a well-demarcated window defect with a mild increase of hyperfluorescence in the late phase. On ICGA, there may be moderate loss of the choriocapillaris but with preservation of the medium and larger-sized choroidal vessels, depending on the severity of geographic atrophy, and mild scleral staining. OCT shows severe disruption or absence of the external limiting membrane and ellipsoid zone accompanied by enhanced visualization of the choroid. If the geographic atrophy is advanced and involves the outer nuclear layer of the retina, there is retinal thinning with the outer plexiform layer directly in contact with Bruch's membrane.

Neovascular AMD is characterized by choroidal neovascularization (CNV) and/or PED. Choroidal new vessels may grow in a flat cartwheel or sea-fan configuration away from their site of entry beneath the RPE, giving rise to a fibrovascular PED or "occult" (type 1) CNV. When the RPE is breached, there is extension into the subretinal space to form a "classic" (type 2) CNV. Signs of activity can be detected on OCT as subretinal and/or intraretinal fluid along with the CNV, but FFA is the most sensitive method for detection of CNV (Figure 10-2). Classic CNV is characterized by early hyperfluorescence,

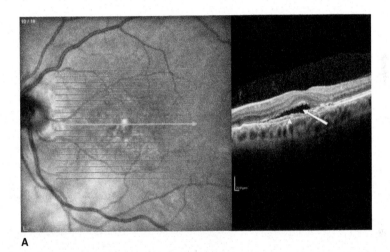

A

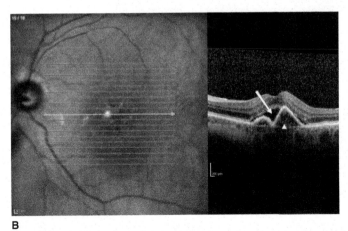

B

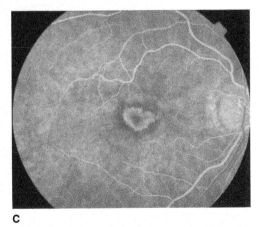

C

▲ **Figure 10-2.** Choroidal neovascularization in age-related macular degeneration (AMD). **A:** Optical coherence tomography (OCT) scan of classic choroidal neovascularization (CNV) **(arrowhead)** with subretinal fluid **(arrow)**. **B:** OCT scan of occult CNV **(arrowhead)** with subretinal fluid **(arrow)**. **C:** Fundus fluorescein angiogram (FFA) of classic CNV showing well-circumscribed, lacy pattern.

which is usually well circumscribed and may have a lacy pattern (Figure 10–2C), and late leakage of fluorescein. Occult CNV is characterized by ill-defined and late hyperfluorescence. For research studies, CNV is subdivided into predominantly classic, in which more than 50% of the lesion has the characteristics of classic CNV; minimally classic, in which less than 50% of the lesion has the characteristics of classic CNV; and pure occult, in which no classic CNV can be identified. Newer imaging techniques such as OCT angiography allow visualization of type 1 and type 2 CNV as organized vascular complexes with branching vessels and anastomoses.

Retinal angiomatous proliferation (RAP) has been termed type 3 CNV. It has been suggested to arise as intraretinal

vessels that extend posteriorly into the choroid in three stages. The first stage is characterized by formation of minute intraretinal new vessels that leads to separation of the neurosensory retina. In the second stage, the intraretinal neovascularization extends into the subretinal space with progression to the third stage of a retinochoroidal anastomosis. Conversely, it has been proposed that the new vessels originate from the choroid, penetrate the RPE, and extend into the retina. Clinically RAP may present with small areas of intraretinal hemorrhages, exudates, and cystoid macular edema (Figure 10–3A). FFA shows bright hyperfluorescence associated with the tip of a retinal vessel during the early phase, increasing fluorescence in the middle phase (Figure 10–3B),

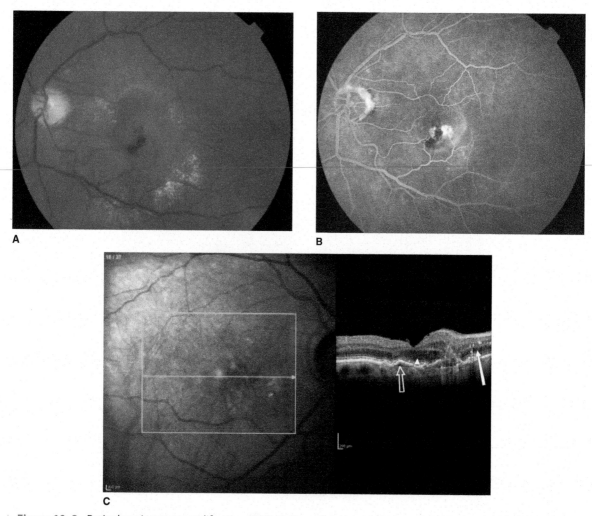

A

B

C

▲ **Figure 10–3.** Retinal angiomatous proliferation (RAP). **A:** Superficial hemorrhage, retinal pigment epithelial detachment, and extensive exudation. **B:** Mid-venous phase of fundus fluorescein angiogram showing focal hyperfluorescence of retinochoroidal anastomosis and diffuse early filling of retinal pigment epithelial detachment. **C:** Optical coherence tomography showing punctuate hyperreflective foci **(arrow)** and intraretinal **(arrowhead)** and subretinal **(outline arrow)** fluid.

and leakage of fluorescein with cystoid macular edema in the late phase. ICGA shows vascular abnormalities and chorio-retinal communication during the middle to late phases with moderate leakage. In the early stages, OCT shows the intra-retinal vascular abnormalities as punctate hyperreflective foci above the external limiting membrane (Figure 10–3C). In the third stage, there is clear visualization of the retino-choroidal anastomosis, along with intraretinal or subretinal fluid as indicators of active disease.

Prophylactic Therapy to Prevent Progression to Late AMD

In patients with bilateral intermediate drusen or unilateral CNV, treatment with oral **vitamins** (vitamin C 500 g and vitamin E 400 IU per day), **antioxidants** (beta-carotene 15 mg/d), zinc (80 mg/d), and copper (2 mg/d) reduces the 5-year risk of progression to late AMD in either eye or in the unaffected eye, respectively. (Smokers and ex-smokers are advised to omit beta-carotene due to an increased risk of development of lung cancer.) Cessation of smoking reduces the rate of progression of AMD, but it takes about 20 years to reduce the risk of development of AMD to that of a non-smoker. Daily exercise lowers the risk of AMD.

Treatment of Neovascular AMD

Vascular endothelial growth factor (VEGF) plays a cru-cial role in development and activity of CNV by inducing angiogenesis and increasing vascular permeability. Repeated intravitreal injections of an anti-VEGF agent is the treatment of choice for neovascular AMD. **Bevacizumab** (Avastin) is a full-length recombinant monoclonal antibody that binds all VEGF isoforms and is approved for intravenous treatment of metastatic colorectal cancer and other cancer types. It has not been developed as an ocular preparation but is widely used off-label with good results. **Ranibizumab** (Lucentis) is a recombinant, humanized Fab fragment of bevacizumab that has been affinity matured and specifically developed for intravitreal injection. **Aflibercept** (Eylea) is a recombi-nant fusion protein consisting of key human VEGF recep-tor (VEGFR) extracellular domains from receptors 1 and 2 (VEGFR1 and VEGFR2) fused to the Fc domain of human IgG1. It has a much higher binding affinity for VEGF-A than either bevacizumab or ranibizumab and, in addition, binds related growth factors such as placental growth factors 1 and 2 (PLGF1 and PLGF2) and VEGF-B. Hence, it has a potentially longer duration of action in the eye. The vitreous half-life of ranibizumab is 4.75 days, aflibercept 7.13 days, and bevacizumab 8.25 days. The standard regimen for anti-VEGF therapy is at least 3 monthly injections until stable visual acuity is attained followed by long-term therapy with less frequent injections for which there are several regimens. (For discussion of such regimens, see later discussion of treatment of diabetic macular edema.) Bevacizumab and ranibizumab have the same efficacy and safety profile. For long-term therapy, aflibercept every 8 weeks is not inferior to ranibizumab. Anti-VEGF agents are more effective in improving and maintaining visual acuity than laser photoco-agulation, photodynamic therapy (PDT), or surgery.

MYOPIC MACULAR DEGENERATION

Pathologic myopia (more than 6 diopters) is one of the leading causes of blindness in the United States and is much more prevalent in the Far East and Japan. It is characterized by· progressive increase in axial length of the eye resulting in thinning and atrophy of the choroid and RPE involving the macula. Characteristic findings on fundoscopy are peri-papillary chorioretinal atrophy (Figure 10–4A), posterior staphyloma, and linear breaks in Bruch's membrane ("lacquer cracks"), which may be complicated by spontaneous retinal hemorrhages unassociated with a CNV. Degenerative changes of the macular RPE may resemble those found in AMD. A characteristic lesion of pathologic myopia is a raised, circular, pigmented macular lesion (Forster-Fuchs spot) caused by growth of fibrovascular tissue from the choroid associated with RPE proliferation. Degenerative macular changes cause a slowly progressive loss of vision in the fifth decade. Rapid loss of visual acuity is usually caused by exudative macu-lar detachment overlying CNV, which occurs in 5–10% of patients. FFA shows delayed filling of choroidal and retinal blood vessel and identifies any CNV. Anti-VEGF therapy is the treatment of choice for subfoveal or juxtafoveal CNV.

The peripheral chorioretinal changes of pathologic myo-pia include paving stone, pigmentary, and lattice degenera-tion that may lead to retinal breaks and retinal detachment. Rhegmatogenous detachment involving the posterior pole also may be caused by a macular hole that may be differenti-ated from myopic CNV by demonstration of the hole on OCT and absence of leakage on FFA. Myopic foveoschisis is a splitting of the neural retina into a thicker inner layer and a thinner outer layer or a compound variant in which there is also splitting of the nerve fiber layer (Figure 10–4B). There may be reasonably good vision, but untreated, there tends to be slow progression to macular hole and/or retinal detach-ment. Treatment is by surgery. Localized posterior choroidal excavation (ectasia) (Figure 10–4C) may involve the outer retinal layers including the external limiting membrane or just the RPE. It may be complicated by CNV.

RETINAL VASCULAR DISEASES

DIABETIC RETINOPATHY

Diabetic retinopathy is the most common microvascular complication of diabetes mellitus and one of the leading causes of blindness in the industrialized world, particularly among individuals of working age. Chronic hyperglycemia,

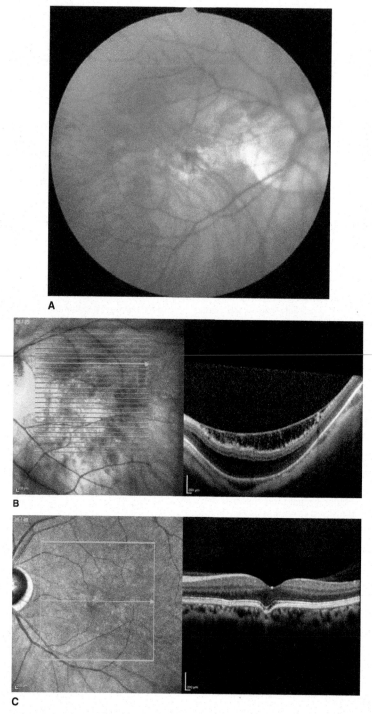

▲ Figure 10–4. Myopic macular degeneration. **A:** Choroidal vessels visible through atrophic retinal pigment epithelium and peripapillary atrophy. **B:** Optical coherence tomography (OCT) of compound myopic foveoschisis showing splitting of the neural retina and the retinal nerve fiber layer. **C:** OCT of myopic choroidal excavation.

systemic hypertension, hypercholesterolemia, and smoking are risk factors for development and progression of retinopathy. Visual impairment is caused by macular edema or the complications of proliferative diabetic retinopathy comprising vitreous hemorrhage, tractional retinal detachment, and neovascular glaucoma. Retinopathy is rare in type 1diabetics prior to puberty, whereas one-third of type 2 diabetics have retinopathy at initial diagnosis. The relative risk for developing diabetic retinopathy is higher in type 1 compared to type 2. The risk of proliferative diabetic retinopathy (PDR) is higher in type 1, whereas diabetic macular edema is more common in type 2.

▶ Screening

Early detection and timely treatment of diabetic retinopathy are essential for prevention of permanent visual loss. Screening should be performed within 3 years from diagnosis in type 1 diabetes, at diagnosis in type 2 diabetes, and annually thereafter in both types. Diabetic retinopathy may progress rapidly during pregnancy, and screening should take place in the first trimester and then at least every 3 months until delivery. Digital fundal photography is an effective and sensitive screening method. Seven-field photography after pupil dilation has been the gold standard, but using two 45° fields, one centered on the macula and the other centered on the disk, has been the method of choice in most screening programs. Recent advances in imaging particularly wide field fundus photography have improved detection of central and peripheral retinopathy.

▶ Pathophysiology

Diabetic retinopathy is a progressive microangiopathy. Chronic hyperglycemia leads to a metabolic response that is mediated by increased glycation end-products, polyols, reactive oxygen species, eicosanoids, nitric oxides, and intercellular adhesion molecules, and activation of the protein kinase C pathway, leading to microvascular endothelial damage, retinal capillary leukostasis, and capillary closure. The resultant inner retinal ischemia triggers release of VEGF, which in turn results in breakdown of inner blood retinal barrier and vascular leakage.

The earliest histopathologic changes are thickening of the capillary endothelial basement membrane and loss of pericytes, leading to outpouchings that form microaneurysms. Superficial flame-shaped hemorrhages in the nerve fiber layer arise from precapillary arterioles, and deep dot and blot hemorrhages arise from the venous end of the capillaries. Cotton-wool spots are evidence of axoplasmic stasis usually due to infarcts of the nerve fiber layer from occlusion of precapillary arterioles.

▶ Classification

Diabetic retinopathy can be broadly classified into nonproliferative retinopathy, maculopathy, and proliferative retinopathy, of which the latter two may coexist.

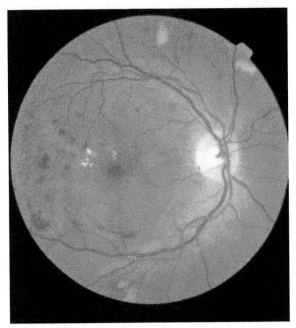

▲ **Figure 10–5.** Moderate nonproliferative diabetic retinopathy showing microaneurysms, deep hemorrhages, flame-shaped hemorrhage, exudates, and cotton-wool spots.

A. NONPROLIFERATIVE DIABETIC RETINOPATHY

Mild nonproliferative diabetic retinopathy (NPDR) is characterized by at least one microaneurysm. In moderate NPDR, there are numerous microaneurysms, intraretinal hemorrhages, venous beading, and/or cotton-wool spots (Figure 10–5). Severe NPDR is characterized by cotton-wool spots, venous beading in two quadrants, and intraretinal microvascular abnormalities (IRMA) either in four quadrants or severe in one quadrant.

B. DIABETIC MACULOPATHY

Diabetic maculopathy manifests as focal or diffuse retinal thickening (edema), caused primarily by a breakdown of the inner blood–retinal barrier at the level of the retinal capillary endothelium that allows leakage of fluid and plasma constituents into the surrounding retina. The criterion for treatment has been clinically significant macular edema (Figure 10–6), which is defined as any retinal thickening within 500 μm of the center of the macula, exudates within 500 μm of the center of the macula with adjacent retinal thickening, or retinal thickening at least one disk area in size, any part of which is within one disk diameter of the center of the macula. With the advent of anti-VEGF treatment,

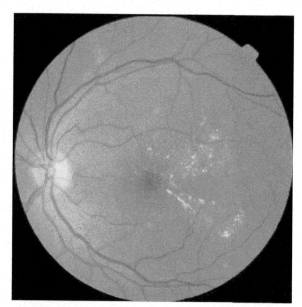

Figure 10–6. Clinically significant macular edema with two circinate rings of exudates.

diabetic macular edema is classified by OCT into center involving and non–center involving.

Maculopathy can also be due to ischemia, which is characterized by edema, deep hemorrhages, and little exudation. FFA shows loss of retinal capillaries with enlargement of the foveal avascular zone (Figure 10–7).

C. PROLIFERATIVE DIABETIC RETINOPATHY

Proliferative diabetic retinopathy (PDR) causes the most severe complications. Retinal ischemia upregulates VEGF, which stimulates angiogenesis, leading to the formation of delicate new vessels and increased vascular permeability with leak of serum proteins. PDR is characterized by new vessels on the optic disk (NVD) (Figure 10–8) or elsewhere in the retina (NVE) (Figure 10–9). High-risk characteristics are NVD extending more than one-third disk diameter, any NVD with vitreous hemorrhage, or NVE extending more than one-half disk diameter with vitreous hemorrhage.

The fragile new vessels proliferate onto the posterior face of the vitreous and become elevated once the vitreous starts to contract away from the retina. If the vessels bleed, vitreous hemorrhage may cause sudden visual loss. There is very little risk of developing neovascularization and vitreous hemorrhage once a complete posterior vitreous detachment has developed. In eyes with proliferative diabetic retinopathy and persistent vitreoretinal adhesions, elevated neovascular fronds may undergo fibrous change and form tight fibrovascular bands, leading to vitreoretinal traction.

This can lead to progressive traction retinal detachment or, if a retinal tear occurs, rhegmatogenous retinal detachment. The retinal detachment may be heralded or concealed by vitreous hemorrhage. Once vitreous contraction is complete, the proliferative retinopathy tends to enter the burnt-out or "involutional" stage. Advanced diabetic eye disease may also be complicated by iris neovascularization (rubeosis iridis) and neovascular glaucoma.

Imaging

OCT is invaluable in the identification and monitoring of macular edema as well as identification of structural changes within the retina. Spectral domain OCT, with increased scan speed and resolution and eye tracking improving reproducibility, enhances assessment.

FFA identifies microvascular abnormalities (Figure 10–10). Filling defects in the capillary beds (capillary nonperfusion), usually most prominent in the mid-periphery (Figure 10–11), show the extent of peripheral retinal and macular ischemia (Figure 10–7), the former being predictive of proliferative retinopathy and the latter being predictive of poor visual prognosis. Fluorescein leakage associated with retinal edema may assume the petalloid configuration of cystoid macular edema (CME) or may be diffuse (Figure 10–12). The distinction helps determine prognosis as well as the required location and extent of laser treatment.

By providing three-dimensional reconstruction of the retinal and choroidal microvasculature without the need for injection of a dye, the new technique of OCT angiography offers more extensive noninvasive assessment. Wide-angle retinal imaging has shown abnormalities outside the standard (Early Treatment Diabetic Retinopathy Study [ETDRS]) fields of assessment in up to 40% of eyes, leading to grading of greater severity in a quarter of such eyes. Presence and increasing extent of lesions outside the ETDRS fields are associated with a three- to five-fold increased risk of progression of retinopathy over 4 years.

Treatment

The mainstay of prevention of progression of retinopathy is tight control of hyperglycemia, systemic hypertension, and hypercholesterolemia.

Ocular treatment depends on the location and severity of the retinopathy. Diabetic macular edema that is not clinically significant is usually monitored closely without treatment. In center-involving macular edema, intravitreal injections of an anti-VEGF agent such as ranibizumab, aflibercept, or bevacizumab improves visual acuity and can maintain the improvement for over 5 years. The treatment regimen consists of a loading phase of three to six monthly injections until visual acuity stabilizes followed by long-term therapy with injections, at potentially longer intervals, either at fixed intervals, as required to treat recurrence of edema

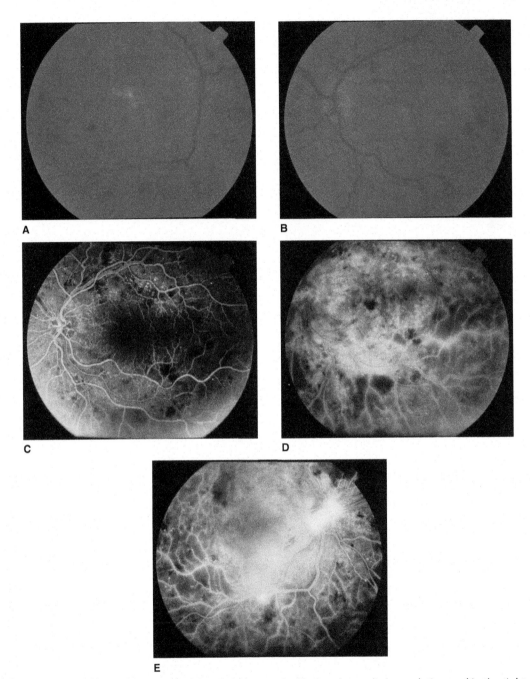

▲ **Figure 10–7.** Diabetic ischemic maculopathy with deep retinal hemorrhages, little exudation, and in the right eye, early optic disk neovascularization. **A:** Right eye. **B:** Left eye. Fundus fluorescein angiogram shows capillary nonperfusion (**arrows**), macular edema, and dye leakage from the optic disk new vessels in the right eye. **C and D:** Left eye early and late phases. **E:** Right eye late phase.

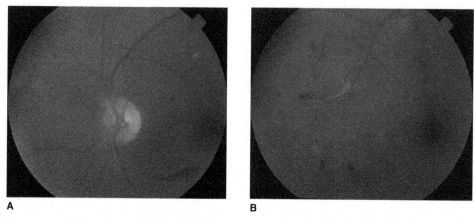

▲ **Figure 10–8.** Diabetic proliferative retinopathy. **A:** Disk new vessels with preretinal hemorrhage. **B:** Peripheral new vessels.

("treat and observe"), or as determined to be adequate to prevent development of edema ("treat and extend"). Laser treatment is reserved for clinically significant edema that is not center involving or in combination with an anti-VEGF agent in center-involving edema.

Panretinal laser photocoagulation (PRP) induces regression of new vessels and reduces the incidence of severe visual loss from proliferative diabetic retinopathy by 50%. Several thousand regularly spaced laser burns are applied throughout the retina outside the vascular arcades to reduce the angiogenic stimulus from ischemic areas (see Chapter 23). Patients at greatest risk of visual loss are those with high-risk characteristics, when it is essential that adequate PRP is performed without delay. Treatment of severe NPDR has not been shown to alter the visual outcome. However, if the patient has type 2 diabetes, poor glycemic control, or cannot be monitored sufficiently carefully, treatment before proliferative disease has developed may be justified.

Vitrectomy removes vitreous hemorrhage and relieves vitreoretinal traction. Twenty percent of eyes with extensive

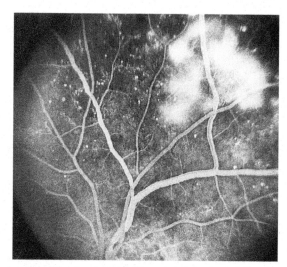

▲ **Figure 10–9.** Fluorescein angiogram of proliferative diabetic retinopathy shows leakage from the neovascular tissue. The pinpoint areas of hyperfluorescence are microaneurysms.

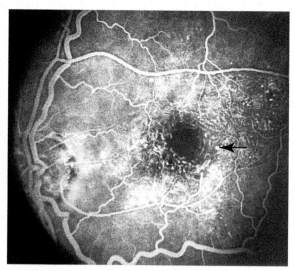

▲ **Figure 10–10.** Fluorescein angiogram in nonproliferative diabetic retinopathy shows microaneurysms (**arrow**) and perifoveal retinal vascular changes.

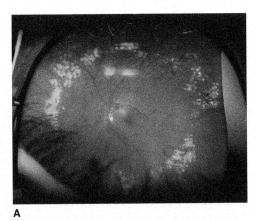 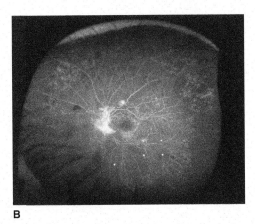

A   B

▲ **Figure 10–11.** Wide-angle images of proliferative diabetic retinopathy. **A:** New vessels on the optic disk (NVD) and peripheral laser scars. **B:** Fluorescein angiogram shows leakage from the NVD and large areas of capillary nonperfusion outside the arcades **(arrowheads)**. (Used with permission from Moorfields Eye Hospital, London.)

vitreous hemorrhage will progress to no perception of light vision within 2 years. Early vitrectomy is indicated for type 1 diabetics with extensive vitreous hemorrhage and severe, active proliferation and poor vision in the contralateral eye, facilitating early visual rehabilitation. Intravitreal anti-VEGF therapy 2 weeks preoperatively reduces the risk of postoperative rebleeding and improves visual outcome. Vitrectomy is also recommended for sight-threatening tractional retinal detachment and for rhegmatogenous retinal detachment

complicating proliferative retinopathy. Complications following vitrectomy include phthisis bulbi, raised intraocular pressure with corneal edema, retinal detachment, and infection.

RETINAL VEIN OCCLUSION

Retinal vein occlusion is a relatively common and easily diagnosed retinal vascular disorder with potentially blinding complications. The patient usually presents with sudden, painless loss of vision at the time of the occlusion, when the clinical appearance varies from a few small, scattered retinal hemorrhages and cotton-wool spots to a marked hemorrhagic appearance with both deep and superficial retinal hemorrhage, which rarely may result in vitreous hemorrhage. The presentation may also be with sudden loss of vision due to vitreous hemorrhage from retinal neovascularization or gradual loss of vision due to macular edema.

In **central retinal vein occlusion** (Figure 10–13), the retinal abnormalities involve all four quadrants of the fundus. In **branch retinal vein occlusion,** typically the abnormalities are confined to one quadrant (Figure 10–14) because the occlusion usually occurs at the site of an arteriovenous crossing, but they may involve the upper or lower half (hemispheric branch retinal vein occlusion) or just the macula (macular branch retinal vein occlusion).

Patients are usually over 50 years of age, and more than 50% have associated cardiovascular disease. Predisposing factors and investigations are discussed in Chapter 15. Raised intraocular pressure should always be excluded (see Chapter 11). The major complications are macular edema, neovascular glaucoma secondary to iris neovascularization, and retinal neovascularization.

▲ **Figure 10–12.** Late-phase fluorescein angiogram shows hyperfluorescence typical of diffuse (noncystoid) diabetic macular edema.

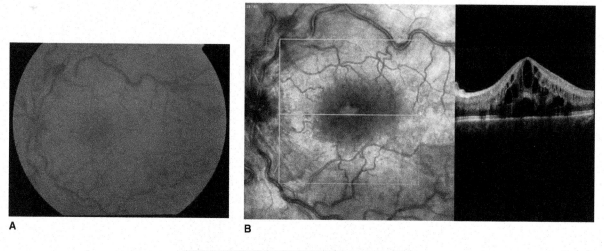

A

B

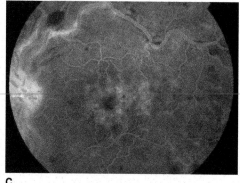

C

▲ **Figure 10–13.** Central retinal vein occlusion. **A:** Retinal hemorrhage in all four quadrants, dilated tortuous veins, and optic disk edema. **B:** Optical coherence tomography shows cystoid macular edema. **C:** Fundus fluorescein angiogram shows late leak with petalloid appearance of macula. (Used with permission from Moorfields Eye Hospital, London.)

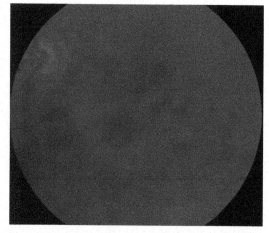

▲ **Figure 10–14.** Branch retinal vein occlusion involving the inferotemporal vein.

1. MACULAR EDEMA IN RETINAL VEIN OCCLUSION

Macular dysfunction occurs in almost all eyes with central retinal vein occlusion. Although some will show spontaneous improvement, most will have persistent decreased central vision due to chronic macular edema, which is also the main cause of persisting reduction of visual acuity in branch retinal vein occlusion.

Intravitreal injection of an anti-VEGF agent is the treatment of choice for macular edema due to central or branch retinal vein occlusion. Monthly injections of ranibizumab or aflibercept have been shown to be effective. Trials are in progress to determine the efficacy of bevacizumab. Intravitreal steroid, either triamcinolone or Ozurdex (Allergan), which is an intravitreal sustained-release implant containing dexamethasone, also is effective but may cause increased intraocular pressure and development or progression of cataract.

Macular edema due to central retinal vein occlusion does not respond to laser treatment. In branch retinal vein occlusion, grid-pattern macular argon laser photocoagulation may be indicated when vision loss due to macular edema persists for several months without any spontaneous improvement.

2. IRIS AND RETINAL NEOVASCULARIZATION IN RETINAL VEIN OCCLUSION

Either initially or subsequently, one-third of central retinal vein occlusions are ischemic, which is associated with visual acuity worse than 20/100 and a relative afferent pupillary defect but is detected best by greater than 10 disk areas of retinal ischemia on FFA. One-half of ischemic eyes will develop anterior segment (iris and/or anterior chamber angle) neovascularization with the risk of progression to neovascular glaucoma. The standard treatment for anterior segment neovascularization is PRP, which may be preceded by an intravitreal anti-VEGF agent.

In branch retinal vein occlusion, retinal neovascularization develops in 40% of eyes with more than five disk areas of retinal ischemia (Figure 10–15). Sectoral retinal laser photocoagulation of the ischemic retina halves the risk of vitreous hemorrhage.

RETINAL ARTERY OCCLUSION

Central retinal artery occlusion causes sudden, severe loss of vision without pain. Antecedent transient visual loss (amaurosis fugax) may be reported and is suggestive of giant cell arteritis or retinal emboli. Visual acuity ranges between counting fingers and light perception in 90% of eyes at initial examination.

Usually there is permanent extensive loss of visual field. Twenty-five percent of eyes have cilioretinal arteries that continue to perfuse the macula, potentially preserving central field and/or visual acuity. An afferent pupillary defect can appear within seconds, preceding any fundus abnormalities, which include opacification of the superficial retina due to infarction and reduced blood flow in the retinal vessels, sometimes visible as segmentation ("cattle trucking") of the blood column in the retinal arterioles. A foveal cherry-red spot (Figure 10–16) develops due to preservation of the relatively normal appearance of the choroidal pigment and RPE through the extremely thin retina overlying the fovea, surrounded by the pale swollen retina of the rest of the macula. The fundal abnormalities resolve within 4–6 weeks, leaving a pale optic disk as the major ocular finding.

Branch retinal artery occlusion also causes sudden painless visual loss but usually manifesting as impairment of visual field that usually is permanent. Visual acuity is reduced only if there is foveal involvement. The extent of the fundal abnormalities, primarily retinal opacification as in central retinal artery occlusion but sometimes accompanied by cotton-wool spots along its border, is determined by the extent of retinal infarction. The cause is often embolic disease, for which clinical evaluation and investigations need to be undertaken (see Chapter 15).

▶ Imaging

In the acute phase of retinal artery occlusion, OCT shows hyperreflectivity with thickening of the inner retina extending to include the outer plexiform layer. The adjacent outer retinal layers are not clearly discernible and are seen as a hyporeflective or widened area, probably due to masking of

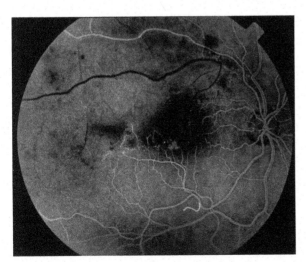

▲ **Figure 10–15.** Fundus fluorescein angiogram of superotemporal branch retinal vein occlusion with extensive retinal ischemia.

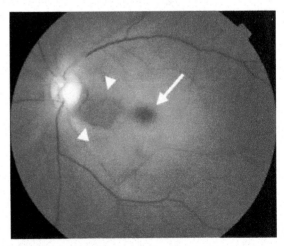

▲ **Figure 10–16.** Acute central retinal artery occlusion with cherry-red spot **(arrow)** and preserved retina due to cilioretinal arterial supply **(arrowheads)**. (Used with permission from Esther Posner.)

the outer layers by the cloudy swelling of the inner retina. Similarly autofluorescence imaging shows reduced autofluorescence due to masking of the normal autofluorescence of the RPE. Resolution of the cloudy swelling leads to recovery of normal autofluorescence, except in areas of very thin inner retina where there may be increased autofluorescence due to a "window defect." FFA in the acute phase shows delayed filling of the involved artery and prolonged retinal arteriovenous transit time. Complete lack of filling of the retinal artery is seen in less than 2% of cases. After a variable interval of time, the retinal circulation is reestablished and may even return to normal. Thus FFA, which is an invasive procedure with a risk of anaphylactic reaction, may be indicated in the acute stage, but thereafter, it is unlikely to be appropriate. OCT and FAF usually will establish the diagnosis. FFA and the noninvasive OCT angiography are able to distinguish between the retinal and choroidal circulation, but only the latter is able to distinguish between the superficial and deep capillary plexus, thus providing additional information on the extent of retinal ischemia.

It can be difficult to diagnose long-standing branch retinal artery occlusion. However, on OCT, the characteristic thinning of the inner retinal layers with a well-demarcated junction between the ischemic and normal retina is a useful sign, and the retinal thickness color map shows the extent of retinal damage (Figure 10–17).

▶ Treatment

Irreversible retinal damage occurs within a few hours of retinal artery occlusion. Treatment options include ocular massage, anterior chamber paracentesis, medications to reduce intraocular pressure, vasodilators (sublingual or transdermal nitroglycerin, oral isosorbide dinitrate, breathing a mixture of oxygen and carbon dioxide), and intra-arterial or intravenous thrombolysis. Intra-arterial thrombolysis is most likely to be effective but is often difficult to administer quickly enough to be beneficial, and its risks may not be justifiable especially in branch retinal artery occlusion. Anterior chamber paracentesis is indicated, particularly when an embolus is visible on the optic disk.

▶ Investigations

Investigation of patients with central or branch retinal artery occlusion is discussed fully in Chapter 15. In older patients with central retinal artery occlusion, giant cell arteritis must be excluded and, if necessary, treated immediately with high-dose systemic corticosteroids to avoid loss of vision in the other eye. Investigation for embolic disease by carotid Doppler studies and echocardiography and assessment of risk factors for arteriosclerosis are important in both central and branch retinal artery occlusion. Also vasculitis and congenital or acquired thrombophilia need to be considered.

RETINAL ARTERIAL MACROANEURYSM

Retinal macroaneurysm is a fusiform or round dilation of a retinal arteriole occurring within the first three orders of arteriolar bifurcation. Most cases are unilateral, involving the superotemporal artery. Two-thirds of patients have associated systemic hypertension.

Macroaneurysm may result in retinal edema, exudation, or hemorrhage typically with an "hourglass" configuration due to bleeding deep and superficial to the retina (Figure 10–18). As hemorrhage is usually followed by fibrosis of the macroaneurysm, no further treatment is required. If edema threatens the macula, the macroaneurysm can be treated by confluent laser photocoagulation followed by a direct hit. There is a risk that this direct hit will result in hemorrhage, but this usually settles with fibrosis of the macroaneurysm.

RETINOPATHY OF PREMATURITY

Retinopathy of prematurity (ROP), which is discussed in Chapter 17, is a vasoproliferative retinopathy affecting premature and low-birth-weight infants.

RETINAL DETACHMENT AND RELATED RETINAL DEGENERATIONS

Retinal detachment is the separation of the sensory retina (ie, the photoreceptors and inner retinal layers) from the underlying RPE. There are three main types: rhegmatogenous, traction, and exudative (serous), which may be hemorrhagic.

1. RHEGMATOGENOUS RETINAL DETACHMENT

The most common type, rhegmatogenous retinal detachment is caused by one or more full-thickness breaks in the sensory retina, variable degrees of vitreous traction, and passage of liquefied vitreous through the breaks into the subretinal space. A retinal break ("rhegma") may be a tear, which typically is U-shaped ("horseshoe") and caused by vitreo-retinal traction; a round hole, which may result from vitreo-retinal traction but typically occurs in an area of retinal degeneration such as lattice degeneration and much less frequently results in retinal detachment than a retinal tear; or a retinal dialysis, in which the most peripheral retina separates from the pars plana at the ora serrata often as a result of blunt ocular trauma. Except when due to a retinal dialysis, rhegmatogenous retinal detachment is usually preceded by posterior vitreous detachment that generally is a spontaneous age-related phenomenon but is rendered more likely by myopia, cataract surgery, and ocular trauma. Lattice degeneration of the retina, which is associated with myopia, increases the likelihood of retinal tears and holes and progression to retinal detachment. Binocular indirect ophthalmoscopy with scleral depression (Figure 2–15) or slitlamp examination with a handheld or contact biomicroscopy lens

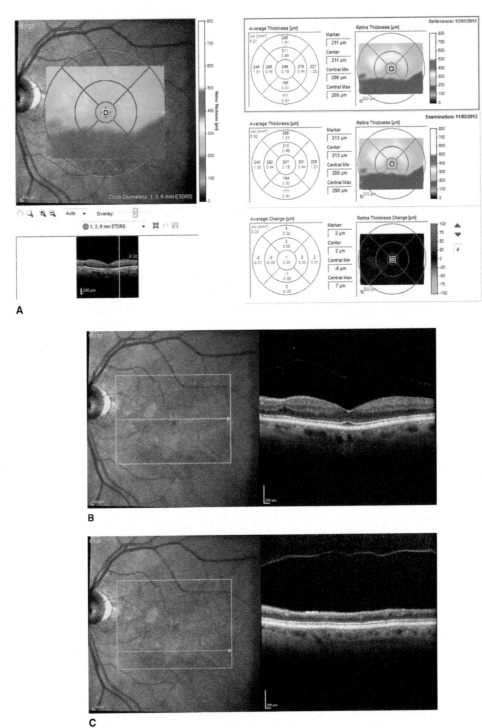

▲ **Figure 10–17.** Optical coherence tomography of branch retinal artery occlusion. **A:** Retinal thickness color image showing well-demarcated thin (blue) inferior retina. **B:** Cross-section through fovea showing normal retinal thickness. **C:** Cross-section of inferior showing inner retinal thinning.

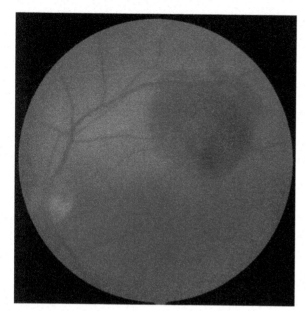

▲ **Figure 10–18.** Retinal macroaneurysm with subretinal, intraretinal, and vitreous hemorrhage.

subretinal fluid away from the retinal break, but external drainage of subretinal fluid may be required. The success rate is 92–94% in suitably selected cases. Complications include change in refractive error, diplopia due to fibrosis or involvement of extraocular muscles in the explant, extrusion of the explant, and possibly increased risk of proliferative vitreoretinopathy.

Pars plana vitrectomy allows relief of vitreo-retinal traction; internal drainage of subretinal fluid, if necessary by injection of perfluorocarbons or heavy liquids; and injection of air or expandable gas to maintain the retina in position or injection of oil if longer-term tamponade of the retina is required. It is used if there are superior, posterior, or multiple retinal breaks; when visualization of the retina is inhibited, such as by vitreous hemorrhage; and if there is significant proliferative vitreoretinopathy. The introduction of 23- and 25-guage rather than 20-gauge vitrectomy instruments has made possible sutureless surgery, with the advantages of reduced operating time, less anterior segment inflammation, improved patient comfort, and more rapid recovery of vision, but with greater risks of postoperative hypotony and endophthalmitis. The 25-gauge system is mainly indicated for macular surgery as there are reports of worse outcome with the 23-gauge system. Postoperative posturing may be required if intraocular air or gas is utilized. Vitrectomy, especially if intraocular air, gas, or oil is used, frequently induces or accelerates cataract formation.

The visual results of surgery for rhegmatogenous retinal detachment primarily depend on the preoperative status of the macula. If the macula has been detached, recovery of central vision is usually incomplete. Thus, surgery should be performed urgently if the macula is still attached. Once the macula is detached, delay in surgery for up to 1 week does not adversely influence visual outcome.

reveals elevation of the translucent detached sensory retina and the retinal breaks. The location of retinal breaks varies according to type; horseshoe tears are most common in the superotemporal quadrant, holes in the temporal quadrants, and retinal dialysis in the inferotemporal quadrant. When multiple retinal breaks are present, they are usually within 90° of one another.

▶ Treatment

Surgery is the only treatment for rhegmatogenous retinal detachment. There are various methods with the intentions of locating all the retinal breaks and treating them by cryotherapy or laser retinopexy to create an adhesion between the RPE and the sensory retina, thus preventing any further influx of fluid into the subretinal space; if necessary draining subretinal fluid, internally or externally; and relieving vitreoretinal traction.

In **pneumatic retinopexy**, air or expandable gas is injected into the vitreous to maintain the retina in position, while the chorioretinal adhesion induced by laser or cryotherapy achieves permanent closure of the retinal break. It has a lower success rate than other methods and is used only when there is a small accessible single retinal break, minimal subretinal fluid, and no vitreoretinal traction.

Scleral buckling maintains the retina in position, while the chorioretinal adhesion forms, by indenting the sclera with a sutured explant in the region of the retinal break. This also relieves vitreo-retinal traction and displaces

2. TRACTION RETINAL DETACHMENT

Traction retinal detachment is most commonly due to proliferative diabetic retinopathy. It can also be associated with proliferative vitreoretinopathy complicating rhegmatogenous retinal detachment, retinal neovascularization following retinal vein occlusion, ROP, or ocular trauma. In comparison to rhegmatogenous retinal detachment, traction retinal detachment has a more concave surface and is likely to be more localized, usually not extending to the ora serrata. The tractional forces actively pull the sensory retina away from the underlying RPE toward the vitreous base. Traction is due to formation of vitreal, epiretinal, or subretinal membranes consisting of fibroblasts and glial and RPE cells. Initially the detachment may be localized along the vascular arcades, but progression may spread to involve the midperipheral retina and the macula. Focal traction from cellular membranes can produce a retinal tear and lead to combined traction-rhegmatogenous retinal detachment.

▶ Treatment

Pars plana vitrectomy allows removal of the tractional elements followed by removal of the fibrotic membranes. Retinotomy and/or injection of perfluorocarbons or heavy liquids may be required to flatten the retina. Gas tamponade, silicone oil, or scleral buckling may be used.

3. EXUDATIVE RETINAL DETACHMENT

Exudative (serous) retinal detachment, which may be hemorrhagic, occurs in the absence of either retinal break or vitreoretinal traction. It is caused primarily by disease of the RPE and choroid. Degenerative, inflammatory, and infectious diseases, including the multiple causes of CNV, may be associated with exudative retinal detachment and are described in an earlier section of this chapter. This type of detachment may also be associated with systemic vascular or inflammatory disease or intraocular tumors (see Chapters 7 and 15).

4. PERIPHERAL RETINAL DEGENERATIONS

▶ Lattice Degeneration

Lattice degeneration is the most important vitreoretinal degeneration that predisposes to retinal detachment. The estimated incidence in the general population is 6–10%, with bilateral disease in up to 50% of cases. It is more commonly found in myopic eyes with some familial tendency. It produces localized round, oval, or linear areas of retinal thinning, with pigmentation, branching white lines, and whitish-yellow flecks, and firm vitreoretinal adhesions at its margins. Lattice degeneration results in retinal detachment in only a small percentage of affected eyes, but 20–30% of eyes with retinal detachment have lattice degeneration. Strong family history of retinal detachment, retinal detachment in the fellow eye, high myopia, and aphakia require the patient to be informed of the risks of retinal detachment and the relevant symptoms but rarely warrant prophylactic treatment with cryosurgery or laser photocoagulation. **Snail-track degeneration**, characterized by groups of white dots, may be a precursor of lattice degeneration.

RETINOSCHISIS AND MICROCYSTOID DEGENERATION

Microcystoid degeneration causes bubbles or vacuoles in the far peripheral retina that may be confused with retinal holes. Degenerative retinoschisis is common and thought to develop from coalescence of microcystoid degeneration. The cystic elevation is most commonly found in the inferotemporal quadrant, followed by the superotemporal quadrant. It develops into one of two forms, typical or reticular, although clinically, the two are difficult to differentiate.

Typical degenerative retinoschisis forms a round or ovoid area of retinal splitting in the outer plexiform layer. Posterior extension and hole formation in the outer layer are uncommon and therefore pose low risk of progression to retinal detachment. **Reticular degenerative retinoschisis** is characterized by round or oval areas of retinal splitting in the nerve fiber layer forming a bullous elevation of an extremely thin inner layer. Retinal holes occur in 23%, and posterior extension or progression to rhegmatogenous retinal detachment may occur and requires treatment.

Degenerative retinoschisis is present in about 4% of the population and is bilateral in approximately 30% of cases. Spontaneous regression occurs in up to 9% of cases. Progression to retinal detachment occurs in up to 2%, with increased risk for those with a family history of retinal detachment. Whether cataract extraction increases the risk of retinal detachment is uncertain. Retinal detachment occurs in one of two ways. A hole in the outer but not the inner retinal layer allows the cystic fluid through the defect. This type is usually not or is only slowly progressive, and therefore, a demarcation line forms. It rarely requires treatment. In the second type, holes form in both the inner and the outer layers. This causes collapse of the schisis and full-thickness retinal detachment forms. Progression is quick, and treatment is required by pneumatic retinopexy, scleral buckle, or vitrectomy, depending on the size and position of the retinal holes and whether there is any proliferative vitreoretinopathy.

There are several features to distinguish retinoschisis from retinal detachment. Retinoschisis causes an absolute scotoma in the visual field, whereas retinal detachment causes a relative scotoma. The cystic elevation of retinoschisis is usually smooth with no associated vitreous pigment cells. The surface of retinal detachment is usually corrugated with pigment cells in the vitreous ("tobacco dust"). Longstanding retinal detachment produces atrophy of the underlying RPE, resulting in a pigmented demarcation line. As the RPE is healthy in retinoschisis, there is no demarcation line. If argon laser photocoagulation to the outer retinal layer, aimed through an inner layer break, creates an equal gray response as in an adjacent area of normal retina, this is thought to be diagnostic of retinoschisis.

BENIGN PERIPHERAL RETINAL DEGENERATIONS

Peripheral chorioretinal atrophy (paving stone degeneration) occurs in nearly one-third of adult eyes. It is thought to be due to choroidal vascular insufficiency and is associated with peripheral vascular disease. The lesions appear as isolated or grouped, small, discrete, yellow-white areas with prominent underlying choroidal vessels and pigmented borders. **White with pressure** and **white without pressure** are characterized by a white appearance of the peripheral retina that is present either with or without scleral depression.

MACULAR HOLE

Macular hole is a full-thickness defect of the central sensory retina. Usually it is idiopathic, developing spontaneously in elderly patients, and is typically unilateral, but it may occur after blunt trauma or rarely in association with rhegmatogenous retinal detachment. Biomicroscopy reveals a full-thickness, round or oval, sharply defined hole measuring one-third disk diameter in the center of the macula, which may be surrounded by a cuff of retinal detachment (Figure 10–19A). Visual acuity is impaired, and metamorphopsia and a central scotoma are present on Amsler grid testing. The Watzke-Allen slit beam test correlates well with the presence of a full-thickness macular hole. A slit beam of light positioned across the macular hole is described by the patient as being either thinned or broken.

Idiopathic macular hole results from tangential traction in the epimacular vitreous cortex. The Gass classification divides its development into four stages. In stage 1, occult hole, there is a yellow spot at the foveola with loss of the foveal reflex (stage 1a) that may be associated with a yellow ring (stage 1b). This stage is reversible if a posterior vitreous detachment occurs. In stage 2, there is a full-thickness hole with diameter less than 400 μm. In stage 3, there is a well-circumscribed full-thickness hole with diameter more than 400 μm that may be surrounded by a cuff of subretinal fluid. In stage 4, the full-thickness hole is associated with a posterior vitreous detachment and an operculum may be

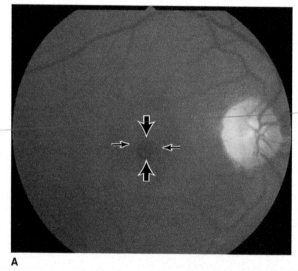

A

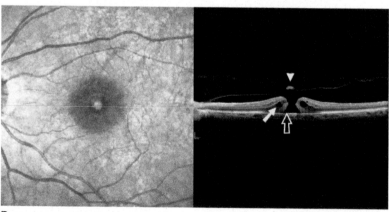

B

▲ **Figure 10–19. A:** Macular hole **(large arrows)** with surrounding sensory retinal detachment **(small arrows)**. (Also (See also Figure 19–12.) **B:** Optical coherence tomography showing intraretinal edema, detachment of the surrounding cuff of retina, and overlying operculum of retina.

identifiable (Figure 10–19B). In the base of a macular hole, there may yellowish white deposits on the RPE.

OCT is the best method of diagnosis and determination of the suitability of surgery as the critical factor is whether there is a partial (lamellar) or full-thickness hole (see Chapter 9). Treatment involves vitrectomy, separation of the posterior hyaloid, removal (peeling) of the retinal internal limiting membrane, and intravitreal injection of gas. For a few days, patients may need to undertake face-down posturing and to avoid sleeping on their back. Cataract due to the intraocular gas develops in most cases, but cataract surgery is often performed at the time of the macular hole surgery, if it has not been performed previously. Use of stains improves visualization of the internal limiting membrane and has greatly improved the rate of closure of macular holes, but the potential toxicity of the stains is debated.

Anatomic closure of macular holes can be achieved in at least 90% of cases, but around 20% of these fail to achieve vision greater than 20/50, particularly in traumatic and chronic holes.

EPIRETINAL MEMBRANES

Fibrocellular membranes may proliferate on the surface of the retina, leading to intraretinal edema and degeneration of the underlying retina. Contraction of such an epiretinal membrane (ERM) involving the macula, an epimacular membrane (EMM), causes varying degrees of visual distortion. Biomicroscopy usually shows wrinkling (striae) of the retina and distortion of retinal vessels (Figure 10–20). Rarely there may be retinal hemorrhages, cotton-wool spots, exudative retinal detachment, and simulation of a macular hole (pseudo-macular hole). Posterior vitreous detachment is nearly always present. OCT is valuable in the identification of EMM and to monitor for development of macular edema. Disorders associated with EMM include retinal tears with or without rhegmatogenous retinal detachment, vitreous inflammatory diseases, trauma, and a variety of retinal vascular diseases.

Visual acuity usually remains stable, suggesting that contraction of EMM is a short-lived and self-limited process. Surgical peeling of severe EMM can be performed to treat visual distortion, but recurrence occurs in some cases (see Chapter 9).

TRAUMATIC AND RELATED MACULOPATHIES

Blunt trauma to the anterior segment of the eye may cause a contrecoup injury to the retina, **commotio retinae.** The retinal whitening in the macular area usually clears completely; however, it may result in a pigmented retinal scar or macular hole with permanent impairment of central vision. Traumatic **choroidal rupture** (Figure 10–21) also may result in permanent visual loss.

Purtscher retinopathy, characterized by bilateral, multiple patches of superficial retinal whitening and hemorrhages, occurs after severe compression injury to the head or trunk. **Terson syndrome,** manifesting as retinal, preretinal, or vitreous hemorrhage, occurs in approximately 20% of patients with intracranial hemorrhage and raised intracranial pressure and is particularly associated with subarachnoid hemorrhage due to rupture of intracranial aneurysm. **Solar retinopathy,** manifesting as sharply demarcated and often irregularly shaped partial-thickness hole or depression in the center of the fovea that is usually bilateral, occurs after sungazing. Foveal injury also can be caused by laser exposure inadvertently during retinal laser treatment, in the industrial

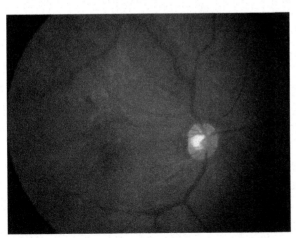

▲ **Figure 10–20.** Epimacular membrane (EMM) with distortion of retinal vessels and retinal striae.

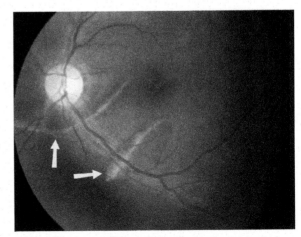

▲ **Figure 10–21.** White sclera visible through two choroidal ruptures.

or military setting, or due to accidental or purposeful exposure to a handheld laser.

CENTRAL SEROUS CHORIORETINOPATHY

Central serous chorioretinopathy (CSCR) is characterized by exudative detachment of the sensory retina due to multifocal areas of hyperpermeability of the choroidal vessels and alteration in the pump function of the RPE. It affects young to middle-aged men and is associated with type A personality, chronic steroid use, and stress. Presentation is with sudden onset of blurred vision, micropsia, metamorphopsia, and central scotoma. Visual acuity is often only moderately decreased and may be improved to near-normal with a small hyperopic correction.

Fundal examination reveals a round or oval area of retinal elevation, variable in size and position, but usually in the macula (Figure 10–22). There may be central yellowish-gray spots representing subretinal exudates. Occasionally there is a exudative RPE detachment in the superior portion. There may be evidence of previous episodes in the form of mild atrophic RPE lesions. Diagnosis is most easily confirmed on OCT. Approximately 80% of eyes with CSCR undergo spontaneous resorption and recovery of normal visual acuity within 6 months after the onset of symptoms. However, despite normal acuity, many patients have a mild permanent visual defect, such as a decrease in color sensitivity, micropsia, or relative scotoma. Approximately 20–30% of patients will have one or more recurrences of the disease. Complications, including CNV and chronic CME, have been described in patients with frequent and prolonged exudative detachments.

Various patterns of abnormality are seen on FFA, of which the most characteristic is a "smokestack" configuration of fluorescein dye leaking from the choriocapillaris followed by accumulation below the RPE or sensory retina (Figures 10–23 A and B). Argon laser photocoagulation to the site of leak significantly shortens the duration of the sensory detachment with quicker recovery of central vision but does not improve final visual outcome. It is not recommended for lesions close to central fixation because scar formation may cause permanent impairment of vision. For such lesions, PDT, including a low-dose (fluence) technique, and micropulse laser have produced encouraging results without the scarring associated with conventional laser treatment. Treatment outcomes are less favorable for any CSCR accompanied by retinal pigment epithelial detachment. In all cases, the duration and location of disease, the condition of the fellow eye, and occupational visual requirements are important considerations in determining treatment recommendations.

MACULAR EDEMA

Macular edema may be due to intraocular inflammatory disease (uveitis), retinal vascular disease such as diabetic retinopathy and retinal vein occlusion, epimacular membrane, intraocular surgery, inherited or acquired retinal degeneration, or drug therapy, or it may be idiopathic. It may present as a diffuse collection of intraretinal fluid or focal accumulation in the honeycomb-like spaces of the outer plexiform

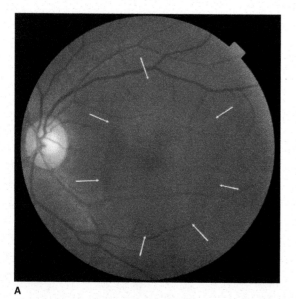

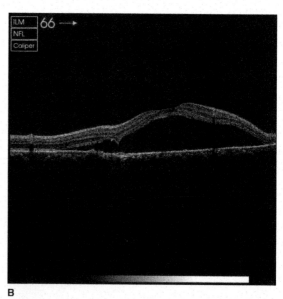

A

B

▲ **Figure 10–22.** Central serous chorioretinopathy. **A:** Circular central retinal elevation (exudative detachment) **(arrows). B:** Optical coherence tomography showing subretinal fluid.

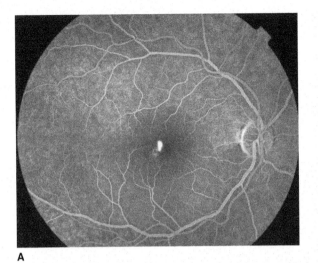

A

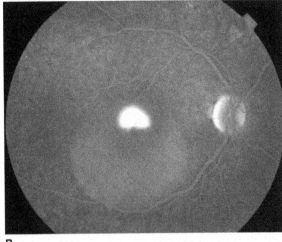

B

▲ **Figure 10–23.** Fundus fluorescein angiogram of central serous chorioretinopathy. **A:** Early phase showing a smoke-stack configuration of dye leakage. **B:** Late phase showing accumulation of dye in the exudative detachment.

and inner nuclear layers, which is known as **cystoid macular edema (CME)** and has a characteristic appearance on OCT, which is a good noninvasive method of monitoring response to treatment (Figure 10–24). On FFA, there is leakage from the perifoveal retinal capillaries and peripapillary region with accumulation in a petalloid pattern around the fovea (Figure 10–25).

The most frequent cause of CME is cataract surgery (Irvine-Gass syndrome), especially if the surgery was complicated or prolonged, or if there is a history of diabetic macular edema or uveitis. Complete posterior vitreous

detachment seems to provide some protection against its development. After routine phacoemulsification surgery, CME is detectable on FFA in approximately 25% of eyes and on clinical examination in about 2%. It usually manifests at 4–12 weeks postoperatively, but in some instances, its onset may be delayed for months or years. Many patients with CME of less than 6 months in duration have self-limited leakage that resolves without treatment. Topical steroid and/or nonsteroidal anti-inflammatory therapy may accelerate improvement in visual acuity in patients with chronic postoperative macular edema. In resistant cases, treatment with

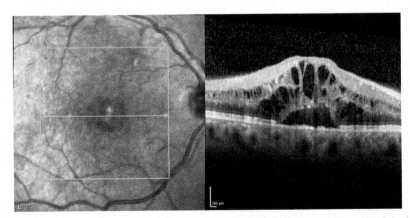

▲ **Figure 10–24.** Optical coherence tomography of cystoid macular edema showing intraretinal thickening with cysts and subretinal fluid.

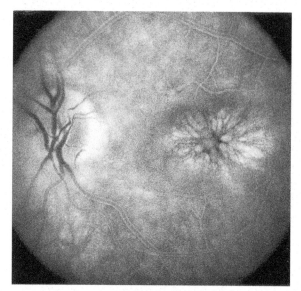

▲ **Figure 10–25.** Flower-petal pattern of fluorescein dye in a patient with cystoid macular edema after cataract surgery.

orbital floor or intravitreal triamcinolone may be beneficial. If there is vitreous traction, early YAG laser vitreolysis (see Chapter 23) or vitrectomy should be considered.

ANGIOID STREAKS

Angioid streaks appear as irregular, jagged tapering lines that radiate from the peripapillary retina into the macula and peripheral fundus (Figure 10–26). The streaks represent linear, crack-like dehiscences in Bruch's membrane. The lesions are rarely noted in children and probably develop in the second or third decade of life. Early in the disease, the streaks are sharply outlined and red-orange or brown. Subsequent fibrovascular tissue growth may partially or totally obscure their margins.

Nearly 50% of patients with angioid streaks have an associated systemic disease, such as pseudoxanthoma elasticum due to mutations in the recessive *ABCC6* gene, Paget disease of bone, Ehlers-Danlos syndrome, hemoglobinopathy, or a hemolytic disorder. Complications that can result in significant visual impairment include direct involvement of the fovea, CNV, and traumatic choroidal rupture. Patients with angioid streaks should be warned of the potential risk of choroidal rupture from even relatively mild eye trauma. Angioid streaks should be suspected in any patient who presents with CNV and no or few drusen in the fellow eye.

▶ Treatment

Retinal laser photocoagulation may be used on extrafoveal CNV, but recurrence is frequent and likely to occur on the

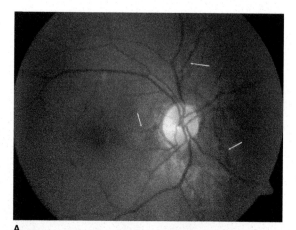

A

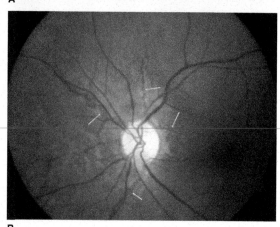

B

▲ **Figure 10–26.** Multiple angioid streaks **(arrows)** extending from the optic nerve. **A:** Right eye. **B:** Left eye.

foveal side of the resultant scar. PDT is unable to prevent the progression of the disease in most patients, and prophylactic treatment of angioid streaks before CNV is not recommended. Intravitreal anti-VEGF therapy stabilizes vision, but recurrence is likely, requiring repeated injections.

INFLAMMATORY DISEASES AFFECTING THE RETINA, RETINAL PIGMENT EPITHELIUM, AND CHOROID

▶ Presumed Ocular Histoplasmosis Syndrome

Presumed ocular histoplasmosis syndrome (POHS) is characterized by exudative possibly hemorrhagic detachments of the macula due to CNV, associated with multiple peripheral atrophic chorioretinal scars (histo spots) and peripapillary chorioretinal scarring (see Chapter 7) in the absence of vitritis. It usually occurs in healthy patients between the third and sixth decades of life, and the scars are probably caused by an antecedent subclinical systemic infection with *Histoplasma capsulatum*. However, only 3% of people with histoplasmosis develop histo spots, which usually remain quiescent, and only 5% of people with histo spots develop CNV. The visual prognosis depends on the proximity of the CNV to the center of the fovea. If it extends inside the foveal avascular zone, only 15% of eyes will retain 20/40 vision. There is a significant risk of CNV in the fellow eye, and patients should be instructed on the frequent use of an Amsler grid and the importance of prompt examination when abnormalities are detected.

▶ Treatment

Treatment options are similar to those for CNV due to AMD. Intravitreal injections have additional risks in younger patients because their posterior vitreous has not detached, but intravitreal bevacizumab produces significant improvement in vision at 1 year. Surgical removal of subfoveal membranes has been disappointing, with stabilization of vision occurring only in those with preoperative visual acuity worse than 20/100.

▶ Acute Posterior Multifocal Placoid Pigment Epitheliopathy

Acute posterior multifocal placoid pigment epitheliopathy (APMPPE) typically affects healthy young patients who develop unilateral subacute moderate visual impairment and photopsia that may proceed to bilateral involvement in a few days or weeks. Fundus examination shows multifocal flat gray-white placoid subretinal lesions involving the RPE (Figure 10–27A). The cause is unknown, but it is associated with a preceding viral illness. The characteristic features of the disease are rapid resolution of the fundus lesions with residual RPE disturbance and a delayed return of visual acuity to near-normal levels but often with small residual paracentral scotomas on careful testing. However, visual acuity remains 6/15 or less in 25% of cases, and recurrence occurs in 50%. Some patients have associated central nervous system (CNS) disease.

On FFA, new lesions show early hypofluorescence and late hyperfluorescence (Figure 10–27 B and C). Old lesions show window defects. On ICGA, new lesions show round hypofluorescent choroidal defects that outnumber those seen on FFA and partially or completely resolve with time. On FAF new lesions show hypoautofluorescence that is replaced by hyperautofluorescence as disease activity subsides. OCT of new lesions may show mild hyperreflectivity anterior to the RPE. Old lesions may show nodular hyperreflectivity at the level of the RPE.

The prognosis in atypical cases, such as unilateral disease or older presentation, is more guarded. Extensive pigmentary changes resulting from APMPPE may mimic widespread retinal degeneration, but the clinical history and normal electrophysiologic findings should lead to the correct diagnosis.

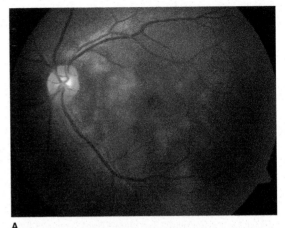

A

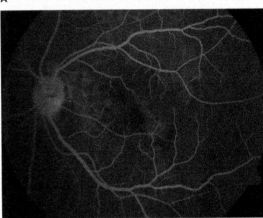

B

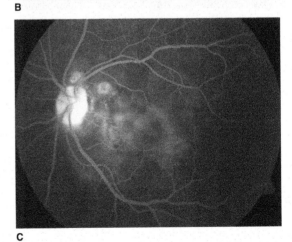

C

▲ **Figure 10–27.** Acute posterior multifocal placoid pigment epitheliopathy. **A:** Multiple macular placoid lesions. **B:** Fundus fluorescein angiogram early phase showing patchy hypofluorescence. **C:** FFA late phase showing dye leakage and pooling.

The condition is self-limiting. Treatment is immunosuppression, either local or systemic, the latter for severe cases involving the macula and for CNS disease.

Serpiginous Choroidopathy

This is a rare, recurrent, and chronically progressive inflammatory disease of unknown cause. Patients tend to be older than in APMPPE and are more often male. There is an association with HLA-B7. It presents with unilateral blurring of central vision, metamorphopsia, or scotoma, but usually, there is asymmetrical bilateral involvement. It characteristically involves the juxtapapillary retina and extends radially to involve the macula and peripheral retina. In the active stage, there are sharply demarcated gray-yellow lesions with irregular borders involving the RPE and choriocapillaris. On FFA, active lesions show early hypofluorescence and late hyperfluorescence. On ICGA, they show marked hypofluorescence throughout all phases. Vitritis may be present. Recurrence is the norm. Unlike APMPPE, recurrence occurs contiguous to the previously affected area and leads to extensive chorioretinal atrophy. The natural history is variable and may correlate with the presence of disease in the fellow eye. Complications are CNV and subretinal fibrosis. Oral or systemic corticosteroid treatment or other immunosuppressants, such as infliximab, may be beneficial during active disease.

Birdshot Chorioretinopathy

This is a chronic, bilateral inflammatory disease. Strong association with HLA-A29 and other features suggest that genetic predisposition and retinal autoimmunity are responsible. In the acute disease, there are diffuse cream-colored patches at the level of the RPE and choroid, retinal vasculitis associated with CME, and vitritis. There are episodes of exacerbation and remission with variable visual outcome. Visual loss may be due to chronic CME, optic atrophy, macular scarring, or CNV. Electroretinography is useful for diagnosis and monitoring disease progression and response to treatment. Treatment with corticosteroids alone does not seem to be effective. Other immunosuppressants may be beneficial.

Acute Macular Neuroretinopathy

Acute macular neuroretinopathy (AMN) is characterized by the acute onset of paracentral scotomas and mild visual acuity loss accompanied by wedge-shaped parafoveal retinal lesions in the deep sensory retina of one or both eyes. The macular lesions are subtle, reddish-brown, and best seen with a red-free light. The patients are usually young adults with a history of acute viral illness. OCT may show hyperreflectivity of the outer nuclear and outer plexiform layers in the acute phase followed by thinning of the outer nuclear layer and focal disruption of the photoreceptor and RPE junction. While the retinal lesions may fade, the scotomas tend to persist. No active treatment is indicated.

Multiple Evanescent White Dot Syndrome

Multiple evanescent white dot syndrome (MEWDS) is an acute and self-limited unilateral disease that affects mainly young women and is characterized clinically by multiple white dots at the level of the RPE, vitreous cells, and transient electroretinographic abnormalities. The cause is unknown. OCT may show disruption at the level of the ellipsoid layer of the inner segments of the photoreceptors. FAF shows hyperfluorescence of the acute lesions. FFA shows hyperfluorescence of the dots in the early phase with staining in the late phase. Occasionally there is staining of the retinal vessels and optic disk. On ICGA, there are hypofluorescent spots, which are more numerous than visible clinically or on FFA. There is no evidence of associated systemic disease. The retinal lesions gradually regress in a matter of weeks, leaving only minor retinal pigment epithelial defects.

Occasionally, MEWDS progresses to become **acute zonal occult outer retinopathy (AZOOR),** with positive visual phenomena, symptomatic reduction of visual field, which typically manifests as enlargement of the blind spot and may be progressive, and angiographic, FAF, and electrophysiologic evidence of retinal dysfunction.

There seems to be overlap between AZOOR, MEWDS, AMN, birdshot chorioretinopathy, serpiginous choroidopathy, APMPPE, and the entities of multifocal choroiditis (MFC), diffuse subretinal fibrosis syndrome, and punctuate inner choroidopathy (PIC), with each being a different manifestation of similar pathophysiologic processes, such that the umbrella term **white dot syndromes** has been suggested. The treatment options for all of them include topical or systemic immunosuppressants and anti-VEGF therapy if there is CNV.

MACULAR DYSTROPHIES

Macular dystrophies are genetically determined, although not usually evident at birth. Usually the disease is restricted to symmetrical macular involvement, but rarely there is associated spinocerebellar ataxia. In the early stages of some macular dystrophies, visual acuity is reduced, but the macular changes are subtle or not visible clinically, such that the patient's symptoms may be dismissed as spurious. In others, the fundoscopic changes are very striking when the patient is still asymptomatic. The more common macular dystrophies can be classified according to the level of retinal involvement (Table 10–1).

X-Linked Juvenile Retinoschisis

This slowly progressive, X-linked, recessively inherited disease affects young males and is characterized by a macular lesion called "foveal schisis." On slitlamp examination, there is a stellate pattern of small superficial retinal cysts with radial striae centered on the fovea (Figure 10–28). Visual acuity begins to fall during the first or second decade of life

Table 10–1. Anatomic Classification of Macular Dystrophies

Inner retina
    X-linked juvenile retinoschisis
Photoreceptors
    Cone-rod dystrophy
Retinal pigment epithelium
    Stargardt disease (fundus flavimaculatus)
    Best disease

and then may remain stable until the fifth or sixth decade but generally reduces to between 20/40 and 20/200 as the disease progresses. Fifty percent of patients have peripheral retinoschisis with peripheral visual field abnormalities. The posterior pole appears normal on FFA, differentiating it from CME. There is a negative electroretinogram (ERG) (normal a-wave amplitude with reduced b-wave amplitude), which is typical of disorders affecting the inner retina but leaving the photoreceptor cells intact. Female carriers have normal ERGs.

X-linked retinoschisis is thought to be due to Muller cell dysfunction. The genetic abnormality is a mutation in the *RS1* gene, which codes for a retina-specific extracellular protein (retinoschisin) that is secreted by photoreceptors but involved in cell–cell interactions and cellular adhesion in the inner retina. Carriers can be identified by DNA analysis.

The main differential diagnosis for foveal schisis is **enhanced S-cone (Goldmann-Favre) syndrome**, which is an autosomal recessive condition with extinguished ERG and characteristic peripheral disk-like pigmentation (Figure 10–29).

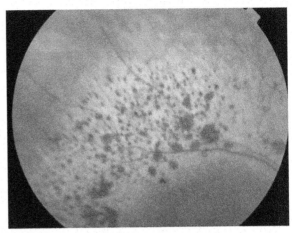

▲ **Figure 10–29.** Enhanced S-cone syndrome showing typical disk-like pigmentation around the vascular arcades.

▶ Cone and Cone-Rod Dystrophies (Cone-Dominant Dystrophies)

Cone and cone-rod dystrophies are relatively rare. Most cases are sporadic, but there may be autosomal dominant, autosomal recessive, or X-linked recessive inheritance. The hallmark is predominant involvement of cone photoreceptors, with presentation in early adulthood with impairment of central vision and color vision, and hemeralopia (intolerance to light). The fundus appearance varies greatly. In many patients, it is normal at initial presentation. There may be optic disk pallor with no obvious macular changes, leading to misdiagnosis of optic nerve disease. FAF is the preferred method of imaging for both diagnosis and monitoring (Figure 10–30A and B). Usually there is patchy central hypoautofluorescence and hyperautofluorescence. OCT shows changes in the outer retinal layers (Figure 10–30C and D). The characteristic bilateral, symmetric bull's-eye pattern of macular depigmentation, visualized on FFA as a zone of hyperfluorescence surrounding a central nonfluorescent spot, is relatively uncommon. If it occurs, chloroquine retinopathy has to be excluded. Electroretinography shows marked loss of cone function and slight to moderate loss of rod function. It is essential for diagnosis and prognosis. There is no specific treatment.

▶ Stargardt Disease and Fundus Flavimaculatus

Stargardt disease (Figure 10–31) is by far the most common macular dystrophy. Gene mutations are identifiable in 50–75% of patients. Usually inheritance is autosomal recessive, with mutations in the *ABCA4* (retina-specific ATP-binding cassette transporter) gene that also are the most common known cause of cone-rod dystrophies (see above),

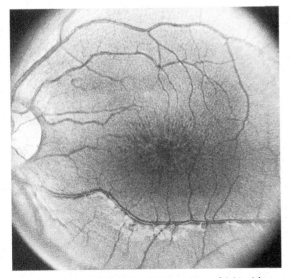

▲ **Figure 10–28.** X-linked juvenile retinoschisis with typical superficial retinal cysts in the fovea.

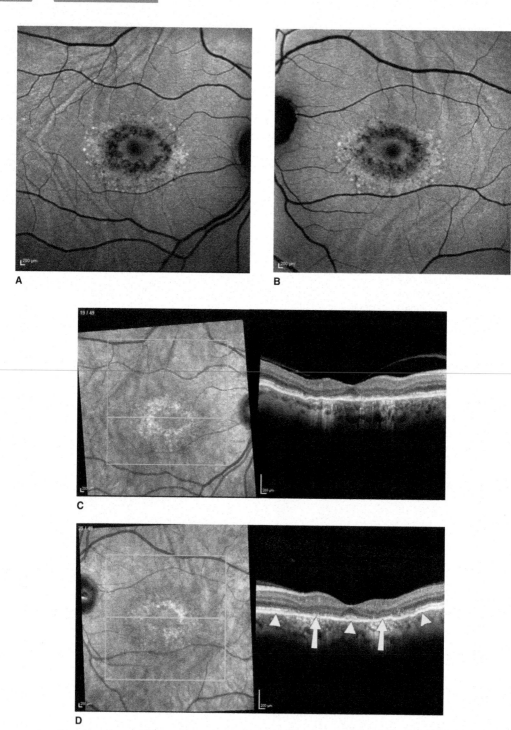

▲ **Figure 10–30.** Cone dystrophy. Fundus autofluorescence showing bull's-eye pattern of macular hypo- and hyperfluorescence. **A:** Right eye. **B:** Left eye. Optical coherence tomography of macula showing parafoveal loss of ellipsoid and external limiting membrane (ELM) **(arrows)** and preserved ellipsoid and ELM in subfoveal **(arrowheads)** and perifoveal areas. **C:** Right eye. **D:** Left eye.

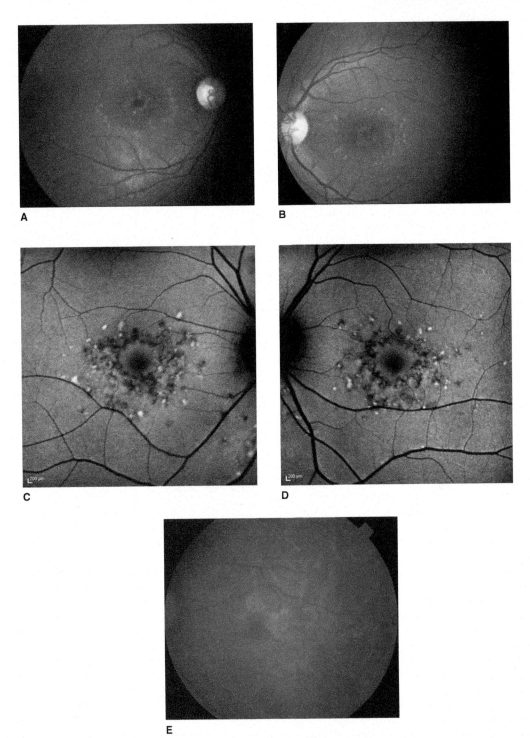

▲ Figure 10–31. Stargardt disease/fundus flavimaculatus. Stargardt disease with multiple irregular fleck lesions involving the macula. **A:** Right eye. **B:** Left eye. Fundus autofluorescence showing hypo- and hyperfluorescent areas. **C:** Right eye. **D:** Left eye. **E:** Fundus flavimaculatus.

or it may be autosomal dominant due to mutations in the *ELOVL4* (elongation of very long chain fatty acids-4) or *PROM1* (prominin 1) gene. **Fundus flavimaculatus**, which is characterized by multiple, variable size and shape, yellow-white fleck lesions of the RPE (Figure 10–31E), is considered to be part of the same spectrum as Stargardt disease.

Stargardt disease typically presents before age 15 with reduced central vision. About one-third of patients present in the first decade of life, one-third in the second decade of life, and one-third over 20 years of age. Initially, there is no macular abnormality clinically, but subsequently, there develops a bronze metal appearance together with mid-peripheral retinal flecks, like those seen in fundus flavimaculatus. FAF shows a range of abnormalities, including hyperautofluorescent flecks and macular hypoautofluorescence, and may be crucial to diagnosis in early cases. Pattern ERG is completely extinguished, even when central vision is good. The full-field ERG is usually normal. Once visual acuity has dropped to 20/40, it usually declines to 20/200 in 5 years.

Patients with fundus flavimaculatus present later than patients with Stargardt disease. They have retinal flecks distributed over the whole of the posterior pole of each eye. Central vision tends to be preserved until after 40 years of age, but full-field ERG changes are more common and are important for predicting prognosis.

Different phenotypes can be partly explained by different mutations of the same genes. Severely pathogenic mutations of the *ABCA4* gene, of which the carrier rate is about 1 in 100, tend to cause cone or cone-rod dystrophies, moderately pathogenic mutations fundus flavimaculatus, and mildly pathogenic mutations Stargardt disease. No specific treatment is available. Protection from excessive, high-energy light exposure may be advisable. Abnormal vitamin A metabolism including high level of vitamin A dimers may play a role in disease progression (eg, acceleration of accumulation of lipofuscin), and hence vitamin A supplementation should be avoided.

Best Vitelliform Macular Dystrophy

Best disease is an autosomal dominant disorder with variable penetrance and expressivity. The genetic abnormality is a mutation in the *BEST1* (VMD2) gene, which encodes a transmembrane calcium-sensitive chloride channel (bestrophin) located on RPE cells. Onset is usually in childhood. The fundoscopic appearance is variable and ranges from a mild pigmentary disturbance within the fovea to the typical vitelliform or "egg yolk" lesion located in the central macula (Figure 10–32). This characteristic cyst-like lesion is generally quite round and well demarcated and contains homogeneous opaque yellow material at the level of the RPE. The "egg yolk" may degenerate, giving rise to the stages described as pseudo-hypopyon by puberty and vitelliruptive when the visual acuity drops. Late-stage disease may be associated

with CNV, subretinal hemorrhage, and extensive macular scarring. Visual acuity often remains good in the early stages, and the ERG is normal. Abnormal electro-oculogram (EOG) is the hallmark of the disease. OCT shows hyperreflective material beneath and within the RPE. FAF shows intense hyperautofluorescence of the yellowish lesions and hypoautofluorescence in atrophic areas.

HEREDITARY RETINAL DEGENERATIONS

▶ Retinitis Pigmentosa (Rod-Dominant Dystrophies)

Retinitis pigmentosa (RP) is a group of heterogeneous hereditary retinal degenerations characterized by progressive dysfunction of the photoreceptors, associated with progressive cell loss and eventual atrophy of several retinal layers. It is the most common hereditary fundus dystrophy, with a reported prevalence of 1 in 5000. RP may occur as a sporadic disorder or be inherited as autosomal recessive, autosomal dominant, or X-linked recessive. Digenic and mitochondrial inheritance may also be possible. The severity of the disease depends on the mode of inheritance. X-linked recessive is the least common but most severe form, with some affected individuals being totally blind by the third or fourth decade. Autosomal recessive disease also can be severe. Sporadic cases may have a more favorable prognosis, with retained central vision until the sixth decade or later. Autosomal dominant disease has the best prognosis. RP may present as an isolated condition (simplex) or in atypical forms associated with other systemic disorders (syndromic).

The hallmark symptoms of retinitis pigmentosa are night blindness (nyctalopia) and gradually progressive peripheral visual field loss as a result of increasing and coalescing ring scotomas. The most characteristic fundoscopic findings are attenuated retinal arterioles, waxy optic disk pallor, mottling of the RPE, and peripheral retinal pigment clumping, referred to as "bone-spicule formation" (Figure 10–33). Although retinitis pigmentosa is a generalized photoreceptor disorder, in most cases, rod function is more severely affected, predominantly leading to poor scotopic vision. The ERG usually shows either markedly reduced or absent retinal function. The EOG lacks the usual light rise.

The most common complication is posterior subcapsular cataract. Other less common complications include open-angle glaucoma, keratoconus, posterior vitreous detachment, intermediate uveitis, and a Coats-like disease with peripheral retinal lipid deposition and exudative retinal detachment. Central visual impairment may be due to macular atrophy, epimacular membrane, or cystoid macular edema.

No specific treatment is available, but regular follow-up may help provide support to patients. High-dose vitamin A has been reported to be marginally beneficial but can be toxic. Patients need to be advised to stop smoking and to

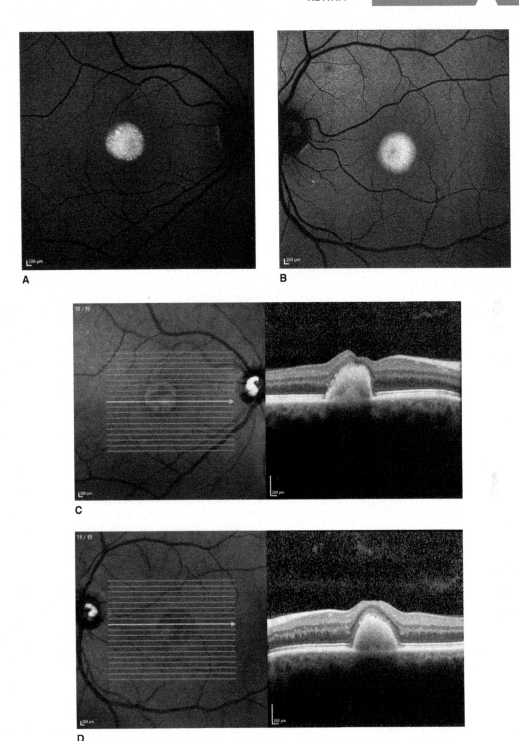

▲ **Figure 10–32.** Best disease. Fundus autofluorescence showing well-demarcated hyperfluorescent lesion. **A:** Right eye. **B:** Left eye. Optical coherence tomography showing hyperreflective subretinal material in the fovea. **C:** Right eye. **D:** Left eye. (Used with permission from Moorfields Eye Hospital, London.)

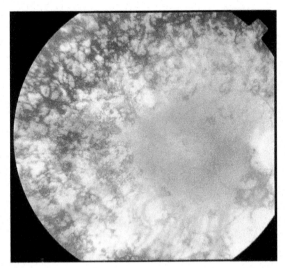

▲ **Figure 10–33.** Retinitis pigmentosa with arteriolar narrowing and peripheral retinal pigment clumping.

avoid other retinotoxic drugs such as hydroxychloroquine, phenothiazine, and vigabatrin. Low-vision aids may be helpful once there is macular involvement. Ongoing trials in gene therapy and retinal prostheses may lead to new treatments.

There has been rapid progress in identification of mutations in retinitis pigmentosa. Relevant genes identified so far can be found on the RetNet website (http://www.sph.uth.tmc.edu/Retnet/). Patients should be referred to specialized centers for genetic counseling and selective mutation analysis. Genetic analysis is useful to identify female carriers in families with X-linked disease and to diagnose dominant disease. In recessive disease, specific features are needed for genetic analysis to be worthwhile.

Fundus Albipunctatus and Retinitis Punctata Albescens

Fundus albipunctatus is an autosomal recessive nonprogressive dystrophy characterized by a myriad of discrete small white dots at the level of the RPE scattered in the posterior pole and midperiphery of the retina. Patients have night blindness, but other parameters such as visual acuity, visual fields, and color vision are normal. Although the ERG and EOG are usually normal, dark adaptation thresholds are markedly raised. Retinitis punctata albescens is the less common progressive variant of this dystrophy. Both conditions are extremely rare.

Familial benign fleck retina syndrome is a very rare autosomal recessive disorder. It is asymptomatic with normal vision and is detected by chance. Multiple, diffuse, yellow-white lesions may be seen throughout the retina with foveal sparing (Figure 10–34). FAF shows increased autofluorescence. The ERG is normal.

Leber Congenital Amaurosis

Leber congenital amaurosis (LCA) is an autosomal recessive disorder of rods and cones and is the most common genetic disorder of pediatric visual impairment. It presents as a triad of severe visual impairment or blindness beginning in the first year of life, nystagmus, and generalized retinal dystrophy. The fundoscopic findings are variable; most patients show either a normal appearance or only subtle retinal pigment epithelial granularity and mild vessel attenuation. A markedly reduced or absent ERG indicates generalized photoreceptor dysfunction, and in infants, this is the only method to confirm the diagnosis.

The condition can present with ocular manifestations only (pure LCA), or there may be extraocular involvement, including mental retardation, oculodigital reflex, seizures, and renal or muscular abnormalities. The division between

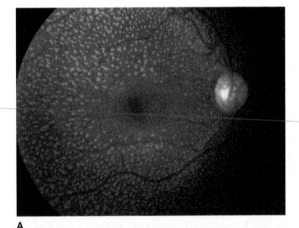

A

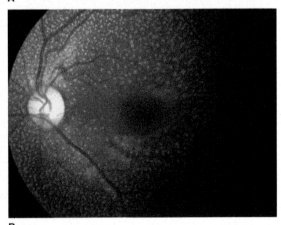

B

▲ **Figure 10–34.** Benign flecked retina syndrome with multiple diffuse yellow-white lesions throughout the retina but sparing the fovea. **A:** Right eye. **B:** Left eye.

these entities is unclear, and they are best classified on a genetic basis. Nine causal genes have been identified, accounting for 65% of cases. The *RPE65* gene mutation has been extensively investigated, including successful gene therapy in dogs, the most famous of which is Lancelot, suggesting that subretinal delivery of the *RPE65* vector in human subjects is feasible. Project 3000 aims to identify and perform genetic testing on all cases of LCA in the United States. Human clinical trials of gene therapy are ongoing in England and the United States.

▶ Gyrate Atrophy

Gyrate atrophy is an autosomal recessive disorder due to reduced activity of ornithine aminotransferase (OAT), a mitochondrial matrix enzyme that catalyzes several amino acid pathways, resulting in raised serum ornithine. The OAT gene has been mapped to chromosome 10. The incidence of this disorder is relatively high in Finland, and the ophthalmologic features are the most prominent manifestations of the disease. Patients initially present with myopia and then develop nyctalopia within the first decade of life, followed by progressive loss of peripheral visual field. Characteristic sharply demarcated circular areas of chorioretinal atrophy develop in the midperiphery of the fundus during the teenage years and become confluent with macular involvement late in the course of the disease. The ERG is decreased or absent, and the EOG is reduced.

Reduction in dietary intake of arginine has been shown to slow progression of the disease. It is most effective when commenced during childhood. Other treatments include pyridoxine supplementation and supplemental dietary lysine.

COLOR VISION DEFECTS

Cone photoreceptors are responsible for color vision, with visual pigments (opsins) in their outer segments absorbing light of wavelengths between 400 and 700 nm. Spectral sensitivity studies have identified blue, green, and red cone photoreceptors. A minimal requirement for color (hue) discrimination is the presence of at least two kinds of cone photopigment (opsin), and normal color vision requires the presence of all three (trichromacy). The red and green cone opsins are encoded by adjacent genes on the X chromosome. The blue cone opsin is encoded on chromosome 7. Color vision testing is described in Chapter 2.

Color vision defects are either congenital (inherited) or acquired. Acquired color vision defects vary in type and severity, depending on the location and source of the ocular pathology, and frequently affect one eye more than the other. Males and females are equally affected.

Congenital color vision defects are constant in type and severity throughout life and affect both eyes equally. They are more common in men than women. The most common congenital color vision defect, red-green color deficiency, is a form of dichromacy, with only two out of three cone opsins functioning normally. It results from mutation in the gene encoding for either the red (**protanopia**) or green (**deuteranopia**) cone opsin. It is X-linked recessive and affects 8% of males and 0.5% of females. Although color discrimination is abnormal, visual acuity is normal. The third type of dichromacy, **tritanopia**, in which there is loss of blue-yellow discrimination due to defect in the blue cone opsin, is a rare autosomal dominant condition resulting from a mutation on chromosome 7.

There are two forms of monochromacy. Although both leave the affected individual completely without color discrimination (achromatopsia), they are two quite separate entities. In the less common **cone monochromacy** (1 in 100,000), visual acuity is normal, but there is no hue discrimination. Only one type of cone photoreceptor is present. It is usually due to **blue cone monochromacy,** an X-linked recessive condition resulting from mutations in the genes encoding for both red and green cone opsins. In **rod monochromacy** (1 in 30,000), an autosomal recessive condition caused by mutations in genes encoding proteins of the photoreceptor cation channel or cone transducin, there are no functioning cones, resulting in achromatic vision, low visual acuity, photophobia, and nystagmus.

10.2. Retinal Tumors

James J. Augsburger, MD, and Zélia M. Corrêa, MD, PhD

This section presents an overview of the most common and most important neoplasms, hamartomas, and choristomas of the retina and ciliary body epithelia. Nonneoplastic lesions and disorders of the fundu (eg, Coats' disease, persistent hyperplastic primary vitreous, ocular toxocariasis, and pars planitis) that can simulate retinoblastoma and other retinal tumors are discussed in other parts of this book.

BENIGN RETINAL TUMORS

Benign neoplasms are acquired tumors composed of cells that are atypical but not sufficiently abnormal to be classified as malignant. They may enlarge slowly but have little or no invasive potential and no metastatic capability. **Hamartomas** are congenital tumors composed of normal or near normal cells and tissues that occur normally at that anatomic site but are present in excess. **Choristomas** are congenital tumors composed of normal cells and tissue elements that do not occur normally at that anatomic site.

Retinal Astrocytoma

Retinal astrocytoma (referred to by some authors as "retinal astrocytic hamartoma" despite the fact that the lesion is rarely present at birth or identified during early childhood) is an acquired benign neoplasm that arises from the astrocytes within the retinal nerve fiber layer. It may be part of an inheritable syndrome, usually tuberous sclerosis, or a noninherited isolated entity. The retinal astrocytomas that occur in tuberous sclerosis frequently are multifocal and bilateral, whereas nonsyndromic retinal astrocytomas are almost exclusively unilateral and unifocal.

Retinal astrocytomas usually become evident during the first or second decade of life. Small lesions appear as ill-defined translucent spots in the inner retina (opalescent patches). Slightly larger lesions appear as discrete, opaque, white nodules of the inner retina (Figure 10–35). Occasional larger, more mature lesions exhibit an irregular nodular character that has been likened to a "white mulberry." Retinal astrocytomas identified early in life typically enlarge slightly,

but most lesions in individuals over the age of 25 years remain stable. Generally, no treatment is indicated unless substantial enlargement is documented. Rarely, a retinal astrocytoma of either the syndromic or isolated variety undergoes substantial progressive enlargement associated with malignant transformation.

Retinal Capillary Hemangioma (von Hippel tumor)

Retinal capillary hemangioma is an acquired benign neoplasm of the retina that is composed of neural retinal cells transformed into poorly differentiated small cells with prominent nuclei and little cytoplasm. It is caused by a mutation of both alleles of the *VHL* gene, which is located on the short arm of chromosome 3 (p25.5 region). It may be part of a syndrome (von Hippel-Lindau disease [VHL]), in which it is likely to be multifocal and bilateral, or an isolated entity, in which it is likely to be solitary and unilateral. In response to angiogenic factors elaborated by its cells, the tumor attracts a dense collection of blood vessels that gives the tumor the appearance of an intraretinal red sphere (hence the name "hemangioma") fed by a dilated, tortuous afferent retinal arteriole and drained by a dilated, tortuous efferent retinal venule (Figure 10–36). The tumor blood vessels tend to be leaky, resulting in progressive accumulation of intraretinal edema and exudates and exudative subretinal fluid around the tumor. As the tumor enlarges, the exudative retinal detachment usually increases in extent and becomes associated with substantial vitreoretinal fibrosis resulting

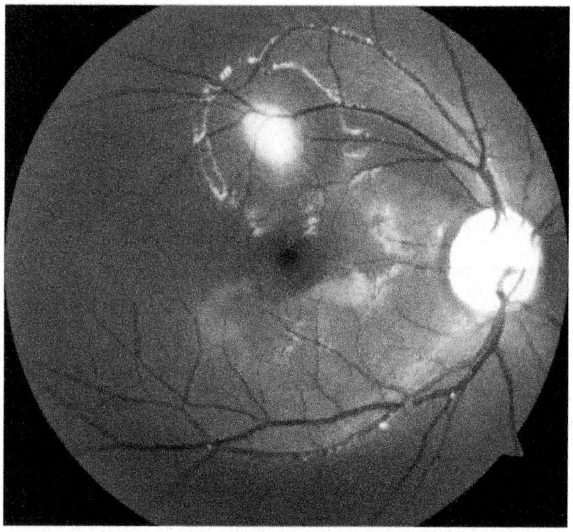

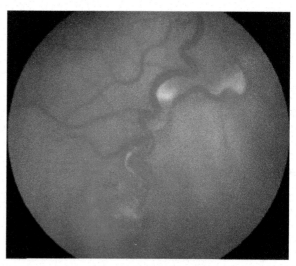

▲ **Figure 10–35.** Solitary retinal astrocytoma just superior to fovea in an 11-year-old boy with tuberous sclerosis.

▲ **Figure 10–36.** Classic retinal capillary hemangioma inferiorly. The tumor is fed and drained by dilated tortuous retinal blood vessels. Note intraretinal and subretinal exudates along the blood vessels.

in tractional retinal detachment. Retinal capillary hemangiomas occur anywhere in the fundus from the optic disk to the peripheral retina but develop most frequently in the equatorial or postequatorial region. They are not present at birth but frequently become evident during the teenage years. Treatment of small von Hippel tumors is usually by laser photocoagulation or cryotherapy, but treatment of larger lesions frequently requires vitreoretinal surgery to address the associated exudative-tractional retinal detachment. Depending on the size and location of the retinal tumors and extent of exudative-tractional retinal detachment when the lesions are first detected, vision in treated eyes can range from excellent to no light perception.

Combined Hamartoma of Retina

Combined hamartoma of retina is a benign congenital malformation composed of overgrown and disorganized normal retinal components. The three typical features of this tumor are deep gray coloration due to involvement of retinal pigment epithelium, superficial white retinal "gliosis," and prominent angulated retinal blood vessels that are incorporated in the lesion (Figure 10–37). It is usually located adjacent to the optic disk (juxtapapillary) or around the optic disk (circumpapillary) and is virtually always unilateral and unifocal. If the macula is involved, vision usually is impaired. This lesion frequently is associated with neurofibromatosis type 2, so affected children generally should be screened for

related abnormalities, particularly vestibular schwannomas. No treatment is indicated for this lesion.

Congenital Hypertrophy of Retinal Pigment Epithelium

Congenital hypertrophy of retinal pigment epithelium (CHRPE) is a benign focal congenital malformation of the retinal pigment epithelium characterized pathologically by increased size (hypertrophy) and increased number (hyperplasia) of retinal pigment epithelial cells in a localized region of the fundus. The abnormal RPE cells tend to be densely packed with large melanin granules. The lesion is always present at birth but usually not identified until late childhood or adulthood. CHRPE occurs in three distinct clinical patterns.

Typical unifocal CHRPE appears as a nummular flat black lesion that is most frequently located in the peripheral fundus (Figure 10–38). It ranges in size from a tiny dot of black pigment to a geographic lesion 5 mm or more in diameter with well-defined smooth margins. It may undergo focal or diffuse depigmentation. Rarely it gives rise to an adenoma or adenocarcinoma of the retinal pigment epithelium, so it should be re-evaluated at least every few years.

The **typical multifocal clustered CHRPE** (grouped pigmentation of the retina, retinal "bear tracks") is characterized by multiple small- to intermediate-size oval to cigar-shaped CHRPE lesions clustered in one region of the fundus of one

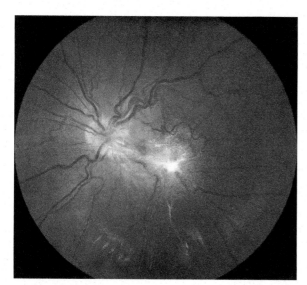

▲ **Figure 10–37.** Combined hamartoma of retina involving macula. Tumor exhibits deep gray color due to retinal pigment epithelial involvement, superficial white color due to retinal gliosis, and angulated intralesional retinal blood vessels.

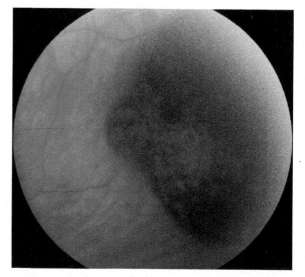

▲ **Figure 10–38.** Typical unifocal peripheral congenital hypertrophy of retinal pigment epithelium (CHRPE). Despite the appearance of the lesion suggesting considerable thickness, B-scan ultrasonography showed no measurable thickness.

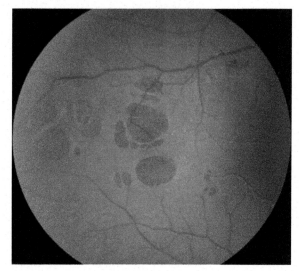

▲ **Figure 10–39.** Typical unilateral clustered congenital hypertrophy of the retinal pigment epithelium (CHRPE). This appearance is commonly referred to as "bear tracks" in the fundus.

eye (Figure 10–39). These lesions do not affect vision and do not appear to have any potential to give rise to RPE neoplasms.

Atypical multifocal bilateral nonclustered CHRPE tends to occur in individuals with Gardner's syndrome and related familial colonic polyposis–carcinoma disorders. The individual lesions tend to be angulated in basal shape and sometimes have distinct areas of depigmentation. They are not clustered in a single area of the fundus but are scattered. They are also frequently bilateral. Lesions of this type have never been reported to give rise to RPE neoplasm. Affected individuals need to be screened for polyps and cancer of the colon. Those with colonic abnormalities generally are advised to undergo colectomy.

RETINAL TUMORS OF INTERMEDIATE CHARACTER

The tumors described in the following paragraphs are categorized as neoplasms of borderline malignancy (ie, ones that no clinician can categorize reliably as unequivocally benign or malignant). If biopsy of a tumor in this category is performed, pathologic study of the tumor cells may reveal benign cells, malignant cells, or cells deemed to be borderline even by cytologic criteria.

Retinoma

Retinoma is a spontaneously arrested form of retinoblastoma (see below). Classified as a "retinocytoma," pathologically it consists of benign-appearing neuroepithelial cells. It arises

within the first few years of life but may not be detected until older childhood or even adulthood. Usually the tumor is unilateral and unifocal, but bilateral multifocal retinomas have been reported.

The classic retinoma appears as an opalescent or off-white retinal tumor of limited size (usually less than 7 mm in diameter and less than 2 mm in thickness) (Figure 10–40). Usually it exhibits few if any fine blood vessels on its surface and is not associated with dilated tortuous afferent and efferent retinal blood vessels. Chorioretinal atrophy is evident along the margins of some lesions, and foci of calcification are frequently present.

While many retinomas remain stable throughout life, some eventually transform into active retinoblastoma, so affected individuals probably should be monitored at least yearly for life.

Medulloepithelioma

Medulloepithelioma is a benign to malignant intraocular neoplasm that usually arises from the primitive neuroepithelium of the ciliary body during embryologic development. Rare cases have arisen from the retina and optic disk, but the cells of origin in such cases are uncertain. Intraocular medulloepithelioma is almost exclusively a unilateral, unifocal tumor. Because the tumor arises from immature neuroepithelial cells, the vast majority of cases occur in children less than 10 years old. The typical lesion is characterized by cords of primitive neuroepithelial cells and multiple

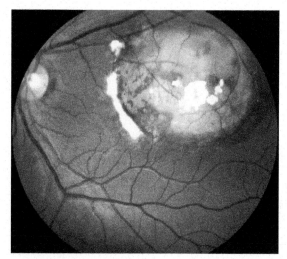

▲ **Figure 10–40.** Macular retinoma in a man whose young son had viable retinoblastoma in each eye. This oval fundus lesion exhibits paracentral calcification, central translucency, extensive clumping of the retinal pigment epithelium, and chorioretinal atrophy along its nasal margin.

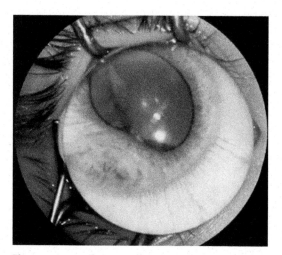

▲ **Figure 10–41.** Congenital medulloepithelioma of the ciliary body and peripheral iris. Note the associated lens coloboma due to the tumor's effect on the zonule in its meridian.

epithelial-lined cysts. The fluid within the cysts stains as vitreous. Occasional medulloepitheliomas exhibit heterotopic elements such as cartilage, glandular tissue, and hair follicles, and such tumors are classified as "teratoid." The component tumor cells tend to be rather bland in most cases, and malignancy of such tumors is generally defined by the presence and extent of invasion of adjacent tissues histopathologically.

The typical medulloepithelioma appears as a white to pink ciliary body tumor that not infrequently invades the peripheral iris (Figure 10–41). Often intralesional cysts are a prominent feature. The tumor is probably present at birth in many cases but is frequently not detected until the child is between 2 and 6 years old. It tends to grow slowly and progressively. It stimulates abrupt development of iris neovascularization with visible iris discoloration, ocular pain (due to neovascular glaucoma), and a red congested eye.

Treatment options include transcleral tumor resection, plaque radiation therapy, and enucleation. Although a few benign ciliary body medulloepitheliomas have been excised successfully, most malignant tumors of this type have recurred locally following attempted excision. Plaque radiation therapy has been used with limited success in some cases, but most eyes containing a medulloepithelioma ultimately come to enucleation. Metastasis from intraocular medulloepithelioma is extremely rare.

MALIGNANT INTRAOCULAR TUMORS

The component cells of malignant retinal tumors and the tissue they form are clearly abnormal morphologically. Invasive clinical and pathologic features are generally evident, and regional and distant metastasis may occur.

▶ Retinoblastoma

Retinoblastoma is a primary malignant intraocular neoplasm that arises from immature neuroepithelial cells of the developing retina (retinoblasts). Most develop within the first few years of life. Some are present at birth, and occasionally, they have been identified by prenatal imaging.

Pathologically, retinoblastoma is composed of small round neoplastic cells that invade and replace the normal retina. Individual tumor cells tend to have a large nucleus and disproportionately small amount of cytoplasm. Intralesional necrosis and foci of calcification are usually evident. Clinically retinoblastoma can affect one eye (usually unifocal) or both eyes (usually multifocally). Most individuals with bilateral and/or multifocal retinoblastoma have a functionally significant mutation or deletion involving one allele of the retinoblastoma gene (a tumor suppressor gene localized to the long arm of chromosome 13 that is normally responsible for production of a nuclear phosphoprotein with DNA binding activity) in most, if not all, of their cells, in which case retinoblastoma is transmitted as an autosomal dominant condition with approximately 90–95% penetrance. Thus, children of such individuals have a nearly 50% chance of having the disease, and regular screening until the child has been shown by genetic testing not to be at risk is important in the early detection of tumors. In contrast, most individuals with unilateral, unifocal retinoblastoma do not have a germline mutation in the retinoblastoma gene and will not transmit the disease to their offspring. Recognized risk factors for occurrence of retinoblastoma include a positive family history and chromosome 13q deletion syndrome. Unaffected parents who have produced one child with retinoblastoma have a 4–7% risk of having a subsequent child with the disease. Sequencing of the gene allows identification of carriers and hence more specific genetic counseling. The cumulative lifetime incidence of retinoblastoma has been estimated to be about 1 in 15,000 to 1 in 18,000 individuals in most Western countries.

The typical small retinoblastoma appears as a translucent to dull white retinal nodule (Figure 10–42). As the tumor gets larger, it attracts dilated tortuous afferent and efferent retinal blood vessels and develops a fine network of capillaries on its surface (Figure 10–43). Larger discrete retinal tumors tend to develop intralesional foci of degenerative calcification, which usually can be detected by B-scan ultrasonography and computed tomography scanning. Exudative retinal detachment develops around the tumor and can become extensive. Eventually tumor cells are shed from the surface of the tumor into the surrounding subretinal fluid and/or overlying vitreous (Figure 10–44), and these tumor "seeds" can implant on the retina, ciliary body, zonule, or posterior surface of the iris, and even extend into the anterior chamber to implant on the anterior surface of the iris and trabecular meshwork. In eyes with extensive retinoblastoma,

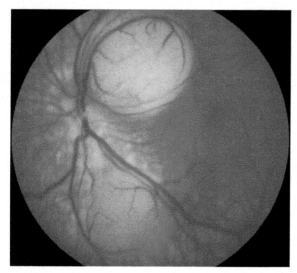

▲ **Figure 10–42.** Two discrete intraretinal retinoblastoma tumors in the left eye of a child with bilateral retinoblastoma. The slightly larger superior tumor is more opaque while the smaller inferior tumor is more translucent.

secondary iris neovascularization and neovascular glaucoma develop frequently. Retinoblastoma has a tendency to invade the optic disk and extend into the orbital optic nerve, invade the choroid with possible hematogenous dissemination, and extend transsclerally to the orbit via scleral vascular and

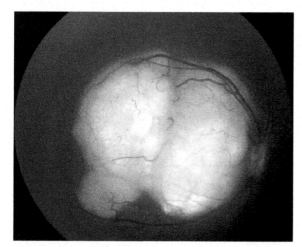

▲ **Figure 10–43.** Multinodular macular intraretinal retinoblastoma tumor formed by coalescence of three distinct tumors. Note the prominent retinal blood vessels on the surface of the tumor.

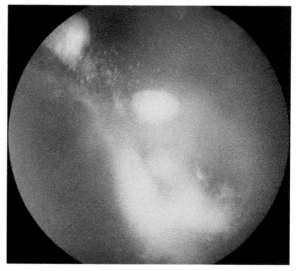

▲ **Figure 10–44.** Finely dispersed and clumped retinoblastoma seeds in vitreous.

neural foramina into the orbit. Once retinoblastoma extends outside the eye, it tends to grow aggressively in the periocular tissues, extend via the optic nerve to the brain, and rapidly metastasize widely. Untreated, children with metastatic retinoblastoma rarely survive for more than 1 year.

Retinoblastoma in children with a positive family history is frequently identified by screening examinations when the extent of intraocular disease is limited (ie, few tumors, small tumors, and no vitreous seeds). In contrast, retinoblastoma in children with unilateral and/or nonfamilial retinoblastoma is usually not detected until the parents or pediatrician note a white pupil ("leukocoria"; Figure 10–45) due

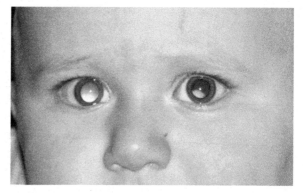

▲ **Figure 10–45.** White pupillary reflection (leukocoria) in each eye (more pronounced in the right eye) due to bilateral retinoblastoma.

to external light reflecting off the white intraocular tumor, strabismus due to impaired vision in one or both eyes, or discoloration of the iris due to iris neovascularization. In most developed countries, the median age at initial diagnosis of retinoblastoma is about 12 months for bilateral cases and about 24 months for unilateral cases. In countries with limited health care services, the median age at detection of both groups tends to be substantially higher.

A number of systems (Reese-Ellsworth classification, Essen prognosis classification, International Classification of Intraocular Retinoblastoma) have been used over the years to categorize eyes with intraocular retinoblastoma into ordinal categorical subgroups having distinct probabilities of disease eradication with ocular preservation using available therapies. None was intended as a staging system for patient survival. Nevertheless, because more extensive intraocular disease is likely to be associated with higher probabilities of extraocular tumor extension and metastasis, patients categorized by these systems to have more advanced intraocular disease tend to have a worse survival prognosis. Systems to classify disease according to probability of cure or death also have been developed (American Joint Committee on Cancer-Retinoblastoma, International Staging System for Retinoblastoma).

For a child with purely intraocular retinoblastoma, the recommended initial treatment depends on the number, size, locations, and types (primary intraretinal tumors, tumor seeds, implantation tumors) of intraocular tumors; the visual status and potential of the affected eye(s); whether the disease is unilateral or bilateral; the types and severity of secondary abnormalities of the eye (eg, retinal detachment, iris neovascularization); the general health of the child; and available technologies and resources. Because some children with familial and/or bilateral-multifocal retinoblastoma develop an independent retinoblastoma-like malignant neoplasm in the brain (pineoblastoma or ectopic intracranial retinoblastoma) and because of the propensity for retinoblastoma to extend extraocularly via the optic nerve and sclera, if available, magnetic resonance imaging of the orbits and brain is performed routinely prior to treatment. Children with one or a few small discrete extramacular tumors, without associated tumor seeding or subretinal fluid, are typically managed by focal laser therapy (postequatorial tumors) and/or focal cryotherapy (peripheral tumors). Children with a solitary medium-sized intraretinal tumor in one or both eyes may be managed initially by plaque radiation therapy. Most children with one or more larger tumors, macular or juxtapapillary tumor, extensive nonrhegmatogenous retinal detachment, and/or subretinal and/or intravitreal tumor seeds at baseline are currently treated initially by intravenous chemotherapy or selective ophthalmic artery infusion chemotherapy, supplemented by focal obliterative therapies to the residual tumors once the original tumors have shrunken

and the retinal detachment has diminished or resolved. Fractionated external beam radiation therapy (EBRT), once the mainstay of treatment for bilateral retinoblastoma, is now generally reserved for eyes with residual or recurrent retinoblastoma following intravenous chemotherapy or selective ophthalmic artery infusion chemotherapy supplemented by local obliterative therapies and possibly intravitreal injections of chemotherapeutic drugs. Some eyes with extensive intraocular retinoblastoma, particularly ones that are blind and painful, have neovascular glaucoma or have extensive intraocular bleeding and/or ocular congestion, and eyes that have failed to respond to eye-preserving therapies are managed by enucleation. Any eye enucleated for retinoblastoma must undergo histopathologic examination for optic nerve invasion, transscleral tumor extension to the orbit, massive choroidal invasion, and other adverse prognostic factors for subsequent orbital tumor relapse or metastasis that may prompt postenucleation adjuvant chemotherapy or orbital radiotherapy.

Initial treatment for a child with regional extraocular extension of retinoblastoma but no intracranial invasion or evident metastasis is being determined by a number of cooperative oncology group studies. Currently the most common treatment is enucleation of the affected eye followed by intensive chemotherapy and orbital irradiation.

Initial treatment for children with metastatic retinoblastoma or retinoblastoma-associated pineoblastoma is intensive intravenous chemotherapy, surgical debulking of the residual intracranial and/or extracranial tumor(s), focal adjuvant radiation therapy to residual disease, and bone marrow transplantation. Although there have been some lasting cures of children with extracranial metastasis, there have been few, if any, cures of children with intracranial extension or metastasis of retinoblastoma or pineoblastoma.

▶ Nonophthalmic Primary Cancer Metastatic to Retina

Occasional nonophthalmic primary cancers give rise to metastatic infiltrates and tumors of the retina, optic disk, and/or vitreous. Although metastatic lesions to these sites are substantially less common than metastatic tumors to the uvea (see Chapter 7), they represent a distinct subgroup of malignant intraocular lesions that should be recognized by ophthalmologists. They usually occur in middle-aged or older individuals with a history or other evidence of a nonophthalmic primary cancer capable of metastasizing. Metastases to the retina of most types of cancer tend to appear as patchy pale infiltrative lesions obscuring the retinal blood vessels (Figure 10–46). Retinal metastasis from primary skin melanoma usually appears dark brown to black. Metastatic tumors to the optic disk tend to appear as white infiltrates invading and replacing the disk tissue. Metastatic vitreous cells are

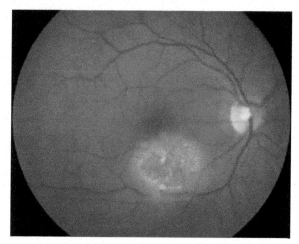

▲ **Figure 10–46.** Metastasis of primary breast cancer to retina just below the macula of right eye.

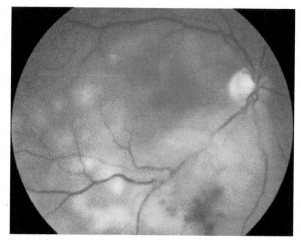

▲ **Figure 10–47.** Primary vitreoretinal lymphoma in right eye. Fundus features include vitreous haze due to intravitreal cells, ill-defined retinal infiltrate of lymphoma cells inferotemporal to the optic disk, associated patch of intraretinal blood, and scattered yellow subretinal retinal pigment epithelial infiltrates temporally and inferotemporally.

indistinguishable from inflammatory vitreous cells and must be suspected on the basis of the clinical history. As with metastatic tumors to the uvea, metastases to the retina, optic disk, and vitreous must be regarded as equivalent to metastases to the brain, with corresponding unfavorable prognosis for survival. Treatment options for retinal and optic disk metastases include EBRT and chemotherapy appropriate to the cancer type. Metastatic cancer cells in the vitreous can be removed by posterior vitrectomy, but then the eye usually must be treated by EBRT to prevent reaccumulation.

▶ Primary Vitreoretinal Lymphoma

Primary vitreoretinal lymphoma is a distinct subtype of **primary intraocular lymphoma.** It is characterized by diffuse infiltration of the vitreous by malignant lymphoid cells and geographic accumulations of malignant lymphoid cells beneath the retinal pigment epithelium. Some patients also develop scattered malignant lymphoid infiltrates within the sensory retina (Figure 10–47). Commonly primary vitreoretinal lymphoma is associated with independent (nonmetastatic) foci of lymphoma within the brain and cerebrospinal fluid (primary CNS lymphoma) in the absence of systemic lymphoma. The malignant lymphoid cells in this disorder are usually of B-cell lineage, and the CNS and intraocular tumors are typically characterized histopathologically as diffuse large-cell lymphoma. Middle-aged to elderly individuals are usually affected with involvement of both eyes, simultaneously or sequentially, in 80% of cases.

Primary vitreoretinal lymphoma is frequently misdiagnosed as uveitis and treated unsuccessfully for a number of months before its true nature is recognized. Diagnosis of primary vitreoretinal lymphoma requires cytopathologic

and immunocytochemical analysis of the lymphoid cells within the vitreous obtained by posterior vitrectomy (or, in rare cases, by fine-needle aspiration biopsy or endoincisional biopsy of discrete geographic subretinal pigment epithelial infiltrates) or pathologic confirmation of primary CNS lymphoma in the context of characteristic intraocular features in one or both eyes. Ocular treatment depends on whether one or both eyes are affected, whether there is concurrent active primary CNS lymphoma, how and when any prior primary CNS lymphoma had been treated, and the general health and survival prognosis of the patient. If vitreous cells are a prominent feature of the condition, a posterior vitrectomy can be performed (on one or both eyes) for both diagnostic and therapeutic purposes. Specific treatment options for residual primary vitreoretinal lymphoma include intravenous chemotherapy (usually a methotrexate-based regimen), EBRT to one or both eyes (and the brain if it is involved clinically), and a series of intravitreal injections of methotrexate. Discrete lymphoid infiltrates in the eye typically regress rapidly in response to these treatments, and long-term remissions frequently but not always occur following these therapies. Unfortunately, median patient survival following diagnosis of primary vitreoretinal lymphoma is generally about 3 years, with death usually caused by relapse and progression of the CNS lymphoma.

Rarely, predominantly vitreoretinal disease can be caused by systemic B-cell lymphoma, but this usually causes uveal infiltration (see Primary Uveal Lymphoma in Chapter 7).

REFERENCES

Retina & Retinal Disorders

Age-Related Eye Disease Study 2 (AREDS2) Research Group et al: Secondary analyses of the effects of lutein/zeaxanthin on age-related macular degeneration progression: AREDS2 report No. 3. JAMA Ophthalmol 2014;132:142. [PMID: 24310343]

Andersen N et al: The Danish registry of diabetic retinopathy. Clin Epidemiol 2016;8:613. [PMID: 27822108]

Ashraf M et al: Central retinal vein occlusion: modifying current treatment protocols. Eye (Lond) 2016;30:505. [PMID: 26869163]

Bernstein PS et al: Lutein, zeaxanthin, and meso-zeaxanthin: The basic and clinical science underlying carotenoid-based nutritional interventions against ocular disease. Prog Retin Eye Res 2016;50:34. [PMID: 26541886]

Bhatnagar A et al: Diabetic retinopathy in pregnancy. Curr Diabetes Rev 2009;5:151. [PMID: 19689249]

Bhavsar KV et al: Multimodal imaging in handheld laser-induced maculopathy. Am J Ophthalmol 2015;159:227. [PMID: 25448992]

Bonini Filho MA et al: Optical coherence tomography angiography in retinal artery occlusion. Retina 2015;35:2339. [PMID: 26457398]

Brown DM et al: Intravitreal aflibercept injection for macular edema secondary to central retinal vein occlusion: 1-year results from the phase 3 COPERNICUS study. Am J Ophthalmol 2013;155:429. [PMID: 23218699]

Campochiaro PA et al: Intravitreal aflibercept for macular edema following branch retinal vein occlusion: The 24-week results of the VIBRANT study. Ophthalmology 2015;122:538. [PMID: 25315663]

Chan CK et al: SCORE Study report #11: Incidences of neovascular events in eyes with retinal vein occlusion. Ophthalmology 2011;118:1364. [PMID: 21440942]

Chan SY et al: Optical coherence tomographic angiography in central serous chorioretinopathy. Retina 2016;36:2051. [PMID: 27164548]

Chen G et al: Subthreshold micropulse diode laser versus conventional laser photocoagulation for diabetic macular edema: A meta-analysis of randomized controlled trials. Retina 2016;36:2059. [PMID: 27096529]

Chong V: Ranibizumab for the treatment of wet AMD: A summary of real-world studies. Eye (Lond) 2016;30:270. [PMID: 26634711]

Coscas G et al: Optical coherence tomography angiography during follow-up: Qualitative and quantitative analysis of mixed type I and II choroidal neovascularization after vascular endothelial growth factor trap therapy. Ophthalmic Res 2015;54:57. [PMID: 26201877]

Cugati S et al: Treatment options for central retinal artery occlusion. Curr Treat Options Neurol 2013;15:63. [PMID: 23070637]

Cunningham ET Jr et al: The creeping choroiditides: Serpiginous and multifocal serpiginoid choroiditis. Ocul Immunol Inflamm. 2014;22:345. [PMID: 25229161]

Daniel E et al: Outcomes in eyes with retinal angiomatous proliferation in the Comparison of Age-Related Macular Degeneration Treatments Trials (CATT). Ophthalmology. 2016;123:609. [PMID: 26681392]

Diabetic Retinopathy Clinical Research Network et al: Five year outcomes of ranibizumab with prompt or deferred laser versus laser or triamcinolone plus deferred ranibizumab for diabetic macular edema. Am J Ophthalmol 2016;164:57. [PMID: 26802783]

Diabetic Retinopathy Clinical Research Network et al: Aflibercept, bevacizumab, or ranibizumab for diabetic macular edema. N Engl J Med 2015;372:1193. [PMID: 25692915]

di Lauro R et al: Intravitreal bevacizumab for surgical treatment of severe proliferative diabetic retinopathy. Graefes Arch Clin Exp Ophthalmol 2010;248:785. [PMID: 20135139]

Duncker T et al: Quantitative fundus autofluorescence and optical coherence tomography in best vitelliform macular dystrophy. Invest Ophthalmol Vis Sci 2014;55:1471. [PMID: 24526438]

Eleftheriadou M et al: Long-term outcomes of aflibercept treatment for neovascular age-related macular degeneration in a clinical setting. Am J Ophthalmol 2017;174:160. [PMID: 27746298]

Ferris FL 3rd et al: Clinical classification of age-related macular degeneration. Ophthalmology 2013;120:844. [PMID: 23332590]

Garcia-Horton A et al: Retinal vein thrombosis: The internist's role in the etiologic and therapeutic management. Thromb Res 2016;148:118. [PMID: 27838473]

Gohil R et al: Myopic foveoschisis: A clinical review. Eye (Lond) 2015;29:593. [PMID: 25744445]

Hashimoto H et al. Ultra-wide-field fundus autofluorescence in multiple evanescent white dot syndrome. Am J Ophthalmol 2015;159:698. [PMID: 25634532]

Hayreh SS. Ocular vascular occlusive disorders: Natural history of visual outcome. Prog Retin Eye Res 2014;41:1. [PMID: 24769221]

Heier JS et al: Intravitreal aflibercept injection for macular edema due to central retinal vein occlusion: Two-year results from the COPERNICUS study. Ophthalmology 2014;121:1414. [PMID: 24679444]

Heier JS et al: Intravitreal aflibercept for diabetic macular edema: 148-week results from the VISTA and VIVID studies. Ophthalmology 2016;123:2376. [PMID: 27651226]

Ho M et al: Retinal vein occlusions, from basics to the latest treatment. Retina 2016;36:432. [PMID: 26716954]

Hornan D et al: Use of pegaptanib for recurrent and non-clearing vitreous haemorrhage in proliferative diabetic retinopathy. Eye 2010;24:1315. [PMID: 20224599]

Inoue R et al: Association between the efficacy of photodynamic therapy and indocyanine green angiography findings for central serous chorioretinopathy. Am J Ophthalmol 2010;149:441. [PMID: 20172070]

Jacobson SG et al: Improvement in vision: A new goal for treatment of hereditary retinal degenerations. Expert Opin Orphan Drugs 2015;3:563. [PMID: 26246977]

Joachim N et al: The incidence and progression of age-related macular degeneration over 15 Years: The Blue Mountains Eye Study. Ophthalmology 2015;122:2482. [PMID: 26383995]

Johnston T et al: Current understanding of the genetic architecture of rhegmatogenous retinal detachment. Ophthalmic Genet 2016;37:121. [PMID: 26757352]

Keenan TD et al: United Kingdom National Ophthalmology Database Study: Diabetic Retinopathy; Report 1: Prevalence of centre-involving diabetic macular oedema and other grades of maculopathy and retinopathy in hospital eye services. Eye (Lond) 2013;27:1397. [PMID: 24051410]

Kuehlewein L et al: Optical coherence tomography angiography of type 1 neovascularization in age-related macular degeneration. Am J Ophthalmol 2015;160:739. [PMID: 26164826]

Lawrenson JG et al: Controversies in the use of nutritional supplements in ophthalmology. Curr Pharm Des 2015;21:4667. [PMID: 26350529]

Lee GD et al: Retinal injury after inadvertent handheld laser exposure. Retina 2014;34:2388. [PMID: 25380069]

Lee R et al: Epidemiology of diabetic retinopathy, diabetic macular edema and related vision loss. Eye Vis (Lond) 2015;2:17. [PMID: 26605370]

Marsiglia M et al: Expanded clinical spectrum of multiple evanescent white dot syndrome with multimodal imaging. Retina 2016;36:64. [PMID: 26166804]

Meuer SM et al: The epidemiology of vitreoretinal interface abnormalities as detected by spectral-domain optical coherence tomography: The Beaver Dam Eye Study. Ophthalmology 2015;122:787. [PMID: 25556116]

Mrejen S et al: Acute zonal occult outer retinopathy: A classification based on multimodal imaging. JAMA Ophthalmol 2014;132:1089. [PMID: 24945598]

Nagiel A et al: Type 3 neovascularization: Evolution, association with pigment epithelial detachment, and treatment response as revealed by spectral domain optical coherence tomography. Retina 2015;35:638. [PMID: 25650713]

Ogura S et al: Wide-field fundus autofluorescence imaging to evaluate retinal function in patients with retinitis pigmentosa. Am J Ophthalmol 2014;158:1093. [PMID: 25062603]

Oishi M et al: Wide-field fundus autofluorescence abnormalities and visual function in patients with cone and cone-rod dystrophies. Invest Ophthalmol Vis Sci 2014;55:3572. [PMID: 24845635]

Park YG et al: One year results of intravitreal ranibizumab monotherapy for retinal angiomatous proliferation: A comparative analysis based on disease stages. BMC Ophthalmol 2015;15:182. [PMID: 26691185]

Payne JF et al: Randomized trial of treat and extend ranibizumab with and without navigated laser for diabetic macular edema: TREX-DME 1 year outcomes. Ophthalmology 2017;124:74. [PMID: 27836430]

Raoof N et al: "Toy" laser macular burns in children: 12-month update. Eye (Lond) 2016;30:492. [PMID: 26611842]

Salomão DR et al: Vitreoretinal presentation of secondary large B-cell lymphoma in patients with systemic lymphoma. JAMA Ophthalmol 2013;131:1151. [PMID: 23744124]

Sarwar S et al: Aflibercept for neovascular age-related macular degeneration. Cochrane Database Syst Rev 2016;2:CD011346. [PMID: 26857947]

Schmitz-Valckenberg S et al: Natural history of geographic atrophy progression secondary to age-related macular degeneration (Geographic Atrophy Progression Study). Ophthalmology 2016;123:361. [PMID: 26545317]

Schrag M et al: Intravenous fibrinolytic therapy in central retinal artery occlusion: A patient-level meta-analysis. JAMA Neurol 2015;72:1148. [PMID: 26258861]

Scripsema NK et al: Lutein, zeaxanthin, and meso-zeaxanthin in the clinical management of eye disease. J Ophthalmol 2015;2015:865179. [PMID: 26819755]

Semeraro F et al: Diabetic retinopathy: Vascular and inflammatory disease. J Diabetes Res 2015;2015:582060. [PMID: 26137497]

Silva PS et al: Peripheral lesions identified on ultrawide field imaging predict increased risk of diabetic retinopathy progression over 4 Years. Ophthalmology 2015;122:949. [PMID: 25704318]

Stitt AW et al: The progress in understanding and treatment of diabetic retinopathy. Prog Retin Eye Res 2016;51:156. [PMID: 26297071]

Toda J et al: The effect of pregnancy on the progression of diabetic retinopathy. Jpn J Ophthalmol 2016;60:454. [PMID: 27456842]

van Lookeren Campagne M et al: Age-related macular degeneration: Complement in action. Immunobiology 2016;221:733. [PMID: 26742632]

Varma DD et al: A review of central retinal artery occlusion: Clinical presentation and management. Eye 2013;27:688. [PMID: 23470793]

Wells JA et al: Diabetic Retinopathy Clinical Research Network. Aflibercept, bevacizumab, or ranibizumab for diabetic macular edema. N Engl J Med 2015;372:1193. [PMID: 25692915]

Wyłęgała A et al: Optical coherence angiography: A review. Medicine (Baltimore) 2016;95:e4907. [PMID: 27741104]

Zając-Pytrus HM et al: The dry form of age-related macular degeneration (AMD): The current concepts of pathogenesis and prospects for treatment. Adv Clin Exp Med 2015;24:10994. [PMID: 26771984]

Retinal Tumors

Abramson DH et al: A phase I/II study of direct intraarterial (ophthalmic artery) chemotherapy with melphalan for intraocular retinoblastoma. Initial results. Ophthalmology 2008;115:1398. [PMID: 18342944]

Arnold AC et al: Solitary retinal astrocytoma. Surv Ophthalmol 1985;30:173. [PMID: 4081977]

Brodie SE et al: Persistence of retinal function after selective ophthalmic artery chemotherapy infusion for retinoblastoma. Doc Ophthalmol 2009;119:13. [PMID: 19169884]

Chantada G et al: A proposal for an international retinoblastoma staging system. Pediatr Blood Cancer 2006;47:801. [PMID: 16358310]

Cohn AD et al: Surgical outcomes of epiretinal membranes associated with combined hamartoma of the retina and retinal pigment epithelium. Retina 2009;29:825. [PMID: 19276871]

Coupland SE et al: Understanding intraocular lymphomas. Clin Experiment Ophthalmol 2008;36:564. [PMID: 18954321]

Eagle RC et al: Malignant transformation of spontaneously regressed retinoblastoma, retinoma/retinocytoma variant. Ophthalmology 1989;96:1389. [PMID: 2780006]

Edge SB et al (eds): AJCC Cancer Staging Manual, 7th ed. Springer; 2009.

Elizalde J et al: Adenoma of the nonpigmented ciliary epithelium. Eur J Ophthalmol 2006;16:630. [PMID: 16952109]

Findeis-Hosey JJ et al: Von Hippel-Lindau disease. J Pediatr Genet 2016;5:116. [PMID: 27617152]

Gallie BL et al: Retinoma: Spontaneous regression of retinoblastoma or benign manifestation of the mutation? Br J Cancer 1982;45:513. [PMID: 7073943]

Gallie BL et al: Significance of retinoma and phthisis bulbi for retinoblastoma. Ophthalmology 1982;89:1393. [PMID: 7162783]

Holdt M et al: Intraocular medulloepithelioma: Series of 10 cases and review of the literature. Klin Monbl Augenheilkd 2009;226:1017. [PMID: 20108196]

Hungerford JL et al: External beam radiotherapy for retinoblastoma. I. Whole eye technique. Br J Ophthalmol 1995;79:109. [PMID: 7696227]

Linn Murphree A: Intraocular retinoblastoma: The case for a new group classification. Ophthalmol Clin North Am 2005;18:41. [PMID: 15763190]

Margo C et al: Retinocytoma. A benign variant of retinoblastoma. Arch Ophthalmol 1983;101:1519. [PMID: 6626001]

Meyer CH et al: Grouped congenital hypertrophy of the retinal pigment epithelium follows developmental patterns of pigmentary mosaicism. Ophthalmology 2005;112:841. [PMID: 15878064]

Murphree AL et al: Chemotherapy plus local treatment in the management of intraocular retinoblastoma. Arch Ophthalmol 1996;114:1348. [PMID: 8906025]

PDQ Pediatric Treatment Editorial Board: Retinoblastoma treatment (PDQ®): Health professional version. PDQ Cancer Information Summaries [Internet] 2016 Sep 19. [PMID: 26389442]

Pe'er J et al: Clinical review: Treatment of vitreoretinal lymphoma. Ocul Immunol Inflamm 2009;17:299. [PMID: 19831557]

Reichstein D. Primary vitreoretinal lymphoma: An update on pathogenesis, diagnosis and treatment. Curr Opin Ophthalmol 2016;27:177. [PMID: 26859131]

Roarty JD et al: Incidence of second neoplasms in patients with bilateral retinoblastoma. Ophthalmology 1988;95:1583. [PMID: 3211467]

Shields CL et al: Solitary congenital hypertrophy of the retinal pigment epithelium: Clinical features and frequency of enlargement in 330 patients. Ophthalmology 2003;110:1968. [PMID: 14522773]

Shields CL et al: Combined hamartoma of the retina and retinal pigment epithelium in 77 consecutive patients. Visual outcome based on macular versus extramacular tumor location. Ophthalmology 2008;115:2246. [PMID: 18995912]

Shields JA et al: Adenoma of the ciliary body epithelium. Arch Ophthalmol 1999;117:592. [PMID: 10326955]

Singh AD et al: Observations on 17 patients with retinocytoma. Arch Ophthalmol 2000;118:199. [PMID: 10676785]

Smith BJ et al: The genetics of retinoblastoma and current diagnostic testing. J Pediatric Ophthalmol Strabismus 1996;33:120. [PMID: 8965236]

Soliman SE et al: Knowledge of genetics in familial retinoblastoma. Ophthalmic Genet 2016;18:1–7. [PMID: 27427836]

Touriño R et al: Value of the congenital hypertrophy of the retinal pigment epithelium in the diagnosis of familial adenomatous polyposis. Int Ophthalmol 2004;25:101. [PMID: 15290889]

Trichopoulos N et al: Adenocarcinoma arising from congenital hypertrophy of the retinal pigment epithelium. Graefes Arch Clin Exp Ophthalmol 2006;244:125. [PMID: 15983818]

Ulbright TM et al: Astrocytic tumors of the retina. Differentiation of sporadic tumor from phakomatosis-associated tumors. Arch Pathol Lab Med 1984;108:160. [PMID: 6421263]

Watkins LM et al: Metastatic tumors of the eye and orbit. Int Ophthalmol Clin 1998;38:117. [PMID: 9532476]

Wong WT et al: Clinical characterization of retinal capillary hemangioblastomas in a large population of patients with von Hippel–Lindau disease. Ophthalmology 2008;115:181. [PMID: 17543389]

Wong WT et al: Ocular von Hippel–Lindau disease: Clinical update and emerging treatments. Curr Opin Ophthalmol 2008;19:213. [PMID: 18408496]

Wong WT et al: Intravitreal ranibizumab therapy for retinal capillary hemangioblastoma related to von Hippel-Lindau disease. Ophthalmology 2008;115:1957. [PMID: 18789534]

Zimmer-Galler IE et al: Long-term observations of retinal lesions in tuberous sclerosis. Am J Ophthalmol 1995;119:318. [PMID: 7872393]

Glaucoma

John F. Salmon, MD, FRCS

Glaucoma is an acquired chronic optic neuropathy characterized by optic disk cupping and visual field loss. It is usually associated with raised intraocular pressure. There are different types of glaucoma, which helps to explain, for example, why one patient with glaucoma may have no symptoms, while another experiences sudden pain and inflammation. In the majority of cases, there is no associated ocular disease (primary glaucoma) (Table 11–1).

About 60 million people have glaucoma. An estimated 3 million Americans are affected, and of these cases, about 50% are undiagnosed. About 6 million people are blind from glaucoma, including approximately 100,000 Americans, making it the leading cause of preventable blindness in the United States. Primary open-angle glaucoma, the most common form among blacks and whites, causes insidious asymptomatic progressive bilateral visual loss that is often not detected until extensive field loss has already occurred. Blacks are at greater risk than whites for early onset, delayed diagnosis, and severe visual loss. The most important risk factors are raised intraocular pressure, age, and genetic predisposition. Angle-closure glaucoma accounts for 10–15% of cases in whites. This percentage is much higher in Asians and the Inuit. Primary angle-closure glaucoma may account for over 90% of bilateral blindness due to glaucoma in China. Normal-tension glaucoma is the most common type in Japan.

The mechanism of raised intraocular pressure in glaucoma is impaired outflow of aqueous resulting from abnormalities within the drainage system of the anterior chamber angle (open-angle glaucoma) or impaired access of aqueous to the drainage system (angle-closure glaucoma) (Table 11–2). Treatment is directed toward reducing the intraocular pressure and, when possible, correcting the underlying cause. Although in normal-tension glaucoma intraocular pressure is within the normal range, reduction of intraocular pressure may still be beneficial.

Intraocular pressure can be reduced by decreasing aqueous production or increasing aqueous outflow, using medical, laser, or surgical treatments. Medications, usually administered topically, are available to reduce aqueous production or increase aqueous outflow. Surgically bypassing the drainage system is useful in most forms of glaucoma if there is a failure to respond to medical treatment. In recalcitrant cases, laser or cryotherapy can be used to ablate the ciliary body to reduce aqueous production. Improving access of aqueous to the anterior chamber angle in angle-closure glaucoma may be achieved by peripheral laser iridotomy or surgical iridectomy if the cause is pupillary block, miosis if there is angle crowding, or cycloplegia if there is anterior lens displacement. In the secondary glaucomas, consideration must always be given to treating the primary abnormality.

In all patients with glaucoma, the necessity for treatment and its effectiveness are assessed by regular determination of intraocular pressure (tonometry), inspection of optic disks, and measurement of visual fields.

The management of glaucoma is best undertaken by an ophthalmologist, but detection of asymptomatic cases is dependent on the cooperation and assistance of all medical personnel, particularly optometrists. Ophthalmoscopy to detect optic disk cupping and tonometry to measure intraocular pressure should be part of the routine ophthalmologic examination of all patients over 35 years of age. This is especially important in patients with a family history of glaucoma and in high-risk groups such as blacks, who should undergo regular screening every 2 years from age 35 and annually from age 50.

PHYSIOLOGY OF AQUEOUS HUMOR

Intraocular pressure is determined by the rate of aqueous production and the resistance to outflow of aqueous from the eye.

Table 11–1. Glaucoma Classified According to Etiology

A. Primary glaucoma
1. Open-angle glaucoma
   a. Primary open-angle glaucoma (chronic open-angle glaucoma, chronic simple glaucoma)
   b. Normal-tension glaucoma (low-tension glaucoma)
2. Angle-closure glaucoma

B. Congenital glaucoma
1. Primary congenital glaucoma
2. Glaucoma associated with other developmental ocular abnormalities
   a. Anterior chamber cleavage syndromes
      Axenfeld-Rieger syndrome
      Peter syndrome
   b. Aniridia
3. Glaucoma associated with extraocular developmental abnormalities
   a. Sturge-Weber syndrome
   b. Marfan's syndrome
   c. Neurofibromatosis 1
   d. Lowe syndrome
   e. Congenital rubella

C. Secondary glaucoma
1. Pigmentary glaucoma
2. Exfoliation syndrome
3. Due to lens change (phacogenic)
   a. Dislocation
   b. Intumescence
   c. Phacolytic
4. Due to uveal tract changes
   a. Uveitis
   b. Posterior synechiae (seclusio pupillae)
   c. Tumor
   d. Ciliary body swelling
5. Iridocorneal endothelial (ICE) syndrome
6. Trauma
   a. Hyphema
   b. Angle contusion and/or recession
   c. Peripheral anterior synechiae
7. Postoperative
   a. Ciliary block glaucoma (malignant glaucoma)
   b. Peripheral anterior synechiae
   c. Epithelial downgrowth
   d. Following corneal graft surgery
   e. Following retinal detachment surgery
8. Neovascular glaucoma
   a. Diabetes mellitus
   b. Central retinal vein occlusion
   c. Intraocular tumor
9. Raised episcleral venous pressure
   a. Carotid-cavernous fistula
   b. Sturge-Weber syndrome
10. Steroid-induced

D. Absolute glaucoma: The end result of any uncontrolled glaucoma is a hard, sightless, and often painful eye.

Table 11–2. Glaucoma Classified According to Mechanism of Intraocular Pressure Rise

A. Open-angle glaucoma
1. Pretrabecular membranes: All of these may progress to angle-closure glaucoma due to contraction of the pretrabecular membranes.
   a. Neovascular glaucoma
   b. Epithelial downgrowth
   c. Iridocorneal endothelial (ICE) syndrome
2. Trabecular abnormalities
   a. Primary open-angle glaucoma
   b. Congenital glaucoma
   c. Pigmentary glaucoma
   d. Exfoliation syndrome
   e. Steroid-induced glaucoma
   f. Hyphema
   g. Angle contusion and/or recession
   h. Anterior uveitis (iridocyclitis)
   i. Phacolytic glaucoma
3. Posttrabecular abnormalities
   a. Raised episcleral venous pressure

B. Angle-closure glaucoma
1. Pupillary block (iris bombé)
   a. Primary angle-closure glaucoma
   b. Posterior synechiae (seclusio pupillae)
   c. Intumescent lens
   d. Anterior lens dislocation
   e. Hyphema
2. Anterior lens displacement
   a. Ciliary block glaucoma
   b. Central retinal vein occlusion
   c. Posterior scleritis
   d. Following retinal detachment surgery
3. Angle crowding
   a. Plateau iris
   b. Intumescent lens
   c. Mydriasis for fundal examination
4. Peripheral anterior synechiae
   a. Chronic angle closure
   b. Secondary to flat anterior chamber
   c. Secondary to iris bombé
   d. Contraction of pretrabecular membranes

▶ Composition of Aqueous

The aqueous is a clear liquid that fills the anterior and posterior chambers of the eye. Its volume is about 250 μL, and its rate of production, which is subject to diurnal variation, is about 2.5 μL/min. The osmotic pressure is slightly higher than that of plasma. The composition of aqueous is similar to that of plasma except for much higher concentrations of ascorbate, pyruvate, and lactate and lower concentrations of protein, urea, and glucose.

Formation & Flow of Aqueous

Aqueous is produced by the ciliary body. An ultrafiltrate of plasma produced in the stroma of the ciliary processes is modified by the barrier function and secretory processes of the ciliary epithelium. Entering the posterior chamber, the aqueous passes through the pupil into the anterior chamber (Figure 11–1) and then to the trabecular meshwork in the anterior chamber angle. During this period, there is some differential exchange of components with the blood in the iris.

Intraocular inflammation or trauma causes an increase in the protein concentration. This is called plasmoid aqueous and closely resembles blood serum.

Outflow of Aqueous

The trabecular meshwork is composed of beams of collagen and elastic tissue covered by trabecular cells that form a filter with a decreasing pore size as the canal of Schlemm is approached. Contraction of the ciliary muscle through its insertion into the trabecular meshwork increases pore size in the meshwork, and hence the rate of aqueous drainage. Passage of aqueous into Schlemm's canal depends on cyclic formation of transcellular channels in the endothelial lining. Efferent channels from Schlemm's canal (about 30 collector channels and 12 aqueous veins) conduct the fluid directly into the venous system. Some aqueous passes between the bundles of the ciliary muscle into the suprachoroidal space and then into the venous system of the ciliary body, choroid, and sclera (uveoscleral flow) (Figure 11–1).

The major resistance to aqueous outflow from the anterior chamber is the juxtacanalicular tissue adjacent to the endothelial lining of Schlemm's canal, rather than the venous system. But the pressure in the episcleral venous network determines the minimum level of intraocular pressure that can be achieved by medical therapy.

PATHOPHYSIOLOGY OF GLAUCOMA

So far, 11 genes and multiple loci have been identified to contribute to the development of glaucoma with their effects being influenced by age and environment. The major mechanism of visual loss in glaucoma is retinal ganglion cell apoptosis, leading to thinning of the inner nuclear and nerve fiber layers of the retina and axonal loss in the optic nerve. The optic disk becomes atrophic, with enlargement of the optic cup (see later in the chapter).

The pathophysiology of intraocular pressure elevation—whether due to open-angle or to angle-closure mechanisms—will be discussed as each disease entity is considered (see later in the chapter). The effects of raised intraocular pressure are influenced by the time course and magnitude of the rise in intraocular pressure. In acute angle-closure glaucoma, the intraocular pressure reaches 60–80 mm Hg,

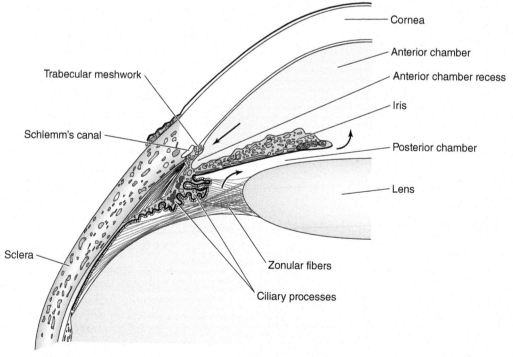

▲ **Figure 11–1.** Anterior segment structures. Arrows indicate direction of flow of aqueous.

resulting in acute ischemic damage to the iris with associated corneal edema and optic nerve damage. In primary open-angle glaucoma, the intraocular pressure does not usually rise above 30 mm Hg and retinal ganglion cell damage develops over a prolonged period, often many years. In normal-tension glaucoma, retinal ganglion cells may be susceptible to damage from intraocular pressures in the normal range, or the major mechanism of damage may be optic nerve head ischemia.

CLINICAL ASSESSMENT IN GLAUCOMA

▶ Tonometry

Tonometry is measurement of intraocular pressure. The most widely used instrument is the Goldmann applanation tonometer, which is attached to the slitlamp and measures the force required to flatten a fixed area of the cornea. Corneal thickness influences the accuracy of measurement. Intraocular pressure is overestimated in eyes with thick corneas and underestimated in eyes with thin corneas. This difficulty may be overcome by the Pascal dynamic contour tonometer. Other applanation tonometers are the Perkins tonometer and the Tono-Pen, both of which are portable, and the pneumatotonometer, which can be used with a soft contact lens in place when the cornea has an irregular surface. The Schiotz tonometer is portable and measures the corneal indentation produced by a known weight. (For further discussion of tonometry, see Chapter 2; for tonometer disinfection techniques, see Chapter 20.)

The normal range of intraocular pressure is 11–21 mm Hg (Figure 11–2). The distribution is Gaussian, but with the curve skewed to the right. In the elderly, average intraocular pressure is higher, giving an upper limit of 24 mm Hg. The intraocular pressure is subject to diurnal

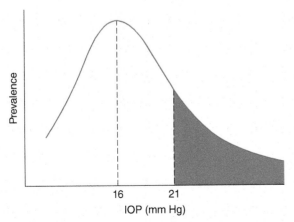

▲ **Figure 11–2.** Distribution of intraocular pressure (IOP) in individuals over the age of 40 years.

fluctuation throughout the day. In primary open-angle glaucoma, 32–50% of affected individuals will have a normal intraocular pressure when first measured. Conversely, isolated raised intraocular pressure does not necessarily mean that the patient has primary open-angle glaucoma, since other evidence in the form of a glaucomatous optic disk or visual field changes is necessary for diagnosis. If the intraocular pressure is consistently raised in the presence of normal optic disks and visual fields (ocular hypertension), the patient should be observed periodically as a glaucoma suspect.

▶ Gonioscopy (see also Chapter 2)

The anterior chamber angle is formed by the junction of the peripheral cornea and the iris, between which lies the trabecular meshwork (Figure 11–3). The configuration of this angle, whether it is wide (open), narrow, or closed, has an important bearing on the outflow of aqueous. The anterior chamber angle width can be estimated by oblique illumination with a penlight (Figure 11–4) or by slitlamp observation of the depth of the peripheral anterior chamber, but it is best determined by gonioscopy, which allows direct visualization of the angle structures (Figure 11–3). If it is possible to visualize the full extent of the trabecular meshwork, the scleral spur, and the iris processes, the angle is open. Being able to see only Schwalbe's line or a small portion of the trabecular meshwork means that the angle is narrow. Being unable to see Schwalbe's line means that the angle is closed.

Large myopic eyes have wide angles, and small hyperopic eyes have narrow angles. Enlargement of the lens with age narrows the angle and accounts for some cases of angle-closure glaucoma.

▶ Optic Disk Assessment

The normal optic disk has a central depression—the physiologic cup—whose size depends on the bulk of the fibers that form the optic nerve relative to the size of the scleral opening through which they must pass. In hyperopic eyes, the scleral opening is small, and thus the optic cup is small; the reverse is true in myopic eyes. The earliest sign of glaucoma is thinning of the retinal nerve fiber layer in the region surrounding the optic disk. Glaucomatous optic atrophy produces specific disk changes characterized chiefly by loss of disk substance, manifesting as enlargement of the cup of the optic disk, and pallor in the area of cupping. Other forms of optic atrophy cause widespread pallor without increased disk cupping.

In glaucoma, there may be concentric enlargement of the optic cup or preferential superior and inferior cupping with focal notching of the rim of the optic disk (Figure 11–5). The optic cup also increases in depth as the lamina cribrosa is displaced backward. As cupping develops, the retinal vessels on

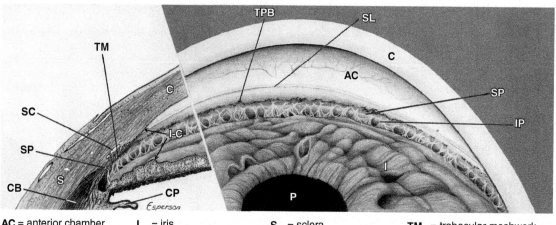

AC = anterior chamber	I = iris	S = sclera	TM = trabecular meshwork
C = cornea	I-C = iris-corneal angle	SC = Schlemm's canal	TPB = trabecular pigment band
CB = ciliary body	IP = iris processes	SL = Schwalbe's line	
CP = ciliary process	P = pupil	SP = scleral spur	

Figure 11–3. Composite illustration showing anatomic **(left)** and gonioscopic **(right)** view of normal anterior chamber angle. (Used with permission from R. Shaffer.)

the disk are displaced nasally. The end result of glaucomatous cupping is the so-called "bean-pot" cup in which no neural rim tissue is apparent (Figure 11–6). Optic disk asymmetry is often suggestive of glaucoma.

Clinical assessment of the optic disk can be performed by direct ophthalmoscopy or by examination with the 78-diopter lens or special corneal contact lenses that give a 3-dimensional view (see also Chapter 2).

Other clinical evidence of neuronal damage in glaucoma is atrophy of the retinal nerve fiber layer, which precedes the development of optic disk changes. It is detectable by

ophthalmoscopy or fundal photography, both aided by using red-free light, optical coherence tomography (see Figure 2–32), scanning laser polarimetry, or scanning laser tomography.

▶ **Visual Field Examination**

Regular visual field examination is essential to the diagnosis and follow-up of glaucoma. Glaucomatous field loss is not in itself specific, since it consists of nerve fiber bundle defects that may be seen in other forms of optic nerve disease; but the pattern of

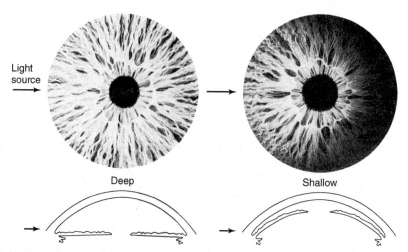

Figure 11–4. Estimation of depth of anterior chamber by oblique illumination (diagram). (Used with permission from R. Shaffer.)

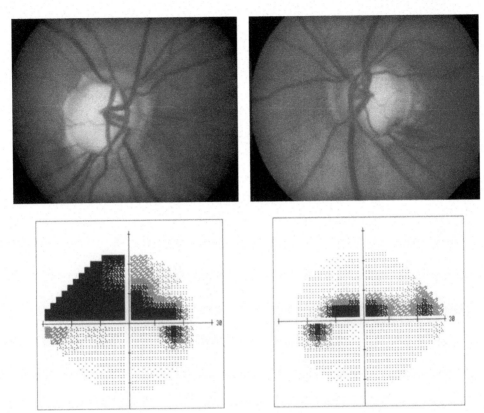

▲ **Figure 11–5.** Typical glaucomatous changes in the inferior neuroretinal rim of the optic disk and a flame-shaped hemorrhage. The visual field defect is close to fixation and there is a nasal "step."

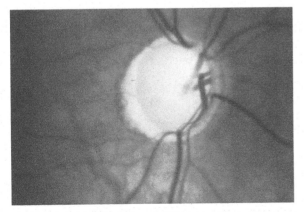

▲ **Figure 11–6.** Glaucomatous ("bean-pot") cupping of the optic disk with nasal displacement of the retinal vessels and completely hollowed-out appearance of the optic disk.

field loss, the nature of its progression, and the correlation with changes in the optic disk are characteristic of the disease.

Glaucomatous field loss involves mainly the central 30° of field (Figure 11–5). Contiguous extension of the blind spot into Bjerrum's area of the visual field—at 15° from fixation—produces a Bjerrum scotoma and then an arcuate scotoma. Focal areas of more pronounced loss within Bjerrum's area are known as Seidel scotomas. Double arcuate scotomas—above and below the horizontal meridian—are often accompanied by a nasal step (of Roenne) because of differences in size of the two arcuate defects. Peripheral field loss tends to start in the nasal periphery as a constriction of the isopters. Subsequently, there may be connection to an arcuate defect, producing peripheral breakthrough. The temporal peripheral field and the central 5–10° are affected late in the disease. Central visual acuity is not a reliable index of progress of the disease. In advanced glaucoma, the patient may have 20/20 visual acuity but only 5° of visual field in each eye and thus be legally blind.

Various ways of testing the visual fields in glaucoma include the automated perimeter (for example, Humphrey, Octopus, or Henson), the Goldmann perimeter, the Friedman field analyzer, and the tangent screen. (For testing techniques, see Chapter 2.) Conventional automated perimetry, most commonly using the Humphrey perimeter, employs a white stimulus on a white background (white-on-white perimetry). Visual field defects are not detected until there is about 40% retinal ganglion loss. Refinements to detect earlier visual field changes include blue-on-yellow perimetry, also known as short-wavelength automated perimetry (SWAP), frequency-doubling perimetry (FDP), and high-pass resolution perimetry.

TREATMENT OF RAISED INTRAOCULAR PRESSURE

▶ Medical Treatment (see also Chapter 22)

A. Facilitation of Aqueous Outflow

The **prostaglandin analogs**, **bimatoprost** 0.003%, **latanoprost** 0.005%, **tafluprost** 0.0015%, and **travoprost** 0.004% solutions, each once daily at night, and **unoprostone** 0.15% solution twice daily, increase uveoscleral outflow of aqueous. They are highly effective as first-line therapy and, when available and affordable, are the preferred first-line agent for most patients; as adjunctive therapy, they are available (except for unoprostone) combined with timolol 0.5% (see later in this section) in the same solution for once-daily use. All the prostaglandin analogs may produce conjunctival hyperemia, hyperpigmentation of periorbital skin, eyelash growth, and permanent darkening of the iris (particularly in green-brown and yellow-brown irides). They have also been rarely associated with reactivation of uveitis and herpes keratitis, and in predisposed individuals, they can cause macular edema after ophthalmic surgery.

Parasympathomimetic agents increase aqueous outflow by action on the trabecular meshwork through contraction of the ciliary muscle. **Pilocarpine** is rarely used since the availability of prostaglandin analogs but can be useful in some patients. It is given as 1–4% solution instilled up to four times a day or as 4% gel instilled at bedtime. Parasympathomimetic agents produce miosis with dimness of vision, particularly in patients with cataract, and accommodative spasm that may be disabling to younger patients. Retinal detachment is a serious but rare occurrence.

B. Suppression of Aqueous Production

Topical **beta-adrenergic blocking agents** may be used alone or in combination with other drugs. **Betaxolol** 0.25% and 0.5%, **carteolol** 1%, **levobunolol** 0.5%, **metipranolol** 0.3%, and **timolol** maleate 0.25% and 0.5% solutions twice daily and timolol maleate 0.25% and 0.5% gel once daily in the morning are the currently available preparations. The major contraindications to their use are chronic obstructive airway disease—particularly asthma—and cardiac conduction defects. Betaxolol, with its relatively greater selectivity for beta-1 receptors, less often produces respiratory side effects, but it is also less effective at reducing intraocular pressure. Depression, confusion, and fatigue may occur with the topical beta-blocking agents. The frequency of systemic effects and the availability of other agents have reduced the popularity of the beta-adrenergic blocking agents.

Apraclonidine (0.5% solution three times daily and 1% solution before and after laser treatment) is an α_2-adrenergic agonist that decreases aqueous humor formation without effect on outflow. It is particularly useful for preventing rise of intraocular pressure after anterior segment laser treatment and can be used on a short-term basis in refractory cases. It is not suitable for long-term use because of tachyphylaxis (loss of therapeutic effect over time) and a high incidence of allergic reactions.

Brimonidine (0.2% solution twice daily) is an α-adrenergic agonist that primarily inhibits aqueous production and secondarily increases aqueous outflow. It may be used as a first-line or adjunctive agent, but allergic reactions are common. It is available combined with timolol in the same solution.

Dorzolamide hydrochloride 2% solution and **brinzolamide** 1% (two or three times daily) are topical carbonic anhydrase inhibitors that are especially effective when employed adjunctively, although not as effective as systemic carbonic anhydrase inhibitors. The main side effects are a transient bitter taste and allergic blepharoconjunctivitis. Both drugs are available combined with timolol in the same solution.

Systemic **carbonic anhydrase inhibitors, acetazolamide** being the most widely used, are used in chronic glaucoma when topical therapy is insufficient and in acute glaucoma when very high intraocular pressure needs to be controlled quickly. They are capable of suppressing aqueous production by 40–60%. Acetazolamide can be administered orally in a dosage of 125–250 mg up to four times daily or as Diamox Sequels 500 mg once or twice daily, or it can be given intravenously (500 mg). The carbonic anhydrase inhibitors are associated with major systemic side effects that limit their usefulness for long-term therapy.

Hyperosmotic agents influence aqueous production as well as dehydrate the vitreous body (see below).

C. Reduction of Vitreous Volume

Hyperosmotic agents render the blood hypertonic, thus drawing water out of the vitreous and causing it to shrink. This is in addition to decreasing aqueous production. Reduction in vitreous volume is helpful in the treatment of acute angle-closure glaucoma and in malignant glaucoma when anterior displacement of the crystalline lens (caused by volume changes in the vitreous or choroid) produces angle closure (secondary angle-closure glaucoma).

Oral **glycerin (glycerol)**, 1 mL/kg of body weight in a cold 50% solution mixed with lemon juice, is the most commonly used agent, but it should be used with care in diabetics. Alternatives are oral isosorbide and intravenous mannitol (see Chapter 22 for dosages).

D. Miotics, Mydriatics, and Cycloplegics

Constriction of the pupil is fundamental to the management of primary angle-closure glaucoma and the angle crowding of plateau iris. Pupillary dilation is important in the treatment of angle closure secondary to iris bombé due to posterior synechiae.

When angle closure is secondary to anterior lens displacement, cycloplegic/mydriatic agents (cyclopentolate and atropine) are used to relax the ciliary muscle and thus tighten the zonular apparatus in an attempt to draw the lens backward.

▶ Surgical & Laser Treatment

A. Peripheral Iridotomy, Iridectomy, and Iridoplasty

Pupillary block in angle-closure glaucoma is most satisfactorily overcome by forming a direct communication between the anterior and posterior chambers that removes the pressure difference between them. Laser peripheral iridotomy is best done with the neodymium:YAG laser, although the argon laser may be necessary in dark irides. Surgical peripheral iridectomy is performed if YAG laser iridotomy is ineffective. YAG laser iridotomy is preventive when used in patients with narrow angles before closure attacks occur.

In some cases of acute angle closure when it is not possible to control the intraocular pressure medically or YAG laser iridotomy cannot be performed, argon laser peripheral iridoplasty (ALPI) can be undertaken. A ring of laser burns on the peripheral iris contracts the iris stroma, mechanically pulling open the anterior chamber angle.

B. Laser Trabeculoplasty

Application of laser (either argon or frequency-doubled Q-switched Nd:YAG) burns via a goniolens to the trabecular meshwork facilitates aqueous outflow by virtue of its effects on the trabecular meshwork and Schlemm's canal or cellular events that enhance the function of the meshwork. The technique is applicable to many forms of open-angle glaucoma, and the results are variable depending on the underlying cause. The pressure reduction usually allows decrease of medical therapy and postponement of glaucoma surgery. Treatments can be repeated (see Chapter 23). Laser trabeculoplasty may be used in the initial treatment of primary open-angle glaucoma. In most cases, the intraocular pressure gradually returns to the pretreatment level 2–5 years later.

The outcome of subsequent glaucoma drainage surgery may be adversely affected.

C. Glaucoma Drainage Surgery

The increased effectiveness of medical and laser treatment has reduced the need for glaucoma drainage surgery, but surgery is able to produce a more marked reduction in intraocular pressure.

Trabeculectomy is the procedure most commonly used to bypass the normal drainage channels, allowing direct access from the anterior chamber to the subconjunctival and orbital tissues (Figure 11–7). The major complication is fibrosis in the episcleral tissues, leading to closure of the new drainage pathway. This is most likely to occur in young patients, in blacks, in patients with secondary glaucoma, and in those who have previously undergone glaucoma drainage surgery or other surgery involving the episcleral tissues. Perioperative or postoperative adjunctive treatment with antimetabolites such as 5-fluorouracil and mitomycin C (in low dosage) reduces the risk of bleb failure and is associated with good intraocular pressure control but may lead to bleb-related complications like persistent ocular discomfort, bleb infection, or maculopathy from persistent ocular hypotony. Trabeculectomy markedly accelerates cataract formation.

Implantation of a silicone tube without a valve (Baerveldt or Molteno tube) or with a valve (Ahmed valve) to form a permanent conduit for aqueous flow out of the eye is an alternative procedure for eyes that are unlikely to respond to trabeculectomy. **Viscocanalostomy** and **deep sclerectomy with collagen implant** avoid full-thickness incisions into the eye. The intraocular pressure reduction is not as good as that achieved with trabeculectomy, but there is less potential for complications. They are technically difficult to perform.

There are a number of novel surgical procedures for glaucoma, including microelectrocautery to ablate a strip of

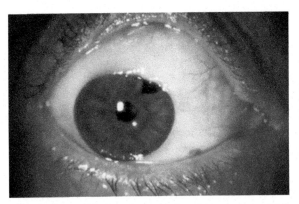

▲ **Figure 11–7.** Trabeculectomy showing an upper nasal "bleb" and peripheral iridectomy.

trabecular meshwork, micro-stents, and canaloplasty, that result in modest reduction of intraocular pressure without the formation of a bleb, but as yet, there are no long-term results and no randomized trials.

Goniotomy and **trabeculotomy** are useful techniques in treating primary congenital glaucoma, in which there appears to be an obstruction to aqueous drainage in the internal portion of the trabecular meshwork.

D. Cyclodestructive Procedures

Failure of medical and surgical treatment in advanced glaucoma may lead to consideration of laser or surgical destruction of the ciliary body to control intraocular pressure. Cryotherapy, thermal mode neodymium:YAG laser, or diode laser can all be used to destroy the ciliary body. Treatment is usually applied externally through the sclera, but endoscopic laser application systems are available.

▼ PRIMARY GLAUCOMA

PRIMARY OPEN-ANGLE GLAUCOMA

Primary open-angle glaucoma is the most common form in blacks and whites. In the United States, 1.29%–2% of persons over age 40, rising to 4.7% of persons over age 75, are estimated to have primary open-angle glaucoma. The disease is four times more common and six times more likely to cause blindness in blacks. There is a strong familial tendency in primary open-angle glaucoma, and close relatives of affected individuals should undergo regular screening.

The chief pathologic feature of primary open-angle glaucoma is a degenerative process in the trabecular meshwork, including deposition of extracellular material within the meshwork and beneath the endothelial lining of Schlemm's canal. This differs from the normal aging process. The consequence is a reduction in aqueous drainage leading to a rise in intraocular pressure.

Juvenile-onset open-angle glaucoma (a familial primary open-angle glaucoma with early onset), about 5% of familial cases of primary open-angle glaucoma, and about 3% of non-familial cases of primary open-angle glaucoma are associated with mutations in the myocilin gene on chromosome 1.

Raised intraocular pressure precedes optic disk and visual field changes by months to years. Although there is a clear association between the level of intraocular pressure and the severity and rate of progression of visual loss, there is great variability between individuals in the effect on the optic nerve of a given pressure elevation. Some eyes tolerate raised intraocular pressure without developing disk or field changes (ocular hypertension; see later in the chapter); others develop glaucomatous changes with consistently "normal" intraocular pressure (low-tension glaucoma; see later in the chapter). Nevertheless, higher levels of intraocular pressure are associated with greater field loss at presentation. When there is glaucomatous field loss on first examination, the risk of further progression is much greater. Since intraocular pressure is the only treatable risk factor, it remains the focus of therapy. There is strong evidence that control of intraocular pressure slows disk damage and field loss. For each 1-mm Hg reduction of intraocular pressure, there is an approximately 10% decreased risk of progression of glaucoma.

If there are extensive disk changes or field loss, it is advisable to reduce the intraocular pressure as much as possible, preferably to less than 15 mm Hg. A patient with only a suspicion of disk or field changes may need less vigorous treatment. In all cases, the inconveniences and possible complications of treatment must be considered. Many glaucoma patients are old and frail and may not tolerate vigorous treatment. In order to gain a perspective on the need for treatment, an initial period of observation without treatment may be necessary to determine the rate of progression of disk and field changes. There is no justification for subjecting an elderly patient to extremes of treatment when the likelihood of their developing significant visual loss during their lifetime is small.

▶ Diagnosis

The diagnosis of primary open-angle glaucoma is established when glaucomatous optic disk or field changes are associated with raised intraocular pressures, a normal-appearing open anterior chamber angle, and no other reason for intraocular pressure elevation. At least one-third of patients with primary open-angle glaucoma have a normal intraocular pressure when first examined, so repeated tonometry can be helpful.

▶ Screening for Glaucoma

The major problem in detection of primary open-angle glaucoma is the absence of symptoms until relatively late in the disease. When patients first notice field loss, substantial optic nerve damage has already occurred. If treatment is to be successful, it must be started early in the disease, and this depends on an active screening program. Unfortunately, glaucoma screening programs are hampered by the unreliability of a single intraocular pressure measurement in the detection of primary open-angle glaucoma and the complexities of relying on optic disk or visual field changes. At present, it is necessary to rely for early diagnosis predominantly on regular ophthalmologic assessment of first-degree relatives of affected individuals.

▶ Course & Prognosis

Without treatment, open-angle glaucoma may progress insidiously to complete blindness. If antiglaucoma drops control the intraocular pressure in an eye that has not suffered extensive glaucomatous damage, the prognosis is good (although visual field loss may progress despite normalized intraocular pressure). When the process is detected early, most glaucoma patients can be successfully managed medically. Trabeculectomy is a good option in patients who progress despite medical treatment.

NORMAL-TENSION GLAUCOMA (LOW-TENSION GLAUCOMA)

Some patients with glaucomatous optic disk or visual field changes have an intraocular pressure consistently below 21 mm Hg. These patients have normal-tension (low-tension) glaucoma. The pathogenesis may involve an abnormal sensitivity to intraocular pressure because of vascular or mechanical abnormalities at the optic nerve head, or this may be a purely vascular disease. There may be an inherited predisposition, with normal-tension glaucoma being particularly common in Japan. A few families with normal-tension glaucoma have an abnormality in the optineurin gene on chromosome 10. Some studies have shown associations with vasospasm and low intracranial pressure. Disk hemorrhages are more frequently seen in normal-tension than in primary open-angle glaucoma and often herald progression of field loss (Figure 11–5).

Before the diagnosis of normal-tension glaucoma can be established, a number of entities must be excluded:

1. Prior episode of raised intraocular pressure, such as caused by anterior uveitis, trauma, or topical steroid therapy.
2. Large diurnal variation in intraocular pressure with significant elevations, usually early in the morning.
3. Postural changes in intraocular pressure with a marked elevation when lying flat.
4. Intermittent elevations of intraocular pressure, such as in subacute angle closure.
5. Underestimation of intraocular pressure due to reduced corneal thickness.
6. Other causes of optic disk and field changes, including congenital disk abnormalities, inherited optic neuropathy, and acquired optic atrophy due to tumors or vascular disease.

Among patients diagnosed with normal-tension glaucoma, approximately 60% have progressive visual field loss, suggesting the possibility of acute ischemic events in the pathogenesis of those without progression. Reduction of intraocular pressure is beneficial in patients with progressive visual field loss, but this may not be achieved with medical therapy. Glaucoma drainage surgery with an antimetabolite may be required. The possibility of a vascular basis for normal-tension glaucoma has led to the use of systemic calcium channel blockers, but definite benefit from this intervention has yet to be demonstrated.

OCULAR HYPERTENSION

Ocular hypertension is raised intraocular pressure without disk or field abnormalities and is more common than primary open-angle glaucoma. The rate at which such individuals develop glaucoma is approximately 1–2% per year. The risk increases with increasing intraocular pressure, increasing age, greater optic disk cupping, a positive family history for glaucoma, and perhaps myopia, diabetes mellitus, and cardiovascular disease. The development of disk hemorrhages in a patient with ocular hypertension also indicates an increased risk for development of glaucoma.

Patients with ocular hypertension are considered glaucoma suspects and should undergo regular monitoring (once or twice a year) of intraocular pressures, optic disks, and visual fields. It is likely that many ocular hypertensives who do not develop glaucoma have relatively thick corneas, producing an overestimation of intraocular pressure. Measurement of central corneal thickness may therefore be useful to determine which patients are at risk of developing glaucoma. Conversely, many individuals with ocular hypertension may have glaucoma, but the retinal ganglion cell damage is not detectable with currently available techniques. Developments in perimetry and retinal nerve fiber layer imaging are addressing this issue.

PRIMARY ANGLE-CLOSURE GLAUCOMA

Primary angle closure occurs in anatomically predisposed eyes without other pathology. Elevation of intraocular pressure is a consequence of obstruction of aqueous outflow by occlusion of the trabecular meshwork by the peripheral iris. The condition may manifest as an ophthalmic emergency or may remain asymptomatic until visual loss occurs. The diagnosis is made by examination of the anterior segment and careful gonioscopy. Primary angle-closure glaucoma is the term that should be used only when primary angle closure has resulted in optic nerve damage and visual field loss. Risk factors include increasing age, female gender, family history of glaucoma, and Southeast Asian, Chinese, or Inuit ethnic background.

1. ACUTE ANGLE CLOSURE

Acute angle closure ("acute glaucoma") occurs when sufficient iris bombé develops to cause occlusion of the anterior chamber angle by the peripheral iris. This blocks aqueous outflow, and the intraocular pressure rises rapidly, causing severe pain, redness, and blurring of vision. Angle closure develops in hyperopic eyes with preexisting anatomic narrowing of the anterior chamber angle, usually when it is exacerbated by enlargement of the crystalline lens associated with aging. The acute attack is often precipitated by pupillary dilation. This occurs spontaneously in the evenings, when the level of illumination is reduced. It may be due to medications with anticholinergic or sympathomimetic activity (eg, atropine for preoperative medication, antidepressants, nebulized bronchodilators, or nasal decongestants). It may occur rarely with pupillary dilation for ophthalmoscopy. If pupillary dilation is necessary in a patient with a shallow anterior chamber (detected by oblique illumination with a penlight [Figure 11–4]), it is best to rely on short-acting mydriatics and avoid constricting the pupil with pilocarpine. The patient should be advised to seek attention immediately in the event of ocular pain or redness or increasingly blurred vision.

Clinical Findings

Acute angle closure is characterized by sudden onset of visual loss accompanied by excruciating pain, halos, and nausea and vomiting. Patients are occasionally thought to have acute gastrointestinal disease. Other findings include markedly increased intraocular pressure, a shallow anterior chamber, a steamy cornea, a fixed, moderately dilated pupil, and ciliary injection. It is important to perform gonioscopy on the fellow eye to confirm the anatomic predisposition to primary acute angle closure.

Differential Diagnosis (see Inside Front Cover)

Acute iritis causes more photophobia than acute glaucoma. Intraocular pressure is usually not raised; the pupil is constricted or irregular in shape and the cornea is usually not edematous. Marked flare and cells are present in the anterior chamber, and there is deep ciliary injection.

Acute conjunctivitis is usually bilateral, and there is little or no pain and no visual loss. There is discharge from the eye and an intensely inflamed conjunctiva but no ciliary injection. The pupillary responses and intraocular pressure are normal, and the cornea is clear.

Complications & Sequelae

If treatment is delayed, the peripheral iris may adhere to the trabecular meshwork (anterior synechiae), producing irreversible occlusion of the anterior chamber angle requiring surgery. Optic nerve damage is common.

Treatment

Acute angle closure is an ophthalmic emergency!

Treatment is initially directed at reducing the intraocular pressure. Intravenous and oral acetazolamide—along with topical agents, such as beta-blockers and apraclonidine, and, if necessary, hyperosmotic agents—will usually reduce the intraocular pressure. Pilocarpine 2% should be instilled one-half hour after commencement of treatment, by which time reduction of iris ischemia and lowering of intraocular pressure allow the sphincter pupillae to respond to the drug.

Topical steroids may also be used to reduce secondary intraocular inflammation. Once the intraocular pressure is under control, laser peripheral iridotomy should be undertaken to form a permanent connection between the anterior and posterior chambers, thus preventing recurrence of iris bombé. This is most often done with the neodymium:YAG laser (see above). Surgical peripheral iridectomy is the conventional treatment if laser treatment is unsuccessful. The fellow eye should always undergo prophylactic laser iridotomy.

2. SUBACUTE ANGLE CLOSURE

The same etiologic factors operate in subacute as in acute angle closure except that episodes of raised intraocular pressure are of short duration and are recurrent. The episodes of angle closure resolve spontaneously, but there is accumulated damage to the anterior chamber angle, with formation of peripheral anterior synechiae. Subacute angle closure will occasionally progress to acute closure.

There are recurrent short episodes of unilateral pain, redness, and blurring of vision associated with halos around lights. Attacks often occur in the evenings and resolve overnight. Examination between attacks may show only a narrow anterior chamber angle with peripheral anterior synechiae. The diagnosis can be confirmed by gonioscopy. Treatment consists of laser peripheral iridotomy.

3. CHRONIC ANGLE-CLOSURE GLAUCOMA

Patients with the anatomic predisposition to anterior-chamber angle closure may never develop episodes of acute rise in intraocular pressure but form increasingly extensive peripheral anterior synechiae accompanied by a gradual rise in intraocular pressure. These patients present in the same way as those with primary open-angle glaucoma, often with extensive visual field loss in both eyes. Occasionally, they have attacks of subacute angle closure.

On examination, there is raised intraocular pressure, narrow anterior chamber angles with variable amounts of peripheral anterior synechiae, and optic disk and visual field changes.

Laser peripheral iridotomy should always be undertaken as the first step in the management of these patients. Intraocular pressure is then controlled medically if possible, but the extent of peripheral anterior synechia formation and sluggish outflow through the remaining trabecular meshwork make pressure control very difficult, so that drainage surgery is often required. Cataract extraction with intraocular lens implantation can be effective in controlling the intraocular pressure, provided no more than two quadrants of synechial angle closure are present. Strong miotics must not be used unless peripheral iridotomy or iridectomy has been performed because they will accentuate angle closure.

4. PLATEAU IRIS

Plateau iris is an uncommon condition in which the central anterior chamber depth is normal but the anterior chamber angle is very narrow because of an anterior position of the ciliary processes. Such an eye has little pupillary block, but dilation will cause bunching up of the peripheral iris, occluding the angle (angle crowding), even if peripheral iridotomy or iridectomy has been performed. Affected individuals present with acute angle closure at a young age, with recurrences after peripheral laser iridotomy or surgical iridectomy. Long-term miotic therapy or laser iridoplasty is required.

5. CONGENITAL GLAUCOMA

Congenital glaucoma is rare. It can be subdivided into (1) primary congenital glaucoma, in which the developmental abnormalities are restricted to the anterior chamber angle; (2) the anterior segment developmental anomalies—Axenfeld-Rieger syndrome and Peters anomaly, in which iris and corneal development are also abnormal; and (3) a variety of other conditions—including aniridia, Sturge-Weber syndrome, neurofibromatosis-1, Lowe (oculo-cerebro-renal) syndrome, and congenital rubella—in which the developmental anomalies of the angle are associated with other ocular or extraocular abnormalities.

▶ Clinical Findings

Congenital glaucoma is manifest at birth in 50%, diagnosed in the first 6 months in 70%, and diagnosed by the end of the first year in 80% of cases. The earliest and most common symptom is epiphora. Photophobia and decreased corneal luster may be present. Increased intraocular pressure is the cardinal sign. Glaucomatous cupping of the optic disk is a relatively early—and the most important—change. Later findings include enlargement of the globe (buphthalmos) (Figure 11–8) with increased corneal diameter (above 11.5 mm is considered significant), corneal epithelial edema,

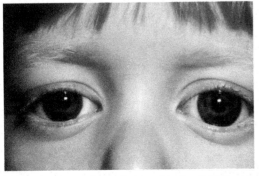

▲ Figure 11–8. Congenital glaucoma (buphthalmos).

tears of Descemet's membrane, and increased depth of the anterior chamber (associated with general enlargement of the anterior segment of the eye), as well as edema and opacity of the corneal stroma.

▶ Course & Prognosis

In untreated cases, blindness occurs early. The eye undergoes marked stretching and may even rupture with minor trauma. Typical glaucomatous cupping occurs relatively soon, emphasizing the need for early treatment. Treatment is always surgical, and either a goniotomy or trabeculectomy can be undertaken.

▼ SECONDARY GLAUCOMA

Increased intraocular pressure occurring as one manifestation of some other eye disease is called secondary glaucoma. These diseases are difficult to classify satisfactorily. Treatment involves controlling intraocular pressure by medical and surgical means but also dealing with the underlying disease if possible.

PIGMENTARY GLAUCOMA

Pigment dispersion syndrome is characterized by abnormal deposition of pigment in the anterior chamber—notably in the trabecular meshwork that presumably impedes outflow of aqueous and on the posterior corneal surface (Krukenberg's spindle)—and iris transillumination defects. Ultrasound studies show a posterior bowing of the iris with contact between the iris and zonules or ciliary processes, suggesting that pigment granules are rubbed off from the back surface of the iris as a result of friction, resulting in the iris transillumination defects. The syndrome occurs most often in myopic males between the ages of 25 and 40 who have a deep anterior chamber with a wide anterior chamber angle.

The pigmentary changes may be present without glaucoma, but such persons must be considered "glaucoma suspects." Up to 10% develop glaucoma within 5 years of presentation and 15% within 15 years.

Both miotic therapy and laser peripheral iridotomy have been shown to reverse the abnormal iris configuration. Laser peripheral iridotomy tends to reduce the intraocular pressure in pigment dispersion syndrome but does not seem to prevent glaucoma. Because the patients are usually young myopes, miotic therapy is poorly tolerated unless administered as pilocarpine once daily, preferably at bedtime.

Both pigment dispersion syndrome and pigmentary glaucoma are notable for a propensity to episodes of markedly raised intraocular pressure—characteristically after exercise or pupillary dilation—and pigmentary glaucoma may progress rapidly. An additional problem is the young age at which pigmentary glaucoma usually develops, increasing the chance that glaucoma drainage surgery will be necessary and that antimetabolite therapy will be required. Laser trabeculoplasty is frequently used in this condition but is unlikely to obviate the need for drainage surgery.

PSEUDOEXFOLIATION GLAUCOMA

In **pseudoexfoliation syndrome,** fine white deposits of a fibrillary material are seen on the anterior lens surface (in contrast to the true exfoliation of the lens capsule caused by exposure to infrared radiation, ie, "glassblower's cataract"), ciliary processes, zonule, posterior iris surface, loose in the anterior chamber, and in the trabecular meshwork (along with increased pigmentation). These deposits can also be detected histologically in the conjunctiva, suggesting a more widespread abnormality. The disease usually occurs in patients over age 65 and is reported to be particularly common in Scandinavia, although this may reflect ascertainment bias. The cumulative risk of developing glaucoma is 5% at 5 years and 15% at 10 years. Two polymorphisms in the coding region of the gene lysyl oxidase-like gene (*LOXL1*, located on chromosome 15q24.1) are associated with pseudoexfoliation glaucoma. Treatment is as for primary open-angle glaucoma. Eyes with pseudoexfoliation syndrome have a greater incidence of complications during cataract surgery.

GLAUCOMA SECONDARY TO CHANGES IN THE LENS

▶ Lens Dislocation

The crystalline lens may be dislocated as a result of trauma or spontaneously, as in Marfan's syndrome. Anterior dislocation may cause obstruction of the pupillary aperture, leading to iris bombé and angle closure. Posterior dislocation into the vitreous is also associated with glaucoma, although the mechanism is obscure. It may be due to angle damage at the time of traumatic dislocation.

In anterior dislocation, the definitive treatment is lens extraction once the intraocular pressure has been controlled medically. In posterior dislocation, the lens is usually left alone and the glaucoma treated as primary open-angle glaucoma.

▶ Intumescence of the Lens

In this rare condition, the lens may take up fluid during cataractous change, increasing markedly in size. It may then encroach upon the anterior chamber, producing both pupillary block and angle crowding and resulting in acute angle closure. Treatment consists of lens extraction once the intraocular pressure has been controlled medically.

▶ Phacolytic Glaucoma

Some advanced cataracts may develop leakiness of the anterior lens capsule, which allows passage of liquefied lens proteins into the anterior chamber. There is an inflammatory reaction in the anterior chamber, and the trabecular meshwork becomes edematous and obstructed with lens proteins, leading to an acute rise in intraocular pressure. Lens extraction is the definitive treatment once the intraocular pressure has been controlled medically and intensive topical steroid therapy has reduced the intraocular inflammation.

GLAUCOMA SECONDARY TO CHANGES IN THE UVEAL TRACT

▶ Uveitis

The intraocular pressure is usually below normal in uveitis because the inflamed ciliary body is functioning poorly. However, elevation of intraocular pressure may also occur through a number of different mechanisms. The trabecular meshwork may become blocked by inflammatory cells from the anterior chamber, with secondary edema, or may occasionally be involved in an inflammatory process specifically directed at the trabecular cells (trabeculitis). One of the most common causes of raised intraocular pressure in individuals with uveitis is the use of topical steroids. Chronic or recurrent uveitis produces permanent impairment of trabecular function, peripheral anterior synechiae, and occasionally angle neovascularization, all of which increase the chance of secondary glaucoma. Seclusio pupillae due to 360° posterior synechiae produces iris bombé and acute angle-closure glaucoma. The uveitis syndromes that tend to be associated with secondary glaucoma are Fuchs' heterochromic cyclists', HLA-B27–associated acute anterior uveitis, and uveitis due to herpes zoster and herpes simplex.

Treatment is directed chiefly at controlling the uveitis with concomitant medical glaucoma therapy as necessary, avoiding miotics because of the increased chance of posterior synechia formation. Long-term therapy, including surgery, is often required because of irreversible damage to the trabecular meshwork.

Acute angle closure due to seclusion of the pupil may be reversed by intensive mydriasis but often requires laser peripheral iridotomy or surgical iridectomy. Any uveitis with a tendency to posterior synechia formation must be treated with mydriatics whenever the uveitis is active to reduce the risk of pupillary seclusion.

▶ Tumor

Uveal tract melanomas may cause glaucoma by anterior displacement of the ciliary body, causing secondary angle closure, direct involvement of the anterior chamber angle, blockage of the filtration angle by pigment dispersion, and angle neovascularization. Enucleation is usually necessary.

▶ Ciliary Body Swelling

Forward rotation of the ciliary body, resulting in anterior displacement of the lens-iris diaphragm and secondary angle-closure glaucoma, may also occur after vitreoretinal surgery or retinal cryotherapy, in posterior uveitis, and with topiramate therapy.

IRIDOCORNEAL ENDOTHELIAL (ICE) SYNDROME (ESSENTIAL IRIS ATROPHY, CHANDLER SYNDROME, IRIS NEVUS SYNDROME)

This rare idiopathic condition of young adults is usually unilateral and manifested by corneal decompensation, glaucoma, and iris abnormalities (corectopia and polycoria).

GLAUCOMA SECONDARY TO TRAUMA

Contusion injuries of the globe may be associated with an early rise in intraocular pressure due to bleeding into the anterior chamber (hyphema). Free blood blocks the trabecular meshwork, which is also rendered edematous by the injury. Treatment is initially medical, but surgery may be required if the pressure remains raised, which is particularly likely if there is a second episode of bleeding.

Late effects of contusion injuries on intraocular pressure are due to direct angle damage. The interval between the injury and the development of glaucoma may obscure the association. Clinically, the anterior chamber is seen to be deeper than in the fellow eye, and gonioscopy shows recession of the angle. Medical therapy is usually effective, but drainage surgery may be required.

Laceration or contusional rupture of the anterior segment is associated with loss of the anterior chamber. If the chamber is not reformed soon after the injury—either spontaneously, by iris incarceration into the wound, or surgically—peripheral anterior synechiae will form and result in irreversible angle closure.

GLAUCOMA FOLLOWING OCULAR SURGERY

▶ Ciliary Block Glaucoma (Malignant Glaucoma)

Surgery upon an eye with markedly increased intraocular pressure and a closed or narrow angle can lead to ciliary block glaucoma. Postoperatively, the intraocular pressure is higher than expected and the lens is pushed forward as a result of the collection of aqueous in and behind the vitreous body. Patients initially become aware of blurred distance vision but improved near vision. This is followed by pain and inflammation.

Treatment consists of cycloplegics, mydriatics, aqueous suppressants, and hyperosmotic agents. Hyperosmotic agents are used to shrink the vitreous body and let the lens move backward.

Posterior sclerotomy, vitrectomy, and even lens extraction may be needed.

▶ Peripheral Anterior Synechiae

Just as with trauma to the anterior segment (see above), surgery that results in a flat anterior chamber will lead to formation of peripheral anterior synechiae. Early surgical reformation of the chamber is required if it does not occur spontaneously.

NEOVASCULAR GLAUCOMA

Neovascularization of the iris (rubeosis iridis) and anterior chamber angle is most often secondary to widespread retinal ischemia such as in advanced diabetic retinopathy and ischemic central retinal vein occlusion. Glaucoma results initially from obstruction of the angle by the fibrovascular membrane, but subsequent contraction of the membrane leads to angle closure.

Treatment of established neovascular glaucoma is difficult and often unsatisfactory. Both the stimulus to neovascularization and the raised intraocular pressure need to be treated. Intravitreal injection of bevacizumab (a monoclonal antibody that inhibits vascular endothelial growth factor) can reverse the iris neovascularization, but in advanced disease, this usually has no effect on intraocular pressure in patients with advanced disease. Topical atropine 1% and intensive topical steroids should be given to reduce inflammation and improve comfort. In many cases, vision is lost and cyclodestructive procedures are necessary to control the intraocular pressure.

GLAUCOMA SECONDARY TO RAISED EPISCLERAL VENOUS PRESSURE

Raised episcleral venous pressure may contribute to glaucoma in Sturge-Weber syndrome, in which a developmental anomaly of the angle is also often present, and carotid-cavernous fistula, which may also cause angle neovascularization due to widespread ocular ischemia. Medical treatment cannot reduce the intraocular pressure below the level of the abnormally raised episcleral venous pressure, and surgery is associated with a high risk of complications.

STEROID-INDUCED GLAUCOMA

Topical, periocular, and intraocular corticosteroids may produce a type of glaucoma that simulates primary open-angle glaucoma, particularly in individuals with a family history of the disease, and will exaggerate the intraocular pressure elevation in those with established primary open-angle glaucoma. Withdrawal of the medication usually eliminates these effects, but permanent damage can occur if the situation goes unrecognized. If topical steroid therapy is absolutely necessary, medical glaucoma therapy will usually control the intraocular pressure. Systemic steroid therapy is less likely to cause a rise in intraocular pressure. It is imperative that patients receiving topical or systemic steroid therapy undergo periodic tonometry and ophthalmoscopy, particularly if there is a family history of glaucoma.

REFERENCES

Baril C et al: Rates of glaucomatous visual field change after trabeculectomy. Br J Ophthalmol 2016 Nov 3. [Epub ahead of print] [PMID: 27811280]

Bengtsson B et al: Lack of visual field improvement after initiation of intraocular pressure reducing treatment in the Early Manifest Glaucoma Trial. Invest Ophthalmol Vis Sci 2016;57:5611. [PMID: 27768797]

Bourne RR et al: Number of people blind or visually impaired by glaucoma worldwide and in world regions 1990-2010: a meta-analysis. PLoS One 2016;11:e0162229. [PMID: 27764086]

Budenz DL: A clinician's guide to the assessment and management of nonadherence in glaucoma. Ophthalmology 2009;116:S43. [PMID: 19837260]

Budenz DL: Thirteen-year follow-up of optic disc hemorrhages in the Ocular Hypertension Treatment Study. Am J Ophthalmol 2017;174:126. [PMID: 27832941]

Busbee BG: Update on treatment strategies for bleb-associated endophthalmitis. Curr Opin Ophthalmol 2005;16:170. [PMID: 15870574]

Chauhan BC et al: Practical recommendations for measuring rates of visual field change in glaucoma. Br J Ophthalmol 2008;92:569. [PMID: 18211935]

Chauhan BC et al: Canadian Glaucoma Study 2. Risk factors for the progression of open-angle glaucoma. Arch Ophthalmol 2008;126:1030. [PMID: 18695095]

Collaborative Normal-Tension Glaucoma Study Group: Comparison of glaucomatous progression between untreated patients with normal-tension glaucoma and patients with therapeutically reduced intraocular pressures. Am J Ophthalmol 1998;126:487. [PMID: 9780093]

Collaborative Normal-Tension Glaucoma Study Group: The effectiveness of intraocular pressure reduction in the treatment of normal-tension glaucoma. Am J Ophthalmol 1998;126:498. [PMID: 9780094]

Doucette LP et al: The interaction of genes, age and environment in glaucoma pathogenesis. Surv Ophthalmol 2015;60:310. [PMID: 25907525]

Foster PJ et al: The definition and classification of glaucoma in prevalence surveys. Br J Ophthalmol 2002;86:238. [PMID: 11815354]

Friedman DS et al: Surgical strategies for coexisting glaucoma and cataract: an evidence-based update. Ophthalmology 2002;190:1902. [PMID: 12359612]

Garway-Heath DF et al: Latanoprost for open-angle glaucoma (UKGTS): a randomised, multicentre, placebo-controlled trial. Lancet 2015;385:1295. [PMID: 25533656]

Gedde SJ et al: Treatment outcomes in the tube versus trabeculectomy (TVT) study after five years of follow-up. Am J Ophthalmol 2012;153:789. [PMID: 22245458]

Heijl A et al: Reduction of intraocular pressure and glaucoma progression: results from the Early Manifest Glaucoma Trial. Arch Ophthalmol 2002;120:1268. [PMID: 12365904]

Heijl A et al: Natural history of open-angle glaucoma. Ophthalmology 2009;116:2271. [PMID: 19854514]

Herndon LW: Central corneal thickness as a risk factor for advanced glaucoma damage. Arch Ophthalmol 2004;122:17. [PMID: 14718289]

Hitchings RA: Glaucoma: an area of darkness. Eye 2009;23:1764. [PMID: 18791552]

Hong CH et al: Glaucoma draining devices: a systemic literature review and current controversies. Surv Ophthalmol 2005;50:48. [PMID: 15621077]

Horsley MB: Anti-VEGF therapy for glaucoma. Curr Opin Ophthalmol 2010;21:112. [PMID: 20040875]

Jampel HD et al: Perioperative complications of trabeculectomy in the Collaborative Initial Glaucoma Treatment Study (CIGTS). Am J Ophthalmol 2005;140:16. [PMID: 15939389]

Johnson DH: Progress in glaucoma: early detection, new treatments, less blindness. Ophthalmology 2003;110:634. [PMID: 12799273]

Jonas JB et al: Facts and myths of cerebrospinal fluid pressure for the physiology of the eye. Prog Retin Eye Research 2015;46:67. [PMID: 25619727]

Kass MA et al: The Ocular Hypertension Treatment Study: a randomized trial determines that topical ocular hypotensive medication delays or prevents the onset of primary open angle glaucoma. Arch Ophthalmol 2002;120:701. [PMID: 12049574]

Kass MA et al: Delaying treatment for ocular hypertension: the ocular hypertension treatment study. Arch Ophthalmol 2010;128:276. [PMID: 20212196]

Kersey JP et al: Corticosteroid-induced glaucoma: a review of the literature. Eye 2006;20:407. [PMID: 15877093]

Kim KE et al: Optic disc hemorrhage in glaucoma: pathophysiology and prognostic significance. Curr Opin Ophthalmol 2017;28:105. [PMID: 27820751]

Konstas AGP et al: Factors associated with long-term progression or stability in exfoliation glaucoma. Arch Ophthalmol 2004;122:29. [PMID: 14718291]

Kotecha A et al: Intravitreal bevacizumab in refractory neovascular glaucoma: a prospective observational case series. Arch Ophthalmol 2011;129:145. [PMID: 21320957]

Lama PJ et al: Antifibrotics and wound healing in glaucoma surgery. Surv Ophthalmol 2003;48:314. [PMID: 12745005]

Leske MC et al: Predictors of long-term progression in the Early Manifest Glaucoma Trial. Ophthalmology 2007;114:1965. [PMID: 17628686]

Medeiros FA et al: Combining structural and functional measurements to improve estimates of rates of glaucomatous progression. Am J Ophthalmol 2012;153:1197. [PMID: 22317914]

Medeiros FA et al: The relationship between intraocular pressure and progressive retinal nerve fibre layer loss in glaucoma. Ophthalmology 2009;116:1125. [PMID: 19376584]

Moghimi S et al: Qualitative evaluation of anterior segment in angle closure disease using anterior segment optical coherence tomography. J Curr Ophthalmol 2016;28:170. [PMID: 27830199]

Monsalve B et al: Diagnostic ability of Humphrey perimetry, octopus perimetry, and optical coherence tomography for glaucomatous optic neuropathy. Eye (Lond) 2016 Nov 11. [Epub ahead of print] [PMID: 27834960]

Morgan WH: Surgical management of glaucoma: a review. Clin Exp Ophthalmol 2012;40:388. [PMID: 22339885]

Musch DC et al: Visual field progression in the Collaborative Initial Glaucoma Treatment Study: the impact of treatment and other baseline factors. Ophthalmology 2009;116:200. [PMID: 19019444]

Musch DC et al: Intraocular pressure control and long-term visual field loss in the Collaborative Initial Glaucoma Treatment Study. Ophthalmology 2011;118:1766. [PMID: 21600658]

Niyadurupola N et al: Pigment dispersion syndrome and pigmentary glaucoma: a major review. Clin Exp Ophthalmol 2009;36:868. [PMID: 19278484]

Nouri-Mahdavi K et al: Predictive factors for glaucomatous visual field progression in the Advanced Glaucoma Intervention Study. Ophthalmology 2004;111:1627. [PMID: 15350314]

Olthoff CM et al: Noncompliance with ocular hypertensive treatment in patients with glaucoma or ocular hypertension: an evidence based review. Ophthalmology 2005;112:953. [PMID: 15885795]

Papadopoulos M et al: Advances in the management of paediatric glaucoma. Eye 2007;21:1319. [PMID: 17914435]

Parrish RK et al: A comparison of latanoprost, bimatoprost, and travoprost in patients with elevated intraocular pressure. A 12-week, randomized, masked-evaluator multicentre study. Am J Ophthalmol 2003;135:688. [PMID: 12719078]

Peters D et al: Lifetime risk of blindness in open angle glaucoma. Am J Ophthalmol 2013;156:724. [PMID: 23932216]

Quigley HA: New paradigms in the mechanisms and management of glaucoma. Eye 2005;19:1241. [PMID: 15543179]

Racette L et al: Primary open-angle glaucoma in blacks: a review. Surv Ophthalmol 2003;48:295. [PMID: 16286617]

Siddiqui Y et al: What is the risk of developing pigmentary glaucoma from pigment dispersion syndrome? Am J Ophthalmol 2003;135:794. [PMID: 12788118]

Sihota R: Classification of primary angle closure disease. Curr Opin Ophthalmol 2011;22:87. [PMID: 21150038]

Sivak-Callcott JA et al: Evidence-based recommendations for the diagnosis and treatment of neovascular glaucoma. Ophthalmology 2001;108:1767. [PMID: 11581047]

Tham CC et al: Phacoemulsification versus trabeculectomy in medically uncontrolled chronic angle-closure glaucoma without cataract. Ophthalmology 2013;120:62. [PMID: 229866111]

Thorleifsson G et al: Common sequence variants in the LOXL1 gene confer susceptibility to exfoliation glaucoma. Science 2007;317:1397. [PMID: 17690259]

van der Valk R et al: Intraocular pressure-lowering effects of all commonly used glaucoma drugs: a meta-analysis of randomized clinical trials. Ophthalmology 2005;112:1177. [PMID: 15921747]

Weinreb RN et al: Primary open-angle glaucoma. Lancet 2004;363:1711. [PMID: 15158634]

Weinreb RN et al: Risk assessment in the management of patients with ocular hypertension. Am J Ophthalmol 2004;138:458. [PMID: 15364230]

Wilkins M et al: Intra-operative mitomycin C for glaucoma surgery. Cochrane Database Syst Rev 2001;1:CD002897. [PMID: 11279773]

Wong MO et al: Systematic review and meta-analysis on the efficacy of selective laser trabeculoplasty in open-angle glaucoma. Surv Ophthalmol 2015;60:36. [PMID: 25113610]

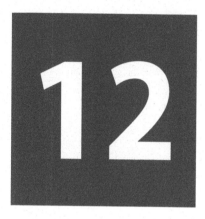

Strabismus

W. Walker Motley, MS, MD

Under normal binocular viewing conditions, the image of the object of regard falls simultaneously on the fovea of each eye (bifoveal fixation), and the vertical retinal meridians are both upright. Strabismus is any ocular misalignment in which only one eye fixates with the fovea on the object of regard. (In everyday language, squint means partial closure of the eye to see more clearly, but sometimes it is used to mean strabismus.) Misalignment of the eyes may be in any direction—inward (eso-), outward (exo-), up (hyper-), down (hypo-), or torsional. The amount of deviation is the angle by which the deviating eye is misaligned. **Tropia (manifest strabismus, heterotropia**; Box 12–1) is strabismus present under binocular viewing conditions. **Phoria (latent strabismus, heterophoria)** is a deviation present only after binocular vision has been interrupted by occlusion of one eye.

Strabismus is present in about 4% of children, and treatment should be started as soon as it is identified to ensure the best possible visual acuity and binocular visual function. Strabismus may also be acquired due to cranial nerve palsies brainstem disease or orbital disease including masses, fractures, and thyroid eye disease.

PHYSIOLOGY

1. MOTOR ASPECTS

▶ Individual Muscle Functions

All six (four rectus and two oblique) extraocular muscles contribute to positioning the globe on its three axes of rotation (Table 12–1). Each muscle has principal (primary) and lesser (secondary and tertiary) actions, and these are determined by its site of attachment to the globe, its site of origin, the orbital connective tissues that regulate its direction of action by acting as its functional mechanical origin (active pulley hypothesis), and the varying orientation of the globe in the orbit.

Even when stationary, the position of the eye is determined by the overall effect of the combined activity of all six extraocular muscles. The **primary position of gaze** is when the eyes are looking straight ahead with the head and body erect. To move the eye into another direction of gaze, the activity of the agonist muscles for the required movement increases and the activity of the antagonist muscles decreases. The **field of action** of a muscle is the direction of rotation of the globe when it contracts (agonist effect). The medial and lateral rectus muscles adduct and abduct the eye, respectively, with little effect on elevation or torsion. The vertical rectus and oblique muscles have both vertical and torsional functions. In general terms, the vertical rectus muscles are the main elevators and depressors of the eyes, and the obliques are mostly involved with torsional positioning. The vertical effects of the superior and inferior rectus muscles are greater when the eye is abducted. The vertical effects of the obliques are greater when the eye is adducted. **Motor fusion** is the process by which activity of the extraocular muscles is adjusted to maintain the ocular alignment necessary for binocular vision.

▶ Synergistic & Antagonistic Muscles (Sherrington's Law)

At any one time, synergistic muscles are those that have the same field of action. Muscles synergistic for one movement of the globe may be antagonistic for another. For vertical gaze, the superior rectus and inferior oblique muscles are synergists as both rotate the globe upward. For torsion, they are antagonists as they intort and extort the globe, respectively. The extraocular muscles, like skeletal muscles, show reciprocal innervation of antagonistic muscles (Sherrington's law). On right gaze, the right lateral and left medial rectus muscles are stimulated, while the right medial and left lateral rectus muscles are inhibited.

BOX 12–1. DEFINITIONS

Angle kappa: Angle between the visual axis and the central pupillary line. When the eye is fixing a light, if the corneal reflection is centered on the pupil, the visual axis and the central pupillary line coincide and the angle kappa is zero. Ordinarily the light reflex is 2–4° nasal to the pupillary center, giving the appearance of slight exotropia (positive angle kappa). A negative angle kappa gives the false impression of esotropia.

Conjugate movement: Movement of the eyes in the same direction at the same time.

Deviation: Magnitude of ocular misalignment usually measured in prism diopters (see later in the chapter) but sometimes measured in degrees.

> Comitant deviation: Deviation not significantly affected by which eye is fixing or direction of gaze, typically a feature of childhood (nonparetic) strabismus.
>
> Incomitant deviation: Deviation varies according to which eye is fixing and direction of gaze, usually a feature of recent-onset extraocular muscle paresis and other types of acquired strabismus.
>
> Primary deviation: Incomitant deviation measured with the normal eye fixing (see Figure 12–2).
>
> Secondary deviation: Incomitant deviation measured with the affected eye fixing.

Ductions: Rotations of one eye with no consideration of the position of the other eye (see Figure 12–3).

Fusion: Formation of one image from the two images seen simultaneously by the two eyes.

> Motor fusion: Adjustments made by the brain to activity of extraocular muscles in order to bring both eyes into bifoveal and torsional alignment.
>
> Sensory fusion: Integration in the visual sensory areas of the brain of information from the two eyes into one image.

Phoria: Ocular misalignment when binocular viewing is interrupted.

Orthophoria: Absence of any tendency of either eye to deviate when binocular viewing is interrupted.

Prism diopter (PD): Unit of angular measurement used to characterize ocular deviations.

Torsion: Physiologic rotation of the eye about its visual axis (see Figure 12–3).

Tropia (manifest strabismus, heterotropia): Abnormal ocular alignment during binocular viewing.

> Esotropia: Convergent manifest deviation ("crossed eyes").
>
> Exotropia: Divergent manifest deviation ("wall eyes").
>
> Hypertropia: Manifest deviation of one eye upward.
>
> Hypotropia: Manifest deviation of one eye upward. By convention, in the absence of specific causation to account for the lower position of one eye, vertical deviations are designated by the higher eye (eg, right hypertropia, not left hypotropia)
>
> Incyclotropia: Manifest rotation of the 12 o'clock meridian of one eye about its visual axis toward the midline of the head.
>
> Excyclotropia: Manifest rotation of the 12 o'clock meridian of one eye about its visual axis away from the midline of the head.

Vergences (disjunctive movements): Normal movement of the two eyes in opposite directions (ie, convergence, divergence).

Versions: Rotations of both eyes in qualitatively the same direction (eg, rightward, leftward, upward).

Table 12–1. Actions of the Extraocular Muscles

Muscle	Primary Action	Secondary Action	Tertiary Action
Lateral rectus	Abduction	None	None
Medial rectus	Adduction	None	None
Superior rectus	Elevation	Intorsion	Adduction
Inferior rectus	Depression	Extorsion	Adduction
Superior oblique	Intorsion	Depression	Abduction
Inferior oblique	Extorsion	Elevation	Abduction

Table 12–2. Yoke Muscle Pairs in Main Directions of Gaze

Right	Right LR, Left MR
Left	Left LR, Right MR
Up and right	Right SR, Left IO
Up and left	Left SR, Right IO
Down and right	Right IR, Left SO
Down and left	Left IR, Right SO

Abbreviations: IO, inferior oblique; IR, inferior rectus; LR, lateral rectus; MR, medial rectus; SO, superior oblique; SR, superior rectus.

Yoke Muscles (Hering's Law)

For movements of both eyes in the same direction, the corresponding agonist muscles receive equal innervation (Hering's law). The pair of agonist muscles that rotate the two eyes in the same direction is called a yoke pair (Table 12–2).

Development of Binocular Movement

The oculomotor system of an infant is immature, and therefore, horizontal ocular deviations are common during the first few months of life. Transient exotropia is the most common. Gradually improving visual acuity and maturating of the ocular motor system typically produces normal ocular alignment by age 2 to 3 months. Ocular misalignment after this age should be investigated by an ophthalmologist.

2. SENSORY ASPECTS

Binocular Vision, Sensory Fusion, & Stereopsis

Binocular vision occurs when the visual information from two eyes viewing the same object is combined into a single image. **Corresponding retinal points** are the retinal locations (one in each eye) where the images of a single object fall. Since the two eyes are not in precisely the same location in space, the images on these retinal points are not exactly the same. **Sensory fusion** is the process whereby disparities between the two images at corresponding retinal points are overcome to allow a single image to be perceived. In reality, there is not absolute correspondence between the retinal points that can be stimulated to produce a single image. Normally, one is capable of fusing a retinal stimulus that strikes sufficiently close to the corresponding retinal point in the other eye. The representation in space of this region of fusible points is called **Panum's area.** It is narrowest at fixation and progressively increases in size with increasing eccentricity in the visual field. Images in the two eyes must be sufficiently similar in size for sensory fusion to occur.

In contradistinction to sensory fusion, **stereopsis** relies upon recognition of the disparities of images that are being fused. It is quantified as the smallest detectable disparity, around 60 seconds of arc being high-grade (fine) stereopsis that is only possible with bifoveal fixation. Although stereopsis is essential for high-grade depth perception, monocular clues such as apparent size of objects, interposition of objects, and motion parallax can also be used to judge depth.

Sensory Phenomena in Strabismus

Strabismus is associated with various abnormal sensory phenomena, including diplopia (double vision), visual confusion, abnormal (anomalous) retinal correspondence, suppression, amblyopia, and eccentric fixation. The occurrence of these phenomena is related to whether the strabismus is present during the development of the visual system, which occurs up to age 7 or 8.

A. Diplopia and Visual Confusion

In the presence of strabismus, each fovea receives a different image. **Diplopia** occurs when the image of the object of regard falls on the fovea of the fixing eye and the object is localized straight ahead, whereas the same image falls on an extrafoveal retinal area in the deviating eye and the object is localized in some other direction, so that the object of regard is perceived to be in two places. **Visual confusion** occurs when the object responsible for the image falling on the fovea of the deviating eye is localized as straight ahead, creating the perception that it and the object of regard (fixated by the fellow eye) are in the same location and therefore appear superimposed. Diplopia is commonly reported in acquired strabismus but not visual confusion.

B. Abnormal Retinal Correspondence

In the presence of manifest strabismus, an extrafoveal retinal point may become the preferred point of fixation in the deviating eye, resulting in **anomalous retinal correspondence (ARC).** There may be exact correlation between the position of this locus and the angle of strabismus (harmonious ARC) or not (unharmonious ARC). ARC is present only under binocular viewing conditions, and therefore if the nondeviating eye is occluded, the deviating eye will shift to foveal fixation. ARC avoids diplopia and visual confusion because the extrafoveal retinal point of fixation in the deviating eye is localized straight ahead during binocular viewing. ARC facilitates low-grade binocular vision.

C. Suppression

Suppression is a common sensory adaptation in childhood strabismus in which there is diminished sensitivity within the visual field of the deviating eye under binocular viewing conditions in order to avoid diplopia and visual confusion.

This **suppression scotoma** is termed a facultative scotoma because it is not present when the suppressing eye is tested alone, contrasting with amblyopia (see below) that persists when the affected eye is tested alone.

In esotropia, the suppression scotoma is usually horizontally elliptical in shape, extending on the retina from just temporal to the fovea to the point in the nasal extrafoveal retina on which the image of the object of regard falls. In exotropia, the suppression scotoma tends to be larger, usually extending from the fovea to include the entire temporal half of the retina. If there is alternating fixation, the suppression scotoma is present in whichever eye is deviating. In the absence of strabismus, a blurred image in one eye may also lead to suppression.

D. Amblyopia

Amblyopia is reduced visual acuity in excess of that explicable by organic disease and is caused by prolonged abnormal visual experience in children under the age of 7. Three main causes of amblyopia are strabismus, **anisometropia** (unequal refractive error), and visual deprivation (eg, media opacity, ptosis).

In strabismus, the eye used habitually for fixation retains normal acuity, whereas acuity is persistently reduced in the deviating eye. In esotropia, amblyopia is common and often severe, whereas in exotropia, it is uncommon and usually mild. If spontaneous alternation of fixation is present, amblyopia does not develop.

E. Eccentric Fixation

In eyes with severe amblyopia, an extrafoveal retinal area may be used for fixation even under monocular viewing conditions, in contrast to ARC (see earlier in the chapter) when the phenomenon only occurs under binocular viewing conditions. Gross eccentric fixation can be readily identified by occluding the preferred eye and asking the patient to look directly at a light source with the nonpreferred eye. An eye with gross eccentric fixation will have an eccentric corneal light reflection. More subtle degrees of eccentric fixation can be detected using an ophthalmoscope that projects a target image onto the retina. The patient is instructed to look directly at the target center. While viewing the fundus, if the examiner observes the target center on an area other than the fovea, eccentric fixation is present.

CLINICAL EVALUATION OF STRABISMUS

1. HISTORY

A careful history is important in the diagnosis of strabismus.

- Laterality. Does the deviation only occur in one eye, or does it alternate?

- Direction. Is the deviation inward, outward, upward, or downward?
- Duration. When was the deviation first noticed? Was the onset gradual or sudden?
- Frequency. Is the deviation constant or intermittent? If intermittent, how often does it occur? Has the frequency increased, decreased, or remained the same since it was first noticed?
- Modifying factors. Is the deviation worse with fatigue, illness, or alcohol use?
- Associated symptoms. Is there diplopia, asthenopia (eyestrain), visual confusion, or headache?
- Past ocular history—including any history of spectacle wear, ocular trauma, or surgery.
- Past medical history—including any history of prematurity, developmental delay, neurological disorder, or thyroid disease.
- Family history—including any history of strabismus, "squint," "cast," amblyopia, "lazy eye," or other ocular disease in the family.

2. EXAMINATION (TABLE 12–3)

▶ Visual Acuity and Refractive Error

Visual acuity must be evaluated in all patients with strabismus (Table 12–3) using a developmentally appropriate acuity test. Refractive error is measured by retinoscopy typically following cycloplegia (see Chapter 17).

Table 12–3. Strabismus Examination

Examination Element	Examples
Visual acuity (developmentally appropriate test)	Snellen (Chapter 2), Lea, HOTV, forced preferential looking, induced tropia test, fixation preference, ability to fixate and follow, objection to occlusion (Chapter 17), presence of nystagmus
Refractive error	Cycloplegic retinoscopy (Chapter 17)
Ocular alignment	Cover test, uncover test, alternate cover test, prism and alternate cover test, Hirschberg method, Krimsky test
Motility	Ductions and versions, presence of nystagmus
Sensory exam	Stereogram test, Worth 4 dot test, red filter test
Anatomic structures (including pupil dilation)	Slitlamp examination and binocular indirect ophthalmoscopy (anterior and posterior segments), penlight (anterior segment) (Chapters 2 and 17)

▶ Inspection and Ocular Examination

Inspection alone may show whether strabismus is constant or intermittent, alternating or nonalternating, and whether it is variable. Associated ptosis and abnormal position of the head should be noted. The quality of fixation of each eye separately and of both eyes together should be assessed. Nystagmus indicates unstable fixation and usually reduced visual acuity. Prominent epicanthal folds that obscure all or part of the nasal sclera may give an appearance of esotropia (pseudostrabismus, see later in chapter).

Dilated eye examination is essential to ensure that strabismus or reduced vision is not due to structural abnormalities. In children, esotropia may be the presenting feature of various diseases, including retinoblastoma, optic nerve hypoplasia, and optic nerve glioma.

▶ Determination of Angle of Strabismus (Angle of Deviation)

A. Cover Testing (Figure 12–1)

All four components of cover testing, (1) the cover test, (2) the uncover test, (3) the alternate cover test, and (4) the prism and alternate cover test, require fixation of a target, which may be in any direction of gaze at distance or near.

1. The **cover test** identifies manifest strabismus. As the examiner observes one eye, a cover is placed in front of the fellow eye to block its view of the target. If the observed eye moves to take up fixation, it was not previously fixing the target, and a manifest strabismus is present. The direction of movement is in the opposite direction to the deviation (eg, if the observed eye moves outward to pick up fixation, then esotropia is present). The cover test is performed on each eye. Childhood strabismus is usually **comitant**, meaning that the magnitude of the manifest strabismus is not significantly influenced by which eye is fixing or the direction of gaze. Recently acquired cranial nerve palsies (paretic strabismus) and other types of acquired strabismus are usually **incomitant,** meaning that the magnitude of the manifest strabismus is less when the normal eye is fixing (**primary deviation**) than when the affected eye is fixing (**secondary deviation**) (Figure 12–2), and the magnitude increases in the field of action of the affected muscles.

2. The **uncover test** provides information on fixation preference if there is manifest strabismus, or identifies latent strabismus if there is no manifest strabismus. As the cover is removed from the eye following the cover test,

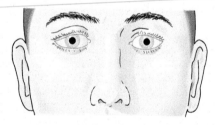

Eyes straight (maintained in position by fusion).

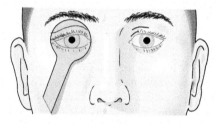

Position of eye under cover in orthophoria (fusion-free position). The right eye under cover has not moved.

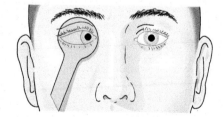

Position of eye under cover in esophoria (fusion-free position). Under cover, the right eye has deviated inward. Upon removal of cover, the right eye will immediately resume its straight-ahead position.

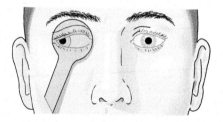

Position of eye under cover in exophoria (fusion-free position). Under cover, the right eye has deviated outward. Upon removal of the cover, the right eye will immediately resume its straight-ahead position.

▲ **Figure 12–1.** Cover testing. The patient is directed to look at a target at eye level 6 m (20 ft) away. Note: In the presence of strabismus, the deviation will remain when the cover is removed.

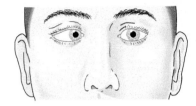 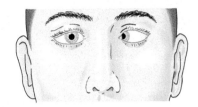

Primary deviation
(left eye fixing)

Secondary deviation (right eye fixing;
"overshoot" of sound left eye)

▲ **Figure 12–2.** Paresis of horizontal muscle (right lateral rectus). Secondary deviation is greater than primary deviation because of Hering's law. With the left eye fixing, the right eye is deviated inward because of the paretic right lateral rectus. For the right eye to fix, the paretic right lateral rectus muscle must receive excessive stimulation. The yoke muscle—the left medial rectus—also receives the same excessive stimulation (Hering's law), which causes "overshoot."

the eye emerging from under the cover is observed by the examiner. If the position of the eye changes, then either (1) a manifest strabismus is present and the eye is once again taking up fixation indicating that it is the preferred eye, or (2) interruption of binocular vision has allowed the eye to deviate and a latent strabismus is revealed. In either case, the direction of corrective movement indicates the type of manifest or latent strabismus, with the same pattern as in the cover test (eg, outward movement reveals esotropia or esophoria). In manifest strabismus, there will also be a movement of the fellow eye. In latent strabismus, there will be no movement of the fellow eye. If the uncover test results in no movement of the uncovered eye, then either (1) a manifest strabismus is present but the fellow eye has maintained fixation, indicating alternating fixation, or (2) orthophoria (absence of any manifest or latent strabismus) is present, but this is rarely seen clinically.

3. The **alternate cover (cross-cover) test** reveals the total deviation (manifest plus latent strabismus). The cover is placed alternately in front of one eye and then the other. It should be moved rapidly from one eye to the other to prevent re-fusion of a latent strabismus.

4. The **prism and alternate cover test** quantifies strabismus. Increasing strength of prism is placed in front of one eye oriented with apex toward the deviation until there is neutralization of the movement on alternate cover testing. For example, to measure the full extent of an esodeviation, the cover is alternated while prisms of increasing base-out strength are placed in front of one eye until there is no horizontal refixational movement. Larger deviations or deviations with horizontal and vertical components may require prisms held before both eyes. Prisms should not be "stacked" before one eye.

B. Other Tests of Alignment

Two other methods commonly used depend on observing the position of the corneal light reflection, but both are less

accurate than cover tests, and their results must be adjusted if the **angle kappa** is abnormal (see Box 12–1).

1. **Hirschberg method.** The patient fixes on a light at a distance of about 33 cm. Decentration of the light reflection is noted in the deviating eye. The angle of deviation may be estimated using a ratio of 18 PD for each millimeter of decentration.

2. **Krimsky test.** The patient fixes on light at a distance of about 33 cm. A prism is placed before the deviating eye, and the strength of the prism required to center the corneal reflection measures the angle of deviation.

▶ Ductions (Monocular Rotations) (Figure 12–3)

With one eye covered, the other eye follows a moving target in all directions of gaze. Any decrease of rotation indicates limitation in the field of action of the respective muscle due to weakness of its contraction or failure of relaxation of its antagonist.

▶ Versions (Conjugate Ocular Movements)

Hering's law states that yoke muscles receive equal stimulation during any conjugate ocular movement. Versions are tested by having the eyes fix a light in the nine cardinal positions: straight ahead, rightward, leftward, upward, downward, up and rightward, down and rightward, up and leftward, and down and leftward (Table 12–2). Difference in rotation of one eye relative to the other is noted as underaction or overaction. By convention, differences in elevation or depression while an eye is adducted are described as under- or overaction of the oblique muscle relative to the yoke muscle of the fellow eye. Fixation by the normal eye in the field of action of a paretic muscle results in underaction of the paretic muscle. Conversely, fixation with the eye with the paretic muscle will lead to overaction of the yoke muscle, since greater than normal contraction of the underacting muscle is required (Figure 12–4).

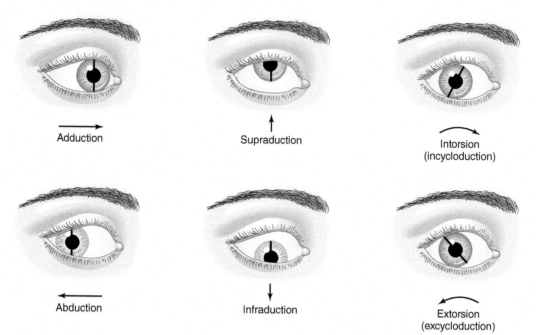

▲ **Figure 12–3.** Ductions (monocular rotations), right eye. Arrows indicate direction of eye movement from primary position.

▶ Disjunctive Movements

A. Convergence (Figure 12–5)

As the eyes follow an approaching object, they must turn inward to maintain alignment of the visual axes with the object of regard. The medial rectus muscles are increasingly stimulated, and the lateral rectus muscles are correspondingly reciprocally inhibited. (Neural pathways of supranuclear control are discussed in Chapter 14.)

Convergence is an active process with a strong voluntary as well as involuntary component and is an important consideration in evaluating the extraocular muscles in strabismus. To test convergence, a small object is slowly brought toward the bridge of the nose. The patient's attention is directed to the object by saying, "Keep the image from going double as long as possible." Convergence can normally be maintained until the object is nearly to the bridge of the nose. An actual numerical value is placed on convergence by measuring the distance from the bridge of the nose (in centimeters) at which the eyes "break" (ie, when the nonpreferred eye swings laterally so that convergence is no longer maintained). This point is termed the **near point of convergence,** and a value of up to 5 cm is considered within normal limits.

Accommodation is the increase of refractive power due to change of shape of the crystalline lens to focus on a near object. The ratio of convergence resulting directly from accommodation (accommodative convergence) to accommodation (AC/A ratio) quantifies the relationship between convergence and accommodation. The result is expressed as prism diopters of convergence per diopter of

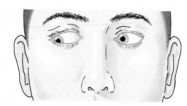
Fixing with normal right eye

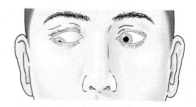
Fixing with paretic left eye

▲ **Figure 12–4.** Testing versions. Example of paretic left superior oblique.

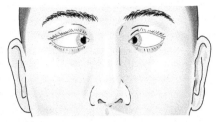

▲ **Figure 12–5.** Convergence. The position of the eyes at the normal near point of convergence (NPC) is shown. The break point is within 5 cm of the bridge of the nose.

accommodation. The normal ratio is about 6, being equal to the interpupillary distance in centimeters. The AC/A ratio is relevant particularly to understand accommodative (refractive) esotropia and its treatment with bifocals and miotics, as described later in this chapter.

B. Divergence

Electromyography has established that divergence is an active process, not merely a relaxation of convergence. Clinically, this function is seldom tested except in considering the amplitudes of fusion.

▶ Sensory Examination

While many tests of binocular vision have been devised, only a few need to be mentioned here. The tests are for stereopsis, suppression, and fusion potential. All require the simultaneous presentation of two targets separately, one to each eye.

A. Binocular Vision and Stereopsis Testing

Binocular vision can be subdivided into **simultaneous perception, fusion** (which requires sensory and motor fusion), and **stereopsis**. Tests for simultaneous perception and fusion involve presentation of a different stimulus to each eye, such as with red/green or polarized glasses, and analysis of how well the stimuli can be fused. Stereopsis is measured by the same technique using animal figures (eg, Titmus/Wirt Fly), shapes (eg, Frisby), or random dot stereograms (TNO, Randot), with the necessary disparity between the images for a three-dimensional form to be seen if stereopsis is present. The images can be presented with a haploscopic system (synoptophore), which, along with random dot stereograms, most effectively minimizes monocular depth clues.

B. Suppression Testing

The presence of suppression is readily demonstrated with the **Worth four-dot test**. Glasses containing a red lens over one eye and a green lens over the other are worn by the patient. A handheld or mounted display of red, green, and white spots is viewed. The color spots are markers for perception through

each eye, and the white dot, potentially visible to each eye, can indicate the presence of diplopia. The separation of the spots and the distance at which the display is presented determine the size of the retinal area tested. Foveal and peripheral areas may be tested at distance and near, respectively.

C. Fusion Potential

In individuals with a manifest deviation, the potential for binocular vision can be determined by the red filter test. A red filter is placed over one eye. The patient is directed to look at a distance or near white light, which is seen as a red light by the eye with the filter and as a white light by the other eye. Prisms are placed over one or both eyes to overcome the manifest deviation. If there is the potential for binocular vision, the two images come together and are seen as a single pink light. If there is no such potential, the one red and one white light still will be seen.

OBJECTIVES & PRINCIPLES OF THERAPY OF STRABISMUS

The main objectives of strabismus treatment in children are to prevent and/or reverse the deleterious sensory effects of strabismus (eg, amblyopia, suppression, loss of stereopsis) and to correct any cosmetically significant manifest deviation. Even when binocular vision is not possible, the psychological and sociologic benefits of straight eyes cannot be overestimated.

▶ Timing of Treatment in Children

A child can be examined at any age, and treatment for amblyopia or strabismus should be instituted as soon as the diagnosis is made. Results are favorably influenced by early realignment of the eyes, preferably by age 2. Good alignment can be achieved later, but normal sensory adaptation becomes more difficult as the child grows older. By age 8, the sensory status is generally so fixed that deficient binocular function cannot be improved and amblyopia treatment is less likely to be successful.

▶ Medical Treatment

Nonsurgical treatment of strabismus includes treatment of amblyopia, the use of optical devices (prisms and glasses), pharmacologic agents, and orthoptics.

A. Treatment of Amblyopia

If amblyopia is present at the time of initial presentation, typically it is treated, along with any nonsurgical strabismus treatment, prior to any surgery. The ocular deviation may lessen—rarely enlarge—with treatment of amblyopia. Although most strabismologists feel that surgical results are more predictable and stable if there is good visual acuity in each eye preoperatively, some have reported equivalent results with earlier surgery and continued amblyopia treatment postoperatively. The two stages of successful amblyopia treatment are (1) initial improvement and (2) maintenance of the improved visual acuity.

1. Initial improvement stage—Two initial treatment options for amblyopia are occlusion and atropine penalization of the better eye in conjunction with spectacle correction of any significant refractive error.

A. OCCLUSION—Occlusion is the "gold standard" for amblyopia treatment. The better eye is covered with a patch for 2 to 14 hours per day to stimulate the amblyopic eye. As a guideline, full-time occlusion (14 hours per day) may be done for as many weeks as the child's age in years without risk of reduced vision in the better eye. Occlusion treatment is continued in some form as long as visual acuity improves. In most cases, if treatment is started early enough, substantial improvement or complete normalization of visual acuity can be achieved. Occasionally, there is no improvement even under ideal conditions. Peeking around a patch or inadequate enforcement of therapy by the parents may limit results.

B. ATROPINE PENALIZATION—Atropine penalization is effective if the better eye is emmetropic or hyperopic. Atropine, as ophthalmic drops or ointment, is instilled in the better eye 2–7 days per week to inhibit its accommodation and promote use of the amblyopic eye during near viewing. Some clinician use atropine penalization as first-line treatment of amblyopia, and others use atropine if a child is unable to tolerate occlusion.

2. Maintenance stage—Following maximum improvement in vision, reduced-intensity occlusion or atropine penalization may be needed to maintain the improved vision beyond an age when amblyopia is likely to recur, which varies from 5 to 13 years.

B. Optical Devices

1. Spectacles—The most important optical device in the treatment of strabismus is accurately prescribed spectacles. Clarification of the retinal image allows the natural fusion mechanisms to operate to the fullest extent. Small refractive errors need not be corrected. If there is significant hyperopia, any esotropia is usually at least partially due to the uncorrected hyperopia (accommodative or refractive esotropia), and prescription of the full hyperopic correction is necessary. If bifocals permit sufficient relaxation of accommodation to allow for near fusion, they should be used as well.

2. Prisms—Prisms overcome ocular deviation by optical redirection of the line of sight. Corresponding retinal elements are brought into line to eliminate diplopia.

Preoperatively, prisms allow prediction of the sensory status following successful strabismus surgery. In children with esotropia, they can predict a postoperative shift in position (prism adaptation test), which can be anticipated by modification of the extent of surgery.

Prisms can be implemented in several ways. Fresnel Press-On® prism is a convenient plastic membrane that can be applied to any spectacle lens for diagnostic and temporary therapeutic purposes. For permanent correction, prisms are ground into spectacle lenses, but the amount is usually limited to about 8 to 10 PD per lens as image degradation is problematic with higher strengths.

C. Botulinum Toxin

The injection of botulinum toxin (type A) (Botox, Dysport) into an extraocular muscle produces a dose-dependent duration of paralysis. The injection is given under electromyographic positional control using a monopolar electrode needle. Several days after botulinum injection, the chemical paralysis of the muscle allows the eye to be moved into the field of action of the antagonist muscle. During the time the eye is deviated, the chemically paralyzed muscle is stretched, whereas the antagonist muscle is contracted. As the paralysis resolves, the eye will gradually return toward its original position but with a new balance of forces that may reduce or eliminate the deviation.

D. Orthoptics

Orthoptic exercises may relieve symptoms in individuals with difficulty maintaining normal convergence with near viewing tasks such as reading (see Convergence Insufficiency).

▶ **Surgical Treatment (Figure 12–6)**

A. Surgical Procedures

A variety of changes in the rotational effect of an extraocular muscle can be achieved with surgery.

1. Muscle weakening and strengthening procedures—Conceptually, the simplest procedures increase or decrease muscle tension in order to cause "weakening" or "strengthening" effects. **Recession** is the standard weakening procedure. The muscle is detached from the eye and resewn to the eye at a measured distance behind its original insertion. Muscle strengthening is achieved by either **resection** or a **tuck**. In resection, the muscle is detached from the eye, shortened by a measured amount, and then resewn to the eye, at the original insertion site. In the tuck procedure, a measured length of muscle or tendon is folded and sutured onto itself or adjacent scleral to shorten the muscle length. Recessions and resections are the usual surgeries performed on rectus muscles. Tuck may be performed on rectus and superior oblique muscles. Superior oblique weakening is

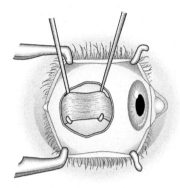

Exposure of lateral rectus

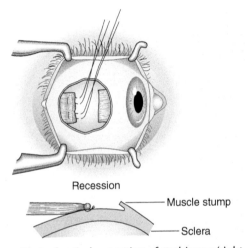

Recession

Muscle stump

Sclera

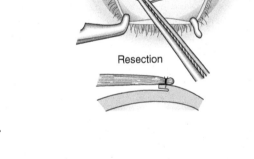

Resection

Figure 12–6. Surgical correction of strabismus (right eye).

accomplished by a tenotomy (complete or partial transection of the tendon) or one of several lengthening procedures. The inferior oblique can be weakened by disinsertion, myectomy, or recession. Repositioning (anterior transposition) of the inferior oblique is used in the treatment of dissociated vertical deviations.

2. Muscle force redirection—In addition to simple strengthening or weakening, the point of attachment of the muscle can be shifted to give the muscle a rotational action it did not previously have. In sixth cranial nerve (abducens) palsy, surgically moving the insertions of both vertical rectus muscles of the same eye toward the insertion of the lateral rectus will passively reduce the inward rotation of the eye in primary gaze and slightly improve abduction. Surgically moving the insertions of horizontal rectus muscles affects the horizontal eye position in upgaze and downgaze. This is used for A or V patterns (see later section in chapter), in which the horizontal deviation is more eso (or less exo) in upgaze or downgaze, respectively. The torsional effect of a

muscle can also be changed. In the Harada-Ito procedure, the anterior fibers of the superior oblique tendon are tightened to increase its incyclotorsional action.

3. Faden procedure—A special operation for muscle weakening is the posterior fixation (Faden) procedure (retroequatorial myopexy) (Figure 12–7), in which a new insertion is created by suturing the muscle well behind the original insertion. This causes mechanical weakening of the muscle as the eye rotates into its field of action without significant alteration of the primary position of the eye. The procedure can be effective on vertical rectus muscles (dissociated vertical deviation) or horizontal muscles (high AC/A ratio, nystagmus, and other less common incomitant muscle imbalances).

B. Choice of Muscles for Surgery

Deciding which muscles to operate on is based on several factors. The first is the amount of misalignment measured in the primary position. Modifications are made for significant

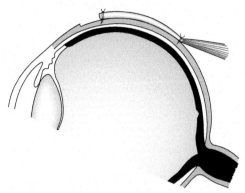

▲ **Figure 12–7.** Posterior fixation (Faden) procedure. The rectus muscle is tacked to the sclera far posterior to its insertion. This prevents unwrapping of the muscle as the eye turns into the muscle's field of action. The muscle is progressively weakened in its field of action. If this procedure is combined with recession, the alignment in primary position is also affected.

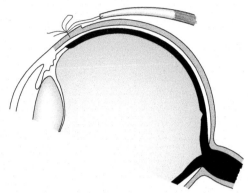

▲ **Figure 12–8.** Adjustable suture. The suture is placed on the sclera at any point that will be accessible to the surgeon. The bow is untied and the position of the muscle changed as desired.

differences in distance and near measurements. The medial rectus muscles have more effect on the angle of deviation for near and the lateral rectus muscles more effect for distance. For esotropia greater at near, both medial rectus muscles should be weakened. For exotropia greater at distance, both lateral rectus muscles should be weakened. For deviations approximately the same at distance and near, bilateral weakening procedures or unilateral recession/resection procedures are equally effective.

C. Adjustable Sutures (Figure 12–8)

The development of adjustable sutures offers an advantage in muscle surgery for reoperations and incomitant deviations. During the operation, the muscle is reattached to the sclera with a slip knot placed so that it is later accessible to the surgeon. After the patient has recovered from the anesthesia to cooperate in the adjustment process, a topical anesthetic drop is placed in the eye and the suture can be tightened or loosened to change the eye position as indicated by cover testing. Adjustable sutures can be used on rectus muscles for recessions or resections and on superior oblique muscle procedures. Although any patient willing to cooperate is suitable, the method is usually not applicable for children under age 12.

ESOTROPIA (CONVERGENT STRABISMUS, "CROSSED EYES")

Esotropia is by far the most common type of strabismus. It is divided into two types: **nonparetic** (comitant) and **paretic** (due to paresis or paralysis of one or both lateral rectus muscles). Nonparetic esotropia is the most common type in infants and children; it may be accommodative, nonaccommodative, or partially accommodative. Most cases of childhood nonaccommodative esotropia are classified as **infantile esotropia,** with onset by age 6 months. Others occur after age 6 months and are classified as **acquired nonaccommodative** esotropia. Nonparetic esotropia has a multifactorial partly genetic basis. Frequently, esophoria and esotropia are an autosomal dominant trait. An accommodative element is sometimes superimposed upon comitant esotropia (partially accommodative). At least half of children with infantile esotropia will later develop an accommodative esotropia as preschoolers, despite successful surgical alignment as infants. Paretic strabismus is uncommon in childhood but accounts for most new cases of strabismus in adults.

NONPARETIC ESOTROPIA

1. NONACCOMMODATIVE ESOTROPIA

A. Infantile Esotropia

Infantile esotropia usually begins by age 6 months, but may present later in the first year. The deviation is comitant, with the angle of deviation being approximately the same in all directions of gaze and usually not affected by accommodation. The cause is not refractive error or paresis of an extraocular muscle. It is likely that the majority of cases are due to faulty innervational control, involving the supranuclear pathways for convergence and divergence and their neural connections to the medial longitudinal fasciculus. A small number are due to anatomic variations such as anomalous insertions of horizontally acting muscles, abnormal check ligaments, or various other fascial abnormalities.

The deviation is often large (≥ 40 PD) in infantile esotropia. Abduction may be limited but can be demonstrated with oculocephalic (doll's head) maneuvers. Vertical deviations may be observed after 18 months of age as a result of overaction of the oblique muscles or dissociated vertical deviation (DVD). Nystagmus, latent or manifest latent, is frequently present (see Chapter 14). The most common refractive error is low to moderate hyperopia.

The eye that appears to be straight is the eye used for fixation. Almost without exception, it is the eye with better vision or lower refractive error (or both). If there is anisometropia, there will probably be some amblyopia as well. If at various times either eye is used for fixation, the patient is said to show spontaneous alternation of fixation, in which case, vision will be equal or nearly equal in both eyes. In large-angle esotropia, the eye preference may be determined by the direction of gaze, with the right eye being used for fixation on left gaze and the left eye on right gaze (cross fixation).

Infantile esotropia is treated surgically. Preliminary nonsurgical treatment may be indicated to ensure the best possible result. Amblyopia should be treated aggressively. Glasses should be tried if there are more than 3 diopters (D) of hyperopia to determine if reducing accommodation has a favorable effect on the deviation.

Surgery is performed after treatment of amblyopia has been completed. Once reproducible measurements are obtained, surgery should be scheduled as early as reasonably possible since there is ample evidence that sensory results are better the sooner the eyes are aligned. Many procedures have been recommended, but the two most popular are (1) recession of both medial rectus muscles and (2) recession of the medial rectus and resection of the lateral rectus on the same eye.

B. Acquired Nonaccommodative Esotropia

This type of nonparetic esotropia develops in childhood, usually after the age of 2 years. There is little or no hyperopia, and the angle of strabismus is often smaller than in infantile esotropia. Infrequently, posterior fossa lesion may cause comitant acquired nonaccommodative esotropia, and neuroimaging should be considered. Treatment is surgical and follows the same guidelines as for infantile esotropia.

2. ACCOMMODATIVE ESOTROPIA

Accommodative esotropia occurs when there is a normal physiologic mechanism of accommodation with an associated overactive convergence response but insufficient relative fusional divergence to hold the eyes straight. There are two pathophysiologic mechanisms at work, singly or together: (1) sufficiently high hyperopia, requiring so much accommodation to clarify the image that esotropia results because of the magnitude of the associated convergence and (2) a high AC/A ratio, accompanied by mild to moderate hyperopia (1.5 D or more).

A. Accommodative Esotropia due to Hyperopia (Figure 12–9)

Accommodative esotropia due to hyperopia typically begins at age 2–3 years but may occur earlier or later. Deviation is variable prior to treatment. Glasses with full cycloplegic refraction allow the eyes to become aligned.

B. Accommodative Esotropia due to High AC/A Ratio

In accommodative esotropia due to a high ratio of accommodative convergence to accommodation (AC/A ratio), the deviation is greater at near than at distance. The refractive error is hyperopic. Treatment is with glasses with full cycloplegic refraction plus bifocals or miotics to relieve excess deviation at near.

3. PARTIALLY ACCOMMODATIVE ESOTROPIA

A mixed mechanism—part muscular imbalance and part accommodative/convergence imbalance—may exist. Although glasses, bifocals, and miotics decrease the angle of deviation,

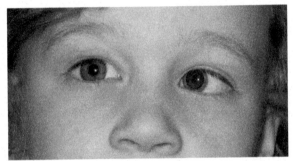

A

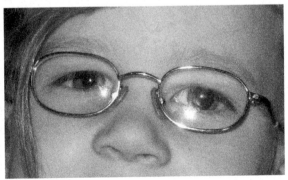

B

▲ **Figure 12–9.** Accommodative esotropia due to hyperopia. **(A)** Hyperopic individual requiring so much accommodation for clear vision that accommodative convergence causes esotropia. **(B)** Normal ocular alignment is achieved with full correction of hyperopia with corrective lenses.

the esotropia is not eliminated. Surgery is performed for the nonaccommodative component of the deviation with the choice of surgical procedure as described for infantile esotropia.

PARETIC (INCOMITANT) ESOTROPIA (SIXTH CRANIAL NERVE PALSY) (FIGURES 12–2 AND 12–10)

Incomitant strabismus results from paresis or restriction of action of one or more extraocular muscles. Incomitant esotropia is usually due to paresis of one or both lateral rectus muscles as a result of unilateral or bilateral sixth cranial (abducens) nerve palsy. Other causes are fracture of the medial orbital wall with entrapment of the medial rectus muscle, Graves' ophthalmopathy causing fibrosis of the medial rectus muscles, and Duane retraction syndrome (see later in the chapter). Sixth cranial nerve palsy is most frequently seen in adults with systemic hypertension or diabetes, in which case spontaneous resolution usually begins within 3 months (see Chapters 14 and 15). It may also be the first sign of intracranial tumor, increased intracranial pressure, or inflammatory disease. Associated neurologic signs are then important clues. Head trauma is another frequent cause.

In sixth cranial palsy, the esotropia is characteristically greater with the affected eye fixing, at distance than at near, and on gaze to the affected side. Thus paresis of the right lateral rectus causes esotropia that is more marked with the right eye fixing, becomes greater on right gaze, and if paresis is mild, with little or no deviation on left gaze. If the lateral rectus muscle is totally paralyzed, the eye will not abduct past the midline. Bilateral sixth cranial palsy causes an esotropia that increases on gaze to either side.

Acquired sixth cranial palsy is initially managed by occlusion of the paretic eye or with prisms. Botulinum toxin injection into the antagonist medial rectus muscle may provide symptomatic relief but does not appear to influence the final outcome. In incomplete palsies, if lateral rectus function has not recovered after 6 months, medial rectus botulinum toxin injections may be used on a long-term basis to allow fusion, abolishing diplopia in primary gaze, or to facilitate prism therapy. However, horizontal rectus muscle surgery (resection of the lateral rectus and recession of the medial rectus of one or both eyes) is usually performed. In complete palsies that have failed to improve after 6 months, transposition of the vertical rectus muscles to the lateral rectus is appropriate (see Transposition in previous section). In conjunction with transposition, the injection of botulinum toxin into the medial rectus may be used when medial rectus restriction is severe. Full abduction cannot be restored, but fusion in primary position, with or without the aid of prisms, and a reasonable field of binocular single vision can usually be achieved. Sixth cranial palsy in infants and children may cause amblyopia, so these patients must be followed carefully and any amblyopia treated appropriately.

▶ Pseudoesotropia

Pseudoesotropia is the illusion of crossed eyes in an infant or toddler when no strabismus is present (Figure 12–11). This appearance is usually caused by a flat, broad nasal bridge, and

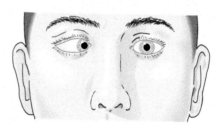

Primary position: right esotropia

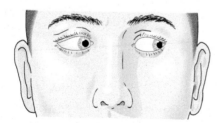

Left gaze: no deviation

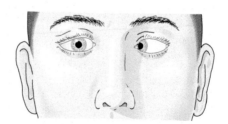

Right gaze: left esotropia

▲ **Figure 12–10.** Incomitant strabismus (paretic). Paresis of right lateral rectus muscle, with left eye fixing.

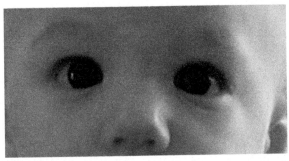

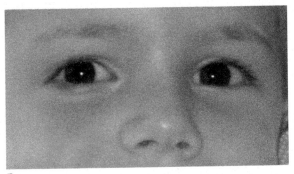

▲ **Figure 12–11. (A)** Toddler with pseudoesotropia. **(B)** Same child 3 years later without any intervention.

prominent epicanthal folds that cover a portion of the nasal sclera. This very common condition may be differentiated from true misalignment by the corneal light reflection appearing in the center of the pupil of each eye when the child fixes a light. With normal facial growth and increasing prominence of the nasal bridge, this pseudoesotropic appearance gradually disappears. Of course, true esotropia may be present in association with this common infantile facial configuration.

▼ EXOTROPIA (DIVERGENT STRABISMUS)

Exotropia is less common than esotropia, but its incidence increases gradually with age. Exotropia often begins as exophoria and progresses to **intermittent exotropia** and finally to **constant exotropia** if no treatment is given. Other cases begin as constant or intermittent exotropia and remain stationary. As in esotropia, there may be a hereditary element. Neurologic impairment and developmental delay are more common than in esotropia.

▶ Descriptive Classification of Exotropia

Exotropia is classified according to whether or not there is an excess of divergence or an insufficiency of convergence, but this does not mean that the underlying cause is understood.

A. Basic Exotropia

Distance and near deviations are approximately equal.

B. Divergence Excess

Distance deviation is significantly larger than near deviation.

C. Pseudodivergence Excess

Distance deviation is significantly larger than near deviation but a +3 diopter lens for near measurement causes the near deviation to become approximately equal to the distance deviation.

D. Convergence Insufficiency

Near deviation is significantly larger than distance deviation.

1. INTERMITTENT EXOTROPIA

▶ Clinical Findings

Intermittent exotropia accounts for well over half of all cases of exotropia. The onset of the deviation may be in the first year, and practically all have presented by age 5. A characteristic sign is closing one eye (squinting) in bright light. The manifest exotropia first becomes noticeable with distance fixation. The patient usually fuses at near, overcoming moderate to large angle exophoria. There is no correlation with a specific refractive error.

Since there is fusion at least part of the time, amblyopia is uncommon, and when present, it is mild. For distance, with one eye deviated, there is suppression of that eye and normal retinal correspondence with little or no amblyopia.

▶ Treatment

A. Medical Treatment

Nonsurgical treatment is largely confined to refractive correction and amblyopia therapy. If the AC/A ratio is high, the use of minus lenses may delay surgery for a while. Antisuppression treatment may be of temporary benefit.

B. Surgical Treatment

Most patients with intermittent exotropia require surgery when their fusional control deteriorates, manifesting over time as increasing duration of manifest exotropia, enlarging angle of deviation, decreasing control for near fixation, and worsening of distance and near binocular function. Surgery may alleviate diplopia or other asthenopic symptoms, but recurrence of exotropia is frequent. The choice of procedure depends on the measurements of the deviation. Bilateral lateral rectus muscle recession is preferred when the deviation is greater at distance. If there is more deviation at near, it is best to undertake resection of a medial rectus muscle and recession of the ipsilateral lateral rectus muscle. Surgery on one or even two additional horizontal muscles may be

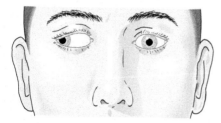

▲ **Figure 12–12.** Right exotropia.

necessary for very large deviations (≥ 50 PD). For best long-term results, it is desirable to obtain slight overcorrection in the immediate postoperative period.

2. CONSTANT EXOTROPIA (FIGURE 12–12)

Constant exotropia is less common than intermittent exotropia. It may be present at birth or may occur when intermittent exotropia progresses to constant exotropia. Because children with infantile exotropia often have neurologic impairment and developmental delays, pediatric neurologic consultation is indicated in all such cases. Exotropia may also have its onset later in life, particularly following loss of vision in one eye (sensory exotropia).

▶ Clinical Findings

Constant exotropia may be of any severity. With chronicity or poor vision in one eye, the deviation can become quite large. Adduction may be limited, and hypertropia also may be present. There is suppression if the deviation was acquired by age 6–8; otherwise, diplopia may be present. If exotropia is due to very poor vision in one eye, there may be no diplopia. Amblyopia is uncommon in the absence of anisometropia, and spontaneous alternation of fixation is frequently observed.

▶ Treatment

Surgery is nearly always indicated. The choice and amount are as described for intermittent exotropia. Slight overcorrection in an adult may result in diplopia. Most patients adjust to this, especially if they have been forewarned of the possibility. If one eye has reduced vision, the prognosis for maintenance of a stable position is less favorable, with the strong possibility that the exotropia will recur following surgery. Botulinum toxin injections can be useful as primary treatment in small deviations or as supplementary treatment in significant surgical overcorrections or undercorrections.

▼ A & V PATTERNS

A horizontal deviation may be vertically incomitant, meaning that its magnitude changes between upgaze and downgaze. An A pattern means more esodeviation or less exodeviation in upgaze compared to downgaze. A V pattern means less esodeviation or more exodeviation in upgaze compared to downgaze. These patterns are frequently associated with overaction of the oblique muscles, inferior obliques for V pattern and superior obliques for A pattern.

When surgically treating an A or V pattern, oblique muscle overaction must be treated if present. If little or no oblique overaction exists, the insertions of the horizontal rectus muscles are surgically transposed vertically by a distance of one tendon width. The insertions of the medial rectus muscles are displaced toward the narrow end of the pattern (in V pattern esotropia, recessed medial rectus muscles are moved downward), and lateral rectus muscles are displaced toward the open end (in V exotropia, the insertions of the recessed lateral rectus muscles are moved upward).

▼ HYPERTROPIA (MANIFEST VERTICAL STRABISMUS) (FIGURE 12–13)

Vertical deviations are customarily named according to the higher eye, regardless of which eye has the better vision and is used for fixation. They are less common than horizontal deviations, commonly present after childhood, and have many causes.

Congenital superior oblique muscle palsy, which is a misleading term as the underlying cause may be a musculofascial anomaly rather than a fourth cranial nerve palsy, is a common cause of pediatric hypertropia, but may not present until adulthood. Congenital anatomic anomalies, such as in craniosynostoses, may result in muscle attachments in abnormal locations. Occasionally, there are anomalous fibrous bands that attach to the eye. The superior oblique is the most commonly paretic vertical muscle because of its susceptibility to closed head trauma. The vertical rectus muscles are commonly involved in orbital trauma, typically entrapment of the inferior rectus in an orbital floor fracture, and in Graves' ophthalmopathy with fibrosis of the inferior rectus limiting the upward movement of the eye and possibly pulling it downward. Orbital tumors, brainstem and other intracranial lesions, including strokes and inflammatory disease such as multiple sclerosis, and even myasthenia gravis can all produce hypertropia. Many of these specific entities are discussed in Chapters 13 and 14.

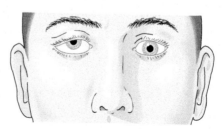

▲ **Figure 12–13.** Right hypertropia.

► Clinical Findings

The clinical findings vary, depending on the cause. The history is particularly important in diagnosis of hypertropia. Diplopia is almost invariably present if strabismus develops past age 6–8. As in other forms of strabismus, sensory adaptation occurs if the onset is before this age range. Suppression and anomalous retinal correspondence may be present in gaze directions where there is manifest strabismus, whereas in gaze directions without manifest strabismus, there may be no suppression and normal stereopsis. Compensatory abnormal head position (AHP) may develop, including head tilt, head turn, or chin depression or elevation, or a combination.

The ocular misalignment usually changes with the direction of gaze because most hypertropias are incomitant. The deviation tends to be greatest in the field of action of one of the four vertically acting muscles and should be quantified by prism and alternate cover test in primary and cardinal positions of gaze before and after correction of any AHP. In hypertropia due to third or fourth cranial nerve palsy, the **three-step test** comprising (1) determination of which eye is higher in primary position, (2) determination of whether the vertical deviation increases on left or right gaze, and (3) the Bielschowsky head tilt test will indicate which muscle is primarily responsible. A fourth step of identification of cyclotorsion in each eye, such as with the double Maddox rod test (see later in the chapter), can be helpful in diagnosis of skew deviation. Observation of ocular rotations for limitations and overactions can also be of great value, but the abnormalities may be subtle. In congenital superior oblique palsy, on gaze to the opposite side, the hypertropia often does not increase on downgaze as would be expected with superior oblique underaction but increases on upgaze due to overaction of the ipsilateral inferior oblique. In longstanding acquired superior oblique palsy, other secondary effects are overaction of the contralateral yoke (inferior rectus) muscle and contracture of the contralateral antagonist (superior rectus) leading to reduction of incomitance (spread of comitance), which can make it difficult to differentiate superior oblique palsy from contralateral superior rectus palsy.

Superior oblique muscle palsy, whether congenital or acquired, typically manifests as hypertropia increasing on gaze to the opposite side and with a head tilt to the opposite side. The **Bielschowsky head tilt test** (Figure 12–14) is particularly useful to confirm the diagnosis. The test exploits the differing effects of each vertical muscle on torsion and elevation. Thus, with a paretic right superior oblique when the head is tilted to the right, the superior rectus and superior oblique contract to intort the eye and maintain the position of the retinal vertical meridian as much as possible. The superior rectus elevates the eye, and the superior oblique depresses the eye. Because of weakness of the superior oblique muscle, the vertical forces do not cancel out as they normally would, and right hypertropia increases. In head tilt to the left, the intorting muscles for the right eye relax, and the right inferior oblique and right inferior rectus both contract to extort the eye. Both the paretic right superior oblique and the right superior rectus relax, and hypertropia

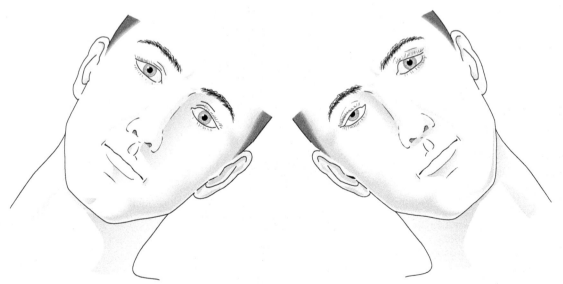

▲ **Figure 12–14.** Head tilt test (Bielschowsky test). Paresis of right superior oblique. **(Left)** Hypertropia is minimized on tilting the head to the sound side. The right eye may then extort and the intorting superior oblique and superior rectus relax. **(Right)** When the head is tilted to the paretic side, the intorting muscles contract together, but their vertical actions do not cancel out as usual, because of superior oblique paresis. Hypertropia is worse with head tilt to the paretic side.

is minimized, which explains the adoption of a head tilt to the opposite side as it reduces the vertical deviation that has to be overcome to achieve fusion. Quantification of the Bielschowsky head tilt test is by measurement by prism and alternate cover test of the hypertropia with the head tilted to either side.

Hypertropia may be accompanied by **cyclotropia**, especially with superior oblique dysfunction. To measure a cyclotropia, the **double Maddox rod test** is used. In a trial frame, a red and white Maddox rod are aligned vertically, one over each eye. With the patient's head held straight and fixing a light, one rod is gradually turned until the observed lines are parallel to each other and to normal horizontal orientation. The angle of tilt is then read from the angular scale on the trial frame. Superior oblique paresis results in excyclotorsion of the affected eye. Skew deviation, which is hypertropia due to a supranuclear lesion, usually caused by brainstem or cerebellar disease, causes conjugate ocular torsion of both eyes, for example, excyclotorsion of the left eye and incyclotorsion of the right eye.

▶ Treatment

A. Medical Treatment

For smaller and more comitant deviations, a prism may be all that is required. For constant diplopia, one eye may need to be occluded, particularly if there is torsional diplopia because this cannot be corrected with a prism. Any underlying cause may require specific treatment.

B. Surgical Treatment

Surgery is often indicated if the deviation, head tilt, and/or diplopia persist (Figure 12–15). The choice of procedure depends on quantitative measurements and the pattern of misalignment.

▼ SPECIAL FORMS OF STRABISMUS

DUANE RETRACTION SYNDROME

Duane retraction syndrome is typically characterized by marked limitation of abduction, mild limitation of adduction, retraction of the globe and narrowing of the palpebral fissure on attempted adduction, and, frequently, upshoot or downshoot of the eye in adduction. It is one type of congenital cranial dysinnervation disorder (CCDD), in which a cranial nerve fails to develop properly and the target muscle is instead abnormally innervated by another cranial nerve.

Duane retraction syndrome is usually monocular, with the left eye more often affected. Most cases are sporadic, although some families with dominant inheritance have been described. A variety of other anomalies may be associated, such as dysplasia of the iris stroma, heterochromia, cataract, choroidal coloboma, microphthalmos, Goldenhar

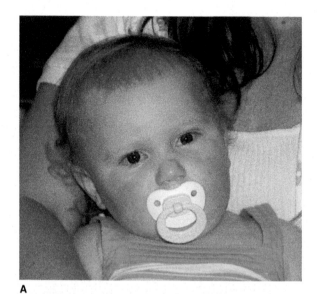

A

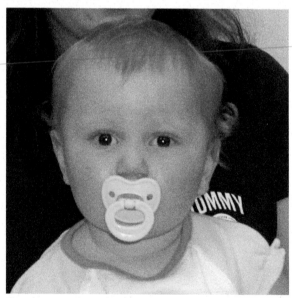

B

▲ **Figure 12–15. (A)** Head tilt due to congenital left superior oblique palsy. **(B)** Resolution of head tilt following extraocular muscle surgery.

syndrome, Klippel-Feil syndrome, cleft palate, and anomalies of the face, ear, or extremities. Most cases can be explained by absence of the sixth cranial nerve with aberrant innervation of the lateral rectus by a branch of the oculomotor nerve. In attempted adduction, the oculomotor nerve is activated causing simultaneous co-contraction of the medial and lateral rectus muscles producing retraction of the globe.

Treatment

Surgery is indicated for primary position misalignment or a significant compensatory head turn. The goal is to obtain straight eyes in the primary position and to horizontally expand the field of single vision. Recession of the medial rectus on the affected side is performed if esotropia is present in the primary position. For more severe cases, temporal transposition of one or both vertical rectus muscles and weakening of the medial rectus muscle is indicated.

DISSOCIATED VERTICAL DEVIATION

Dissociated vertical deviation (DVD) is frequently associated with infantile esotropia and rarely with an otherwise normal muscle balance. The exact cause is not known, but it is likely to be abnormal supranuclear innervation.

Clinical Findings

When covered, the eye drifts upward, frequently with extorsion and abduction. DVD does not obey Hering's law as the eye returns to its resting binocular position when the cover is removed without any vertical shift in position of the fellow eye. Occasionally, the upward drifting will occur spontaneously without occlusion, causing a noticeable vertical misalignment. Most cases are bilateral, although asymmetry of involvement is common.

Treatment

Treatment is indicated if the appearance of vertical deviation is unacceptable. Nonsurgical treatment is limited to refractive correction to maximize motor fusion. A popular and relatively successful procedure is graded recession of the superior rectus, occasionally combined with posterior fixation (Faden) sutures. Anterior transposition of the inferior oblique insertion to the lateral border of the inferior rectus muscle is indicated when there is associated inferior oblique muscle overaction.

BROWN SYNDROME (SUPERIOR OBLIQUE TENDON SHEATH SYNDROME)

Brown syndrome is due to fibrous adhesions or inflammation in the superior nasal quadrant of the orbit involving the superior oblique tendon and trochlea, which mechanically limit elevation of the eye. Limitation of elevation is most marked in the adducted position, and improvement in elevation occurs gradually as the eye is abducted. The condition is usually unilateral and idiopathic, although rarely it may be due to trauma, inflammation, or tumor.

Surgical treatment is limited to those cases where there is an AHP to compensate for hypotropia or cyclotropia of the involved eye. The objective is to lessen the mechanical restriction via a superior oblique tenotomy. Normalization of the head position may occur, but restoration of full motility is seldom achieved.

HETEROPHORIA

Heterophoria is deviation of the eyes that is held in check by binocular vision. Almost all individuals have some degree of heterophoria. Symptoms correlate with the level of effort required by the individual to maintain fusion.

Clinical Findings

The symptoms of heterophoria may be clear-cut (intermittent diplopia) or vague ("eyestrain" or asthenopia, fatigue, headache, aversion to reading). There is no degree of heterophoria that is clearly abnormal, although larger amounts are more likely to be symptomatic. Except for hyperopia, high AC/A ratios, and mild cases of muscle paresis not resulting in frank heterotropia, the fundamental causes of heterophorias are unknown.

Asthenopia is sometimes caused by uncorrected refractive errors as well as by muscle imbalance. One possible mechanism is **aniseikonia,** in which an image seen by one eye is a different size and shape from that seen by the other eye, preventing sensory fusion. Spectacles with unequal lens powers in the two eyes can cause asthenopia by creating prismatic displacement of the image in one eye for gaze away from the optic axis that is too large to control (induced prism). Another mechanism that may produce symptoms is a change in spatial perception due to the curvature of the lenses or astigmatic corrections (see Chapter 21). Anisometropia is more likely to cause symptoms when its onset is sudden, such as scleral buckle procedure for retinal detachment causing myopia.

Diagnosis

The diagnosis of heterophoria is based on prism and cover measurements. Relative fusional vergence amplitudes are measured. While the patient views an accommodative target at distance or near, prisms of increasing strength are placed in front of one eye. The fusional vergence amplitude is the amount of prism the patient is able to overcome and still maintain single vision. Measurements are done with base-out, base-in, base-up, and base-down prisms. The important feature is the size of the amplitudes in comparison to the angle of heterophoria. While one cannot give exact norms for normal relative fusion vergence, guidelines for typical normal findings are as follows: at distance, convergence 14 PD, divergence 6 PD, and vertical 2.5 PD; at near, convergence 35 PD, divergence 15 PD, and vertical 2.5 PD.

Treatment

Heterophoria requires treatment only if symptomatic. Untreated heterophoria or asthenopia does not cause any permanent damage to the eyes. Treatment methods are all aimed at reducing the effort required to achieve fusion or at changing muscle mechanics so that the muscle imbalance itself is reduced.

A. Medical Treatment

1. Accurate refractive correction—Occasionally, poor visual acuity is the cause of symptomatic heterophoria. Refractive correction to optimize clarity of vision may be all that is needed to alleviate symptoms, with the clearer image allowing fusional capacity to function fully.

2. Manipulation of accommodation—In general, esophorias are treated with antiaccommodative therapy and exophorias by stimulating accommodation. Plus lenses often work well for esophoria, especially if hyperopia is present, by reducing accommodative convergence. A high AC/A ratio may be effectively treated with plus lenses, sometimes combined with bifocals or miotics.

3. Prisms—The use of prisms requires the wearing of glasses that may not be tolerated. Plastic Fresnel press-on prisms should be tried before ground-in prisms are ordered. Optical distortion and thickness limit the usefulness of higher strength prisms. Correction of one-third to one-half of the measured deviation is usually sufficient to enable comfortable fusion. Prisms can be useful for esophoria, exophoria, and vertical phorias as well.

4. Botulinum toxin type A (Botox, Dysport) injection—This treatment is well suited to producing small to moderate shifts in ocular alignment and has been used as a substitute for surgical weakening of one muscle. The main disadvantage is that the resulting effect may be variable or wear off completely months later.

B. Surgical Treatment

Surgery should be performed only once other treatments have failed. Muscles are chosen for correction according to the measured deviation at distance and near in various directions of gaze. Sometimes only one muscle needs adjustment. Adjustable sutures can be very helpful (Figure 12–8).

REFERENCES

Adams GG et al: Is strabismus the only problem? Psychological issues surrounding strabismus surgery. J AAPOS 2016;20:383. [PMID: 27651232]

Astudillo PP et al: The effect of achieving immediate target angle on success of strabismus surgery in children. Am J Ophthalmol 2015;160:913. [PMID: 26210862]

Clark RA: The role of extraocular muscle pulleys in incomitant non-paralytic strabismus. Middle East Afr J Ophthalmol 2015;22:279. [PMID: 26180464]

Erbağcı I et al: Using liquid crystal glasses to treat amblyopia in children. J AAPOS 2015;19:257. [PMID: 26059673]

Graeber CP et al: Changes in lateral comitance after asymmetric horizontal strabismus surgery. JAMA Ophthalmol 2015;133:1241. [PMID: 26291652]

Gunton KB et al: Treatment of sixth nerve palsy. J Pediatr Ophthalmol Strabismus 2015;52:198. [PMID: 26214719]

Guo CX et al: Binocular treatment of amblyopia using videogames (BRAVO): study protocol for a randomised controlled trial. Trials 2016;17:504. [PMID: 27756405]

Hatt SR et al: Interventions for dissociated vertical deviation. Cochrane Database Syst Rev 2015;11:CD010868. [PMID: 26587695]

Hatt SR et al: Symptoms in children with intermittent exotropia and their impact on health-related quality of life. Strabismus 2016;24:139. [PMID: 27835070]

Holmes JM et al: Effect of a binocular iPad game vs part-time patching in children aged 5 to 12 years with amblyopia: a randomized clinical trial. JAMA Ophthalmol 2016;134:1391. [PMID: 27812703]

Irsch K: Optical issues in measuring strabismus. Middle East Afr J Ophthalmol 2015;22:265. [PMID: 26180462]

Jeon H et al: Strabismus in children with white matter damage of immaturity: MRI correlation. Br J Ophthalmol 2016 Jul 15. [Epub ahead of print] [PMID: 27422974]

Kalevar A et al: Duane syndrome: Clinical features and surgical management. Can J Ophthalmol 2015;50:310. [PMID: 26257226]

Khan AO: A Modern approach to incomitant strabismus. Middle East Afr J Ophthalmol 2015;22:263. [PMID: 26180461]

Kim MK et al: Hyperopic refractive errors as a prognostic factor in intermittent exotropia surgery. Eye (Lond) 2015;29:1555. [PMID: 26293140]

Koller HP et al: Diagnosis and treatment of fourth nerve palsy. J Pediatr Ophthalmol Strabismus 2016;53:70. [PMID: 27018877]

Koo EB et al: Treatment of amblyopia and amblyopia risk factors based on current evidence. Semin Ophthalmol 2017;32:1. [PMID: 27748640]

Lavrich JB: Intermittent exotropia: continued controversies and current management. Curr Opin Ophthalmol 2015;26:375. [PMID: 26204476]

Lueder GT: Orbital causes of incomitant strabismus. Middle East Afr J Ophthalmol 2015;22:286. [PMID: 26180465]

Olitsky SE et al: Complications of strabismus surgery. Middle East Afr J Ophthalmol 2015;22:271. [PMID: 26180463]

Park MJ et al: Ocular findings in patients with spastic type cerebral palsy. BMC Ophthalmol 2016;16:195. [PMID: 27821110]

Peragallo JH et al: Diplopia: an update. Semin Neurol 2016;36:357. [PMID: 27643904]

Piano ME et al: Perceptual visual distortions in adult amblyopia and their relationship to clinical features. Invest Ophthalmol Vis Sci 2015;56:5533. [PMID: 26284559]

Schnall BM: Is there anything new in strabismus? Curr Opin Ophthalmol 2015;26:352. [PMID: 26196096]

Stager D Jr et al: Uses of the inferior oblique muscle in strabismus surgery. Middle East Afr J Ophthalmol 2015;22:292. [PMID: 26180466]

Tailor V et al: Binocular versus standard occlusion or blurring treatment for unilateral amblyopia in children aged three to eight years. Cochrane Database Syst Rev 2015;8:CD011347. [PMID: 26263202]

Wang X et al: Effectiveness of strabismus surgery on the health-related quality of life assessment of children with intermittent exotropia and their parents: a randomized clinical trial. J AAPOS 2015;19:298. [PMID: 26235788]

Weiss AH et al: Crouzon syndrome: relationship of eye movements to pattern strabismus. Invest Ophthalmol Vis Sci 2015;56:4394. [PMID: 26176876]

Xiao O et al: Prevalence of amblyopia in school-aged children and variations by age, gender, and ethnicity in a multi-country refractive error study. Ophthalmology 2015;122:1924. [PMID: 26278861]

Orbit

M. Reza Vagefi, MD

Orbital disease usually arises within the bony confines of the orbit or by spread from adjacent structures, particularly the paranasal sinuses. The etiology may be inflammation, infection, neoplasia, or vascular anomaly. An orbital mass may also be a metastatic tumor and hence a harbinger of a serious and sometimes life-threatening entity.

PHYSIOLOGY OF SYMPTOMS

An increase in orbital volume results in displacement of the globe. Since the orbit has rigid bony walls (see Chapter 1), such displacement usually manifests predominantly as forward protrusion of the globe (**proptosis**), which is a hallmark of orbital disease. Pathology within the muscle cone displaces the globe anteriorly (**axial proptosis**). Pathology outside the muscle cone also causes vertical and/or lateral displacement (**nonaxial proptosis**). Bilateral involvement generally indicates systemic disease, such as autoimmune hyperthyroidism (Graves' disease). The proptosis in Graves' ophthalmopathy is often termed **exophthalmos**.

Pulsating proptosis may be due to carotid-cavernous fistula, arterial orbital vascular malformation, or transmission of cerebral pulsations due to a bone defect such as in the sphenoid dysplasia of type 1 neurofibromatosis. Proptosis that increases on bending the head forward or with Valsalva maneuver can be a sign of venous orbital vascular malformation (orbital varices) or bone defect. **Intermittent proptosis** may be the result of a sinus mucocele. The Hertel exophthalmometer (see Chapter 2) is the standard method of quantifying the magnitude of proptosis. Serial measurements are most accurate if performed by the same individual with the same instrument. **Pseudoproptosis** is apparent proptosis in the absence of orbital disease. It may be due to an enlarged globe from high myopia or buphthalmos, lid retraction, extraocular muscle weakness or paralysis, asymmetrical orbital size, or posterior displacement (**enophthalmos**) of the contralateral globe.

Proptosis does not impair vision unless there are corneal changes due to corneal exposure. However, any orbital process that arises from, involves, or compresses the optic nerve, can result in an optic neuropathy that may manifest as a relative afferent pupillary defect or reduction of color vision before there is reduction of visual acuity. In addition, visual impairment may be caused by compression of the globe resulting in distortion of the retina and possible elevation of intraocular pressure.

Limitation of ocular movements resulting in binocular diplopia (double vision) may be due to direct involvement of the extraocular muscles, interference with their mechanisms of action, or dysfunction of the third (oculomotor), fourth (trochlear), or sixth (abducens) cranial nerves. Pain may occur as a result of rapid expansion or inflammation or the orbital tissues or infiltration of sensory nerves.

Disease involving the superior orbital fissure produces a characteristic combination (**superior orbital fissure syndrome**) of diplopia (third, fourth, and/or sixth cranial nerves), corneal and facial anesthesia (first [ophthalmic] division of fifth [trigeminal] cranial nerve), and possible proptosis. Disease at the orbital apex also causes visual impairment because of second (optic) cranial nerve dysfunction (**orbital apex syndrome**). In the **cavernous sinus syndrome,** there is diplopia (third, fourth, and/or sixth cranial nerves) and fifth cranial nerve dysfunction, potentially involving all three divisions. There may be proptosis due to venous congestion. Vision is spared unless there is sufficient expansion to compress the intracranial optic nerve or the optic chiasm.

DIAGNOSTIC STUDIES

▶ Computed Tomography and Magnetic Resonance Imaging

Computed tomography (CT) uses x-rays to create cross-sectional, two-dimensional images of the body (Figures 13–1 and 13–2). Modern-day scanners use spiral or helical technology where the x-ray source rotates continuously in one direction within a ring of detectors as the patient is moved

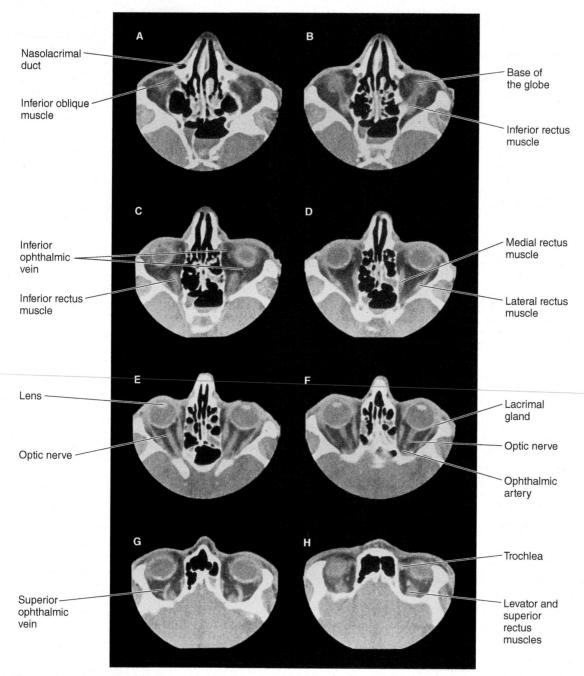

Nasolacrimal duct

Inferior oblique muscle

Base of the globe

Inferior rectus muscle

Inferior ophthalmic vein

Inferior rectus muscle

Medial rectus muscle

Lateral rectus muscle

Lens

Optic nerve

Lacrimal gland

Optic nerve

Ophthalmic artery

Superior ophthalmic vein

Trochlea

Levator and superior rectus muscles

▲ **Figure 13–1.** Normal computed tomography scan—axial sections (1.5 mm) demonstrating the anatomy of the orbit. **A–H:** Sequence of sections from inferior to superior orbit. Note the clear delineation of individual muscles, optic nerve, and major veins within the orbital fat.

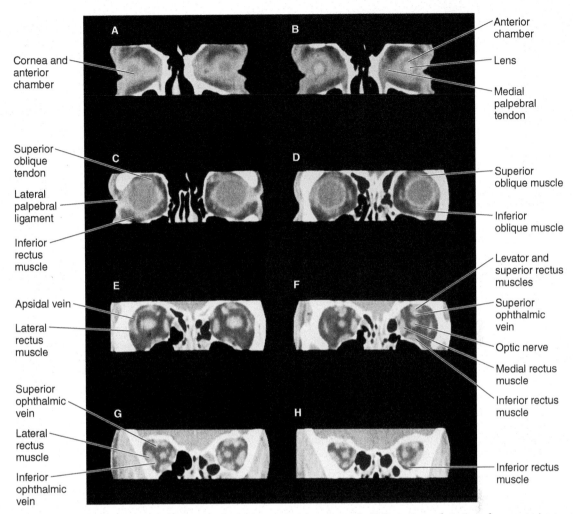

Cornea and anterior chamber
Anterior chamber
Lens
Medial palpebral tendon
Superior oblique tendon
Lateral palpebral ligament
Inferior rectus muscle
Superior oblique muscle
Inferior oblique muscle
Apsidal vein
Lateral rectus muscle
Levator and superior rectus muscles
Superior ophthalmic vein
Optic nerve
Medial rectus muscle
Inferior rectus muscle
Superior ophthalmic vein
Lateral rectus muscle
Inferior ophthalmic vein
Inferior rectus muscle

▲ Figure 13–2. Normal computed tomography scan—coronal sections. **A–H:** Sequence of sections from anterior to posterior orbit. Note the detailed demonstration of ocular and orbital structures.

forward through the ring. The data for the images are acquired quickly and as a continuous volume, allowing for a reduction of motion artifacts. Using complex algorithms, three-dimensional reconstructions can be rendered. The diagnostic capabilities of CT are essential to daily practice and have largely replaced the use of plain x-rays, especially for orbital trauma. **Magnetic resonance imaging** (MRI) generates cross-sectional images by taking advantage of the magnetic properties of atomic nuclei. Soft tissue visualization within the orbit is superior with this modality because of the near absence of signal created by bone and because resonance signals from different tissues can be manipulated to enhance contrast differentiation. Moreover, technological developments allow for suppression of the increased fat

signal in the orbit and thus provide better visualization of pathology. MRI is contraindicated in the presence of a suspected or known intraorbital or intracranial foreign body. It is the preferred study of choice in children to avoid unneeded radiation exposure when trauma is not of concern.

▶ **Ultrasonography**

CT and MRI have largely supplanted the use of ultrasonography in the diagnosis of orbital disease. Although it is a noninvasive and inexpensive form of imaging, its usefulness is limited to the anterior portion of the orbit. It is of greatest value in the hands of the clinician-ultrasonographer capable of interpreting "real-time" images. It can provide a noninvasive method of diagnosing carotid artery–cavernous sinus fistula and extraocular muscle enlargement due to Graves' ophthalmopathy.

Fine-Needle Aspiration Biopsy

Fine-needle aspiration biopsy is an invasive procedure that has proved useful in orbital diagnosis. Cytology specimens can be aspirated from a lesion, the exact location of which is determined by orbital imaging. Definitive pathological diagnosis is made more than 75% of the time.

DISEASES & DISORDERS OF THE ORBIT

INFLAMMATORY DISORDERS

1. GRAVES' OPHTHALMOPATHY (SEE ALSO CHAPTER 15)

Graves' ophthalmopathy (GO) (thyroid eye disease [TED], Graves' orbitopathy, thyroid-associated ophthalmopathy or orbitopathy) is an autoimmune disorder believed to result from activation of orbital fibroblasts by antibodies initially directed at the thyrotropin receptor of thyroid follicular endothelial cells. Once activated, these fibroblasts increase the production of mucopolysaccharides that accumulate in the extraocular muscles. In addition, differentiation of the fibroblasts to adipocytes and myoblasts results in expansion of orbital fat and fibrosis, respectively. GO usually occurs in association with autoimmune hyperthyroidism (Graves' disease), but the same disease process can occur in the euthyroid or hypothyroid states. It is associated with other autoimmune diseases, including myasthenia gravis, and can be exacerbated by cigarette smoking and radioactive iodine (RAI) therapy.

Clinical Findings

Some degree of mild eye disease, typically including upper eyelid retraction, occurs in a high percentage of hyperthyroid patients. Severe disease with marked proptosis and restricted ocular motility occurs in about 5–10% of cases of Graves' disease (Figure 13–3).

GO is the most common cause of unilateral or bilateral proptosis in adults. The accompanying upper eyelid retraction, manifesting as disproportionately greater exposure of sclera superiorly than inferiorly, and lid lag (von Graefe sign), manifesting as impaired descent of the upper eyelid on downward gaze, usually distinguish it from other causes of proptosis.

Ocular surface discomfort is common in all stages of the disease, in some cases due to superior limbic keratoconjunctivitis (see Chapter 5). Incomplete eyelid closure (lagophthalmos) results from proptosis and lid retraction, and corneal

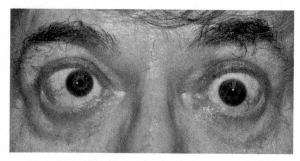

▲ **Figure 13–3.** Graves' ophthalmopathy.

exposure may be present even in mild cases. Ptosis in association with GO usually is due to coexistent myasthenia gravis, which may also contribute to ocular motility disturbance.

The extraocular muscle involvement of GO begins with lymphocytic infiltration and edema of the rectus muscles, typically the inferior and medial recti (Figure 13–4). The inflamed muscles subsequently may become fibrotic. Diplopia usually begins in the upper field of gaze due to asymmetric tethering of the inferior recti that also may cause elevation of intraocular pressure on upgaze or in primary gaze in severe cases. All extraocular muscles eventually may be involved with diplopia in all directions of gaze.

If the extraocular muscles become markedly enlarged, there may be compression of the optic nerve at the orbital apex that is not necessarily accompanied by significant proptosis. Early signs include a relative afferent pupillary defect and impairment of color vision, followed by reduction of visual acuity. Blindness may develop if the compression is not relieved.

Treatment

In the treatment of hyperthyroidism, the risk of GO is increased by untreated hypothyroidism; is less after thyroidectomy than after RAI; and seems to be reduced by statin therapy. After RAI, about 15% of patients develop new GO or have progression of pre-existing disease. This risk is decreased by a course of oral steroids after the RAI. There is negligible risk of exacerbation of inactive GO with RAI. RAI should be avoided in active smokers.

Management of GO should be multidisciplinary. An endocrinologist should manage the thyroid status, because optimal control is crucial to preventing more severe eye disease. GO activity should be graded using defined clinical activity scores. Therapy is adjusted according to disease severity.

Mild GO often manifests as ocular surface problems that usually can be controlled with topical lubricants. Oral selenium slows disease progression in mild active GO.

In moderate to severe GO, immunosuppressant therapy may be required. Pulsed intravenous glucocorticoid therapy is more efficacious with less adverse effects than oral or

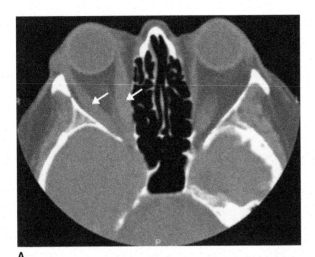

A

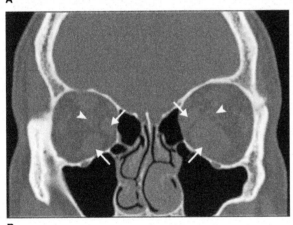

B

▲ **Figure 13–4.** Computed tomography scan of Graves' ophthalmopathy. **A:** Axial section demonstrates markedly enlarged medial and lateral recti of the right orbit **(arrows)**. **B:** Coronal section demonstrates optic nerves **(arrowheads)** and markedly enlarged medial and inferior recti in both orbits **(arrows)**.

retrobulbar steroids. Rituximab, a biologic that targets B cells, potentially provides better therapeutic outcomes than steroids. The benefit of orbital radiotherapy is less clear. It may offer more rapid improvement of inflammation and decrease the severity of diplopia. It is contraindicated in diabetic patients with retinopathy. For immediate treatment of exposure keratitis due to severe proptosis, lateral tarsorrhaphy or chemodenervation with botulinum toxin injection of the levator palpebrae superioris muscle may be considered.

Sight-threatening, compressive optic neuropathy or proptosis with severe exposure keratitis uncontrolled by lubricants requires emergency treatment initially with high-dose

systemic steroids ideally using pulsed intravenous glucocorticoids. If this is unsuccessful, surgical decompression of the orbit is usually performed.

GO is presumed to be a self-limiting disease but characterized by an active course of exacerbations and remissions, lasting months to years. Once disease activity has settled and a euthyroid state has been maintained for at least 6 months, surgical rehabilitation may be considered. Surgery is approached in a staged manner. When indicated, orbital decompression for proptosis is considered first, followed by strabismus surgery to correct ocular deviations and concluded by eyelid surgery to address malpositions.

Orbital decompression is indicated for proptosis resulting in keratitis that cannot be medically controlled or an unacceptable aesthetic appearance. Several techniques have been devised using external or transnasal endoscopic approaches. All aim to expand the orbital volume by removal of the bony walls, usually the medial wall, lateral wall, and/or floor. Because the primary goal of surgery is to shift the position of the globe more posteriorly in the orbit, there is a risk of causing or exacerbating diplopia. Thus, if decompression surgery is required, it is performed before strabismus surgery.

Double vision may not be sufficiently bothersome to require treatment. While the ophthalmopathy is active, prisms or eye occlusion may be helpful. As with decompression, strabismus surgery should not be undertaken until the ophthalmopathy is inactive and the ocular motility disturbance has been stable for at least 6 months. Tight muscles, usually the inferior and medial recti, are recessed. Most patients can achieve an area of binocular vision without diplopia in primary gaze. Botulinum toxin is rarely helpful in the acute or chronic stages of the disease. Some patients have intractable diplopia despite all attempts at correction.

Eyelid retraction may result in exposure keratitis and often in an aesthetically unappealing appearance. Orbital decompression may improve lid retraction, but some patients may forego this type surgery and opt for surgical correction of lid retraction only since it offers a lower risk profile and faster recovery and can camouflage proptosis to some extent. Small amounts (2 mm) of lid retraction can be corrected by disinserting the retractors from the upper tarsal border. For larger degrees of retraction, a graded full-thickness blepharotomy can be performed, or insertion of a spacer graft, such as banked scleral tissue, to lengthen the upper and lower lid can be considered.

2. NONSPECIFIC ORBITAL INFLAMMATION

Nonspecific orbital inflammation (NSOI) (idiopathic orbital inflammation or orbital inflammatory syndrome) is typically a unilateral process of rapid onset that presents with pain, periocular and conjunctival edema, proptosis, and diplopia. (The previous term *orbital pseudotumor* to indicate an orbital mass simulating a neoplasm with inflammatory histology is a confusing anachronism.) In the pediatric population, it more often presents as bilateral disease with accompanying uveitis, disk edema, and eosinophilia.

NSOI is characterized by a pleomorphic inflammatory response involving several cell types (eg, lymphocytes, fibroblasts, histiocytes, and/or plasma cells). The inflammatory process can be diffuse or localized, specifically involving any orbital structure (eg, myositis, dacryoadenitis, superior orbital fissure syndrome, or optic perineuritis). There may be extension to involve the cavernous sinuses and intracranial meninges. MRI helps to identify the involved tissues. The differential diagnosis includes GO, orbital lymphoma, and other specific types of orbital inflammation including sarcoidosis, granulomatosis with polyangiitis (Wegener's granulomatosis) and IgG4-related disease. Laboratory testing may sometimes indicate a more specific cause for inflammation.

Systemic treatment with glucocorticosteroids is typically the first line. Recurrence or lack of treatment response is common, and alternative nonspecific (eg, cyclophosphamide) or biologic (eg, infliximab) immunosuppressants should be considered. It is unclear if radiotherapy is beneficial as the studies involve small cohorts and different protocols with a significant number of patients having partial or no response. Surgery is reserved for biopsy to establish the diagnosis or rarely for surgical debulking or exenteration in cases of refractory disease once vision has been irreparably lost.

ORBITAL INFECTIONS

1. ORBITAL CELLULITIS AND PRESEPTAL CELLULITIS

Orbital cellulitis is a bacterial infection located posterior to the orbital septum (postseptal). It is the most common cause of proptosis in children. Immediate treatment is essential because delay can lead to blindness due to optic nerve compression or infarction, or rarely death from septic cavernous sinus thrombosis or intracranial sepsis. Although most cases occur in children, elderly and immunocompromised individuals may also be affected.

The majority of cases of childhood orbital cellulitis arise from extension of acute sinusitis through the thin ethmoid bone via emissary veins. The organisms usually responsible are *Staphylococcus aureus* with an increasing number of cases caused by methicillin-resistant *S aureus* (MRSA), *Streptococcus anginosus*, *Streptococcus pneumonia*, and *Streptococcus pyogenes*. *Haemophilus influenzae* type B (Hib) infection is infrequently seen because of Hib immunization. In adolescents and adults, when there is often chronic sinus infection, anaerobic organisms may also be involved, and there is a higher risk of intracranial infection. If there is a history of penetrating trauma, *S aureus*, including MRSA, and *S pyogenes* are commonly responsible.

In comparison, **preseptal cellulitis** is a bacterial infection superficial to the orbital septum. It is usually caused by infection arising within the eyelid from a hordeolum (see Chapter 4), recent lid surgery, traumatic wound, or an insect or animal bite. Predominate pathogens include *S aureus* and *Streptococcus* species.

▶ Clinical Findings

Orbital cellulitis is characterized by fever, pain, eyelid edema and erythema, proptosis, chemosis, limitation of extraocular movements, and leukocytosis (Figure 13–5A). Nonaxial proptosis suggests subperiosteal or intraorbital abscess. Extension to the cavernous sinus can produce contralateral orbital involvement, trigeminal dysfunction, and more marked systemic illness. Intracranial extension can result in subdural empyema and meningitis. Few orbital processes, other than fungal disease, progress as rapidly as bacterial infections.

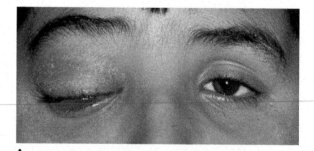

A

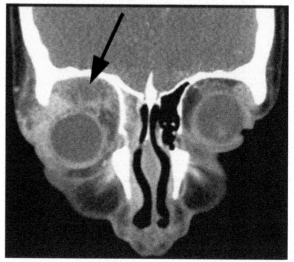

B

▲ **Figure 13–5. A:** Orbital cellulitis secondary to frontal sinusitis. **B:** Coronal computed tomography scan shows right orbital abscess **(arrow).**

Preseptal cellulitis may also mimic the initial stages of orbital cellulitis; however, there is lack of proptosis, chemosis, or limitation of extraocular movements. Other entities to be considered are rhabdomyosarcoma in children, GO, and NSOI.

A CT scan or MRI provides essential information regarding the source and extent of infection (Figure 13–5B). MRI is preferred over CT to detect cavernous sinus thrombosis and organic foreign bodies. Plain x-rays are rarely performed.

▶ Treatment

Treatment of orbital cellulitis should be initiated before the causative organism is identified. As soon as nasal, conjunctival, and blood cultures are obtained, antibiotics should be administered. Intravenous therapy is preferred with a third-generation cephalosporin (eg, cefotaxime or ceftriaxone) or a β-lactamase–resistant drug, such as nafcillin, imipenem, or piperacillin/tazobactam. Vancomycin is also typically administered to cover for MRSA. Possible anaerobic infection requires addition of metronidazole or clindamycin. For patients with penicillin hypersensitivity, vancomycin, levofloxacin, and metronidazole are recommended. Success with oral ciprofloxacin and clindamycin has been reported in uncomplicated cases.

Early consultation with an otolaryngologist is important for sinus infections. Nasal decongestants and vasoconstrictors help drain the paranasal sinuses. Observation for antibiotic response may be considered in children aged less than 9 years with a medial, subperiosteal abscess of modest size and without compromised vision. Otherwise surgical drainage of the abscess should be performed in conjunction with functional endoscopic sinus surgery to address the source of infection.

Preseptal cellulitis can usually be treated with oral antibiotics, such as amoxicillin/clavulanate, but the patient should be monitored closely for development of postseptal involvement. Therapy should be adjusted if there is high likelihood of MRSA infection, for a dirty wound, or if the patient is immunocompromised, in which case gram-negative organisms should be covered.

2. ACUTE FULMINANT INVASIVE FUNGAL SINUSITIS

Acute fulminant invasive fungal sinusitis (AFIFS) (zygomycosis, mucormycosis) occurs predominately in patients with severe immunosuppression. AFIFS is usually due to *Aspergillus* species or fungi from the class Zygomycetes, including *Rhizopus*, *Rhizomucor*, *Absidia*, and *Mucor*. In 80% of diabetic patients, a species of Zygomycetes is responsible, and in 80% of neutropenic patients, *Aspergillus* is responsible. The fungi invade blood vessels, leading to ischemic necrosis. Infection usually begins in the sinuses and spreads into the orbit, resulting in periorbital edema, ptosis, ophthalmoplegia, visual loss, and proptosis. Central nervous system involvement may manifest as decreased mentation. Examination of the nose and palate characteristically reveals black, necrotic mucosa, a smear of which demonstrates branching hyphae.

Without treatment, the infection quickly invades the intracranial space, resulting in meningitis, brain abscess, and death usually within days to weeks. Treatment is fraught with difficulties and often inadequate. It consists of reversing the underlying immunosuppression if possible, administration of intravenous antifungal agents (including amphotericin B, caspofungin, and/or posaconazole) and surgical debridement. Local injections of amphotericin B in the orbit may also be considered.

CYSTIC LESIONS INVOLVING THE ORBIT

1. DERMOID AND EPIDERMOID CYSTS

Dermoid and epidermoid cysts are not true neoplasms but benign choristomas arising from embryonic tissue not usually found in the orbit. They originate from surface ectoderm and are lined by a keratinizing epithelium. A dermoid cyst contains epithelial structures such as keratin, hair, and even sometimes teeth, while an epidermoid cyst is filled with keratin but lacks dermal appendages. The contents of either type of cyst can incite a severe inflammatory reaction if liberated into the orbit. Preseptal dermoid and epidermoid cysts most commonly occur at the lateral brow at the frontozygomatic suture, but may develop at any suture line (Figure 13–6). Cysts that are within the orbit typically occur in the superior temporal quadrant and do not present until adulthood. CT scan demonstrates a sharp, round bony defect from the pressure of a slowly growing mass affixed to the periosteum. En-bloc surgical removal with preservation of the cyst wall during surgery is the treatment of choice.

2. SINUS MUCOCELE

Obstruction of drainage from a paranasal sinus may lead to a benign, expansile, mucus-filled cyst called a sinus mucocele.

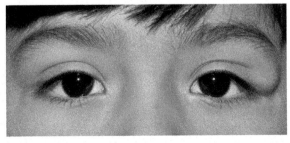

▲ **Figure 13–6.** Dermoid cyst of the left frontozygomatic suture.

Frontal or ethmoid sinus mucoceles typically present with progressive nonaxial proptosis, whereas sphenoid sinus mucoceles present with optic neuropathy (Figure 13–7). Presentation may be rapid if there is associated infection. CT scan is usually diagnostic. MRI may be required to differentiate from a dermoid cyst and to define the extent of the lesion. Preferred treatment is endoscopic sinus surgery performed by otolaryngology to marsupialize the cyst and reestablish sinus drainage.

3. MENINGOCELE

Extension of meninges into the orbital cavity through a congenital dehiscence in the bony sutures creates a cystic mass filled with cerebrospinal fluid known as a meningocele. If there is also brain tissue, it is known as a meningoencephalocele.

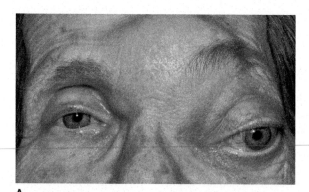

A

B

▲ **Figure 13–7. A:** Frontoethmoidal mucocele involving left orbit. **B:** Axial computed tomography scan.

The resultant fluctuant mass in the superior medial orbit typically enlarges with Valsalva maneuver. Most cases are present at birth, but those arising from the sphenoid bone may not become apparent until adolescence. Surgical treatment typically involves a multidisciplinary approach for resection and dural reconstruction.

VASCULAR ABNORMALITIES INVOLVING THE ORBIT

1. ARTERIOVENOUS MALFORMATION

Arteriovenous malformations are an uncommon cause of proptosis. Orbital venous anomalies (varices) produce intermittent proptosis, sometimes associated with pain and transient reduction of vision. There may be acute exacerbations due to hemorrhage. On examination, some degree of proptosis can be induced with Valsalva maneuver or by placing the head in a dependent position. MRI is usually diagnostic. Endovascular embolization is the preferred method of treatment. Surgical excision is very challenging because the anomaly is often intimately associated with orbital structures, and thus, there is risk of permanent visual impairment.

2. CAROTID-CAVERNOUS FISTULA

A carotid-cavernous fistula (CCF) results from an abnormal communication between the carotid artery and the venous cavernous sinus. Direct, high-flow fistulas are from a communication between the internal carotid artery (ICA) and the cavernous sinus. They usually follow severe head trauma and are less commonly due to spontaneous rupture of an intracavernous ICA aneurysm. Physical signs include dilated conjunctival vessels, marked orbital congestion with chemosis, pulsating proptosis, prominent orbital bruit, raised intraocular pressure, retinal hemorrhages, and ophthalmoplegia.

Indirect, low-flow fistulas occur between dural branches of the external or internal carotid artery and the cavernous sinus. They are usually spontaneous, more commonly occurring in elderly females, and can be associated with systemic hypertension, atherosclerotic disease, pregnancy, connective tissue disease, and minor trauma. Diagnosis may be delayed because of confusion with other entities such as chronic conjunctivitis. Orbital congestion, arterializations of episcleral vessels, raised intraocular pressure, mild proptosis, and a possible faint bruit are the typical features.

Orbital ultrasound with color Doppler imaging provides a noninvasive method of diagnosing a CCF by demonstrating arterialized blood flow in the superior ophthalmic vein. CT or magnetic resonance angiography provides more definitive diagnosis. However, the gold standard is by catheter angiography that allows characterization of the fistula's blood supply and drainage. Glaucoma, diplopia, intolerable bruit or headache, and severe proptosis are the main indications for intervention. Direct fistulas generally need to be treated by transarterial or transvenous embolization with coils, particles, glue, or balloons. Many indirect CCFs resolve spontaneously, but embolization may sometimes be required, such as to treat cerebral cortical venous hypertension. Radiotherapy, intermittent manual self-compression of the affected ICA, and occlusion of the ipsilateral ICA have also been described as treatment for indirect CCFs.

PRIMARY ORBITAL TUMORS

CAPILLARY HEMANGIOMA

Capillary hemangiomas are the most common benign orbital tumor in children (Figure 13–8). Superficial lesions involving the eyelid are reddish (strawberry nevus) in color, and deeper lesions of the orbit are more bluish. Over 90% become apparent before the age of 6 months. They tend to enlarge rapidly in the first year of life and regress slowly over 6–7 years. Lesions within the orbit may cause strabismus, proptosis, or compressive optic neuropathy. Involvement of the eyelids may induce astigmatism or occlude vision, resulting in amblyopia.

Systemic or intralesional steroids were the standard first-line therapy. A systemic beta-blocker, typically propranolol, also is effective. Treatment is initially performed in a hospital setting to monitor for potential side effects including shortness of breath, bradycardia, and hypoglycemia. Surgery is typically reserved for refractory cases or those with visual compromise.

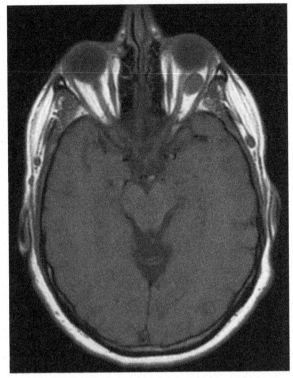

▲ **Figure 13–9.** Axial magnetic resonance imaging of intraconal cavernous hemangioma of left orbit abutting the optic nerve.

CAVERNOUS HEMANGIOMA

Cavernous hemangiomas are the most common benign orbital tumor in adults (Figure 13–9). They more frequently occur in women and most often lie within the muscle cone, producing axial proptosis, hyperopia, and choroidal folds. Unlike capillary hemangiomas, they do not tend to regress spontaneously. Surgical excision is usually successful and is indicated if the patient is symptomatic. Alternatively, for masses involving the orbital apex or extending intracranially that pose a surgical challenge, radiotherapy may be considered.

LYMPHANGIOMA

Lymphangioma is an uncommon tumor of the orbit that presents in the first decade of life. Unlike a capillary hemangioma, the tumor does not regress and is characterized by bouts of intermittent proptosis, especially during upper respiratory illnesses likely because of lymphoid tissue within the tumor. Spontaneous hemorrhage results in large blood cysts that may cause proptosis, diplopia, and compressive optic neuropathy, requiring evacuation.

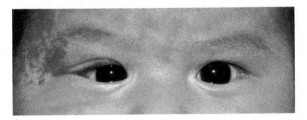

A

B

▲ **Figure 13–8.** Capillary hemangioma with cutaneous and orbital involvement on the right side resulting in esotropia. **A:** Before treatment. **B:** Near resolution after 4 months of treatment with systemic propranolol.

The tumor is often multifocal and frequently also occurs in the soft palate and other areas of the face. It is best visualized with MRI. On histologic examination, it consists of large serum-filled channels lined by endothelial cells and lymphoid follicles scattered in the interstitium. Treatment is either for acute decompression of a hemorrhagic blood cyst or resection of the tumor. Needle aspiration of blood or extirpation of a specific cyst may be temporarily effective. Surgical excision is difficult and seldom satisfactory, as complete resection is often not possible. Percutaneous sclerotherapy has been shown to be a potentially better treatment option.

RHABDOMYOSARCOMA

Rhabdomyosarcoma is the most common primary malignant orbital tumor in childhood. Presentation is before age 10 and rapid growth is characteristic with proptosis and/or downward globe displacement, as two-thirds of these tumors are located in the superonasal orbit (Figure 13–10). The tumor may destroy adjacent orbital bone and spread into the brain. Treatment depends on staging and includes surgery, chemotherapy, and/or radiotherapy. Survival rates have drastically improved for these patients from less than 50%, when orbital exenteration was used, to over 90%.

NEUROFIBROMA

Neurofibromatosis type 1 (NF1) (von Recklinghausen's disease) is an autosomal dominant inherited disease due to mutations in neurofibromin 1, a tumor suppressor gene located on chromosome 17q. Plexiform neurofibromas are characteristic and can distort the eyelids and disfigure the orbit (Figure 13–11). The presence of iris Lisch nodules and cutaneous cafe au lait spots helps confirm the diagnosis. Sphenoid wing dysplasia results in pulsating exophthalmos or enophthalmos. Fifteen percent of patients may develop an optic nerve glioma that can manifest as proptosis and/or visual loss. Some of these patients also develop meningiomas and, rarely, malignant peripheral nerve sheath tumors.

OPTIC NERVE GLIOMA

Approximately 75% of symptomatic optic nerve gliomas become apparent before age 10. Thirty percent are associated with NF1. They are classified as low-grade astrocytomas. Those anterior to the chiasm tend to behave in a benign fashion and may regress spontaneously; those in and posterior to the chiasm may be more aggressive. Visual loss and optic atrophy are the most common signs. Proptosis occurs if the tumor is in the orbit.

Treatment is controversial. Some believe that these tumors do not require treatment, and others advocate surgical excision, radiotherapy, or chemotherapy. If progressive tumor growth and visual loss can be clearly documented, radiotherapy is often effective in stabilizing or even improving vision.

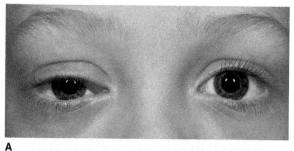

A

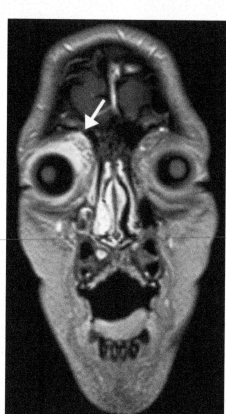

B

▲ **Figure 13–10. A:** Rhabdomyosarcoma of the right orbit. **B:** Coronal magnetic resonance imaging showing tumor in the superonasal orbit **(arrow).**

In blind eyes with marked proptosis, the patient's aesthetic appearance can often be improved by excising the tumor through a lateral orbitotomy.

LACRIMAL GLAND TUMORS

Fifty percent of masses of the lacrimal gland are epithelial tumors, of which 50% are malignant, and the other 50% of masses are inflammatory or lymphoproliferative tumors. The

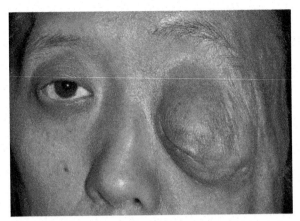

Figure 13–11. Plexiform neurofibroma involving left face, lids, and orbit in neurofibromatosis type 1.

most common benign epithelial tumor is the **pleomorphic adenoma** (benign mixed tumor), which should be excised— not biopsied—because of their propensity for recurrence and malignant transformation.

Of malignant epithelial tumors of the lacrimal gland, 60% are comprised of **adenoid cystic carcinoma**, which typically presents with pain, nonaxial proptosis, and destructive bony changes of the superotemporal fossa on CT scan. Biopsy should be performed through the eyelid to avoid tumor seeding in the orbit. Radical treatment of this highly malignant tumor with orbital exenteration and ostectomy has failed to demonstrate improved long-term survival. Instead, some choose to perform high-dose radiotherapy with exenteration or surgical debulking. Brachytherapy to the lacrimal fossa is another option. Despite these measures, perineural intracranial extension or systemic metastases often occur 10 to 15 years after initial presentation. More recently, a protocol of neoadjuvant intracarotid cytoreductive chemotherapy followed by exenteration, radiotherapy, and systemic chemotherapy has demonstrated improved survival in a small, retrospective, interventional cohort.

LYMPHOMA

Lymphoproliferative tumors of the orbit range from benign reactive lymphoid hyperplasia to malignant lymphoma, the most common of which is extranodal marginal zone lymphoma or mucosa-associated lymphoid tissue (MALT). Lymphoma accounts for 24% of all orbital malignancies in patients greater than 59 years of age. It can appear solely in the orbit or be a manifestation of systemic disease. Presentation is typically of a painless, slowly enlarging orbital mass that can sometime be palpated through the eyelid. Orbital imaging typically reveals an ovoid mass that molds to the globe and orbit without bony erosion. Patients also

require a systemic workup with an oncologist for staging using the World Health Organization classification. Fifty percent of patients with orbital lymphoma will have systemic disease. Biopsy allows for classification of the lymphoma using flow cytometry, immunohistochemical staining, and DNA hybridization. The prognosis for both polyclonal lymphoid proliferations and well-differentiated B-cell monoclonal lesions is excellent. If disease is confined to the orbit, management is with radiation. For systemic lymphoma, treatment is chemotherapy. Among patients with lymphoma confined to the orbit at presentation, the overall risk of systemic lymphoma at 10 years is 33% and more likely if presentation is with bilateral orbital disease.

LANGERHANS CELL HISTIOCYTOSIS

Proliferation of Langerhans cells with characteristic cytoplasmic granules comprises a spectrum of disease that includes what were formerly classified as unifocal and multifocal eosinophilic granuloma, Hand-Schuller-Christian disease (multifocal lytic skull lesion, proptosis, and diabetes insipidus), and Letterer-Siwe disease (cutaneous, visceral, and lymph node involvement). The younger the child is at the time of diagnosis, the greater is the chance of multifocal disease. Unifocal disease of the orbit can be treated with surgical curettement and/or intralesional corticosteroid injections.

METASTATIC TUMORS

Metastatic tumors reach the orbit by hematogenous spread. In adults, breast, lung, and prostate cancer and melanoma are the usual primaries. In children, the most common metastatic tumor is neuroblastoma, which is often associated with spontaneous periocular hemorrhage as the rapidly growing tumor becomes necrotic. Metastatic tumors are much more common in the choroid than in the orbit, probably because of the nature of the blood supply.

Many metastatic orbital tumors respond to radiation and some to chemotherapy. Small localized tumors that are symptomatic can sometimes be completely or partially excised. Neuroblastomas in children under 11 months have a relatively good prognosis. In contrast, adults with orbital metastasis generally have a poor life expectancy.

SECONDARY TUMORS

Basal cell, squamous cell, and sebaceous gland carcinomas may initially invade the anterior orbit and continue to spread posteriorly. Nasopharyngeal carcinomas, most commonly from the maxillary sinus and intracranial meningiomas, can also invade the orbit, the latter by spreading along the optic nerve sheath.

REFERENCES

Acharya SH et al: Radioidoine therapy (RAI) for Graves' disease (GD) and the effect on ophthalmopathy: A systematic review. Clin Endocrinol 2008;69:943. [PMID: 18429949]

Andrew N et al: IgG4-related orbital disease: A meta-analysis and review. Acta Ophthalmol 2013;91:694. [PMID: 22963447]

Andrew NH et al: Lymphoid hyperplasia of the orbit and ocular adnexa: A clinical pathologic review. Surv Ophthalmol 2016;61:778. [PMID: 27127077]

Avery RA et al: Orbital/periorbital plexiform neurofibromas in children with neurofibromatosis type 1: Multidisciplinary recommendations for care. Ophthalmology 2017;124:123. [PMID: 27817916]

Bahn RS: Graves' ophthalmopathy. N Engl J Med 2010;362:726. [PMID: 20181974]

Bartalena L et al: The 2016 European Thyroid Association/European Group on Graves' Orbitopathy guidelines for the management of Graves' orbitopathy. Eur Thyroid J 2016;5:9. [PMID: 27099835]

Bhatti MT et al: Thyroid eye disease: Therapy in the active phase. J Neuroophthalmol 2014;34:186. [PMID: 24821102]

Boboridis KG et al: Surgical orbital decompression for thyroid eye disease. Cochrane Database Syst Rev 2011;12:CD007630. [PMID: 22161415]

Bradley EA et al: Orbital radiation for Graves' ophthalmopathy: A report by the American Academy of Ophthalmology. Ophthalmology 2008;115:398. [PMID: 18082885]

Cannon PS et al: Our experience using primary oral antibiotics in the management of orbital cellulitis in a tertiary referral centre. Eye 2009;23:612. [PMID: 18309335]

Carruth BP et al: Inflammatory modulators and biologic agents in the treatment of idiopathic orbital inflammation. Curr Opin Ophthalmol. 2012;23:420. [PMID: 22729181]

Demirci H et al: Orbital lymphoproliferative tumors: Analysis of clinical features and systemic involvement in 160 cases. Ophthalmology 2008;115:1626. [PMID: 18440641]

Dodgshun AJ et al: Long-term visual outcome after chemotherapy for optic pathway glioma in children: Site and age are strongly predictive. Cancer 2015;121:4190. [PMID: 26280460]

Dolman PJ et al: Orbital radiotherapy for thyroid eye disease. Curr Opin Ophthalmol 2012;23:427. [PMID: 22729183]

Esmaili N et al: Langerhans cell histiocytosis of the orbit: Spectrum of disease and risk of central nervous system sequelae in unifocal cases. Ophthal Plast Reconstr Surg 2016;32:28. [PMID: 25689784]

European Group on Graves' Orbitopathy (EUGOGO): Outcome of orbital decompression for disfiguring proptosis in patients with Graves' orbitopathy using various surgical procedures. Br J Ophthalmol 2009;93:1518. [PMID: 19028743]

Gao Y et al: Lacrimal gland masses. AJR Am J Roentgenol 2013;201:W371. [PMID: 23971467]

Gerring RC et al: Orbital exenteration for advanced periorbital non-melanoma skin cancer: Prognostic factors and survival. Eye (Lond) 2016 Oct 21. [Epub ahead of print] [PMID: 27768120]

Gorovoy IR et al: Fungal rhinosinusitis and imaging modalities. Saudi J Ophthalmol 2012;26:419. [PMID: 23961027]

Hill RH 3rd, et al: Percutaneous drainage and ablation as first line therapy for macrocystic and microcystic orbital lymphatic malformations. Ophthal Plast Reconstr Surg 2012;28:119. [PMID: 22366666]

Kang IG et al: Effect of endoscopic marsupialization of paranasal sinus mucoceles involving the orbit: A review of 27 cases. Eur Arch Otorhinolaryngol 2014;271:293. [PMID: 23644998]

Karra E et al: Clinical assessment of patients with thyroid eye disease. Br J Hosp Med (Lond) 2016;77:C2. [PMID: 26903467]

Karra E et al: Management of patients with thyroid eye disease. Br J Hosp Med (Lond) 2016;77:C6. [PMID: 26903468]

Léauté-Labrèze C et al. Propranolol for severe hemangiomas of infancy. N Engl J Med 2008;358:2649. [PMID: 18550886]

Liao JC et al: Subperiosteal abscess of the orbit: Evolving pathogens and the therapeutic protocol. Ophthalmology 2015;122:639. [PMID: 25439602]

Lowery AJ et al: Graves' ophthalmopathy: The case for thyroid surgery. Surgeon 2009;7:290. [PMID: 19848063]

Marcocci C et al: European Group on Graves' Orbitopathy. Selenium and the course of mild Graves' orbitopathy. N Engl J Med 2011;364:1920. [PMID: 21591944]

McKinsley SH et al: Microbiology of pediatric orbital cellulitis. Am J Ophthalmol 2007;144:497. [PMID: 17698020]

Nassiri N et al: Orbital lymphaticovenous malformations: Current and future treatments. Surv Ophthalmol 2015;60:383. [PMID: 26077629]

Pakdaman MN et al: Orbital inflammatory disease: Pictorial review and differential diagnosis. World J Radiol 2014;6:106. [PMID: 24778772]

Patel P et al: Recurrent thyroid eye disease. Ophthal Plast Reconstr Surg 2015;31:445. [PMID: 25621464]

Payne SJ et al: Acute invasive fungal rhinosinusitis: A 15-year experience with 41 patients. Otolaryngol Head Neck Surg 2016;154:759. [PMID: 26884367]

Ponto KA et al: The tale of radioiodine and Graves' orbitopathy. Thyroid 2010;20:785. [PMID: 20578895]

Rajendram R et al: Orbital radiotherapy for adult thyroid eye disease. Cochrane Database Syst Rev 2012;7:CD007114. [PMID: 22786503]

Raney RB et al: Results of the Intergroup Rhabdomyosarcoma Study Group D9602 protocol, using vincristine and dactinomycin with or without cyclophosphamide and radiation therapy, for newly diagnosed patients with low-risk embryonal rhabdomyosarcoma: a report from the Soft Tissue Sarcoma Committee of the Children's Oncology Group. J Clin Oncol 2011;29:1312. [PMID: 21357783]

Rootman DB et al: Stereotactic fractionated radiotherapy for cavernous venous malformations (hemangioma) of the orbit. Ophthal Plast Reconstr Surg 2012;28:96. [PMID: 22410657]

Rose GE et al: Acute presentation of vascular disease within the orbit: A descriptive synopsis of mechanisms. Eye 2013;27:299. [PMID: 23370421]

Salvi M et al: Efficacy of B-cell targeted therapy with rituximab in patients with active moderate to severe Graves' orbitopathy: A randomized controlled study. J Clin Endocrinol Metab 2015;100:422. [PMID: 25494967]

Shapey J et al: Diagnosis and management of optic nerve glioma. J Clin Neurosci 2011;18:1585. [PMID: 22071462]

Shields JA et al: Orbital cysts of childhood: Classification, clinical features, and management. Surv Ophthalmol 2004;49:281. [PMID: 15110666]

Stein JD et al: Risk factors for developing thyroid-associated ophthalmopathy among individuals with Graves disease. JAMA Ophthalmol 2015;133:290. [PMID: 25502604]

Stiebel-Kalish H et al: Treatment modalities for Graves' ophthalmopathy: Systematic review and metaanalysis. J Clin Endocrinol Metab 2009;94:2708. [PMID: 19491222]

Swerdlow SH et al: *WHO Classification of Tumours of Haematopoietic and Lymphoid Tissues*, 4th ed. Lyon: IARC Press, 2008.

Tanda ML et al: Prevalence and natural history of Graves' orbitopathy in a large series of patients with newly diagnosed graves' hyperthyroidism seen at a single center. J Clin Endocrinol Metab 2013;98:1443. [PMID:23408569]

Taubenslag KJ et al: Management of frontal sinusitis-associated subperiosteal abscess in children less than 9 years of age. J AAPOS 2016;20:527. [PMID: 27810421]

Tse DT et al: Long-term outcomes of neoadjuvant intra-arterial cytoreductive chemotherapy for lacrimal gland adenoid cystic carcinoma. Ophthalmology 2013;120:1313. [PMID: 23582989]

Uhumwangho OM et al: Current trends in treatment outcomes of orbital cellulitis in a tertiary hospital in Southern Nigeria. Niger J Surg 2016;22:107. [PMID: 27843275]

Valenzuela AA et al: Orbital metastasis: Clinical features, management and outcome. Orbit 2009;28:153. [PMID: 19839900]

Verity DH et al: Acute thyroid eye disease (TED): Principles of medical and surgical management. Eye 2013;27:308. [PMID: 23412559]

von Holstein SL et al: Epithelial tumours of the lacrimal gland: A clinical, histopathological, surgical and oncological survey. Acta Ophthalmol 2013;91:195. [PMID: 22471335]

Winegar BA et al: Imaging of orbital trauma and emergent non-traumatic conditions. Neuroimaging Clin N Am 2015;25:439. [PMID: 26208419]

Zanaty M et al: Endovascular treatment of carotid-cavernous fistulas. Neurosurg Clin N Am 2014;25:551. [PMID: 24994090]

Zuniga MG et al: Treatment outcomes in acute invasive fungal rhinosinusitis. Curr Opin Otolaryngol Head Neck Surg 2014;22:242. [PMID: 24756031]

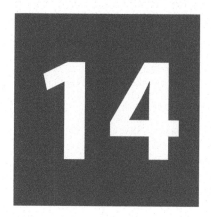

Neuro-Ophthalmology

Paul Riordan-Eva, FRCOphth

The retinas and anterior visual pathways (optic nerves, optic chiasm, and optic tracts) (Figures 14–1 and 14–2) are an integral part of the brain, providing a substantial proportion of its total sensory input. The pattern of visual field loss indicates the site of damage in the visual pathway (Figures 14–3 to 14–5). Eye movement disorders may be due to disease of cranial nerves III, IV, or VI, or a more central lesion. Cranial nerves V and VII are also intimately associated with ocular function.

THE OPTIC NERVE

A wide variety of diseases affect the optic nerve (Table 14–1). Clinical features indicative of optic nerve disease are reduction of visual acuity and field, afferent pupillary defect, poor color vision, and optic disk changes.

Optic disk swelling occurs predominantly in diseases directly affecting the anterior portion of the optic nerve but also occurs with raised intracranial pressure (papilledema) and compression of the intraorbital optic nerve. It is also a feature of central retinal vein occlusion, ocular hypotony, and intraocular inflammation. Peripapillary exudates occur with optic disk swelling due to inflammation (papillitis), ischemic optic neuropathy, raised intracranial pressure, or severe systemic hypertension. The term *neuroretinitis* for retinal exudates, including a macular star, due to optic disk swelling of whatever cause is a misnomer in that there is no inflammation of the retina, the exudates being a response to the anterior optic nerve disease (Figure 14–6A). The term is more reasonably applied if there is inflammation of the retina and optic nerve (Figure 14–6B).

Optic atrophy (Figure 14–7) is a nonspecific response to optic nerve damage from any cause and also occurs in primary retinal disease, such as central retinal artery occlusion or retinitis pigmentosa. In general, in optic nerve disease, there is a correlation between degree of optic disk pallor and loss of acuity, visual field, color vision, and pupillary responses, but the relationship varies according to the underlying etiology.

An important exception to this rule is compressive optic neuropathy, in which optic disk pallor is generally a late manifestation such that the optic disk may be normal even when there is severe reduction of visual acuity and field. Hereditary optic neuropathies usually produce bilateral temporal disk pallor with preferential loss of papillomacular axons.

Excavation of the optic nerve head (optic disk cupping) is generally but not necessarily a sign of glaucomatous optic neuropathy (see Chapter 11).

1. OPTIC NEURITIS (INFLAMMATORY OPTIC NEUROPATHY)

The most common cause of optic neuritis is demyelinative disease, including the typical acute demyelinative optic neuropathy that is associated with multiple sclerosis. Retrobulbar means that the optic disk is normal during the acute stage, whereas papillitis means that the optic disk is swollen. Loss of vision is the cardinal symptom of optic neuritis and is particularly useful in differentiating papillitis (Figure 14–8) from papilledema (Figure 14–9), with which it may be confused on ophthalmoscopic examination.

Because of major differences in management and outcome, optic neuritis is classified as typical or atypical.

Typical Optic Neuritis (Acute Demyelinative Optic Neuropathy)

- **Epidemiology**

  - Usually unilateral

  - Three times more common in women

  - Mostly age 20–40

  - Associated with multiple sclerosis in up to 85% of cases

  - (In children, more likely to be bilateral and parainfectious or postimmunization)

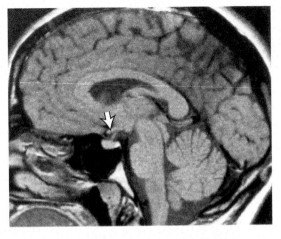
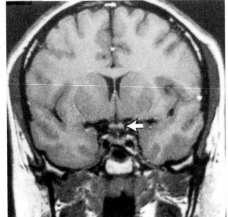
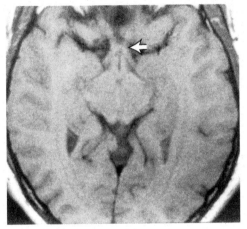

▲ **Figure 14–1.** Magnetic resonance imaging of normal brain in sagittal section **(upper left),** coronal section **(upper right),** and axial section **(lower left).** The white arrows indicate the chiasm.

- **Clinical features**

  - Subacute loss of vision developing over 2–7 days

  - Reduced visual acuity (one-third better than 20/40, one-third worse than 20/200)

  - Visual field defect

  - Reduced color vision

  - Reduced pupillary response to light shone in the affected (relative afferent pupillary defect)

  - Periocular pain in 90%, exacerbated by eye movement in 50%

  - Optic disk

    ○ Normal during acute phase in two-thirds (retrobulbar optic neuritis)

    ○ Mildly swollen in acute phase in one-third (papillitis)

    ○ In children, swollen optic disk in acute phase in two-thirds

    ○ Retinal exudates and cotton-wool spots do not occur and are suggestive of an infectious etiology

  - No associated systemic illness

  - Usually spontaneous recovery of vision with visual acuity better than 20/30 within 2 weeks

- **Differential diagnoses**

  - Retrobulbar optic neuritis

    ○ Optic nerve compression

  - Papillitis

    ○ Anterior ischemic optic neuropathy

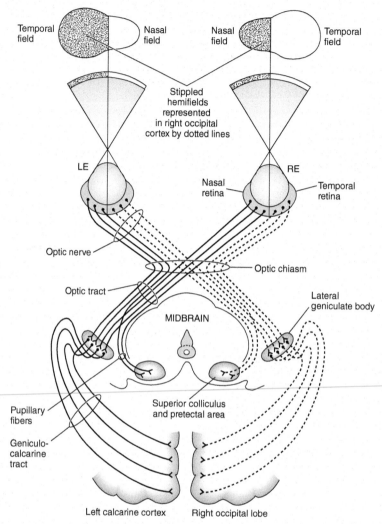

▲ **Figure 14–2.** The optic pathway. The dotted lines represent nerve fibers that carry visual and pupillary afferent impulses from the left half of the visual field.

○ Papilledema

○ Atypical optic neuritis

- **Investigation**
  - If there is the expected recovery of vision, no investigation is needed, but if magnetic resonance imaging (MRI) scans are performed:
    ○ Optic nerve MRI shows gadolinium enhancement, increased signal, and sometimes swelling of the affected nerve.
    ○ Brain MRI may show cerebral, brainstem, and/or cerebellar white matter lesions.

- If continuing deterioration of vision after 2 weeks or no recovery after 6 weeks, investigate for other conditions.

- **Treatment**
  - Steroid therapy (intravenously [methylprednisolone, 1 g/d for 3 days with or without a subsequent tapering course of oral prednisolone] or orally [methylprednisolone, 500 mg/d to 2 g/d for 3–5 days with or without subsequent oral prednisolone, or prednisolone, 1 mg/kg/d tapered over 10–21 days]) accelerates recovery of vision but does not influence the final visual outcome.

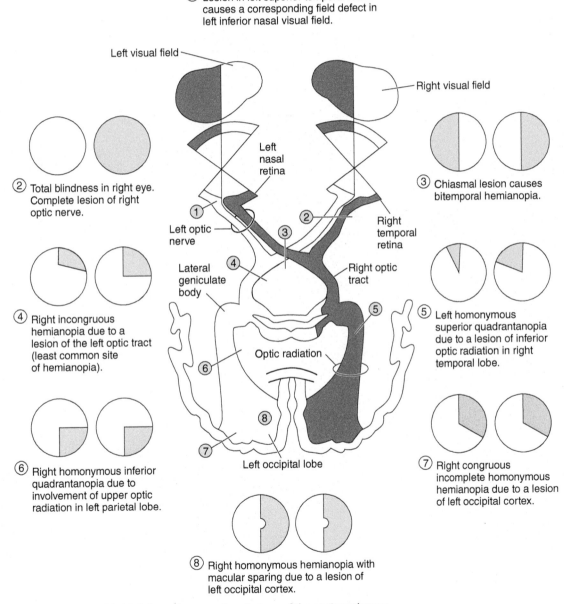

Normal blind spots

① Lesion in left superior temporal retina causes a corresponding field defect in left inferior nasal visual field.

Left visual field

Right visual field

Left nasal retina

② Total blindness in right eye. Complete lesion of right optic nerve.

③ Chiasmal lesion causes bitemporal hemianopia.

Left optic nerve

Right temporal retina

Lateral geniculate body

Right optic tract

④ Right incongruous hemianopia due to a lesion of the left optic tract (least common site of hemianopia).

⑤ Left homonymous superior quadrantanopia due to a lesion of inferior optic radiation in right temporal lobe.

Optic radiation

⑥ Right homonymous inferior quadrantanopia due to involvement of upper optic radiation in left parietal lobe.

Left occipital lobe

⑦ Right congruous incomplete homonymous hemianopia due to a lesion of left occipital cortex.

⑧ Right homonymous hemianopia with macular sparing due to a lesion of left occipital cortex.

▲ **Figure 14–3.** Visual field defects due to various lesions of the optic pathways.

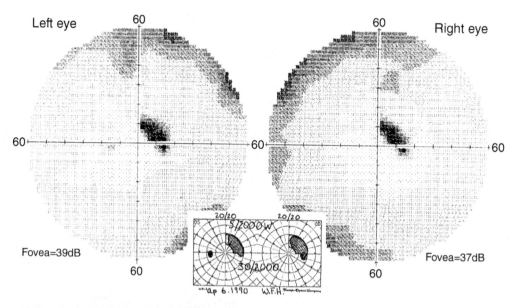

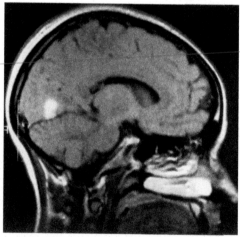

▲ **Figure 14–4.** Occipital lobe abscess. **Top:** Automated perimetry and tangent screen examination showing homonymous, congruous, paracentral scotoma in right upper visual fields. **Bottom:** Parasagittal magnetic resonance imaging showing lesion involving left inferior calcarine cortex. (Reproduced, with permission, from Horton JC, Hoyt WF: The representation of the visual field in human striate cortex. A revision of the classic Holmes map. Arch Ophthalmol 1991;109:816. Copyright © 1991. American Medical Association. All rights reserved.)

- **Prognosis**

  - Vision continues to improve with recovery of acuity to 20/40 or better in over 90% of cases at both 1 year and 15 years from onset.

  - Poorer vision during the acute episode is correlated with poorer visual outcome, but even loss of all perception of light can be followed by recovery of acuity to 20/20.

- If the disease process is sufficiently destructive, the optic disk becomes pale and defects appear in the retinal nerve fiber layer (Figure 14–10).

- There is a 50% 15-year risk of development of multiple sclerosis after first episode with stratification of risk according to brain MRI abnormalities (Figure 14–11), female sex, lack of optic disk swelling, and cerebrospinal fluid oligoclonal bands.

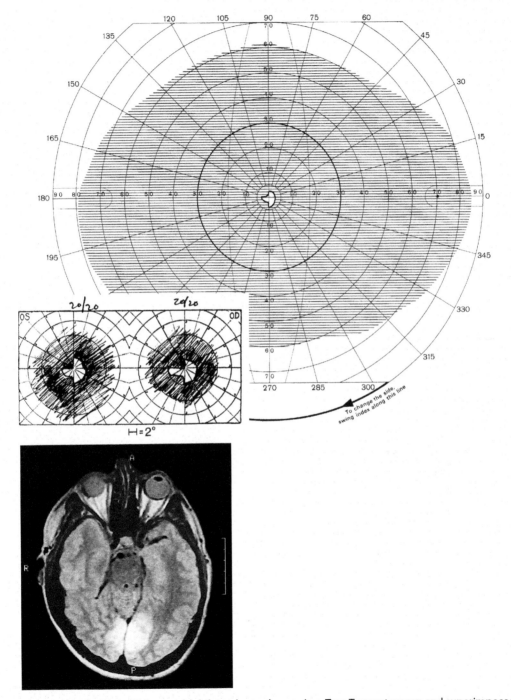

▲ Figure 14–5. Bilateral occipital infarcts with bilateral macular sparing. **Top:** Tangent screen and superimposed Goldmann visual fields of both eyes showing bilateral homonymous hemianopia with macular sparing, greater in the right hemi-field. **Bottom:** Axial magnetic resonance imaging showing sparing of occipital poles. (Reproduced, with permission, from Horton JC, Hoyt WF: The representation of the visual field in human striate cortex. A revision of the classic Holmes map. Arch Ophthalmol 1991;109:816. Copyright © 1991. American Medical Association. All rights reserved.)

Table 14–1. Etiologic Classification of Diseases of the Optic Nerve

Optic neuritis
Typical
  Demyelinative
    Multiple sclerosis
  Acute disseminated encephalomyelitis
    Parainfectious
    Postimmunization
    Idiopathic
Atypical
  Demyelinative
    Neuromyelitis optica (Devic's disease) (anti–aquaporin-4
      antibodies) (AQP4-IgG)
    Anti–myelin oligodendrocyte glycoprotein (MOG) antibodies
  Granulomatous
    Sarcoidosis
    Chronic relapsing inflammatory optic neuropathy (CRION)
    Idiopathic
  Immune-mediated (may cause ischemic optic neuropathy;
    see below)
    Systemic lupus erythematosus
    Antiphospholipid syndrome
    Sjögren's syndrome
  Direct infection
    Herpes zoster
    Syphilis
    Tuberculosis
    Cryptococcosis
    Cytomegalovirus
    Borreliosis (Lyme disease)
    Bartonellosis (cat-scratch disease)
  Contiguous inflammatory disease
    Intraocular inflammation (see Chapter 7)
    Orbital disease (see Chapter 13)
    Sinus disease, including mucormycosis that typically occurs
      in diabetics (see Chapter 13)
    Intracranial disease: meningitis, encephalitis

Ischemic optic neuropathy
Nonarteritic anterior ischemic optic neuropathy
Systemic vasculitis (arteritic anterior ischemic optic neuropathy)
  Large vessel
    Giant cell arteritis
  Medium vessel
    Polyarteritis nodosa
  Small vessel
    Granulomatosis with polyangiitis (Wegener's)
    Eosinophilic granulomatosis with polyangiitis (Churg-Strauss)
  Immune-mediated (also may cause optic neuritis; see above)
    Systemic lupus erythematosus
    Antiphospholipid syndrome
    Sjögren's syndrome
  Diabetic papillopathy
Posterior ischemic optic neuropathy
  Sudden massive blood loss (eg, trauma, gastrointestinal hemorrhage)
  Postoperative visual loss (POVL)
    Prolonged prone position lumbar spine surgery
    Cardiac surgery
  Radiation optic neuropathy

Raised intracranial pressure (papilledema)
Intracranial mass or cerebral swelling
  Tumor
  Abscess
Subdural or extradural hemorrhage
Encephalitis
Obstruction to flow of cerebrospinal fluid (obstructive
  hydrocephalus)
  Aqueduct stenosis
Obstruction to drainage of cerebrospinal fluid (communicating
  hydrocephalus)
  Meningitis
  Subarachnoid hemorrhage
  Cerebral venous sinus or jugular vein occlusion including
    thrombosis
  Congenital Chiari type I malformation
  Chiari type II (Arnold-Chiari) malformation
  Raised cerebrospinal fluid (CSF) protein
    Spinal tumor
    Acute idiopathic polyneuropathy (Guillain-Barré
      syndrome)
Mixed mechanism
  Arteriovenous malformation
  Craniosynostosis
  Mucopolysaccharidosis
Uncertain mechanism (pseudotumor cerebri)
  Idiopathic intracranial hypertension
  Tetracyclines
  Obstructive sleep apnea
  Respiratory failure
  Steroid therapy or withdrawal
  Vitamin A (retinoid) therapy or toxicity
  Uremia
  Hypoparathyroidism

Optic nerve compression
Intracranial disease: meningioma, pituitary adenoma,
  craniopharyngioma, supraclinoid internal carotid aneurysm,
  meningeal carcinomatosis, basal meningitis
Orbital disease: dysthyroid eye disease, idiopathic orbital
  inflammatory disease, orbital neoplasm, orbital abscess
Optic nerve sheath meningioma

Nutritional or toxic
Vitamin deficiencies: vitamin B_{12} (pernicious anemia), vitamin B_1
  (thiamin), folate
Tobacco-alcohol amblyopia
Heavy metals: lead, mercury (high consumption of red snapper
  and/or tuna), cobalt (metal on metal joint prostheses), thallium
  (depilatory creams), arsenic
Drugs: ethambutol, isoniazid, linezolid, disulfiram, tamoxifen,
  quinine, chloramphenicol, amiodarone, chemotherapeutic
  agents (especially high-dose or intra-arterial therapy)
Chemicals: methanol, ethylene glycol

Trauma
Direct optic nerve injury
Indirect optic nerve injury
Optic nerve avulsion

(continued)

Table 14–1. Etiologic Classification of Diseases of the Optic Nerve (*Continued*)

Hereditary optic atrophy
    Leber's hereditary optic neuropathy (mitochondrial inheritance)
    Autosomal hereditary optic atrophy
        Dominant (juvenile) optic atrophy
        Recessive (infantile) optic atrophy
        Wolfram's syndrome (DIDMOAD: diabetes insipidus, diabetes
            mellitus, optic atrophy, deafness)
    Inherited neurodegenerative diseases
        Hereditary spinocerebellar ataxia (Friedreich's ataxia)
        Hereditary motor and sensory neuropathy (Charcot-Marie-Tooth
            disease)
        Lysosomal storage disorders
 	
Neoplastic infiltration
    Glioma, leukemia, lymphoma, meningeal carcinomatosis,
        astrocytic hamartoma (tuberous sclerosis complex),
        melanocytoma, hemangioma
	Optic nerve anomalies
	    Hypoplasia
	    Dysplasia (including "morning glory syndrome," coloboma, and
	        optic nerve pit)
	    Tilted disks, including situs inversus, and scleral crescents
	    Megalopapilla
	    Myelinated nerve fibers
	    Persistent hyaloid system
	    Prepapillary vascular loops
	    Optic nerve head drusen
	    Hyperopic pseudopapilledema
	
	Glaucomatous optic neuropathy (see Chapter 11)
	Optic atrophy secondary to retinal disease

2. MULTIPLE SCLEROSIS

Multiple sclerosis is typically a chronic relapsing and remitting demyelinating disorder of the central nervous system. The cause is unknown. Some patients develop a chronically progressive form of the disease, either following a period of relapses and remissions (secondary progressive) or, less commonly, from the outset (primary progressive). Characteristically, the lesions occur at different times and in noncontiguous locations in the nervous system (dissemination in time and space). Onset is usually in young adult life; the disease rarely begins before 15 years or after 55 years of age. There is a tendency to involve the optic nerves and chiasm, brainstem, cerebellar peduncles, and spinal cord, although no part of the central nervous system is protected. The peripheral nervous system is seldom involved.

▶ Clinical Features

Optic neuritis may be the first manifestation. There may be recurrent episodes, and the other eye usually becomes involved. The overall incidence of optic neuritis in multiple

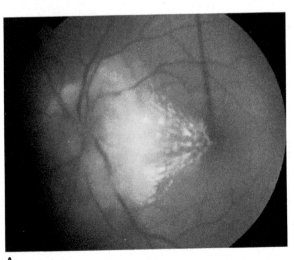
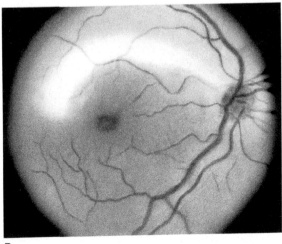

A   **B**

▲ **Figure 14–6. A:** Retinal exudates due to optic disk swelling. **B:** Arcuate neuroretinitis due to acute retinal necrosis syndrome. (B: Reproduced, with permission, from Margolis T et al: Acute retinal necrosis syndrome presenting with papillitis and arcuate neuroretinitis. Ophthalmology 1988;95:937. Copyright © 1988 American Academy of Ophthalmology, Inc. Published by Elsevier Inc.)

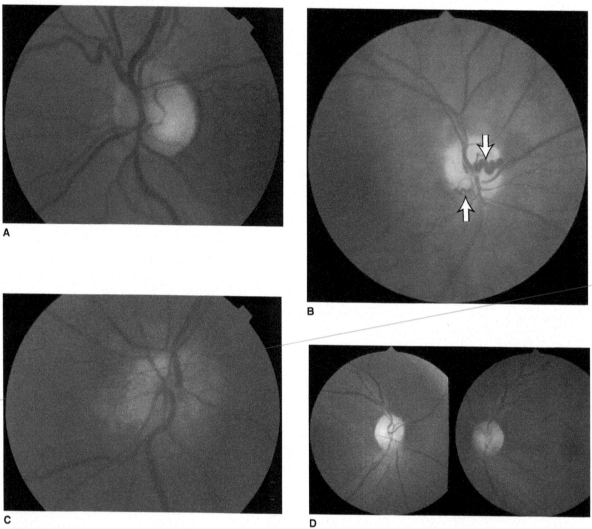

▲ **Figure 14–7.** Examples of optic atrophy. **A:** Primary optic atrophy due to nutritional amblyopia. **B:** Secondary optic atrophy with retinochoroidal collaterals **(arrows)** due to optic nerve sheath meningioma. **C:** Optic atrophy with optic disk drusen. **D:** Pallor (atrophy) of right optic disk due to nerve compression by sphenoid meningioma. The left disk is normal.

sclerosis is 90%, and the identification of symptomatic or subclinical optic nerve involvement is an important diagnostic clue.

Diplopia is a common early symptom, due most frequently to internuclear ophthalmoplegia that is frequently bilateral (Figure 14–12). Less common causes are lesions of the sixth or third cranial nerve within the brainstem.

Nystagmus is a common sign, and unlike most manifestations of the disease (which tend toward remission), it is often permanent (70%).

Intraocular inflammation may occur, particularly subclinical peripheral retinal venous sheathing, which can be highlighted by fluorescein angiography.

▶ **Investigation**

Diagnosis of multiple sclerosis traditionally relied upon clinical evidence of white matter disease of the central nervous system disseminated in time and space (Schumacher criteria), subsequently supported by MRI and cerebrospinal fluid abnormalities (Poser criteria). Increasingly, emphasis is

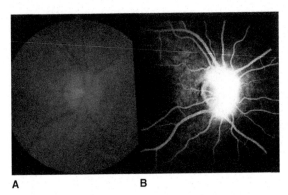

A B

▲ **Figure 14–8.** Mild disk swelling **(A)** in demyelinative papillitis, with disk leakage on fluorescein angiography **(B)**.

being placed on MRI abnormalities, in the brain and spinal cord, supported by clinical features and cerebrospinal fluid abnormalities, to establish dissemination in time and space (McDonald criteria), thus facilitating earlier diagnosis.

Cerebrospinal fluid oligoclonal bands that are not present in the serum—representing intrathecal production of immunoglobulins—are characteristic but not diagnostic. There may be cerebrospinal fluid lymphocytosis or a mildly raised cerebrospinal fluid protein concentration during an acute relapse.

Retinal optical coherence tomography scans and visual evoked responses detect optic nerve involvement even in patients who have not had symptoms of optic neuritis.

▶ Course, Treatment, & Prognosis

The course of disease is unpredictable. Optic neuritis rather than brainstem or spinal cord disease as the initial

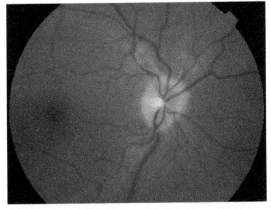

▲ **Figure 14–9.** Mild papilledema. The disk margins are blurred superiorly and inferiorly by the thickened layer of nerve fibers entering the disk.

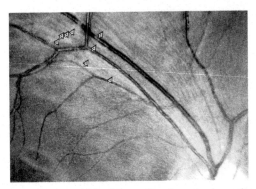

▲ **Figure 14–10.** Retinal nerve fiber layer in demyelinating optic neuropathy of multiple sclerosis. The upper temporal nerve fiber bundles show multiple slit-like areas of thinning **(arrows)** representing retrograde axonal atrophy from subclinical disease in the optic nerve. Vision in the eye was 20/20.

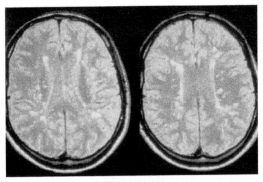

▲ **Figure 14–11.** Cerebral hemisphere white matter lesions on magnetic resonance imaging in a patient with a first episode of acute demyelinative optic neuropathy (typical optic neuritis).

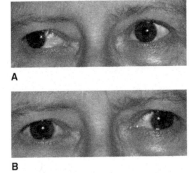

A

B

▲ **Figure 14–12.** Bilateral internuclear ophthalmoplegia due to multiple sclerosis. **(A)** Reduced adduction of the left eye on rightward gaze. **(B)** Reduced adduction of the right eye on leftward gaze.

manifestation is associated with a better prognosis. Relapses and remissions are characteristic, with permanent disability tending to increase with each relapse. Pregnancy or the number of pregnancies has no effect on disability, but there is an increased risk of relapse just after delivery. Onset during pregnancy has a more favorable outcome than onset unrelated to pregnancy. Elevation of body temperature may exacerbate disability (Uhthoff phenomenon), particularly visual impairment.

Steroid treatment, usually oral or intravenous methylprednisolone, is useful in hastening recovery from acute relapses but does not influence the final disability or the frequency of subsequent relapses. Disease-modifying drugs such as β-interferon, glatiramer acetate, teriflunomide, dimethyl fumarate, mitoxantrone, natalizumab, and fingolimod reduce the frequency and severity of relapses and slow the progression of brain MRI abnormalities, but the effect on long-term disability is still being determined. Many treatments have been tested for progressive disease with no significant benefit.

3. ACUTE DISSEMINATED ENCEPHALOMYELITIS

Acute disseminated encephalomyelitis for the most part is a monophasic illness that is more common in children than adults. Typically it occurs 1–2 weeks following a viral infection or immunization, but there may be no precipitating event. Bilateral optic neuritis is a common feature. The severity of the encephalomyelitis is variable. Generally, prognosis is good, aided by steroid and other treatments. There is no association with subsequent development of multiple sclerosis, but recurrent disease may occur.

▶ Atypical Optic Neuritis

- **Diagnostic clues**
  - Marked pain
  - Continuing deterioration of vision after 2 weeks
  - No recovery of vision after 6 weeks
  - Progression of loss of vision for more than 2 weeks
  - Complete loss of vision (no light perception)
  - Lack of recovery of vision after 6 weeks from its onset
  - Simultaneous or rapidly sequential onset
- **Investigation**
  - Optic nerve and brain MRI
    - Exclude optic nerve compression
    - Optic chiasmal as well as optic nerve abnormalities suggest neuromyelitis optica but rarely can be due to malignant glioma

  - Exclude orbital, sinus, and intracranial disease (computed tomography [CT] of head and orbits also may be helpful)
- Lumbar puncture with cerebrospinal fluid analysis including oligoclonal bands
- Investigations for sarcoidosis, immune-mediated disease, and infections (particularly relevant in the immunocompromised)
- Aquaporin-4 antibodies (AQP4-IgG)
- Anti–myelin oligodendrocyte glycoprotein (MOG) antibodies
- **Treatment**
  - Steroid therapy (intravenous methylprednisolone, 1 g/d for 3 days, followed by oral prednisolone, 1 mg/kg/d)
  - Plasmapheresis if poor response to steroid therapy

4. NEUROMYELITIS OPTICA

Neuromyelitis optica (Devic's disease) is characterized by recurrent optic neuritis and transverse myelitis that may resemble severe multiple sclerosis, but lesions on brain MRI are atypical for multiple sclerosis; spinal cord lesions are long and necrotic; there may be a cellular cerebrospinal fluid response; severe disability is common; and there is a specific probably pathogenic serum autoantibody to the water channel aquaporin-4 (anti-aquaporin-4 antibodies [AQP4-IgG]). The clinical outcome is variable. Approximately 50% of patients progress to death within the first decade due to the paraplegia, but the remainder may have a prolonged remission and, ultimately, a better prognosis than patients with multiple sclerosis. Treatment is with systemic steroids or, if necessary, plasmapheresis for the acute episodes, followed by long-term immunosuppression, primarily targeted at humoral immunity, according to disease activity. There is overlap with the neurologic disease of Sjögren's syndrome.

Relapsing and bilateral optic neuritis, acute disseminated encephalomyelitis, and transverse myelitis occur in demyelinative inflammatory neurologic disease associated with antibodies to myelin oligodendrocyte glycoprotein (anti-MOG antibodies). The treatment is the same as for neuromyelitis optica.

5. ISCHEMIC OPTIC NEUROPATHY

Ischemic optic neuropathy is caused by infarction of the optic nerve. Anterior ischemic optic neuropathy is caused by infarction of the retrolaminar optic nerve (the region just posterior to the lamina cribrosa) from occlusion (eg, giant cell arteritis), thrombosis, or more commonly, decreased perfusion (eg, nonarteritic type) of the short posterior ciliary arteries. It causes acute loss of vision with optic disk swelling in all cases

(Figure 14–13). In the rare posterior ischemic optic neuropathy due to infarction of the retrobulbar optic nerve, there are no optic disk changes in the acute stage. Optic atrophy develops after both anterior and posterior ischemic optic neuropathy.

Nonarteritic Anterior Ischemic Optic Neuropathy

- **Epidemiology**
  - Usually unilateral but with 15% risk of future fellow eye involvement
  - Usually sixth or seventh decade but can occur throughout adulthood
  - Associated with diabetes, hypertension, hyperlipidemia, and end-stage renal disease
  - Risk factors
    - Small (crowded) optic disk ("disk at risk")
    - Obstructive sleep apnea
    - Nocturnal hypotension including treatment of hypertension
    - Phosphodiesterase inhibitors

- **Clinical features**
  - Sudden (occasionally progressive over 2 weeks) loss of vision
  - Visual acuity normal or reduced
  - Visual field defect (typically inferior altitudinal)
  - Color vision normal or reduced
  - Reduced pupillary response to light shone in the affected eye (relative afferent pupillary defect)
  - Painless
  - Swollen optic disk often with peripapillary splinter hemorrhages
  - Recovery of visual acuity in 40% of eyes by 6 months

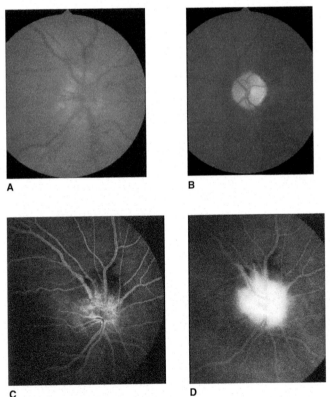

A   B

C   D

▲ **Figure 14–13.** Pseudo-Foster Kennedy syndrome due to sequential anterior ischemic optic neuropathy. **A:** Swollen right optic disk with hemorrhages due to current ischemic episode. **B:** Atrophy of left optic disk due to previous ischemia. **C:** Early phase of fluorescein angiogram of right eye showing poor perfusion of optic disk and dilated superficial disk capillaries. **D:** Late phase of fluorescein angiogram showing disk leakage.

- **Main differential diagnoses**
  - Arteritic anterior ischemic optic neuropathy due to giant cell arteritis
  - Optic neuritis
  - Papilledema
  - Mild, chronic, usually bilateral disk swelling with little change in visual function
    - Diabetic papillopathy
    - Amiodarone optic neuropathy
- **Investigations**
  - In most cases, investigation is limited to assessment of vascular risk factors.
  - In younger patients, consider systemic vasculitis and acquired or inherited thrombophilia.
- **Treatment**
  - No treatment is generally accepted to be beneficial, but systemic steroids may be used.
  - Low-dose aspirin therapy may reduce the risk of future fellow eye involvement.

Arteritic Anterior Ischemic Optic Neuropathy due to Giant Cell Arteritis (GCA)

- **Epidemiology**
  - Age over 50 with increasing incidence with increasing age
- **Clinical features**
  - Usually severe visual loss with risk of complete blindness without prompt treatment
  - Other ocular manifestations of GCA
    - Central retinal artery occlusion
    - Cilioretinal artery occlusion
    - Retinal cotton-wool spots
    - Ophthalmic artery occlusion
    - Diffuse ocular ischemia
  - Nonocular manifestations of GCA
    - Headache
    - Swollen, tender, typically pulseless superficial temporal arteries
    - Jaw pain on chewing (jaw claudication)
    - General malaise, weight loss
    - Muscle aches and pains (polymyalgia rheumatica)

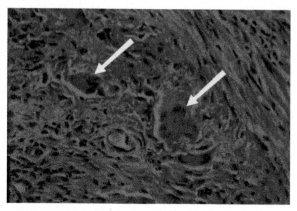

▲ **Figure 14–14.** Giant cell arteritis. Positive temporal artery biopsy with giant cells **(arrows)**.

- **Investigations**
  - Erythrocyte sedimentation rate (ESR) and C-reactive protein (CRP) are usually raised.
  - Temporal artery biopsy for definitive diagnosis (inflammatory cell infiltration, often but not always including giant cells, and prominent disruption of the internal elastic lamina) (Figure 14–14) within 2 weeks after commencement of steroid therapy.
  - Temporal and other artery ultrasound may be helpful.
  - Positron emission tomography scans show large vessel arteritis.
- **Treatment**
  - High-dose systemic steroids as soon as a clinical diagnosis is made
    - Oral prednisolone 1–1.5 mg/kg/d
    - Intravenous hydrocortisone, 250–500 mg, if delay of oral therapy
    - Intravenous methylprednisolone, 500–1000 mg/d for 3 days
      - Bilateral disease, including transient visual loss in the fellow eye
      - Progression of visual loss or persistence of systemic manifestations and/or raised ESR/CRP despite oral therapy
    - Oral prednisolone usually reduced to 40 mg/d over 4 weeks and then more gradually tapered and discontinued after 9–12 months overall as long as no recurrence of disease activity
    - 30% of patients require long-term steroid therapy

▶ Posterior Ischemic Optic Neuropathy

- Sudden visual loss due to optic neuropathy
- No optic disk swelling during the acute stage
- Specific causes

  - Massive blood loss, such as from trauma or bleeding peptic ulcer

  - Nonocular surgery, particularly lumbar spine surgery in the prone position or cardiac surgery

  - Radiotherapy, usually treatment for skull base or sinus tumors 12–18 months previously with characteristic pattern of gadolinium enhancement on MRI and possible benefit from early hyperbaric oxygen therapy

  - Giant cell arteritis

  - Mucormycosis, which usually occurs in diabetics

- Unless clear precipitating cause, investigation is required, particularly head imaging (CT or MRI), to exclude optic nerve compression.

6. PAPILLEDEMA (FIGURES 14–9 AND 14–15 TO 14–17)

Papilledema is, by definition, optic disk swelling due to raised intracranial pressure (see Table 14–1). In ophthalmology practice, a frequent cause is **idiopathic intracranial hypertension.** This is characterized by raised intracranial pressure, no neurologic or neuroimaging abnormality except for anything attributable to the raised intracranial pressure, such as sixth cranial nerve palsy, and normal cerebrospinal fluid constituents. It is a diagnosis of exclusion, and other causes of raised intracranial pressure, such as cerebral venous sinus occlusion, tetracycline or vitamin A (retinoid) therapy, and particularly in men obstructive sleep apnea, can have similar clinical features.

For papilledema to occur, the subarachnoid space around the optic nerve must be patent to allow transmission of the raised intracranial pressure in the intracranial subarachnoid space to the anterior (retrolaminar) optic nerve. Slow and fast axonal transport is blocked, resulting in axonal distention, which is first apparent in the peripapillary retinal nerve fiber layer at the superior and inferior poles of the optic disk and causes blurring of the margin of the optic disk. Hyperemia of the disk with dilated surface capillaries is an important feature. Spontaneous venous pulsation is usually absent. There may be retinal folds usually circumferential around the optic disk (Paton lines). In acute papilledema (Figure 14–15), probably as a consequence either of markedly raised or rapidly increasing intracranial pressure, there are hemorrhages and cotton-wool spots on and around the optic disk, indicating vascular and axonal decompensation with the attendant risk of acute optic nerve damage

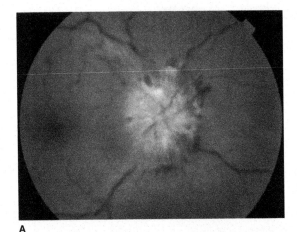

A

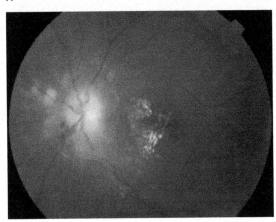

B

▲ **Figure 14–15.** Acute papilledema. **(A)** Optic disk swelling with cotton-wool spots and hemorrhages. **(B)** Retinal exudates.

and visual field defects. There may also be retinal edema, which can extend to the macula and may have a subretinal component, retinal exudates, and choroidal folds. In chronic papilledema (Figure 14–16), which is likely to be the consequence of prolonged, moderately raised intracranial pressure, a process of compensation limits the optic disk changes such that there are few if any hemorrhages or cotton-wool spots. With persistent raised intracranial pressure, the optic disk gradually becomes increasingly pale as a result of astrocytic gliosis and neural atrophy with secondary constriction of retinal blood vessels, leading to atrophic papilledema (Figure 14–17). There may also be retinochoroidal collaterals (previously known as opticociliary shunts) linking the central retinal vein and the peripapillary choroidal veins, which develop when the retinal venous circulation is obstructed in the prelaminar region of the optic nerve. (Other causes of retinochoroidal collaterals are central retinal vein occlusion,

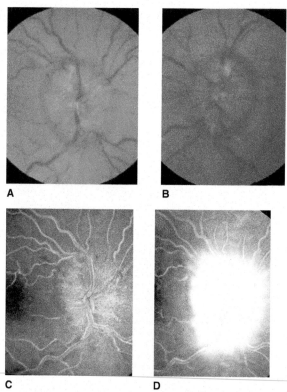

A   B

C   D

▲ **Figure 14–16.** Chronic papilledema with prominent disk swelling, capillary dilation, and retinal folds but few hemorrhages or cotton-wool spots **(A)** and **(B).** Fluorescein angiography demonstrates the capillary dilation in its early phase **(C)** and marked disk leakage in its late phase **(D).**

optic nerve sheath meningioma [Figure 14–7], optic nerve glioma, and optic nerve head drusen.) The presence of glistening deposits within the swollen optic nerve head, which indicates that the swelling is likely to have been present for several months, characterizes vintage papilledema.

It takes 24–48 hours for early papilledema to occur and 1 week to develop fully. It takes 6–8 weeks for fully developed papilledema to resolve following return of intracranial pressure to normal. Transient visual obscurations are a characteristic symptom of papilledema. Acute papilledema may reduce visual acuity by causing hyperopia and occasionally is associated with optic nerve infarction, but in most cases, vision is normal apart from blind spot enlargement. Chronic, particularly atrophic or vintage, papilledema is associated with gradual constriction of the peripheral visual field, particularly inferonasal loss. Sudden reduction of intracranial pressure or systolic perfusion pressure may precipitate severe visual loss in any stage of papilledema.

Papilledema is often asymmetric and may be unilateral. It occurs late in glaucoma and will not occur at all if there is optic atrophy or if the optic nerve sheath is not patent. The Foster Kennedy syndrome is papilledema on one side with optic atrophy due to optic nerve compression on the other, commonly due to skull-base meningioma. It is mimicked (pseudo-Foster Kennedy syndrome) by ischemic optic neuropathy when optic disk swelling due to a new episode of ischemic optic neuropathy is associated with optic atrophy in the fellow eye due to a previous episode (Figure 14–13).

Papilledema can be mimicked by buried optic nerve head drusen, small hyperopic disks, and myelinated nerve fibers (Figure 14–18).

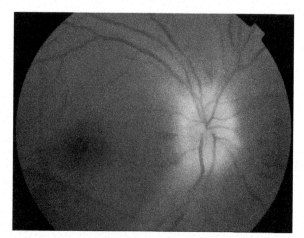

▲ **Figure 14–17.** Atrophic papilledema in idiopathic intracranial hypertension. The disk is pale and mildly raised with blurred margins. The white areas surrounding the macula are reflected light from the vitreoretinal interface.

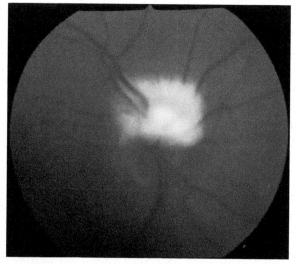

▲ **Figure 14–18.** Large patch of myelinated nerve fibers originating from superior edge of the optic disk.

The treatment of papilledema must be directed to the underlying cause. **Idiopathic intracranial hypertension** generally affects obese young women and maintained weight loss is then an important treatment objective. The major morbidity is visual loss, but headaches may also be troublesome. Oral acetazolamide—usually 250 mg one to four times daily but up to 1 g four times daily in severe cases—or diuretics such as furosemide are usually effective. Cerebrospinal fluid shunting or optic nerve sheath fenestration may be undertaken if there is severe or progressive loss of vision or if medical therapy is not tolerated. Repeated lumbar punctures are rarely indicated except as a temporary measure prior to surgical therapy. Headaches usually respond to control of intracranial pressure, but other treatments may be required. It is essential that patients with idiopathic intracranial hypertension undergo regular visual field assessments by perimetry.

7. OPTIC NERVE COMPRESSION

Optic nerve compression is often amenable to treatment, and early recognition is vital to optimal outcome. Optic nerve compression should be considered in any patient with signs of optic neuropathy or visual loss not explained by an intraocular lesion. Optic disk swelling may occur with intraorbital optic nerve compression, but in many cases, particularly when the optic nerve compression is intracranial, the optic disk shows no abnormality until optic atrophy develops or there is papilledema from associated raised intracranial pressure. Investigation of possible optic nerve compression requires early imaging by MRI or CT. If no structural lesion is identified and meningeal disease is suspected, it may be necessary to proceed to lumbar puncture for cerebrospinal fluid examination.

Intracranial meningiomas that may compress the optic nerve include those arising from the sphenoid wing, the tuberculum sellae/planum sphenoidale (suprasellar meningioma), and the olfactory groove. Sphenoid wing meningiomas also produce proptosis, ocular motility disturbance, and fifth nerve sensory loss (Figure 14–19). Surgical excision is generally effective in debulking intracranial meningiomas, but complete excision is often very difficult to achieve. Radiotherapy may be indicated as adjuvant or primary treatment. Pituitary adenoma and craniopharyngioma are discussed in the section on chiasmal disease (see later in the chapter). The management of orbital causes of optic nerve compression is discussed in Chapter 13.

Primary optic nerve sheath meningioma is a rare tumor most commonly presenting, like other types of meningioma, in middle-aged women (Figure 14–20). Five percent of cases are bilateral. Visual loss is slowly progressive. The classic clinical features are a pale, slightly swollen optic disk with retinochoroidal collaterals (Figure 14–7), but in most cases, the collateral vessels are not present. Stereotactic fractionated radiotherapy is the preferred treatment.

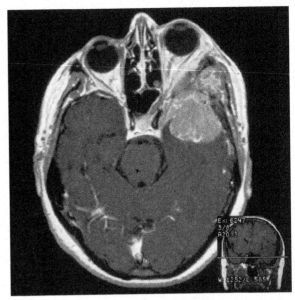

▲ **Figure 14–19.** Axial magnetic resonance imaging of sphenoid wing meningioma causing proptosis.

8. NUTRITIONAL & TOXIC OPTIC NEUROPATHIES

The usual clinical features of nutritional and toxic optic neuropathy are subacute, progressive, symmetrical visual loss, with reduction of visual acuities, central field defects including both fixation and the blind spot (centrocecal scotoma) (Figure 14–21), poor color vision, and the development of

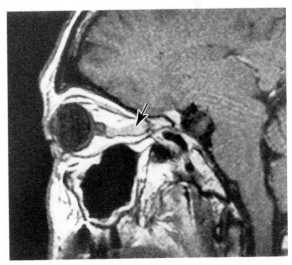

▲ **Figure 14–20.** Magnetic resonance imaging of tubular optic nerve sheath meningioma.

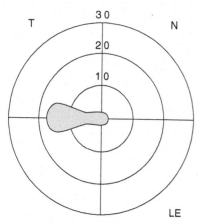

▲ **Figure 14–21.** Nutritional amblyopia showing centro-cecal scotoma. VA = 20/200.

temporal disk pallor (Figure 14–7). The differential diagnosis includes Leber's hereditary optic neuropathy, autosomal dominant optic atrophy, the rare chronic optic neuropathy of progressive multiple sclerosis, and macular disease. Correction of the nutritional deficiency or withdrawal of the toxic agent is the primary treatment.

Tobacco-Alcohol Amblyopia

Nutritional amblyopia is probably a more accurate term for this entity. Usually it occurs in individuals with poor dietary habits, heavy alcohol consumption, and/or heavy smoking. Strict vegetarianism without vitamin supplementation may contribute. Adequate diet plus thiamine, folic acid, and vitamin B_{12} supplements may be effective if presentation is not delayed. Withdrawal of tobacco and alcohol is advisable and may hasten the cure, but adequate nutrition or vitamin B_{12} supplements can be effective despite continued excessive intake of alcohol or tobacco. Improvement usually begins within 1–2 months, although in occasional cases, significant improvement may not occur for 1 year. Visual function can but may not return to normal. Permanent optic atrophy or at least temporal disk pallor can occur depending on the stage of disease at the time treatment was started (Figure 14–7).

Drug-Induced Optic Neuropathy

Ethambutol optic neuropathy is dependent on dose, body weight, and renal function. Patients should be warned to report immediately any deterioration of vision. Recovery of vision often takes many months after cessation of ethambutol and may be accelerated by oral copper and zinc supplements. Quinine overdose produces optic neuropathy, narrowed retinal arterioles, and irregular, poorly reactive pupils. Amiodarone generally causes chronic bilateral optic disk swelling

with relatively mild reduction of vision, but distinction from nonarteritic anterior ischemic optic neuropathy can be difficult. It also causes vortex keratopathy.

Methanol Poisoning

Absorption, usually oral, of methanol, which is used widely in the chemical industry as antifreeze, solvent varnish, or paint remover, causes visual impairment, sometimes progressing to complete blindness. Whitish, striated edema of the peripapillary retina is a characteristic sign.

Treatment consists of correction of the acidosis with intravenous sodium bicarbonate and oral or intravenous administration of ethanol to compete with, and thus prevent, the slower metabolism of methanol into its by-products. Hemodialysis is indicated for blood methanol levels over 50 mg/dL.

9. OPTIC NERVE TRAUMA

Direct optic nerve injury occurs in penetrating orbital trauma, including local anesthetic injections for ocular surgery, and in mid-facial fractures involving the optic canal. Visual loss due to indirect optic nerve trauma, which refers to optic nerve damage secondary to distant skull injury, occurs in approximately 1% of all head injuries. The site of injury is usually the forehead, often without skull fracture, and the probable mechanism of optic nerve injury is transmission of shock waves through the orbital walls to the orbital apex. Optic nerve avulsion usually results from an abrupt rotational injury to the globe, such as from being poked forcibly in the eye with a finger.

Surgery may be indicated to relieve orbital, subperiosteal, or optic nerve sheath hemorrhage or to treat orbital fractures. High-dose systemic steroids for direct or indirect optic nerve injury and decompression of the bony optic canal for indirect injury have been advocated, but their value is uncertain. There is no effective treatment for optic nerve avulsion.

10. HEREDITARY OPTIC ATROPHY

Leber's Hereditary Optic Neuropathy

Leber's hereditary optic neuropathy (LHON) is a rare disease characterized by sequential subacute optic neuropathy usually in males aged 11–30 years. The underlying genetic abnormality is a point mutation in mitochondrial DNA (mtDNA), with over 90% of affected families harboring a mutation at position 11778, 14484, or 3460. mtDNA is exclusively derived from the mother, and thus, in accordance with the general pattern of mitochondrial (maternal) inheritance (see Chapter 18), the mutation is transmitted through the female line. However, the disease rarely manifests in carrier females. Matrilineal nephews (any sons of the affected individual's sisters) are particularly at risk of visual loss.

Blurred vision and a central scotoma usually appear first in one eye and later—within days, weeks, or months—in the other eye. During the acute episode, there may be swelling of the optic disk and peripapillary retina with dilated telangiectatic small blood vessels on their surface, but characteristically, there is no leak from the optic disk during fluorescein angiography. Both optic nerves eventually become atrophic, and vision is usually between 20/200 and counting fingers. The 14484 mutation is associated with recovery of vision but not until many months after the initial onset of visual loss. Total loss of vision or recurrences of visual loss usually do not occur. LHON may be associated with a multiple sclerosis–like illness (particularly in affected females), cardiac conduction defects, and dystonia.

Diagnosis is by identification of a pathogenic mtDNA point mutation. No treatment is definitely effective. Because high tobacco and alcohol consumption may precipitate visual loss in susceptible individuals, carriers of a pathogenic mutation, particularly males, should be advised not to smoke and to avoid high alcohol consumption.

Optic atrophy also occurs in other mitochondrial disorders, either as a manifestation of primary optic neuropathy—for example, myoclonic epilepsy and ragged red fibers (MERRF) and mitochondrial myopathy, lactic acidosis, and stroke-like episodes (MELAS)—or secondary to retinal degeneration, for example, Kearns-Sayre syndrome. Wolfram's syndrome (see later in the chapter) is also probably the result of a mitochondrial disorder.

▶ Autosomal Hereditary Optic Atrophy

Autosomal dominant (juvenile) optic atrophy generally has an insidious onset in childhood, with slow progression of visual loss throughout life. It is often detected as mild reduction of visual acuity by childhood vision screening programs. There is characteristically a centrocecal scotoma with impaired color vision. Temporal optic disk pallor is usually present, although often mild, and mild disk cupping is occasionally seen. Diagnosis is by identification of other affected family members. The majority of affected families have a mutation of the OPA1 gene on chromosome 3. Rarely, the disease is associated with congenital or progressive deafness or ataxia.

Autosomal recessive (infantile) optic atrophy manifests as severe visual loss, present at birth or within 2 years and accompanied by nystagmus. It can be associated with progressive hearing loss, spastic quadriplegia, and dementia, although an inborn error of metabolism must first be considered. Wolfram's syndrome consists of juvenile diabetes insipidus, diabetes mellitus, optic atrophy, and deafness (DIDMOAD). Although there is a recessive pattern of inheritance, with the gene defect localized to chromosome 4, the underlying metabolic abnormality is probably a defect in cellular energy production, as in the mitochondrial diseases.

11. OPTIC NERVE ANOMALIES

Congenital optic nerve anomalies may be associated with other anomalies of the head since closure of the fetal fissure, ocular melanogenesis, and development of the optic disks occur at the same time as development of the skull and face.

Optic nerve hypoplasia, dysplasia, and coloboma have all been associated with basal encephaloceles and with varying intracranial anomalies, including agenesis of the corpus callosum (de Morsier's syndrome) and pituitary-hypothalamic dysfunction (especially growth hormone deficiency). Hypoplastic optic nerves are small, with normal-sized retinal blood vessels (Figure 14–22). They are associated with a wide range of visual acuities, astigmatism, a peripapillary halo that may have a pigmented rim (double-ring sign), and various visual field defects. Superior segmental optic nerve hypoplasia (topless optic disk) usually occurs in children born to mothers with type 1 diabetes. It is characterized by superior disk entrance of the central retinal artery, superior disk pallor (Figure 14–23), and inferior visual field loss. Dysplastic optic disks usually are associated with poor vision and show abnormal vasculature, retinal pigment epithelium, and glial tissue. They are often surrounded by a chorioretinal pigmentary disturbance. They have been reported in trisomy 4q. The papillorenal syndrome has been reported with dysplastic disks and colobomas. Colobomas of the optic nerve have been called "pseudoglaucoma" because of their resemblance to glaucomatous cupping (Figure 14–24). Disk colobomas or hypoplasia when associated with chorioretinal lacunae,

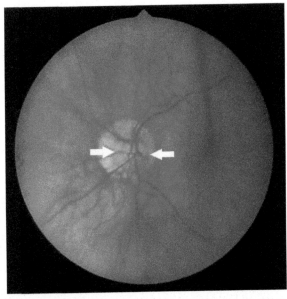

▲ **Figure 14–22.** Optic nerve hypoplasia. (**Arrows** indicate optic disk margins.)

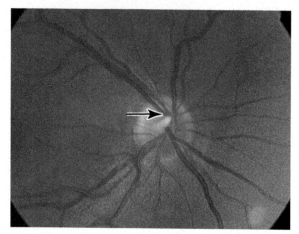

▲ **Figure 14–23.** Superior segmental optic nerve hypoplasia with superior entrance of central retinal artery **(arrow)**.

absence of the corpus callosum, and focal seizures constitute Aicardi's syndrome. This can also include retrobulbar cysts. Optic disk pits are usually not associated with any visual symptoms, but they can be mistaken for glaucomatous cupping, particularly if there is an associated field defect. Optic disk pits may present later in life as a consequence of serous detachment of the macula.

Tilted disks, which occur in 3% of normal subjects, may also be seen with hypertelorism or the craniofacial dysostoses (Crouzon's disease, Apert's disease). They are oval disks with usually an inferior scleral crescent and an associated area of fundus hypopigmentation (Figure 14–25). They

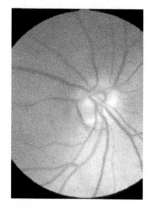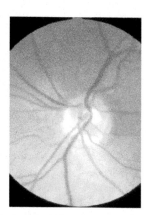

▲ **Figure 14–25.** Bilateral tilted optic disks.

may be mistaken for papilledema. They may also produce predominantly upper temporal field defects, which may be mistaken for bitemporal loss due to chiasmal dysfunction. Scleral crescents are particularly common in myopic eyes.

Megalopapilla may be mistaken for optic atrophy due to the prominence of the lamina cribrosa. Myelinated nerve fibers usually extend into the retina from the disk (Figure 14–18) but occasionally are just seen in the retinal periphery. They always follow the course of the retinal nerve fiber layer. Remnants of the embryonic hyaloid system range from tissue fragments on the optic disk (Bergmeister's papilla) to strands extending to the posterior lens capsule. Prepapillary vascular loops are distinct from the hyaloid system and occasionally become obstructed, leading to branch retinal artery occlusion.

Optic nerve head drusen are clinically apparent in about 0.3% of the population but are found on ultrasound or histopathologic studies in up to 2%. They are exclusively found in white individuals. In children, they are usually buried within the disk substance, and thus are not visible on clinical examination but cause elevation of the disk surface and mimic papilledema. The optic disk is characteristically small, with no physiologic cup and an anomalous pattern of the retinal vessels. With increasing age and loss of overlying axons, optic nerve head drusen become exposed, being apparent as "lumpy-bumpy" yellow crystalline excrescences, highlighted by retroillumination of the disk substance (Figure 14–7). On fluorescein angiography, exposed drusen are autofluorescent (Figure 14–26) and result in accumulation of dye within the disk substance. Buried drusen are best diagnosed by orbital ultrasound, thin-slice CT scanning that detects their associated calcification, or optical coherence tomography. Optic nerve head drusen are usually bilateral. They can rarely cause visual loss, either by optic neuropathy or choroidal neovascularization. Hyperopic eyes may also have small raised disks, resembling buried optic nerve head drusen and similarly mimicking papilledema (pseudo-papilledema).

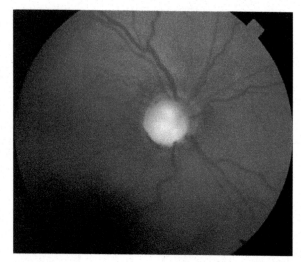

▲ **Figure 14–24.** Optic disk coloboma.

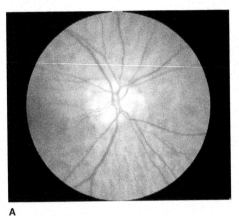 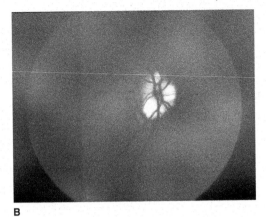

A   B

▲ **Figure 14–26.** Optic nerve head drusen **(A)** exhibiting autofluorescence **(B).**

▼ THE OPTIC CHIASM

Lesions of the chiasm typically cause bitemporal hemianopic visual field defects (Figure 14–3). Initially these defects are incomplete and are often asymmetric. As the disease progresses, the temporal hemianopia becomes complete but central visual acuity is preserved until there is also loss of the nasal visual fields or associated optic nerve dysfunction. Most diseases that affect the chiasm are neoplastic. Vascular and inflammatory chiasmal diseases are uncommon.

PITUITARY TUMORS

The anterior lobe of the pituitary gland is the site of origin of pituitary tumors (Figure 14–27), which manifest as pituitary dysfunction with a mass arising from the pituitary sella and extending into the suprasellar and/or parasellar regions, respectively causing loss of vision and cranial nerve palsies including extraocular muscle palsies.

Visual assessment, especially documentation of visual fields, is vital to decisions about management. Prolactinomas are generally treated medically in the first instance with dopamine agonists such as cabergoline, bromocriptine, or pergolide. Other pituitary macroadenomas generally undergo transsphenoidal hypophysectomy. Radiotherapy may be used as an adjuvant to surgery or for recurrent disease. Visual acuity and visual fields may improve dramatically after the chiasm is decompressed. The initial appearance of the optic nerve head does not predict the ultimate visual outcome, but optic atrophy is a poor prognostic sign.

CRANIOPHARYNGIOMA

Craniopharyngiomas arise from epithelial remnants of Rathke's pouch and characteristically become symptomatic between the ages of 10 and 25 years but occasionally not until the 60s and 70s. They are usually suprasellar (Figure 14–28) but occasionally intrasellar. The signs and symptoms vary tremendously with the age of the patient and the exact location of the tumor as well as its rate of growth. When a suprasellar tumor occurs, asymmetric chiasmatic or tract field defects are prominent. Papilledema is more common than in pituitary tumors. Optic nerve hypoplasia can be seen with tumors presenting in infancy. Pituitary deficiency may result, and involvement of the hypothalamus may cause stunted growth. Calcification of parts of the tumor contributes to a characteristic radiologic appearance, especially in children.

Treatment consists of surgical removal—as complete as possible but limiting damage to the hypothalamus. Adjunctive radiotherapy is often used, particularly if there has been incomplete surgical removal.

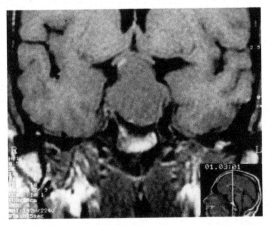

▲ **Figure 14–27.** Coronal magnetic resonance imaging showing large pituitary adenoma elevating and distorting the optic chiasm.

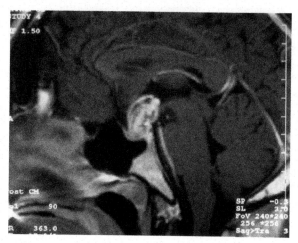

▲ **Figure 14–28.** Contrast-enhanced sagittal magnetic resonance imaging showing suprasellar craniopharyngioma.

SUPRASELLAR MENINGIOMAS

Suprasellar meningiomas arise from the meninges covering the tuberculum sellae and the planum sphenoidale, with a high proportion of patients being female. Visual loss, due to involvement of the optic chiasm and nerves, is often the presenting feature. Diagnosis is usually possible on the neuroimaging appearance. Treatment consists of surgical removal, possibly combined with adjuvant radiotherapy if there has been incomplete excision or the histopathology shows an aggressive tumor.

CHIASMATIC & OPTIC NERVE GLIOMAS

Gliomas of the anterior visual pathway, more commonly arising in the optic nerve but sometimes arising in the optic chiasm, are rare, usually indolent disorders of children, particularly associated with neurofibromatosis 1 (see later in the chapter). About 70% of cases present before the age of 7 years, with visual loss, proptosis, strabismus, or nystagmus. Occasionally onset is sudden, with rapid loss of vision. There may be optic disk swelling, but optic atrophy is more common. Visual field defects reveal an optic nerve or chiasmal syndrome. Neuroimaging may reveal optic nerve expansion or a mass in the region of the chiasm and hypothalamus. Treatment depends on the location of the tumor and its clinical course. Chemotherapy can be given during a tumor growth spurt, with irradiation being avoided in children because of adverse effects on the developing brain, and optic nerve resection can be carried out when an optic nerve tumor aggressively starts to extend intracranially toward the chiasm, but generally management is conservative.

Malignant glioma of the anterior visual pathways is rare with rapid progression to bilateral blindness and death due to invasion of the base of the brain. There is no effective treatment.

THE RETROCHIASMATIC VISUAL PATHWAYS

Cerebrovascular disease and tumors are responsible for most lesions of the retrochiasmatic visual pathways.

Retrochiasmatic lesions produce contralateral homonymous visual field defects (Figure 14–3). Anterior partial lesions, in the optic tract, lateral geniculate nucleus, or geniculocalcarine tract (optic radiation), tend to produce incongruous (or dissimilar) visual field defects. Posterior partial lesions, in the geniculocalcarine tract or occipital cortex, tend to produce more congruous visual field defects. Once any retrochiasmatic lesion becomes complete, incongruity cannot be assessed, and this sign loses its localizing ability. Any unilateral retrochiasmatic lesion should spare visual acuity since the contralateral visual pathway is intact.

Lesions of the optic tract or lateral geniculate nucleus are uncommon. After several weeks to months, the disks may become pale, more marked in the contralateral eye, with corresponding retinal nerve fiber layer defects. In optic tract lesions, there may be a contralateral relative afferent pupillary defect. The optic tract and lateral geniculate nucleus have at least a dual blood supply, so that primary vascular lesions are uncommon. Most cases are due to trauma, tumors, and arteriovenous malformations.

Lesions involving the geniculocalcarine tract do not result in optic atrophy (due to the synapse at the geniculate nucleus) unless the lesion is longstanding, usually congenital. The inferior portion of the geniculocalcarine tract passes through the temporal lobe and the superior portion through the parietal lobe, with macular function between them. Lesions of the inferior and superior portions result in predominantly superior and inferior visual field defects, respectively. Processes affecting the anterior and midtemporal lobes are commonly neoplastic; posterior temporal lobe and parietal processes can be either vascular or neoplastic. An insidious onset with mild and multiple neurologic deficits would be more typically neoplastic, whereas an acute event would be more typically vascular.

Vascular lesions of the occipital lobe are common and account for over 80% of cases of isolated homonymous visual field loss in patients over age 50 years. Macular function is represented at the most posterior tip of each occipital lobe, the representation of increasingly peripheral visual field lying increasingly anterior. Due to the frequent presence of a dual blood supply, vascular occlusions may selectively spare the posterior cortex to produce homonymous defects with central (macular) sparing (Figures 14–3 and 14–5), or conversely involve the posterior occipital cortex to produce homonymous congruous central or paracentral scotomas (Figure 14–4). The cortical centers involved in the generation of optokinetic nystagmus lie in the area between the occipital and temporal lobes and in the posterior parietal area, which are within the vascular territory of the middle cerebral artery. Optokinetic nystagmus asymmetry characteristically occurs in parietal lesions but not in occipital lesions. An asymmetric optokinetic nystagmus combined with an occipital visual field defect indicates a process not respecting vascular territories, and thus suggests a tumor (Cogan sign). Posterior reversible encephalopathy syndrome, which can be due to severe systemic hypertension, such as in eclampsia, diabetic hyperglycemia, or drugs, including cyclosporin and tacrolimus, characteristically involves the posterior cerebral hemispheres, causing homonymous hemianopia, or even cortical blindness, and visual perceptual abnormalities. CT and MRI demonstrate structural cerebral lesions with remarkable clarity (Figures 14–4, 14–5, 14–29, and 14–30). Visual disturbance with dementia is suggestive of the predominantly visual variants of Alzheimer's disease and sporadic Creutzfeldt-Jakob disease, both characterized by a paucity of imaging changes initially.

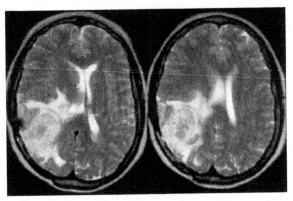

▲ **Figure 14–30.** Axial magnetic resonance imaging of parietal meningioma with secondary cerebral edema.

▼ THE PUPIL

The size of the normal pupil varies from person to person and with age, emotional state, alertness, accommodation, and ambient lighting. The normal pupillary diameter is 3–4 mm, is smaller in infancy, and tends to be larger in childhood and again progressively smaller with advancing age. Pupillary size relates to varying interactions between the parasympathetically (third nerve) innervated iris sphincter muscle that causes constriction (miosis) and the sympathetically innervated iris dilator muscle that causes dilation (mydriasis), with supranuclear control from the frontal (alertness) and occipital lobes (accommodation). Thirty percent of normal patients have a slight difference in pupil size (physiologic anisocoria), usually less than 1 mm. Mydriatic agents work more effectively on blue eyes than on brown eyes.

▶ Pupillary Light Reflex (Figure 14–31)

The pupillary response to light is a pure reflex with an entirely subcortical pathway. Whereas previously retinal photoreceptors were thought to be the sole receptors for the pupillary light reflex, intrinsically photosensitive retinal ganglion cells in the inner retina are now known to be involved.

Light shone into the right eye produces a direct response in the right eye and a consensual response in the left eye (Figure 14–32). The intensity of the response in each eye is proportionate to the light-carrying ability of the directly stimulated optic nerve.

▶ Pupillary Near Response

When the eyes look at a near object, three responses occur—accommodation to focus on the object, convergence so that both eyes are directed at the target, and miosis of the pupils. Although the three components are closely associated, the near response is not a pure reflex, as each component can be

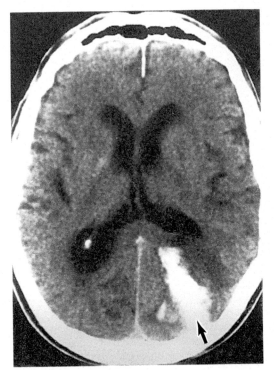

▲ **Figure 14–29.** Axial computed tomography showing occipital hematoma (**arrow**) resulting from a bleeding arteriovenous malformation. This lesion produced homonymous hemianopia and headache.

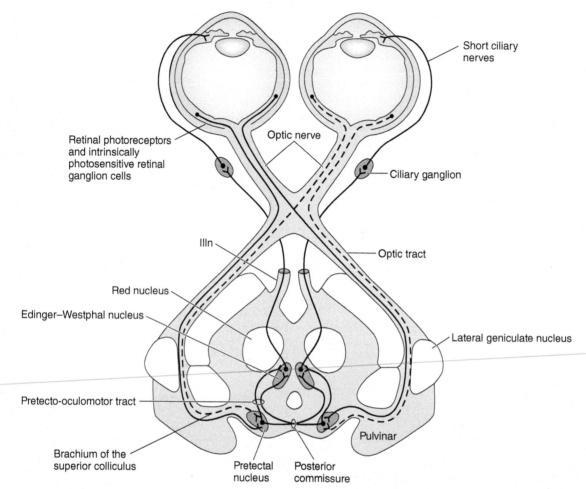

Short ciliary
nerves

Retinal photoreceptors
and intrinsically
photosensitive retinal
ganglion cells

Optic nerve

Ciliary ganglion

IIIn

Red nucleus

Edinger–Westphal nucleus

Optic tract

Lateral geniculate nucleus

Pretecto-oculomotor tract

Pulvinar

Brachium of the
superior colliculus

Pretectal   Posterior
nucleus   commissure

▲ **Figure 14–31.** Diagram of the path of the pupillary light reflex. (Reproduced, with permission, from Walsh FB, Hoyt WF: Clinical Neuro-Ophthalmology, 3rd ed. Vol 1. Williams & Wilkins, 1969.)

neutralized while leaving the other two intact—that is, by lenses (neutralizing accommodation), by prisms (neutralizing convergence), and by weak pupil-dilating (mydriatic) drugs (neutralizing miosis). It can be elicited in a blind person by asking the person to look at his thumb while it is held in front of his nose.

AFFERENT PUPILLARY DEFECT

One of the most important assessments in a patient complaining of decreased vision is whether it is due to an ocular problem (eg, cataract) or to a potentially more serious optic nerve problem. If an optic nerve lesion is present, the pupillary light response (both the direct response in the stimulated eye and the consensual response in the fellow eye) is less intense when the involved eye is stimulated than when the normal eye is stimulated. This phenomenon is called a relative afferent pupillary defect (RAPD) (Figure 14–33). It is made more obvious by alternate stimulation of one eye then the other ensuring that the intensity and duration of stimulation of each eye are the same (swinging penlight test). It will be present also if there is a large retinal or severe macular lesion, but even dense cataract does not impair the pupillary light response. Other causes of unilateral decreased vision without an RAPD include refractive error, media opacity other than cataract such as corneal opacity or vitreous hemorrhage, amblyopia, and functional visual loss. In a lesion of the brachium of the superior colliculus, it is possible for an RAPD to be present when visual function is normal.

Light stimulus

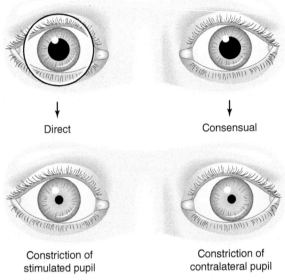

Direct   Consensual

Constriction of   Constriction of
stimulated pupil   contralateral pupil

▲ **Figure 14–32.** Normal pupillary light reflex.

Diffuse illumination

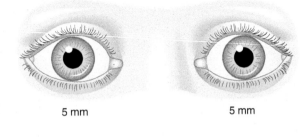

5 mm   5 mm

Light on normal eye

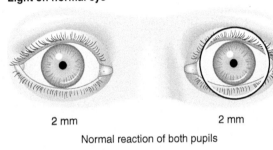

2 mm   2 mm

Normal reaction of both pupils

Light on eye with afferent defect

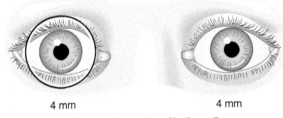

4 mm   4 mm

Decreased reaction of both pupils

▲ **Figure 14–33.** Relative afferent pupillary defect.

Absolute afferent pupillary defect is the absence of pupillary response to light stimulation of a completely blind (amaurotic) eye. Light shone into the normal eye would still induce a consensual response in the blind eye (Figure 14–34).

An afferent pupillary defect can still be identified if one pupil is either not visible, due to corneal disease, or is unable to respond due to structural damage or damage to its innervation, for example, third nerve palsy, by examination of the normal pupil as light is shone into the normal and then into the abnormal eye.

PUPILLARY LIGHT-NEAR DISSOCIATION

The light reflex normally produces more miosis than the near response. The reverse is known as pupillary light-near dissociation. This is most commonly due to an afferent pupillary defect (such as in optic nerve disease) because the pupillary light reflex to stimulation of the affected eye is reduced but the near response is normal. It occurs also in lesions of the ciliary ganglion or of the midbrain, in which the light reflex pathway is relatively dorsal and the near response pathway relatively ventral. Causes include tonic pupil (see later in the chapter), midbrain tumors and infarcts, diabetes, chronic alcoholism, encephalitis, and central nervous system degenerative disease.

Argyll Robertson pupils, which are usually bilateral, are typically small (less than 3 mm in diameter), commonly irregular and eccentric, do not respond to light stimulation but do respond to a near stimulus, and dilate poorly with

mydriatics as a consequence of concomitant iris atrophy. Typically they occur in central nervous system syphilis.

TONIC PUPIL

Tonic pupil is characterized by light-near dissociation, delayed dilation after a near stimulus (tonic near response), segmental iris constriction, and constriction in response to a weak (0.1%) solution of pilocarpine (denervation hypersensitivity). It results from damage to the ciliary ganglion or the short ciliary nerves. In the acute stage, the pupil is dilated, and accommodation is impaired. The pattern of recovery is influenced by fibers in the short ciliary nerves subserving the near response outnumbering those subserving the light reflex by 30:1. Accommodation usually recovers fully, but

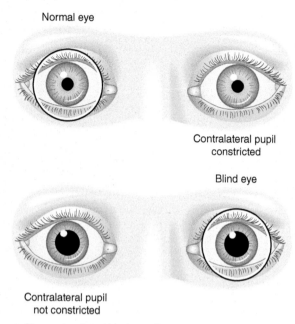

Normal eye

Contralateral pupil
constricted

Blind eye

Contralateral pupil
not constricted

▲ **Figure 14–34.** Absolute afferent (amaurotic) pupillary defect.

incomplete reinnervation of the iris results in segmental iris constriction and pupillary light-near dissociation. The pupil usually becomes smaller than the pupil in the fellow eye.

Tonic pupil is usually an isolated benign entity, presenting in young women. It may be associated with loss of deep tendon reflexes (Adie's syndrome). Subsequent involvement of the other eye over a period of 10 years occurs in 50% of individuals, but bilateral tonic pupils may be due to autonomic neuropathy. Tonic pupil may occur after retinal laser photocoagulation.

HORNER'S SYNDROME

Horner's syndrome is caused by a lesion of the sympathetic pathway either (1) in its **central portion,** which extends from the posterior hypothalamus through the brainstem to the upper spinal cord (C8–T2); or (2) in its **preganglionic portion,** which exits the spinal cord and synapses in the superior cervical (stellate) ganglion; or (3) in its **postganglionic portion,** from the superior cervical ganglion via the carotid plexus and the ophthalmic division of the fifth nerve, by which it enters the orbit. The sympathetic fibers then follow the nasociliary branch of the ophthalmic division of the fifth nerve and the long ciliary nerves to the iris and innervate Müller muscle and the iris dilator. Iris dilator muscle paresis causes miosis, which is more evident in dim light. Melanocyte maturation in the iris depends on sympathetic innervation; thus, a less pigmented (bluer) iris occurs

in congenital or longstanding acquired Horner's syndrome. Paresis of Müller muscle produces ptosis. Sweating on the ipsilateral face and neck is reduced in central and preganglionic lesions, whereas it is normal in postganglionic lesions because the relevant nerve fibers follow the external rather than the internal carotid artery.

Central Horner's syndrome may be due to brainstem infarction, particularly lateral medullary infarction (Wallenberg's syndrome), syringomyelia, or cervical cord tumor. Preganglionic Horner's syndrome may be due to cervical rib, cervical vertebral fractures, apical pulmonary lesions—particularly bronchogenic carcinoma (Pancoast's syndrome)—or brachial plexus injuries. Postganglionic Horner's syndrome may be due to carotid artery dissection, skull base tumors, or cluster headache. The localization of central and preganglionic Horner's syndrome is often apparent from the associated clinical features. Sudden-onset isolated painful Horner's syndrome, particularly with a recent history of neck trauma or associated with pain in the neck or jaw, necessitates urgent investigation for carotid dissection, which may lead to thrombotic or embolic stroke. Horner's syndrome associated with chronic facial pain, particularly if associated with fifth, sixth, third, fourth, or second cranial nerve palsy, requires investigation for skull-base tumor. In most cases of isolated congenital Horner's syndrome, no etiology is identified. Birth trauma is a commonly identified cause, and neuroblastoma is occasionally responsible. Unexplained acquired Horner's syndrome in infants requires imaging for neuroblastoma.

Pharmacologic testing with apraclonidine drops confirms Horner's syndrome by reversal of the anisocoria, with the affected pupil becoming larger than the normal pupil. Hydroxyamphetamine drops differentiate central and preganglionic from postganglionic lesions, but they are difficult to obtain.

▼ EYE MOVEMENTS

The neural control of eye movements is ultimately due to alterations in activity in the nuclei and nerve fibers of the third, fourth, and sixth cranial nerves. These are referred to as the nuclear and infranuclear pathways. Coordination of eye movements requires connections between these ocular motor nuclei, the internuclear pathways. The supranuclear pathways are responsible for generation of the commands necessary for the execution of the appropriate movement, whether it be voluntary or involuntary.

▶ Classification & Generation of Eye Movements

Eye movements are classified as fast or slow (Table 14–2). The generation of a fast eye movement involves a **pulse** of increased innervation to move the eye in the required

Table 14–2. Classification of Eye Movements

Fast eye movements
Refixation (saccades)
    Reflexive (involuntary refixation to a target)
    Voluntary (refixation to command)
    Remembered (refixation to a remembered target)
    Anti-saccade (refixation in the opposite direction to a target)
Fast phases of jerk nystagmus
    Vestibular nystagmus
    Optokinetic nystagmus
    Pathological nystagmus (see later in chapter)

Slow eye movements
Pursuit (following)
Slow phases of nystagmus (see later in chapter)
Responses to rotational head movement (doll's head maneuver)
    Rapid head movement, or slow head movement in darkness
        or in coma (vestibulo-ocular response)
    Slow head movement (predominantly pursuit response)
    Vergence (response to target movement toward or away from
        the subject)
    Convergence
    Divergence

direction and a **step** increase in tonic innervation to maintain the new position in the orbit by counteracting the viscoelastic forces working to return the eye to the primary position. The pulse is produced by the **burst cells of the saccadic generator.** The step change in tonic innervation is produced by the **tonic cells of the neural integrator,** so called because it effectively integrates the pulse to produce the step. There is a close relationship between the amplitude of movement and its peak velocity, with larger movements having greater peak velocities. The generation of a slow eye movement involves a maintained increase of tonic innervation of magnitude correlating with the required velocity of movement.

For the most part, the supranuclear control systems of horizontal and vertical fast eye movements are distinct, whereas the systems for vertical and torsional fast eye movements are closely related, with the vertical system being subsidiary to the torsional (Table 14–3). Table 14–4 describes the generation and abnormalities of slow eye movements.

ABNORMALITIES OF EYE MOVEMENTS

Due to the multiplicity of pathways involved in the supranuclear control of eye movements, with origins in different areas of the brain and an anatomic separation in the brainstem of the horizontal and vertical eye movement systems, disorders of the supranuclear pathways characteristically produce a dissociation of effect upon the various types of eye movements. Thus, the clinical clues to a supranuclear lesion are a differential effect on horizontal and vertical eye

movements or upon saccadic, pursuit, and vestibular eye movements. In diffuse brainstem disease, such features may not be apparent, and differentiation from disease at the neuromuscular junction or within the extraocular muscles on clinical grounds can be difficult.

Disease of the internuclear pathways results in a disruption of the conjugacy of eye movements. In infranuclear disease, the pattern of eye movement disturbance reflects the involvement of one or more cranial nerves or their nuclei.

1. SPECIFIC LESIONS OF THE SUPRANUCLEAR PATHWAYS

Dorsal midbrain syndrome (Parinaud's syndrome) is characterized by loss of upward fast eye movements, convergence-retraction nystagmus (see later in the chapter), pupillary light-near dissociation (see earlier in the chapter), and eyelid retraction (Collier sign). There may also be insufficiency or spasm of convergence and/or accommodation and loss of downward fast eye movements. Conjugate horizontal ocular movements are usually not affected. The syndrome results from damage to the dorsal midbrain usually involving the posterior commissure. Pineal tumor, hydrocephalus, midbrain infarct or arteriovenous malformation, and trauma may be responsible.

▶ Spasm of the Near Response

Spasm of the near response, also known as convergence or accommodative spasm, is usually caused by functional disease, but it may be caused by a midbrain lesion. It is characterized by convergent strabismus with diplopia, miotic pupils, and spasm of accommodation (induced myopia). In functional disease, the features are usually intermittent and provoked by eye movement examination. Cyclopentolate 1%, one drop in each eye twice daily, with reading glasses to compensate for loss of accommodation may be helpful. Psychiatric consultation may be indicated.

▶ Convergence Insufficiency

Convergence insufficiency is characterized by diplopia for near vision in the absence of any impairment of adduction on monocular testing, with refractive error, particularly presbyopia, also having been excluded. It is caused by functional disease or dysfunction of the supranuclear pathway for convergence in the midbrain. In organic lesions, pupillary miosis may still occur when convergence is attempted, whereas in functional disease, it does not.

2. INTERNUCLEAR OPHTHALMOPLEGIA

The medial longitudinal fasciculus is an important fiber tract extending from the rostral midbrain to the spinal cord. It contains many pathways connecting nuclei within

Table 14–3. Generation and Abnormalities of Fast Eye Movements

		Location	Effect of Dysfunction
Saccade generator (burst cells/pulse generator)		Horizontal movements	
		Pons Paramedian pontine reticular formation (PPRF)	Slow ipsilateral horizontal fast eye movements (horizontal saccade palsy)
		Torsional and vertical movements	
		Midbrain Rostral interstitial nucleus of the medial longitudinal fasciculus (riMLF)	Slow ipsilateral torsional and vertical fast eye movements (torsional and vertical saccade palsy)
Neural integrator (tonic cells/step generator)		Horizontal movements	
		Pons Nucleus of the prepositus hypoglossi	Ipsilateral horizontal gaze-paretic nystagmus
		Torsional and vertical movements	
		Midbrain Interstitial nucleus of Cajal **Medulla** Vestibular nuclei	Ocular tilt reaction (OTR) (conjugate ocular torsion and vertical ocular misalignment [skew deviation]), vertical gaze-paretic nystagmus
Neural pathways		Horizontal movements	
	Supranuclear	**Voluntary** Frontal lobe (frontal eye field area 8) via anterior limb of the internal capsule and basal ganglia to contralateral PPRF	Unilateral frontal lobe: ipsilateral horizontal gaze deviation with loss of contralateral fast eye movements (frontal gaze palsy) until recovery from substitution of function by the contralateral frontal eye field (preservation of contralateral slow eye movements including pursuit) [Frontal lobe excitatory (seizure) focus: horizontal contralateral gaze deviation]
		Reflexive (involuntary) Visual cortical centers and subcortical pathway to contralateral PPRF with involvement of superior colliculus	Bilateral frontal lobe: impaired horizontal and vertical fast eye movements (acquired ocular apraxia)
	Internuclear	Medial longitudinal fasciculus (MLF) between sixth nerve nucleus and medial rectus subnucleus of contralateral third nerve nucleus	Impaired adduction of ipsilateral eye and abducting nystagmus in contralateral eye with preserved convergence except in midbrain lesions and upbeating nystagmus if bilateral
	Nuclear	Sixth nerve nucleus	Impairment of all ipsilateral horizontal movements
		Torsional and vertical movements	
	Supranuclear	As for horizontal movements except that the destinations of the pathways are the riMLFs in the midbrain	
	Internuclear	Connections to the ocular motor nuclei including by pathways that decussate in the posterior commissure or anterior to the aqueduct	Posterior commissure: impaired upward fast eye movements (Parinaud's syndrome) Midbrain lesion dorsal and medial to the red nuclei (anterior to the aqueduct): impaired downward fast eye movements
	Nuclear	Third nerve nucleus	Ipsilateral third nerve palsy plus contralateral superior rectus palsy, contralateral ptosis, and possibly contralateral dilated unreactive pupil
		Fourth nerve nucleus	Contralateral fourth nerve palsy

Table 14–4. Generation and Abnormalities of Slow Eye Movements

	Stimulus	Pathway	Effect of Dysfunction
Vestibular	Velocity signal resulting from neural integration of neural signal produced by semicircular canals in response to acceleration of the head	From semicircular canals via vestibular nuclei directly to ocular motor nuclei along the medial longitudinal fasciculus (MLF) and other brainstem pathways	Unilateral: nystagmus with slow phase direction determined by pattern of vestibule-ocular pathway dysfunction (see later in the chapter) Bilateral: instability of vision (oscillopsia) during head motion
Pursuit	Target motion	From visual (occipital) cortical center via the posterior limb of the internal capsule to midbrain and ipsilateral paramedian pontine reticular formation (PPRF)	Posterior cerebral hemisphere: impaired ipsilateral pursuit with substitution by fast eye movements ("saccadic pursuit") PPRF: impaired ipsilateral pursuit (as well as ipsilateral horizontal saccade palsy [see Table 14–3]) with preservation of ipsilateral vestibular movements
Optokinetic	Target and background motion	From visual cortical centers including motion detection center (area V5 [middle temporal] at junction of occipital and temporal lobes) and subcortical pathway passing with pursuit pathways to brainstem and then involving vestibulo-ocular pathways	Parietal lobe: asymmetry of optokinetic nystagmus with impaired of ipsilateral slow phases
Vergence	Retinal disparity (stimulation of noncorresponding retinal loci)	From occipital cortex via posterior limb of internal capsule to midbrain nuclei and then directly to medial rectus subnuclei of third nerve nuclei and then via MLFs to contralateral sixth nerve nuclei	Midbrain: impaired convergence sometimes with preservation of pupillary miosis, or spasm of the near response

the brainstem, particularly those concerned with eye movements. The typical manifestation of damage to the medial longitudinal fasciculus is an internuclear ophthalmoplegia, in which conjugate horizontal eye movements are disrupted due to failure of coordination between the sixth nerve nucleus in the pons and the third nerve nucleus in the midbrain. On horizontal eye movements, abduction of each eye is normal, whereas adduction of the eye ipsilateral to the lesion of the brainstem is impaired (ie, there is incoordination of gaze to the contralateral side). (The ipsilateral eye is affected because the pathway connecting the sixth nerve nucleus to the contralateral third nerve nucleus decussates in the pons, and thus the majority of its course is on the same side of the brainstem as the third nerve nucleus to which it connects.) In the mildest form of internuclear ophthalmoplegia, the clinical abnormality is restricted to a slowing of saccades in the adducting eye, producing transient diplopia on lateral gaze. In the most severe form, there is complete loss of adduction on horizontal gaze, producing constant diplopia on lateral gaze (Figure 14–12). Convergence is characteristically preserved in internuclear ophthalmoplegia except when the lesion is in the midbrain, when the convergence

mechanisms may also be affected. Another feature of internuclear ophthalmoplegia is nystagmus in the abducting eye on attempted horizontal gaze, which is at least in part a result of compensation for the failure of adduction in the other eye. In bilateral internuclear ophthalmoplegia, there may also be an upbeating nystagmus on upgaze due to failure of control of gaze holding in the upward direction, and the eyes may be divergent, in which case it is known as the wall-eyed bilateral internuclear ophthalmoplegia (WEBINO) syndrome.

Internuclear ophthalmoplegia may be due to multiple sclerosis (usually in young adults), brainstem infarction (usually in older adults), tumor, arteriovenous malformation, Wernicke's encephalopathy, and encephalitis. Bilateral internuclear ophthalmoplegia is most commonly due to multiple sclerosis.

A horizontal gaze palsy combined with an internuclear ophthalmoplegia, due to a lesion of the sixth nerve nucleus or paramedian pontine reticular formation extending into the ipsilateral medial longitudinal fasciculus, affects all horizontal eye movements in the ipsilateral eye and adduction in the contralateral eye. This is known as a "one-and-a-half syndrome," or paralytic pontine exotropia.

3. NUCLEAR & INFRANUCLEAR CONNECTIONS

▶ Ocular Motor Cranial Nerve Palsies

Ocular motor cranial nerve palsies result in impairment of eye movements, with the pattern being determined by which extraocular muscles are involved; ocular misalignment, which at least in the acute stage also varies in severity with different gaze positions according to which muscles are paretic; and ptosis in third nerve palsy due to palsy of the levator palpebrae superioris muscle. Misalignment of the visual axes results in diplopia, unless there is suppression that more commonly develops in children than adults. Dizziness or disequilibrium may occur but disappears with monocular patching. There may be an abnormal head posture (head turn to the same side in sixth nerve palsy or head tilt to the opposite side in fourth nerve palsy). Paresis of an extraocular muscle can be simulated by restriction of action of the yoke muscle; for example, limitation of abduction may be due to medial rectus restriction rather than lateral rectus paresis. Assessment of velocity of saccades may be helpful, but forced duction tests may need to be performed. Velocity of saccades may also help identify which muscle is paretic, for instance in differentiating superior oblique from inferior rectus palsy.

There is wide variation in the site of damage and etiology in ocular motor cranial nerve palsies. Nuclear lesions have specific localizing features. Fascicular lesions within the brainstem resemble peripheral nerve lesions but usually can be differentiated on the basis of other brainstem signs. Any extraocular muscle palsy that occurs with minor head trauma (subconcussive injuries) should be investigated for an intracranial lesion. In ischemic (microvascular) palsies, recovery by 4 months is the rule. Palsies that have not started to recover by then—especially those involving the sixth nerve—should be evaluated for another cause, particularly a structural lesion. Urgent investigation should be undertaken when there is evidence of multiple cranial nerve dysfunction or for any extraocular muscle palsy in a young adult. Assessment of any ocular motor nerve palsy must include assessment of second, fifth, and seventh cranial nerve function.

▶ Third Cranial (Oculomotor) Nerve (III)

The motor fibers arise from a group of nuclei in the central gray matter ventral to the cerebral aqueduct at the level of the superior colliculus. The midline central caudal nucleus innervates both levator palpebrae superioris muscles. The paired superior rectus subnuclei each innervate the contralateral superior rectus. The efferent fibers decussate immediately and pass through the opposite superior rectus subnucleus. The subnuclei for the medial rectus, inferior rectus, and inferior oblique muscles are also paired structures but innervate the ipsilateral muscles. The fascicle of the third nerve courses through the red nucleus and the inner side of the substantia nigra to emerge on the medial side of the cerebral peduncles. The nerve runs alongside the sella turcica, in the outer wall of the cavernous sinus, and through the superior orbital fissure to enter the orbit. The superior branch innervates the levator palpebrae and superior rectus muscles and the inferior branch of all other muscles and the sphincter.

The parasympathetics arise from the Edinger-Westphal nucleus just rostral to the motor nucleus of the third nerve and pass via the inferior division of the third nerve to the ciliary ganglion. From there, the short ciliary nerves are distributed to the sphincter muscle of the iris and to the ciliary muscle.

A. Third Nerve Palsy

Lesions of the third nerve nucleus typically affect the ipsilateral medial and inferior rectus and inferior oblique muscles, both levator muscles, and both superior rectus muscles. There will be bilateral ptosis and bilateral limitation of elevation as well as limitation of adduction and depression ipsilaterally.

From the fascicle of the nerve in the midbrain to its eventual termination in the orbit, third nerve palsy produces purely ipsilateral dysfunction. The exact pattern depends on the extent of the palsy, but in general, the ipsilateral eye is turned out by the intact lateral rectus muscle and slightly depressed by the intact superior oblique muscle. The eye may only be moved laterally. (Incyclotorsion from the action of the intact superior oblique muscle can be observed by watching a small blood vessel on the medial conjunctiva as depression of the eye is attempted.) There can be a dilated fixed pupil, absent accommodation, and ptosis of the upper lid, often severe enough to cover the pupil. The pattern of pupil abnormality may be influenced by concomitant Horner's syndrome (sympathetic paresis), resulting in a relatively small unreactive pupil or aberrant regeneration (see later in the chapter).

Ischemia, intracranial aneurysm, head trauma, and intracranial tumor are the most common causes of third nerve palsy in adults. Causes of ischemic (microvascular) palsy include diabetes mellitus, hypertension, hyperlipidemia, and systemic vasculitis. Aneurysm usually arises from the junction of the internal carotid and posterior communicating arteries. Intracranial tumor may cause third nerve palsy by direct damage to the nerve or due to mass effect. Pupillary dilation, initially unilateral and then bilateral, is an important sign of herniation of the medial temporal lobe through the tentorial hiatus (tentorial herniation) due to a rapidly expanding supratentorial mass. Bilateral peripheral third nerve palsies can be caused by an interpeduncular lesion, such as basilar artery aneurysm.

A useful guide clinically is that in ischemic lesions pupil function is preserved, whereas in compression, including aneurysmal, pupil function is abnormal, with initially loss of reactivity and then also dilation. Less than 5% of vascular third nerve palsies are associated with complete pupillary palsy, and in only 15%, there is partial pupillary palsy. Painful isolated third nerve palsy with pupillary involvement necessitates emergency investigation for ipsilateral posterior communicating artery aneurysm. Such investigation may also be indicated in painful isolated third nerve palsy without pupillary involvement and in young patients with painless isolated third nerve palsy with pupillary involvement.

Monocular elevator paralysis—inability to elevate one eye in both abduction (superior rectus) and adduction (inferior oblique)—can be due to paresis of the superior division of the third nerve, such as due to tumor, sinusitis, or after a virus, but it also occurs as a congenital defect or in Graves' ophthalmopathy, orbital myositis, orbital floor fracture, myasthenia, and midbrain stroke.

Third nerve palsies in children may be congenital or may be due to ophthalmoplegic migraine or meningitis or occur after a virus.

B. Oculomotor Synkinesis (Aberrant Regeneration of the Third Nerve)

This phenomenon is characterized by inappropriate activation of muscles innervated by the third nerve, including (1) lid dyskinesias due to inappropriate activation of levator palpebrae superioris either on horizontal gaze (eyelid elevates on attempted adduction) or on vertical gaze (eyelid elevates on attempted depression; "pseudo-Graefe sign"); (2) adduction or retraction on attempted upgaze due to inappropriate activation of medial rectus or inferior rectus; (3) pupillary constriction on attempted adduction or depression; and (4) a monocular vertical optokinetic nystagmus response (due to coactivation of superior rectus, inferior oblique, and inferior rectus muscles fixing the involved eye, allowing only the normal eye to respond to the moving target).

Oculomotor synkinesis most commonly occurs in congenital third nerve palsy or during recovery from acute third nerve palsy due to trauma or aneurysmal compression (secondary oculomotor synkinesis). It may also occur as a primary phenomenon in chronic compression, usually due to an internal carotid aneurysm or meningioma in the cavernous sinus. Oculomotor synkinesis is not a feature of ischemic third nerve palsy.

C. Cyclic Third Nerve Palsy

Cyclic third nerve palsy can complicate congenital third nerve palsy. It is a rare, predominantly unilateral event, with a typical third nerve palsy showing cyclic spasms every 10–30 seconds. During these intervals, ptosis improves and accommodation increases. This phenomenon continues unchanged throughout life but decreases with sleep and increases with greater arousal.

D. Marcus Gunn Phenomenon (Jaw-Winking Syndrome)

This rare usually congenital condition consists of elevation of a ptotic eyelid upon movement of the jaw. Acquired cases occur after damage to the third nerve with subsequent innervation of the lid (levator palpebrae superioris) by a branch of the fifth cranial nerve.

▶ Fourth Cranial (Trochlear) Nerve (IV)

Motor (entirely crossed) fibers arise from the fourth nerve nucleus just caudal to the third nerve nucleus at the level of the inferior colliculus; they then run posteriorly, decussate in the anterior medullary velum, and wind around the cerebral peduncles. The fourth nerve travels near the third nerve along the wall of the cavernous sinus to the orbit, where it supplies the superior oblique muscle. The fourth nerve is unique among the cranial nerves in arising from the dorsal brainstem.

A. Fourth Nerve Palsy

Congenital fourth nerve palsy is probably not usually neurogenic in origin but due to developmental anomaly within the orbit. It may present in childhood with an abnormal head posture (see later in the chapter) or in childhood or adult life with eyestrain or diplopia due to reduced ability to overcome the vertical ocular deviation (decompensation). Acquired fourth nerve palsy is commonly traumatic. The nerve is vulnerable to injury at the site of exit from the dorsal aspect of the brainstem. Both nerves may be damaged by severe trauma as they decussate in the anterior medullary velum. Acquired fourth nerve palsy may also be ischemic (microvascular) or secondary to posterior fossa surgery. Rarely, posterior fossa tumors may present with an isolated fourth nerve palsy.

Superior oblique palsy results in upward deviation (hypertropia) of the eye, which increases when the patient looks down and to the opposite side. In addition, in acquired palsy, there is excyclotropia; therefore, one of the diplopic images will be tilted with respect to the other. Thus, torsional diplopia indicates an acquired palsy, and lack of torsional symptoms indicates a congenital palsy. Tilting the head toward the involved side increases the vertical ocular deviation (Bielschowsky head tilt test). Tilting the head away from the side of the involved eye may relieve the diplopia, and patients frequently adopt such a head tilt. History of an abnormal head posture during childhood, which may be confirmed by review of family photographs, and a large vertical prism fusion range are strong clues that a fourth nerve palsy is congenital. In bilateral traumatic palsy, there is usually a chin-down head posture. Strabismus surgery is effective in decompensated congenital palsy not controlled by prisms and for unresolved acquired palsy.

B. Superior Oblique Myokymia

Contrary to its name, this is an acquired tremor of the superior oblique muscle, affecting only one eye. The patient complains of episodes of torsional and/or vertical oscillopsia or double vision, which may be precipitated by looking down, such as when reading. Various anticonvulsants, typically carbamazepine, or β-blocker eye drops can be beneficial. Superior oblique muscle surgery may be undertaken. The cause may be compression of the fourth nerve by an aberrant artery, for which intracranial surgery may be successful.

▶ Sixth Cranial (Abducens) Nerve (VI)

Motor (entirely uncrossed) fibers arise from the nucleus in the floor of the fourth ventricle in the lower portion of the pons near the internal genu of the facial nerve. Piercing the pons, the fibers emerge anteriorly, with the nerve running a long course over the tip of the petrous portion of the temporal bone into the cavernous sinus. It enters the orbit with the third and fourth nerves to supply the lateral rectus muscle.

A. Sixth Nerve Nucleus Lesion

The sixth nerve nucleus contains the motor neurons to the ipsilateral lateral rectus and the cell bodies of interneurons innervating the motor neurons to the contralateral medial rectus. It is the final common relay point for all horizontal conjugate eye movements, and a lesion within the nucleus will produce an ipsilateral horizontal gaze palsy affecting all types of eye movement, including vestibular movements. This contrasts with a lesion of the paramedian pontine reticular formation, in which vestibular movements are preserved.

B. Sixth Nerve Palsy (see also Chapter 12)

This is the most common single extraocular muscle palsy. Abduction of the eye is reduced or absent; esotropia is present in the primary position and increases with distance fixation and upon gaze to the affected side. Ischemia (arteriosclerosis, diabetes, migraine, and hypertension) is a common cause. However, increased intracranial pressure, in which the sixth nerve palsy is a false localizing sign, intracranial tumor, particularly at the base of the skull, trauma, meningitis, demyelination, dural arteriovenous fistula, and intracranial hypotension including after lumbar puncture are other causes. Infections can produce sixth nerve palsy from direct involvement, as in middle ear infection, ischemia, or meningitis. Arnold-Chiari malformation (congenital downward displacement of the cerebellar tonsils) can produce sixth nerve palsy due to traction but can also produce a distance esotropia without limitation of abduction due to cerebellar dysfunction. A child with a sixth nerve palsy should be evaluated for a brainstem tumor (glioma) or inflammation if trauma was not present or if trauma was minimal. Möbius' syndrome (congenital facial diplegia) can be associated with a sixth nerve or conjugate gaze palsy. Mimics of sixth nerve paly include Duane's syndrome, spasm of the near response, Graves' ophthalmopathy, myasthenia, and medial rectus entrapment in an ethmoid fracture.

C. Duane's Syndrome

Duane's syndrome is uncommon (< 1% of cases of strabismus) and in almost all cases congenital. It is a stationary, nearly always unilateral condition characterized by complete or partial deficiency of abduction, with retraction of the globe and narrowing of the lid fissure on adduction. Congenital absence of the sixth nerve with coinnervation of the lateral rectus by a branch of the third nerve is the likely cause in most cases, and other congenital anomalies are common. The visual handicap is seldom severe. Visual acuity is usually normal. Unless there is a marked abnormal head posture, strabismus surgery is best avoided.

D. Gradenigo's Syndrome

Gradenigo's syndrome is characterized by pain in the face (from irritation of the fifth nerve) and sixth nerve palsy. The syndrome is produced by disease of the tip of the petrous bone and most often occurs as a complication of otitis media with mastoiditis or petrous bone tumors.

▶ Syndromes Affecting Cranial Nerves III, IV, & VI

A. Superior Orbital Fissure Syndrome

All the ocular motor nerves pass through the superior orbital fissure and can be affected by tumor, inflammation, or trauma involving the fissure.

B. Orbital Apex Syndrome

This syndrome is similar to the superior orbital fissure syndrome with the addition of optic nerve signs and usually greater proptosis. It is also caused by tumor, inflammation, or trauma.

C. Sudden Complete Ophthalmoplegia

Complete ophthalmoplegia of sudden onset can be due to extensive brainstem vascular disease, Wernicke's encephalopathy, Fisher's syndrome, bulbar poliomyelitis, pituitary apoplexy, basilar aneurysm, meningitis, diphtheria, botulism, or myasthenic crisis.

4. THE CEREBELLUM

The cerebellum has an important modulating influence on the function of the neural integrators. Thus, it is involved in gaze holding and the control of saccades, particularly the relationship between the pulse and the step of saccade generation. Cerebellar dysfunction produces gaze-evoked nystagmus, by its influence on gaze holding, and abnormalities of saccades, including saccadic dysmetria in which the saccadic amplitude is inaccurate, and postsaccadic drift due to a mismatch between the pulse and step of the saccade.

The cerebellum is also important in the control of pursuit eye movements, and cerebellar dysfunction may thus result in broken (saccadic) pursuit. It may also result in ocular misalignment, either vertical due to skew deviation or horizontal.

MYASTHENIA GRAVIS

Myasthenia (gravis) is characterized by abnormal fatigability of striated muscles after repetitive contraction that improves after rest and often manifests as weakness of the extraocular muscles. Unilateral fatiguing ptosis is a frequent first sign, with subsequent bilateral involvement of extraocular muscles, so that diplopia is often an early symptom. Unusual ocular presentations may simulate gaze palsy, internuclear ophthalmoplegia, vertical nystagmus, and progressive external ophthalmoplegia. Generalized weakness of the arms and legs, difficulty in swallowing, weakness of jaw muscles, and difficulty in breathing may follow rapidly in untreated cases. The weakness often worsens as the day progresses but can be improved by rest. There are no sensory changes.

The incidence of the disease is in the range of 1:30,000 to 1:20,000. Myasthenia usually presents in young adults aged 20–40 (70% are under 40 years of age), although it may occur at any age and can be misdiagnosed as functional, especially because the weakness can be greater in exciting or embarrassing situations. Older patients are more commonly male and are more likely to have a thymoma.

The onset may follow an upper respiratory infection, stress, pregnancy, or any injury, and the disease has been noted as a transitory condition in newborn infants of myasthenic mothers. Drugs, including β-blockers (eg, propranolol), penicillamine, statins, lithium, aminoglycoside antibiotics, chloroquine, and phenytoin, may induce, unmask, or exacerbate the disease. Myasthenia is associated with hyperthyroidism (5%), thyroid abnormalities (15%), autoimmune diseases (5%), and diffuse metastatic carcinoma (7%).

In about one-third of cases, the disease is confined to the extraocular muscles at onset. In about two-thirds of these cases, the disease will become generalized with time, usually within the first year.

The differential diagnosis includes chronic progressive external ophthalmoplegia (see later in the chapter), oculopharyngeal muscular dystrophy, myotonic dystrophy, ocular motor cranial nerve palsies, and brainstem lesions including encephalitis, botulism, and multiple sclerosis.

The disease has its origin at the neuromuscular junction, especially at the postsynaptic site, primarily due to antibodies against it and the presynaptic site. Anti-acetylcholine receptor antibodies are diagnostic. They are present in 80–90% of patients with systemic myasthenia and 40–60% of patients with pure ocular myasthenia, but the titers do not correlate with severity of disease. Antibody-positive patients should undergo chest CT or MRI to detect thymic enlargement.

Thymomas occur in 15% of patients. A large proportion of patients with generalized myasthenia without acetylcholine receptor antibodies have antibodies against muscle-specific receptor tyrosine kinase (MuSK). These patients tend to be female, with predominant cranial and bulbar muscle involvement, frequent respiratory crises, and poorer response to treatment. MuSK antibody myasthenia may also present with pure ocular disease.

Cholinesterase destroys acetylcholine at the neuromuscular junction, and cholinesterase-inhibiting drugs such as pyridostigmine may improve myasthenia by increasing the amount of acetylcholine available to the damaged postsynaptic site. Intravenous edrophonium or intramuscular neostigmine can be used for diagnosis. In the edrophonium (Tensilon) test, pretreatment with intravenous atropine is recommended. Edrophonium, 2 mg (0.2 mL), is given intravenously over 15 seconds. If no response occurs in 30 seconds, an additional 5–7 mg (0.5–0.7 mL) is given. The test is most helpful when marked ptosis is present. Significant improvement in muscle function constitutes a positive response and confirms the diagnosis of myasthenia. Slightly positive edrophonium tests can occur in neurogenic palsies, and there may be false-negative results when myasthenia is complicated by muscle wasting. Improvement of ptosis with rest or application of ice can be helpful for diagnosis.

Repetitive nerve stimulation, especially of the facial or proximal muscles, can demonstrate abnormal muscle fatigability (more than 10% decrease in the response is diagnostic of myasthenia). Variation in size and shape of motor unit potentials is noted on needle electromyography of affected muscles, and single-fiber studies show increased variability (jitter) in the temporal pattern of action potentials from muscle fibers of the same motor unit. Orbicularis oculi single-fiber electromyography is particularly useful in diagnosis of ocular myasthenia.

Myasthenia can be treated with pyridostigmine, systemic steroids, other immunosuppressants such as azathioprine, immunoglobulins, and plasmapheresis according to the severity of disease. During severe exacerbations, artificial ventilation may be necessary. Thymectomy may be indicated in patients with thymoma (although it may not influence the severity of the myasthenia) and in patients with early-onset generalized disease without evidence of thymoma—in one-third of whom it may produce complete remission without the need for immunosuppressants. Ocular myasthenia tends to respond less well to anticholinesterase agents than generalized disease, but the response to systemic steroids is usually good. Extraocular muscle surgery can be undertaken but should be delayed until the ocular motility deficit has been stable for a long time.

Myasthenia is generally a chronic disease with a tendency to pursue a relapsing and remitting course. The prognosis depends on the extent of the disease, the response to medication and thymectomy, and the careful management of severe exacerbations.

CHRONIC PROGRESSIVE EXTERNAL OPHTHALMOPLEGIA

Chronic progressive external ophthalmoplegia (CPEO) is characterized by ptosis and slowly progressive inability to move the eyes with normal pupillary responses. It may begin at any age and progresses over a period of 5–15 years to complete external ophthalmoplegia. It is a form of mitochondrial myopathy and may be associated with other manifestations of mitochondrial disease, such as pigmentary degeneration of the retina, deafness, cerebellar-vestibular abnormalities, seizures, cardiac conduction defects, and peripheral sensorimotor neuropathy, in which case the term "ophthalmoplegia-plus" may be applied. Onset before 15 years of age of CPEO, heart block, and pigmentary retinopathy constitute the Kearns-Sayre syndrome. CPEO is associated with deletions of mitochondrial DNA, which are more frequent and more extensive in the cases with nonocular manifestations.

NYSTAGMUS (TABLE 14–5)

Nystagmus is defined as repetitive, rhythmic oscillations of one or both eyes in any or all fields of gaze, initiated by a slow eye movement. The waveform may be pendular, in which the movements in each direction have equal speed, amplitude, and duration; or jerk, in which the slow movement in one direction is followed by a rapid corrective return to the original position (fast component). By convention, the direction of jerk nystagmus is given as the direction of the corrective fast phase and not the direction of the primary slow phase.

Jerk nystagmus is classified as grade I, present only with the eyes directed toward the fast component; grade II, present also with the eyes in primary position; or grade III, present even with the eyes directed toward the slow component. The movements of pendular or jerk nystagmus may be horizontal, vertical, torsional, oblique, circular, or a combination of these. The direction may change depending on the direction of gaze.

The **amplitude** of nystagmus is the extent of the movement; the **rate** of nystagmus is the frequency of oscillation. Generally speaking, the faster the rate, the smaller is the amplitude and vice versa. Nystagmus is usually conjugate but is occasionally dysconjugate, as in convergence-retraction nystagmus and seesaw nystagmus.

Nystagmus is also occasionally dissociated (more marked in one eye than the other), as in internuclear ophthalmoplegia, spasmus nutans, monocular visual loss, and acquired pendular nystagmus and with asymmetric muscle weakness in myasthenia.

Physiology of Symptoms

Reduced visual acuity is caused by inability to maintain steady fixation. The patient may complain of illusory movement of objects (oscillopsia), which is usually indicative

Table 14–5. Classification of Nystagmus

Physiologic nystagmus
End-point nystagmus
Optokinetic nystagmus
Stimulation of semicircular canals (physiologic vestibular nystagmus)
Rotatory
Caloric
Pathologic nystagmus
Congenital nystagmus
CN type
With sensory abnormality
Without sensory abnormality (congenital idiopathic motor)
Latent nystagmus (LN)
Manifest latent nystagmus (MLN)
Acquired pendular nystagmus
Infantile visual deprivation
Spasmus nutans
Oculopalatal myoclonus
Vestibular nystagmus
Peripheral vestibular nystagmus
Central vestibular nystagmus
Downbeat nystagmus
Upbeat nystagmus
Gaze-evoked nystagmus
Gaze-paretic nystagmus
Convergence-retraction nystagmus
Seesaw nystagmus
Periodic alternating nystagmus
Mimics of nystagmus
Saccadic intrusions
Spontaneous eye movements in coma
Voluntary nystagmus

of acquired rather than congenital nystagmus and is particularly severe in vestibular disease. Head tilting is usually involuntary, to decrease the nystagmus. The head is turned toward the fast components in jerk nystagmus or set so that the eyes are in a position that minimizes ocular movement in pendular nystagmus. Head nodding may occur in congenital nystagmus and is a characteristic feature of spasmus nutans. Nystagmus is noticeable and cosmetically disturbing except when excursions of the eye are very small.

PHYSIOLOGIC NYSTAGMUS

Three types of nystagmus can be elicited in the normal person.

End-Point (End-Gaze) Nystagmus

Normal individuals may have nystagmus on extreme horizontal gaze, which disappears when the eyes are moved centrally by a few degrees. It is primarily horizontal but may have a slight torsional component and greater amplitude in the abducting eye.

Optokinetic Nystagmus

This type of nystagmus may be elicited in all normal individuals, usually with a rotating drum with alternating black and white lines but by any repetitive targets in the visual field, such as repetitive telephone poles as seen from a window of a fast-moving vehicle. The slow component follows the object, and the fast component moves rapidly in the opposite direction to fixate on the succeeding object. A unilateral or asymmetric horizontal response usually indicates a deep parietal lobe lesion, especially a tumor. It occurs as a result of a deficit in the slow (pursuit) phase. Anterior cerebral (ie, frontal lobe) lesions may inhibit this response only temporarily when an acute saccadic gaze palsy is present, which suggests the presence of a compensatory mechanism that is much greater than for lesions situated farther posteriorly. Asymmetry of response in the vertical plane suggests a brainstem lesion. Since it is an involuntary response, this test is especially useful in detecting functional visual loss. A large mirror filling the patient's central field at near can be rotated from side to side and will induce an optokinetic nystagmus if vision is present.

Stimulation of Semicircular Canals

The three semicircular canals of each inner ear sense movements of the head in space, being primarily sensitive to acceleration. The neural output of the vestibular system, after processing within the vestibular and related brainstem nuclei, is a velocity signal. This is transmitted, principally via the medial longitudinal fasciculus on each side of the brainstem, to the ocular motor nuclei to produce the necessary compensatory eye movements (vestibulo-ocular response [VOR]) for maintaining a stable position of the eyes in space, and hence optimal vision. Vestibular signals also pass to the cerebellum and cerebral cortex.

Stimulation of the semicircular canals results in a compensatory eye movement. In the unconscious subject with an intact brainstem, this leads to a tonic deviation of the eyes, whereas in the conscious subject, a superimposed corrective fast-phase movement, returning the eyes back toward the straight-ahead position, results in a jerk nystagmus. These tests are useful methods of investigating vestibular function in conscious subjects and, in the case of caloric stimulation, brainstem function in comatose patients.

A. Rotatory Physiologic Nystagmus (Bárány Rotating Chair)

When the head is tilted 30° forward, the horizontal semicircular canals lie horizontally in space. Rotation, such as in a Bárány chair, then leads to horizontal jerk nystagmus with the compensatory slow-phase eye movement opposite to the direction of turning and the corrective fast phase in the direction of turning. Due to impersistence of the vestibular signal during continued rotation, the nystagmus abates. Once the rotation stops, there is a vestibular tone in the opposite direction, which

results in a jerk nystagmus with the fast phase away from the original direction of turning (postrotatory nystagmus). Since the subject is stationary, postrotatory nystagmus is often easier to analyze than the nystagmus during rotation.

B. Caloric Stimulation

With the head tilted 60° backward, the horizontal semicircular canals lie vertically in space. Water irrigation of the auditory canal generates convection currents predominantly within the horizontal rather than the vertical semicircular canals. Cold water irrigation induces a predominantly horizontal jerk nystagmus with a fast phase opposite to the side of irrigation, and warm water irrigation induces a similar jerk nystagmus with a fast phase toward the side of irrigation. (The mnemonic device is "COWS": cold-opposite, warm-same.) Caloric nystagmus is made more obvious by the patient wearing Frenzel spectacles, which eliminate patient fixation and provide a magnified view for the examiner. It is important to verify that the tympanic membrane is intact before performing irrigation of the external auditory canal.

PATHOLOGIC NYSTAGMUS

A. Congenital Nystagmus

Congenital nystagmus is nystagmus present within 6 months after birth. Ocular instability is usual at birth, due to poor visual fixation, but this abates during the first few weeks of life. The presence of spontaneous nystagmus is always pathologic.

Congenital impairment of vision or visual deprivation due to lesions in any part of the eye or optic nerve can result in nystagmus at birth or soon thereafter. Causes include corneal opacity, cataract, albinism, achromatopsia, bilateral macular disease, aniridia, and optic atrophy. By definition, congenital idiopathic motor nystagmus has no associated underlying sensory abnormality, although visual performance is limited by the ocular instability. Typically it is not present at birth but becomes apparent between 3 and 6 months of age.

At one time it was thought that congenital pendular nystagmus was indicative of an underlying sensory abnormality whereas congenital jerk nystagmus was not. Eye movement recordings have shown this not to be true, with both pendular and jerk waveforms being seen whether or not there is a sensory abnormality. Indeed, in many cases, a mixed pattern of alternating pendular and jerk waveforms is seen. Congenital nystagmus, particularly the idiopathic motor type with its potential for better visual fixation, generally undergoes a progressive change in its waveform during early childhood. There is development of periods of relative ocular stability, that is, relatively slow eye velocity, known as foveation periods since they are thought to be an adaptive response to maximize the potential for fixation, and hence to improve visual acuity. In addition, congenital nystagmus with a jerk nystagmus has a characteristic waveform in which the slow phases have an exponentially increasing velocity. This is known as CN-type waveform, and with very few exceptions, its presence signifies that the nystagmus has been present since early childhood. This can be a particularly useful feature in determining that nystagmus noted in adulthood is not of recent onset.

Congenital nystagmus is usually horizontal and conjugate. Vertical and torsional components are only occasionally present. The direction of any jerk component often varies with the direction of gaze, but an important feature in comparison to many forms of acquired nystagmus is that there is no additional vertical component on vertical gaze. In most patients with congenital nystagmus, there is a direction of gaze (null zone) in which the nystagmus is relatively quiet. If this null zone is away from primary position, a head turn may be adopted to place the eccentric position straight ahead. In a few cases, the position of the null zone varies to produce the congenital type of periodic alternating nystagmus. Congenital nystagmus is usually decreased in intensity by convergence, and some patients will adopt an esotropia (nystagmus blockage). Anxiety and increased "effort to see" will often increase the intensity of congenital nystagmus and thus reduce visual acuity.

Once congenital nystagmus has been noted, it is important to identify any underlying sensory abnormality, if only to determine the visual potential. This may require electrodiagnostic studies. Extraocular muscle surgery is predominantly indicated for patients with a marked head turn. Supramaximal recessions of the horizontal rectus muscles reduce the intensity of congenital nystagmus, but the effect is only temporary. Gabapentin and/or memantine may be beneficial.

Nystagmus with a **latent component** means that it increases in intensity when one eye is covered, which is a characteristic feature of congenital nystagmus. There is also a specific type of latent nystagmus, known as **LN**, which is predominantly seen in infantile esotropia. LN is a horizontal jerk nystagmus with the fast phase toward the side of the fixing eye—with the left eye covered, there is a rightward nystagmus, and with the right eye covered, a leftward nystagmus. LN also becomes more marked when one eye is covered, only then being apparent on clinical examination, but eye movement recordings show that the nystagmus is always present. **Manifest latent nystagmus (MLN)** is a particular type of LN in which the nystagmus is always apparent on clinical examination. It occurs in patients with LN when binocular function is lost, that is, the equivalent of one eye being covered. This may be because of loss of sight in one eye or even from the development of a divergent squint. If binocular function is restored, MLN will revert to LN.

B. Acquired Pendular Nystagmus

Any child who develops bilateral visual loss before 6 years of age may also develop a pendular nystagmus, and indeed the acquisition of a pendular nystagmus during infancy necessitates further investigation. A specific syndrome of acquired pendular nystagmus in childhood is **spasmus nutans.** This is a bilateral, generally horizontal (occasionally vertical), fine, dissociated pendular nystagmus, associated with head nodding and an abnormal head posture. There is a benign form, which may be familial, with onset before age 2 and spontaneous improvement during the third or fourth year. Spasmus nutans may also rarely be the first manifestation of an anterior visual pathway glioma.

In adults, acquired pendular nystagmus is a feature of brainstem disease, usually multiple sclerosis or brainstem stroke. There may be horizontal, vertical, or torsional components or even a combination of components to produce oblique or elliptical trajectories. The syndrome of **oculopalatal myoclonus** characteristically develops several months after a brainstem stroke. There is pendular nystagmus with synchronous movements variably involving the soft palate, larynx, and diaphragm as well as producing head titubation. (The term "myoclonus" is a misnomer since the abnormal movements are a form of tremor.) The associated hypertrophy of the inferior olivary nucleus in the medulla and other evidence suggest a disruption of the dentato-rubro-olivary pathway between the brainstem and the cerebellum as the underlying pathogenesis. Various drug treatments have been tried for adult acquired pendular nystagmus, of which gabapentin, memantine, and baclofen have produced the best, although still limited, results. Base-out prisms may also be tried.

C. Vestibular Nystagmus

Abnormalities of vestibular tone result in abnormal activation of the vestibulo-ocular pathways and abnormal neural drive to the extraocular muscles. Loss of function in the left horizontal semicircular canal is equivalent to activation of the right horizontal semicircular canal, as would normally be produced by a rightward head turn. The eye movement response is conjugate leftward slow-phase movement of the eyes. The corrective fast-phase response is rightward in direction, and a right-beating horizontal nystagmus is thus generated. The pattern of response to dysfunction of one or more semicircular canals can be similarly derived to give the full possible range of **peripheral vestibular nystagmus,** although in clinical practice, it is the effect of dysfunction of the horizontal canals that usually predominates. As a general rule, peripheral vestibular lesions are destructive, and the fast phase of the resulting nystagmus is away from the side of the lesion. Since the neural signal of the vestibulo-ocular pathways is a velocity signal, the slow phase of peripheral vestibular nystagmus has a constant velocity. This gives rise to the characteristic saw-tooth waveform on eye movement recordings.

Peripheral vestibular nystagmus is not dependent on visual stimuli and thus is still present in the dark or with the eyes closed, as well as in blind individuals. It is, however, inhibited by visual fixation or, conversely, accentuated by wearing Frenzel spectacles, and this is an important factor in the normal dampening over 2–3 weeks of peripheral vestibular nystagmus. Head position does not usually influence peripheral vestibular nystagmus except in benign paroxysmal positional vertigo, in which elicitation of the characteristic pattern of nystagmus with the Hallpike maneuver is a specific diagnostic feature. Other clinical features associated with peripheral vestibular disease are vertigo, tinnitus, and deafness, the latter two reflecting the close association between the vestibular and auditory systems. Causes of peripheral vestibular disease are labyrinthitis, Ménière's disease, trauma (including surgical destruction of one labyrinth), and vascular, inflammatory, or neoplastic lesion of the vestibular nerve.

Central vestibular nystagmus is an acquired jerk nystagmus due to disease in the central vestibular pathways of the brainstem and cerebellum. It has a variety of forms, but characteristic types are a purely torsional or vertical jerk nystagmus and the syndromes of downbeat and upbeat nystagmus, which result from imbalance in vestibular tone from the vertical semicircular canals. Central vestibular nystagmus is frequently elicited or enhanced by specific head positions, presumably as a result of modulation by input from the peripheral vestibular apparatus. It is not dampened by visual fixation and does not spontaneously abate in intensity with time. Other clinical features reflect the associated brainstem and cerebellar dysfunction and include abnormalities of smooth pursuit eye movements other than those due to the nystagmus itself. Causes of central vestibular nystagmus include lesion of the vestibular nuclei (brainstem demyelination, including multiple sclerosis, inflammation, and stroke, particularly thrombosis of the posteroinferior cerebellar artery leading to lateral medullary infarction—Wallenberg's syndrome).

Downbeat nystagmus is a downward-beating nystagmus, usually present in primary position. It is often most obvious on gaze down and to the side, when the nystagmus becomes oblique, with the horizontal component in the direction of lateral gaze. Downbeat nystagmus is characteristically associated with lesions at the cervicomedullary junction, notably Chiari malformation and basilar invagination, and all patients should undergo MRI to exclude such lesions. Other causes are cerebellar degeneration, demyelinating disease, hydrocephalus, anticonvulsants, and lithium. Clonazepam or aminopyridines may be beneficial.

Upbeat nystagmus is characterized by an upward-beating nystagmus in primary position, which usually increases, although it may reduce in intensity on upgaze. It is virtually always the result of brainstem disease but occasionally reflects cerebellar disease. It is seen in brainstem encephalitis, demyelination, and tumor and also as a toxic side effect of barbiturates, alcohol, and anticonvulsants. Baclofen or aminopyridines may be beneficial.

D. Gaze-Evoked & Gaze-Paretic Nystagmus

Maintenance of steady eccentric gaze is dependent on the neural integrator system, which produces the tonic extraocular muscle activity necessary to overcome the viscous and elastic orbital forces acting to return the globe to primary position. Reduction in activity of the neural integrator results in eccentric gaze being negated by a slow drift of the globe toward primary position. Since the force acting to produce this central drift reduces with decreasing eccentricity, this slow drift has an exponentially decreasing velocity. Additional corrective fast eye movements, returning the eye to the desired eccentric position, result in nystagmus beating in the direction of gaze, whether it is horizontal, vertical, or oblique.

End-point nystagmus (see earlier in the chapter) is the physiologic manifestation of the inability of the neural integrator to maintain steady eye position in extreme eccentric gaze. Gaze-evoked nystagmus is the result of pathologic failure of the neural integrator system. In its mildest form, it manifests only on moderate horizontal gaze, whereas in its most severe form, nystagmus is present with any movement away from primary position. In many cases of gaze-evoked nystagmus, there is also **rebound nystagmus**—following return of the eyes to primary position from a position of eccentric gaze, a jerk nystagmus beating away from the direction of the eccentric gaze develops after a latent period and lasts for a short period.

The neural integrator is situated in the brainstem but is highly dependent on cerebellar inputs. Thus, gaze-evoked nystagmus may be a manifestation of either brainstem or, especially, cerebellar disease. Often there are other cerebellar eye movement abnormalities, such as saccadic dysmetria and disruption of smooth pursuit. The most common causes of gaze-evoked nystagmus are cerebellar diseases, sedatives, and anticonvulsants. Cerebellopontine angle neoplasms, such as vestibular schwannoma (acoustic neuroma), may produce a combination of gaze-evoked nystagmus and a peripheral vestibular nystagmus beating toward the opposite side (Brun's nystagmus).

Reduction of the supranuclear input into the neural integrator or in the ability of the peripheral eye movement system to facilitate its function will lead to nystagmus with the same basic characteristics as gaze-evoked nystagmus. Thus, many conditions such as gaze palsy, ocular motor cranial nerve palsies, myasthenia, and extraocular muscle disease can manifest with nystagmus on eccentric gaze in the direction of the affected eye movements. This is termed gaze-paretic nystagmus and should be excluded whenever the possibility of a gaze-evoked nystagmus is being considered so as to avoid misdirected investigation.

E. Convergence-Retraction Nystagmus

Convergence-retraction nystagmus is a feature of the dorsal midbrain (Parinaud's) syndrome either from intrinsic lesion (tumor, hemorrhage, infarction, or inflammation) or extrinsic lesion, particularly pineal tumor and hydrocephalus. On attempted upgaze, which is usually defective, the eyes undergo rapid convergent movements with retraction of the globes. This is best elicited as the patient watches downward-moving stripes on an optokinetic tape or drum. Electromyographic studies have shown cocontraction of extraocular muscles and loss of normal agonist–antagonist reciprocal innervation. Convergence-retraction nystagmus may represent asynchronous, opposed, adducting saccades due to inappropriate activation of the medial rectus muscles.

F. Seesaw Nystagmus

Seesaw nystagmus is characterized by rising intorsion of one eye and falling extorsion of the other—and then the reverse. It may have a pendular or jerk waveform. Although it is uncommon, it occurs with acquired and congenital chiasmal lesions in association with a bitemporal hemianopia, and midbrain lesions. There does not appear to be a single underlying pathogenesis, but it is likely that dysfunction of the interstitial nucleus of Cajal or the rostral interstitial nucleus of the medial longitudinal fasciculus is important in the cases with midbrain disease.

G. Periodic Alternating Nystagmus

This is a horizontal jerk nystagmus regularly alternating between leftward and rightward directions, with each phase lasting approximately 2 minutes. The acquired form usually results from cerebellar disease, such as cerebellar degeneration; congenital hindbrain anomaly, such as Chiari malformation; multiple sclerosis; or anticonvulsant therapy. It characteristically responds to baclofen. It may also occur with bilateral blindness and be suppressed if vision is restored. Periodic alternation may also be a feature of congenital nystagmus (see earlier in the chapter).

MIMICS OF NYSTAGMUS

Abnormal spontaneous eye movements may be the result of unwanted saccadic eye movements (saccadic intrusions), which include square-wave jerks, macrosaccadic oscillations, ocular flutter, and opsoclonus. These are generally due to cerebellar disease. There is also a variety of abnormal eye movements that occur in coma, including ocular bobbing, ocular dipping, and ping-pong gaze. Superior oblique myokymia (see earlier in the chapter) is a tremor of the superior oblique muscle leading to episodic monocular vertical or torsional oscillopsia. About 5% of normal individuals can generate short bursts of ocular oscillations (voluntary nystagmus) that resemble small-amplitude, fast, horizontal

pendular nystagmus. Eye movement recordings show the movements to be rapidly alternating saccades. Recognition of the entity is important to avoid unnecessary investigation.

CEREBROVASCULAR DISORDERS OF OPHTHALMOLOGIC IMPORTANCE

▶ Vascular Insufficiency & Occlusion of the Internal Carotid Artery

Transient episodes of visual loss most often result from retinal emboli (amaurosis fugax), usually from carotid disease but possibly from cardiac valvular disease or cardiac arrhythmia (see Chapter 15). They also occur in thrombotic disorders such as hyperviscosity states or antiphospholipid syndrome and from other causes of impaired ocular or cerebral perfusion such as giant cell arteritis, migraine, vertebrobasilar ischemia (see later in the chapter), severe hypotension, or shock. The visual loss from retinal emboli is characteristically described as a curtain descending across the vision of one eye, with complete loss of vision for 5–10 minutes, and then complete recovery. There may be associated transient ischemic attacks or completed strokes of the ipsilateral cerebral hemisphere. In other causes of transient visual loss, there may be constriction of the visual field from the periphery to the center, "graying" rather than complete loss of vision, and involvement of both eyes simultaneously. Fleeting episodes of visual loss that last a few seconds (transient visual obscurations) may occur in papilledema, affecting one or both eyes together, or monocularly with orbital tumors.

Cholesterol, platelet-fibrin, and calcific are the three main types of retinal emboli. Cholesterol emboli (Hollenhorst plaques) may be visible with the ophthalmoscope as small, glistening, yellow-red crystals at bifurcations of the retinal arteries. The nonreflective gummy white plugs filling retinal vessels, which characterize platelet-fibrin emboli, are less commonly seen because they quickly disperse and traverse the retinal circulation. Calcific emboli, which usually originate from damaged cardiac valves, have a duller, white-gray appearance compared with cholesterol emboli. Retinal emboli may also produce branch or, particularly in the case of calcific emboli, central retinal arterial occlusions.

Amaurosis fugax is the ocular equivalent of cerebral hemisphere transient ischemic attack and requires the same urgent assessment and treatment to reduce the risk of cerebral hemisphere stroke and retinal artery occlusion. Most patients require antiplatelet agent, usually low-dose (81 mg/d) aspirin, and may require treatment to reduce blood pressure and serum lipids. High-grade (70–99%) stenosis of the internal carotid artery, as determined by ultrasound or angiographic studies, is an indication for urgent carotid endarterectomy or possibly carotid artery stenting. Incidentally noted cholesterol retinal emboli in asymptomatic individuals are associated with a tenfold increased risk of cerebral infarction, but the role of carotid endarterectomy in such individuals is uncertain.

In the acute stage of embolic retinal arterial occlusion, treatment with ocular massage, anterior chamber paracentesis, rebreathing into a paper bag to increase inhaled CO_2 level, and intravenous acetazolamide may lead to displacement of the embolus and recovery of vision. After 12 hours, the clinical picture is usually irreversible, although many exceptions to this rule have been reported. Visual acuity better than counting fingers on presentation has a better prognosis with vigorous treatment. Embolic retinal arterial occlusion has a poorer 5-year survival rate due to attendant cardiac disease or stroke than occlusion due to thrombotic disease.

Slow flow (venous stasis) retinopathy is a sign of generalized ocular ischemia and indicative of severe carotid disease, usually with complete occlusion of the ipsilateral internal carotid artery. It is characterized by venous dilation and tortuosity, retinal hemorrhages, macular edema, and eventual neovascular proliferation. It resembles diabetic retinopathy, but the changes occur more in the retinal midperiphery than the posterior pole. In more severe cases, there may be vasodilation of the conjunctiva, iris neovascularization, neovascular glaucoma, and frank anterior segment ischemia with corneal edema, anterior uveitis, and cataract. Diagnosis is most easily confirmed by demonstration of reversal of blood flow in the ipsilateral ophthalmic artery using orbital ultrasound, but further investigation by angiography is usually required to determine the full extent of arterial disease. Carotid endarterectomy may be indicated but carries a risk of precipitating or exacerbating intraocular neovascularization. The role of panretinal laser photocoagulation in treating intraocular neovascularization is uncertain.

Occlusion of the Middle Cerebral Artery

This disorder may produce severe contralateral hemiplegia, hemianesthesia, and homonymous hemianopia. The lower quadrants of the visual fields (upper radiations) are most apt to be involved. Aphasia may be present if the dominant hemisphere is involved.

Vascular Insufficiency of the Vertebrobasilar Arterial System

Brief episodes of transient bilateral blurring of vision commonly precede a basilar artery stroke. An attack seldom leaves any residual visual impairment, and the episode may be so minimal that the patient or doctor does not heed the warning. The blurring is described as a graying of vision just as if the house lights were being dimmed at a theater. Episodes seldom last more than 5 minutes (often only a few seconds) and may be associated with other transient symptoms of vertebrobasilar insufficiency. Antiplatelet drugs can decrease the frequency and severity of vertebrobasilar symptoms.

Occlusion of the Basilar Artery

Complete or extensive thrombosis of the basilar artery nearly always causes death. With partial occlusion or basilar "insufficiency" due to arteriosclerosis, a wide variety of brainstem and cerebellar signs may be present. These include nystagmus, supranuclear eye movement abnormalities, and involvement of third, fourth, sixth, and seventh cranial nerves.

Prolonged anticoagulant therapy has become the accepted treatment of partial basilar artery thrombotic occlusion.

Occlusion of the Posterior Cerebral Artery

Occlusion of the posterior cerebral artery seldom causes death. Occlusion of the cortical branches (most common) causes homonymous hemianopia, usually superior quadrantic (the artery supplies primarily the inferior visual cortex). Lesions on the left in right-handed persons can cause aphasia, agraphia, and alexia if extensive with parietal and occipital involvement. Involvement of the occipital lobe and splenium of the corpus callosum can cause alexia (inability to read) without agraphia (inability to write); such a patient would not be able to read his or her own writing. Occlusion of the proximal branches may produce the thalamic syndrome (thalamic pain, hemiparesis, hemianesthesia, choreoathetoid movements), and cerebellar ataxia.

Subdural Hemorrhage

Subdural hemorrhage results from tearing or shearing of the veins bridging the subdural space from the pia mater to the dural sinus. It leads to an encapsulated accumulation of blood in the subdural space, usually over one cerebral hemisphere. It is nearly always caused by head trauma. The trauma may be minimal and may precede the onset of neurologic signs by weeks or even months.

In infants, subdural hemorrhage produces progressive enlargement of the head with bulging fontanelles. Ocular signs include strabismus, pupillary changes, papilledema, and retinal hemorrhages. In adults, the symptoms of chronic subdural hematoma are severe headache, drowsiness, and mental confusion, usually appearing hours to weeks (even months) after trauma. Symptomatology is similar to that of cerebral tumors. Papilledema is present in 30–50% of cases. Retinal hemorrhages occur in association with papilledema. Ipsilateral dilation of the pupil is the most common and most serious sign and is an urgent indication for immediate surgical evacuation of blood. Unequal, miotic, or mydriatic pupils can occur, or there may be no pupillary signs. Other signs, including vestibular nystagmus and cranial nerve palsies, also occur. Many of these signs result from herniation and compression of the brainstem, and therefore often appear late with stupor and coma.

CT scan or MRI confirms the diagnosis.

Treatment of acute large subdural hematoma consists of surgical evacuation of the blood; small hematomas may be simply followed with careful observation. Without treatment, the course of large hematomas is progressively downhill to coma and death. With early and adequate treatment, the prognosis is good.

Subarachnoid Hemorrhage

Subarachnoid hemorrhage most commonly results from ruptured congenital berry aneurysm of the circle of Willis in the subarachnoid space. It may also result from trauma, birth injury, intracranial hemorrhage, hemorrhage associated with tumor, arteriovenous malformation, or systemic bleeding disorder.

The most prominent symptom of subarachnoid hemorrhage is sudden, severe headache, usually occipital and often associated with signs of meningeal irritation (eg, stiff neck). Drowsiness, loss of consciousness, coma, and death may occur rapidly.

Treatment of intracranial aneurysm prior to rupture greatly improves prognosis. An expanding posterior communicating artery aneurysm may present with painful isolated third nerve palsy with pupillary involvement (see earlier in the chapter), which thus necessitates emergency investigation. Third nerve palsy with associated numbness and pain in the distribution of the ipsilateral fifth nerve may be caused by supraclinoid, internal carotid, or posterior communicating artery aneurysm. Subarachnoid hemorrhage with optic nerve dysfunction suggests an ophthalmic artery aneurysm. If it occurs, papilledema develops after subarachnoid hemorrhage has occurred. Various types of intraocular hemorrhage occur infrequently (preretinal hemorrhages are the most common—Terson's syndrome) and carry a poor prognosis for life when they are both early and extensive, since they reflect rapid severe elevation of intracranial pressure.

Subarachnoid hemorrhage may be diagnosed by CT scan or cerebrospinal fluid examination. CT angiography (CTA) or magnetic resonance angiography (MRA) may identify intracranial aneurysm and will exclude other causes of subarachnoid hemorrhage, but cerebral angiography is usually necessary to determine appropriate treatment, of which endovascular therapy or surgical ligation of the aneurysm neck or of the parent arterial trunk are the main options. Supportive treatment, including control of blood pressure and vasodilator therapy, is important during the acute phase of subarachnoid hemorrhage.

Migraine

Migraine is a common episodic illness of unknown cause and varied symptomatology characterized by unilateral headache (which usually alternates sides), visual disturbances, nausea, and vomiting. There is usually a family history. The disease usually manifests between ages 15 and 30 years. It is more common and more severe in women. Many factors, including emotional ones, may predispose or contribute to attacks.

Photophobia is common during a migraine attack. Visual auras characteristically consist of a repeating triangular-colored pattern ("fortification spectrum"), beginning in the center of vision and moving with increasing speed across the same side of the visual field of each eye. The whole episode usually lasts 15–30 minutes. It may be followed by a homonymous hemianopia on the same side that lasts for several hours. Permanent visual field loss rarely develops. It may be due to cerebral infarction but should also arouse suspicion of an underlying arteriovenous malformation. Migrainous visual auras frequently have a less typical pattern. Migraine sufferers may also suffer episodes of transient monocular visual loss (see earlier in the chapter) thought to be due to either retinal or choroidal vasospasm.

PHAKOMATOSES

The phakomatoses are a group of diseases characterized by multiple hamartomas occurring in various organ systems and at variable times.

NEUROFIBROMATOSIS

Neurofibromatosis is a generalized hereditary disease characterized by multiple tumors of the skin, central nervous system, peripheral nerves, and nerve sheaths. Other developmental anomalies, particularly of the bones, may be associated. There are two distinct dominant conditions, both due to inactivating mutations of tumor suppressor genes. **Neurofibromatosis type 1 (NF1)** is associated with tumors primarily of astrocytes and neurons, whereas **neurofibromatosis type 2 (NF2)** is associated with tumors of the meninges and Schwann cells. There is no racial predominance. The manifestations may be present at birth but often become apparent during pregnancy, during puberty, and at menopause.

NF1 is characterized by multiple café au lait spots (six or more greater than 1.5 cm in diameter) (99%), peripheral neurofibromas, which are usually nodular but may be diffuse (plexiform) and usually cutaneous but may involve deep structures, axillary freckling, and Lisch nodules (iris hamartomas) (93%). Its gene lies on chromosome 17. The frequency is 1:3000 live births, with 100% penetrance but variable expressivity. When lesions are confined to the skin, the prognosis is good. The disease tends to be fairly stationary, with only slow progression over long periods of time. Neurofibromas may need to be removed, for instance to relieve spinal nerve root compression. They may undergo sarcomatous degeneration.

A defining feature of NF2 is bilateral vestibular schwannoma (Figure 14–35), but unilateral vestibular schwannoma, other intracranial or spinal schwannoma, multiple intracranial or intraspinal meningiomas, or gliomas may occur.

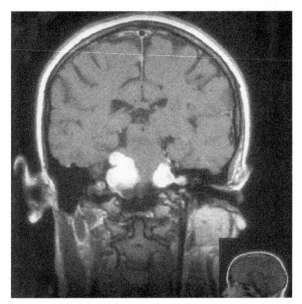

▲ **Figure 14–35.** Coronal magnetic resonance imaging of bilateral acoustic neuromas in neurofibromatosis type 2.

Café au lait spots and peripheral neurofibromas may be present. Its gene lies on chromosome 22. The frequency is 1:35,000.

Ophthalmic Features

In NF1, as well as Lisch nodules, there may be neurofibromas of the lids, either cutaneous nodular or subcutaneous plexiform (rubbery "bag of worms"). Corneal nerves are often prominent. There may be congenital glaucoma. Anterior visual pathway glioma (see earlier in the chapter) is particularly associated with NF1, with bilateral optic nerve disease being pathognomonic, and many are asymptomatic (30–80%). A subgroup of patients with nerves having a thickened nerve core and a low-density perineural proliferation are more likely to be symptomatic. Treatment depends on disease location and progression, which is probably less severe than in patients without NF1.

About 75% of patients with NF2 have early posterior subcapsular lens opacities. Epiretinal membranes, combined pigment epithelial and retinal hamartomas, optic disk gliomas, and optic nerve sheath meningiomas occur with increased frequency.

VON HIPPEL-LINDAU DISEASE

Usually presenting in the second decade and rarely after age 45, von Hippel-Lindau disease is due to a mutation on chromosome 3. Inheritance is autosomal dominant with high penetrance. The incidence is approximately 1:40,000. The most common manifestation is retinal capillary hemangioma.

Other manifestations are cerebellar hemangioblastoma; cysts of the kidneys, pancreas, and epididymis; pheochromocytoma; and renal cell carcinoma.

Retinal capillary hemangioma usually develops in the peripheral retina (see Figure 10–36). Occasionally, it develops adjacent to the optic disk (juxtapapillary). In the peripheral retina, it initially manifests as dilation and tortuosity of retinal vessels, followed by development of an angiomatous lesion with hemorrhages and exudates. A stage of massive exudation, retinal detachment, and secondary glaucoma occurs later and will cause blindness if left untreated. Among all patients with retinal capillary hemangioma, about 80% have von Hippel-Lindau disease, and they usually have multiple lesions. Among patients with solitary retinal capillary hemangioma, the prevalence of von Hippel-Lindau disease is about 45%. The diagnosis is usually obvious by personal or family history but may become apparent after screening for associated lesions or after genetic testing. Sporadic retinal capillary hemangioma not associated with von Hippel-Lindau disease usually presents in the fourth decade. Any patient with bilateral retinal capillary hemangiomas or multiple lesions in eye—either at presentation or developing during follow-up—must be assumed to have von Hippel-Lindau disease.

Treatment & Prognosis

Retinal capillary hemangiomas may be treated with laser photocoagulation, cryotherapy, or plaque radiotherapy. All patients, particularly those with von Hippel-Lindau disease, need regular screening for detection of new lesions. Patients with von Hippel-Lindau disease also need regular screening for development of central nervous system and abdominal disease. Presymptomatic detection of the lesions of von Hippel-Lindau disease greatly improves the prognosis. First-degree relatives of patients with von Hippel-Lindau disease also need to undergo regular screening. Genetic testing increasingly allows identification of individuals specifically at risk.

STURGE-WEBER SYNDROME

This uncommon nonfamilial disease with unknown inheritance is recognizable at birth by a characteristic nevus flammeus (port wine stain or venous angioma) on one side of the face. There is corresponding angiomatous involvement (leptomeningeal angiodysplasia) of the meninges and brain, which causes seizures (85%), mental retardation (60%), and cerebral atrophy. Since the cortical lesions calcify, they can be seen on plain skull x-rays after infancy. Unilateral infantile glaucoma on the affected side frequently develops if there is extensive involvement of the conjunctiva with hemangioma of the episclera and anterior chamber anomalies. Lid or conjunctival involvement nearly always implies ultimate intraocular involvement and glaucoma. Forty percent of patients with a port wine stain on the face develop choroidal hemangioma, usually diffuse rather than circumscribed, on the same side.

Treatment & Prognosis

There is no effective treatment for Sturge-Weber syndrome. The glaucoma is difficult to control. Choroidal hemangioma may require treatment with laser photocoagulation or radiotherapy.

WYBURN-MASON SYNDROME

Wyburn-Mason syndrome is a rare nonhereditary disorder of multiple arteriovenous malformations, variably involving the retina, other portions of the anterior visual pathway, the midbrain, the maxilla, and the mandible, all on the same side of the head.

Headaches and seizures are the common presenting symptoms. Large, tortuous, dilated vessels covering extensive areas of the retina are an important diagnostic clue and can cause cystic retinal degeneration with decreased vision. Optic atrophy without retinal lesions can also occur.

ATAXIA-TELANGIECTASIA

Ataxia-telangiectasia is an autosomal recessive disorder characterized by skin and conjunctival telangiectases, cerebellar ataxia, and recurrent sinopulmonary infections. All signs and symptoms are progressive with time, but the ataxia appears first as the child begins to walk, and the telangiectases appear between 4 and 7 years of age. Mental retardation also occurs. The recurrent infections relate to thymic deficiencies and corresponding T-cell abnormalities as well as to deficiency of immunoglobulins. Saccadic and eventually pursuit abnormalities produce a supranuclear ophthalmoplegia.

TUBEROUS SCLEROSIS COMPLEX

Tuberous sclerosis complex (TSC) is a multisystem genetic disorder characterized by the triad of adenoma sebaceum, epilepsy, and mental retardation, although 40–50% of affected individuals have normal intelligence. Adenoma sebaceum (angiofibromas) occurs in 90% of patients over the age of 4 years, and the number of lesions increases with puberty. These flesh-colored papules are 1–2 mm in diameter and have a butterfly distribution on the nose and malar area; they can also occur in the subungual and periungual areas. Ashleaf-shaped hypopigmented ovals can be present on the skin even of neonates and are best seen under Wood's (ultraviolet) light.

Retinal astrocytomas appear as oval or circular white areas in the peripheral fundus and, like optic nerve astrocytomas, characteristically have a mulberry-like appearance (Figure 10–35). Renal hamartomas occur in 70–80% of patients. Subependymal nodules in the periventricular areas of the brain can calcify and appear as candle-wax gutterings or drippings on radiologic studies. MRI can show actively growing subependymal nodules. These can become astrocytomas. Seizures occur in 70% of patients, often starting within the first year of life.

The disease is caused by mutations in the *TSC1* gene on chromosome 9 and *TSC2* gene on chromosome 16. Eighty percent of cases are sporadic. The estimated prevalence is 1:6000. Vision is generally normal, and progression of retinal hamartomas is rare. The prognosis for life relates to the degree of central nervous system involvement. In severe cases, death can occur in the second or third decade; if there is minimal central nervous system involvement, life expectancy should be normal.

CEREBROMACULAR DEGENERATION

The genetically determined (autosomal recessive) lysosomal storage disorders may affect the neural elements of the retina. The clinical forms are classified by the age at onset and the enzyme deficiency. The pathologic changes are present prenatally. Clinical manifestations occur as a critical level of intraneuronal lipid deposition is reached, resulting in a progressive disease, including dementia, visual disturbance, and neuromotor deterioration.

The striking ocular finding of a cherry-red spot in the macula is seen in a number of lysosomal storage disorders, for example, gangliosidosis (Tay-Sachs disease, Sandhoff's disease, and generalized GM_1), Niemann-Pick type A (sphingomyelin lipidosis), neuraminidase deficiency (sialidosis and Goldberg's syndrome), and Farber's disease. A halo occurs from loss of transparency of the ganglion cell ring of the macula, which accentuates the central red of the normal choroidal vasculature. Optic atrophy is also prominent in Tay-Sachs disease and Niemann-Pick type A. Retinal degeneration without a macular cherry-red spot occurs in mucopolysaccharidoses and in the lipopigment storage disorder, neuronal ceroid lipofuscinosis.

Eye movement disorders occur in the lysosomal storage disorders, Niemann-Pick type C (vertical supranuclear gaze palsy) and juvenile (type 3) Gaucher's disease (horizontal supranuclear gaze palsy), and occasionally in Refsum's disease, a disorder of lipid metabolism, and abetalipoproteinemia; latter two disorders are more typically associated with pigmentary retinopathy.

REFERENCES

Agarwal S, Kushner BJ: Results of extraocular muscle surgery for superior oblique myokymia. J AAPOS 2009;13:472. [PMID: 19716737]

Ajlan AM et al: Meningiomas of the tuberculum and diaphragma sellae. J Neurol Surg B Skull Base 2015;76:74. [PMID: 25685653]

Antonio-Santos AA, Eggenberger ER: Medical treatment options for ocular myasthenia gravis. Curr Opin Ophthalmol 2008;19:468. [PMID: 18854691]

Bartynski WS: Posterior reversible encephalopathy syndrome, part 1: fundamental imaging and clinical features. AJNR Am J Neuroradiol 2008;29:1036. [PMID: 18356474]

Bartynski WS: Posterior reversible encephalopathy syndrome, part 2: controversies surrounding pathophysiology of vasogenic edema. AJNR Am J Neuroradiol 2008;29:1043. [PMID: 18403560]

Beck RW, Gal RL: Treatment of acute optic neuritis. A summary of findings from the Optic Neuritis Treatment Trial. Arch Ophthalmol 2008;126:994. [PMID: 18625951]

Biousse V et al: Retinal and optic nerve ischemia. Continuum (Minneap Minn) 2014;20:838. [PMID: 25099097]

Biousse V et al: Ischemic optic neuropathies. N Engl J Med 2015;372:2428. [PMID: 26083207]

Biswas J et al: Ocular manifestation of storage diseases. Curr Opin Ophthalmol 2008;19:507. [PMID: 18854696]

Bonhomme GR et al: Pediatric optic neuritis: Brain MRI abnormalities and risk of multiple sclerosis. Neurology 2009;72:881. [PMID: 19273821]

Borchert M, Garcia-Filion P: The syndrome of optic nerve hypoplasia. Curr Neurol Neurosci Rep 2008;8:395. [PMID: 18713575]

Brazis PW: Isolated palsies of cranial nerves III, IV, and VI. Semin Neurol 2009;29:14. [PMID: 19214929]

Bruce BB et al: Traumatic homonymous hemianopia. J Neurol Neurosurg Psychiatry 2006;77:986. [PMID: 16574725]

Bruce BB et al: Idiopathic intracranial hypertension in men. Neurology 2009;72:304. [PMID: 18923135]

Bruce BB, Biousse V, Newman NJ: Third nerve palsies. Semin Neurol 2007;27:257. [PMID: 17577867]

Butty Z et al: Horner's syndrome in patients admitted to the intensive care unit that have undergone central venous catheterization: A prospective study. Eye (Lond) 2016;30:31. [PMID: 26381100]

Campbell UB et al. Acute nonarteritic anterior ischemic optic neuropathy and exposure to phosphodiesterase type 5 inhibitors. J Sex Med 2015;12:139. [PMID: 25358826]

Chang YS et al: Risk of nonarteritic anterior ischemic optic neuropathy following end-stage renal disease. Medicine (Baltimore) 2016;95:e3174. [PMID: 27015205]

Chaudhry F et al: Commonly asked questions in transient ischemic attack. Expert Rev Neurother 2013;13:151. [PMID: 23368802]

Chen CS, Miller NR: Ocular ischemic syndrome: Review of clinical presentations, etiology, investigation, and management. Compr Ophthalmol Update 2007;8:17. [PMID: 17394756]

Chi JJ: Management of the eye in facial paralysis. Facial Plast Surg Clin North Am 2016;24:21. [PMID: 26611698]

Chitnis T et al: Clinical features of neuromyelitis optica in children: US Network of Pediatric MS Centers report. Neurology 2016;86:245. [PMID: 26683648]

Comi G et al: Effect of glatiramer acetate on conversion to clinically definite multiple sclerosis in patients with clinically isolated syndrome (PreCISe study): A randomised, double-blind, placebo-controlled trial. Lancet 2009;374:1503. [PMID: 19815268]

Curatolo P et al: Neurological and neuropsychiatric aspects of tuberous sclerosis complex. Lancet Neurol 2015;14:733. [PMID: 26067126]

Dale RC, Brilot, Banwell B: Pediatric central nervous system inflammatory demyelination: Acute disseminated encephalomyelitis, clinically isolated syndromes, neuromyelitis optica, and multiple sclerosis. Curr Opin Neurol 2009;22:233. [PMID: 19434783]

Dickersin K et al: Surgery for nonarteritic anterior ischemic optic neuropathy. Cochrane Database Syst Rev 2015;3:CD001538. [PMID: 25763979]

Dorigo W et al: Urgent carotid endarterectomy in patients with recent/crescendo transient ischaemic attacks or acute stroke. Eur J Vasc Endovasc Surg 2011;41:351. [PMID: 21196126]

Ehrhardt D et al: Medical treatment of acquired nystagmus. Curr Opin Ophthalmol 2012;23:510. [PMID: 23014266]

Fenu G et al: Induction and escalation therapies in multiple sclerosis. Antiinflamm Antiallergy Agents Med Chem 2015;14:26. [PMID: 25938688]

Fraser JA et al: The treatment of giant cell arteritis. Rev Neurol Dis 2008;5:140. [PMID: 18838954]

Galal A et al: Determinants of postoperative visual recovery in suprasellar meningiomas. Acta Neurochir (Wien) 2010;152:69. [PMID: 19707716]

Golnik KC: Cavitary anomalies of the optic disc: Neurologic significance. Curr Neurol Neurosci Rep 2008;8:409. [PMID: 18713577]

Guarino M et al: Short- and long-term stroke risk after urgent management of transient ischaemic attack: The Bologna TIA clinical pathway. Eur Neurol 2015;74:1. [PMID: 26044401]

Hardy TA et al: Atypical inflammatory demyelinating syndromes of the CNS. Lancet Neurol 2016;15:967. [PMID: 27478954]

Hasanreisoglu M et al: Do patients with non-arteritic ischemic optic neuritis have increased risk for cardiovascular and cerebrovascular events? Neuroepidemiology 2013;40:220. [PMID: 23364133]

Hayreh SS: Management of non-arteritic anterior ischemic optic neuropathy. Graefes Arch Clin Exp Ophthalmol 2009;247:1595. [PMID: 19916247]

Hornyak M, Digre K, Couldwell WT: Neuro-ophthalmologic manifestations of benign anterior skull base lesions. Postgrad Med 2009;121:103. [PMID: 19641276]

Iijima K, Shimizu K, Ichibe Y: A study of the causes of bilateral optic disc swelling in Japanese patients. Clin Ophthalmol 2014;8:1269. [PMID: 25031527]

Johnson FR et al: Multiple sclerosis patients' benefit-risk preferences: Serious adverse event risks versus treatment efficacy. J Neurol 2009;256:554. [PMID: 19444531]

Johnston PC et al: Pituitary tumor apoplexy. J Clin Neurosci 2015;22:939. [PMID: 25800143]

Jung JJ, Baek SH, Kim US: Analysis of the causes of optic disc swelling. Korean J Ophthalmol 2011;25:33. [PMID: 21350692]

Kappos L et al: Long-term effect of early treatment with interferon beta-1b after a first clinical event suggestive of multiple sclerosis: 5-year active treatment extension of the phase 3 BENEFIT trial. Lancet Neurol 2009;8:987. [PMID: 19748319]

Kawasaki A, Kardon RH: Intrinsically photosensitive retinal ganglion cells. J Neuro-Ophthalmol 2007;27:195. [PMID: 17895821]

Kawasaki A, Purvin V: Giant cell arteritis: An updated review. Acta Ophthalmol 2009;87:13. [PMID: 18937808]

Kedar S et al: Pediatric homonymous hemianopia. J AAPOS 2006;10:249. [PMID: 16814179]

Kedar S et al: Congruency in homonymous hemianopia. Am J Ophthalmol 2007;143:772. [PMID: 17362865]

Kerr NM, Chew SSSL, Danesh-Meyer HV: Non-arteritic anterior ischaemic optic neuropathy: A review and update. J Clin Neurosci 2009;16:994. [PMID: 19596112]

Kidd D: The optic chiasm. Clin Anat 2014;27:1149. [PMID: 24824063]

Kidd DP et al: Optic neuropathy associated with systemic sarcoidosis. Neurol Neuroimmunol Neuroinflamm 2016;3:e270. [PMID: 27536707]

Kim HJ et al: MRI characteristics of neuromyelitis optica spectrum disorder: An international update. Neurology 2015;84:1165. [PMID: 25695963]

Kim JD et al: Neuroimaging in ophthalmology. Saudi J Ophthalmol 2012;26:401. [PMID: 23961025]

Kitley J et al: Neuromyelitis optica spectrum disorders with aquaporin-4 and myelin-oligodendrocyte glycoprotein antibodies: a comparative study. JAMA Neurol 2014;71:276. [PMID: 24425068]

Koller HP et al: Diagnosis and treatment of fourth nerve palsy. J Pediatr Ophthalmol Strabismus 2016;53:70. [PMID: 27018877]

Komotar RJ, Roguski M, Bruce JN: Surgical management of craniopharyngiomas. J Neurooncol 2009;92:283. [PMID: 19357956]

Kwancharoen R et al: Clinical features of sellar and suprasellar meningiomas. Pituitary 2014;17:342. [PMID: 23975080]

Lee AG: Neuroophthalmological management of optic pathway gliomas. Neurosurg Focus 2007;23:E1. [PMID: 18004957]

Lee J et al: Co-occurrence of acute retinal artery occlusion and acute ischemic stroke: Diffusion-weighted magnetic resonance imaging study. Am J Ophthalmol 2014;157:1231. [PMID: 24503410]

Low L et al: Double vision. BMJ 2015;351:h5385. [PMID: 26581615]

Luneau K, Newman NJ, Biousse V: Ischemic optic neuropathies. Neurologist 2008;14:341. [PMID: 19008740]

Malik A et al: Treatment options for atypical optic neuritis. Indian J Ophthalmol 2014;62:982. [PMID: 25449930]

Martinez-Hernandez E et al: Antibodies to aquaporin 4, myelin-oligodendrocyte glycoprotein, and the glycine receptor α1 subunit in patients with isolated optic neuritis. JAMA Neurol 2015;72:187. [PMID: 25506781]

McLean RJ, Gottlob I: The pharmacological treatment of nystagmus: A review. Exp Opin Pharmacother 2009;10:1805. [PMID: 19601699]

McLean RJ et al: Living with nystagmus: A qualitative study. Br J Ophthalmol 2012;96:981. [PMID: 22517800]

McLean RJ et al: What we know about the generation of nystagmus and other ocular oscillations: Are we closer to identifying therapeutic targets? Curr Neurol Neurosci Rep 2012;12:325. [PMID: 22354547]

Mealy MA et al: Comparison of relapse and treatment failure rates among patients with neuromyelitis optica: Multicenter study of treatment efficacy. JAMA Neurol 2014;71:324. [PMID: 24445513]

Mehta AR et al: The pharmacological treatment of acquired nystagmus. Pract Neurol 2012;12:147. [PMID: 22661344]

Merle H et al: Natural history of the visual impairment of relapsing neuromyelitis optica. Ophthalmology 2007;114:810. [PMID: 17141316]

Miller DH et al: Treatment of clinically isolated syndrome: To be PreCISe. Lancet 2009;374:1475. [PMID: 19815269]

Mortini P et al: Magnetic resonance imaging as predictor of functional outcome in craniopharyngiomas. Endocrine 2016;51:148. [PMID: 26179178]

Mughal M et al: Current pharmacologic testing for Horner syndrome. Curr Neurol Neurosci Rep 2009;9:384. [PMID: 19664368]

Münch M et al: Intrinsically photosensitive retinal ganglion cells: Classification, function and clinical implications. Curr Opin Neurol 2013;26:45. [PMID: 23254557]

Muppidi S, Wolfe GI: Muscle-specific receptor tyrosine kinase antibody-positive and seronegative myasthenia gravis. Front Neurol Neurosci 2009;26:109. [PMID: 19349708]

Mustafa S et al: Approach to diagnosis and management of optic neuropathy. Neurol India 2014;62:599: [PMID: 25591670]

Newman NJ: Perioperative visual loss after nonocular surgeries. Am J Ophthalmol 2008;145:604. [PMID: 18358851]

Ogra S et al: Visual acuity and pattern of visual field loss at presentation in pituitary adenoma. J Clin Neurosci 2014;21:735. [PMID: 2465673]

Ontaneda D, Fox RJ: Progressive multiple sclerosis. Curr Opin Neurol 2015;28:237. [PMID: 25887766]

Optic Neuritis Study Group: Visual function 15 years after optic neuritis: A final follow-up report from the Optic Neuritis Treatment Trial. Ophthalmology 2008;115:1079. [PMID: 17976727]

Optic Neuritis Study Group: Multiple sclerosis risk after optic neuritis. Final Optic Neuritis: Treatment Trial follow-up. Arch Neurol 2008;65:727. [PMID: 18541792]

Pache F et al: MOG-IgG in NMO and related disorders: A multicenter study of 50 patients. Part 4: Afferent visual system damage after optic neuritis in MOG-IgG-seropositive versus AQP4-IgG-seropositive patients. J Neuroinflammation 2016;13:282. [PMID: 27802824]

Pandit L et al: Demographic and clinical features of neuromyelitis optica: A review. Mult Scler 2015;21:845. [PMID: 25921037]

Park HH et al: Use of optical coherence tomography to predict visual outcome in parachiasmal meningioma. J Neurosurg 2015;123:1489. [PMID: 26162035]

Petzold A et al: Embolic and nonembolic transient monocular visual field loss: A clinicopathologic review. Surv Ophthalmol 2013;58:42. [PMID: 23217587]

Pitkänen H et al: Vasospastic transient monocular visual loss: Effect of treatment with different doses of nifedipine. J Neuroophthalmol 2014;34:386. [PMID: 24905274]

Pittock SJ, Lucchinetti CF: Neuromyelitis optica and the evolving spectrum of autoimmune aquaporin-4 channelopathies: A decade later. Ann N Y Acad Sci 2016;1366:20. [PMID: 26096370]

Pohl D et al: Acute disseminated encephalomyelitis: Updates on an inflammatory CNS syndrome. Neurology 2016;87:S38. [PMID: 27572859]

Proulx AA, Strong MJ, Nicolle DA: Creutzfeldt-Jakob disease presenting with visual manifestations. Can J Ophthalmol 2008;43:591. [PMID: 18982039]

Pula JH, Eggenberger E: Posterior reversible encephalopathy syndrome. Curr Opin Ophthalmol 2008;19:479. [PMID: 18854692]

Qiao L et al: The clinical characteristics of primary Sjogren's syndrome with neuromyelitis optica spectrum disorder in China: A STROBE-Compliant Article. Medicine (Baltimore) 2015;94:e1145. [PMID: 26181553]

Quiroga AC et al: Teaching video neuroimages: The hopping lid twitch in myasthenia gravis. Neurology 2016;87:e55. [PMID: 27481465]

Ramanathan S et al: Anti-MOG antibody: The history, clinical phenotype, and pathogenicity of a serum biomarker for demyelination. Autoimmun Rev 2016;15:307. [PMID: 26708342]

Rappoport D et al: Parainfectious optic neuritis: Manifestations in children vs adults. J Neuroophthalmol 2014;34:122. [PMID: 24667772]

Rucker JC: Oculomotor disorders. Semin Neurol 2007;27:244. [PMID: 17577866]

Sakai RE et al: Vision in multiple sclerosis (MS): the story, structure-function correlations, and models for neuroprotection. J Neuroophthalmol 2011;31:362. [PMID: 22089500]

Sato DK et al: Distinction between MOG antibody-positive and AQP4 antibody-positive NMO spectrum disorders. Neurology 2014;82:474. [PMID: 24415568]

Sheldon CA et al: Pediatric idiopathic intracranial hypertension: Age, gender, and anthropometric features at diagnosis in a large, retrospective, multisite cohort. Ophthalmology 2016;123:2424. [PMID: 27692528]

Silverman AL et al: Assessment of optic nerve head drusen using enhanced depth imaging and swept source optical coherence tomography. J Neuro-Ophthalmol 2014;34:198. [PMID: 24662838]

Straube A et al: Nystagmus and oscillopsia. Eur J Neurol 2012;19:6. [PMID: 21906211]

Strömberg S et al: Risk of early recurrent stroke in symptomatic carotid stenosis. Eur J Vasc Endovasc Surg 2015;49:137. [PMID: 25548062]

Strupp M et al: Pharmacotherapy of vestibular and ocular motor disorders, including nystagmus. J Neurol 2011;258:1207. [PMID: 21461686]

Swanton JK et al: Early MRI in optic neuritis: The risk for disability. Neurology 2009;72:542. [PMID: 19204264]

Tamhankar MA et al: Management of acute cranial nerve 3, 4, and 6 palsies: Role of neuroimaging. Curr Opin Ophthalmol 2015;26:464. [PMID: 26367093]

Taylor D: Developmental abnormalities of the optic nerve and chiasm. Eye 2007;21:1271. [PMID: 17914430]

Thurtell MJ et al: Treatment of nystagmus. Curr Treat Options Neurol 2012;14:60. [PMID: 22072056]

Tilikete C et al: Acquired pendular nystagmus in multiple sclerosis and oculopalatal tremor. Neurology 2011;76:1650. [PMID: 21555732]

Traber GL et al: Malignant optic glioma: The spectrum of disease in a case series. Graefes Arch Clin Exp Ophthalmol 2015;253:1187. [PMID: 26004076]

Uehara T et al: Guidelines for management of patients with transient ischemic attack. Front Neurol Neurosci 2014;33:103. [PMID: 2415755]

Volpe NJ: The Optic Neuritis Treatment Trial. A definitive answer and profound impact with unexpected results. Arch Ophthalmol 2008;126:996. [PMID: 18625952]

von Weitzel-Mudersbach P et al: Low risk of vascular events following urgent treatment of transient ischaemic attack: The Aarhus TIA study. Eur J Neurol 2011;18:1285. [PMID: 21645177]

Wall M: Idiopathic intracranial hypertension (pseudotumor cerebri). Curr Neurol Neurosci Rep 2008;8:87. [PMID: 18460275]

Walsh MT et al: Management options for cavernous sinus meningiomas. J Neurooncol 2009;92:307. [PMID: 19357958]

Wang X et al: Giant cell arteritis. Rheumatol Int 2008;29:1. [PMID: 18716781]

Warren FA: Atypical optic neuritis. J Neuroophthalmol 2014;34:e12. [PMID: 25405666]

Wingerchuk DM et al: International consensus diagnostic criteria for neuromyelitis optica spectrum disorders. Neurology 2015;85:177. [PMID: 26092914]

Wingerchuk DM et al: The spectrum of neuromyelitis optica. Lancet Neurol 2007;6:805. [PMID: 17706564]

Wingerchuk DM et al: International consensus diagnostic criteria for neuromyelitis optica spectrum disorders. Neurology 2015;85:177. [PMID: 26092914]

Wolfe GI et al: Randomized trial of thymectomy in myasthenia gravis. N Engl J Med 2016;375:511. [PMID: 27509100]

Yonghong J et al: Detailed magnetic resonance imaging findings of the ocular motor nerves in Duane's retraction syndrome. J Pediatr Ophthalmol Strabismus 2009;46:278. [PMID: 19791724]

Young NP et al: Acute disseminated excephalomyelitis: Current understanding and controversies. Semin Neurol 2008;28:84. [PMID: 18256989]

Yu-Wai-Man P et al: Inherited mitochondrial optic neuropathies. J Med Genet 2009;46:145. [PMID: 19001017]

Zhang C et al: Prediction factors of recurrent ischemic events in one year after minor stroke. PLoS One 2015;10:e0120105. [PMID: 25774939]

Zhang X et al: Homonymous hemianopias: Clinical-anatomic correlations in 904 cases. Neurology 2006;66:906. [PMID: 16567710]

Zhang X et al: Natural history of homonymous hemianopia. Neurology 2006;66:901. [PMID: 16567709]

Zhang X et al: Homonymous hemianopia in stroke. J Neuroophthalmol 2006;26:180. [PMID: 16966935]

Ocular Disorders Associated with Systemic Diseases

Alastair Stuart, BMBS, FRCOphth, and
Edward Pringle, MRCP, FRCOphth

Examination of the eye provides invaluable information for the diagnosis and monitoring of systemic disease. Nowhere else in the body can a microcirculatory system be visualized directly and investigated with such precision or neural tissue be examined so easily, and nowhere else are the results of minute focal lesions so devastating. Many systemic diseases involve the eyes, and therapy demands some knowledge of the vascular, rheologic, and immunologic nature of these diseases.

VASCULAR DISEASE

NORMAL ANATOMY & PHYSIOLOGY

The blood supply to the eye is from the ophthalmic artery, which is the first branch of the internal carotid artery (see Chapter 1). The first branches of the ophthalmic artery are the central retinal artery and the long posterior ciliary arteries. The retina is supplied by the retinal and choroidal circulations that have contrasting anatomic and physiologic characteristics. The retinal arteries correspond to arterioles in the systemic circulation. They function as end arteries and feed a capillary bed consisting of small capillaries (7 μm) with tight endothelial junctions, which forms the blood-retina barrier, and they are autoregulated, there being no autonomic nerve fibers. However, most of the blood within the eye is in the choroidal circulation, which has a high flow rate, autonomic regulation, and an anatomic arrangement of collateral branching and large capillaries (30 μm), all of which have fenestrations in juxtaposition to Bruch's membrane. Examination of the retinal vessels is facilitated by red-free light and fluorescein angiography, whereas indocyanine green angiography highlights the choroidal vessels.

CLINICAL MANIFESTATIONS

Hemorrhages

The sources of fundal hemorrhages may be arteries, capillaries, or veins, and their appearance primarily depends on their location (Table 15–1 and Figure 15–1). They usually indicate abnormality of the retinal or choroidal vascular system, but they may be caused by any condition that alters the efficacy of the endothelial barrier. The contribution of systemic factors should be considered in relation to (1) vessel wall disease (eg, hypertension, diabetes), (2) blood disorders (eg, thrombocytopenia, anemia, leukemia), and (3) reduced perfusion pressure (eg, carotid artery–cavernous sinus fistula, acute blood loss).

Acute Ocular Ischemia

A. Optic Disk Infarction (Anterior Ischemic Optic Neuropathy) (Figure 15–2)

Impairment of blood supply to the optic disk produces sudden visual loss, usually with an altitudinal field defect, and sectoral pallid swelling of the optic disk, sometimes with hemorrhages. Pathologic studies show infarction of the retrolaminar region of the optic nerve, which is supplied by the short posterior ciliary vessels that are part of the choroidal circulation. Fluorescein angiography demonstrates reduced perfusion of the disk and adjacent choroid; dilation of the capillaries, which are part of the retinal circulation, on the surface of its unaffected portion; and late leakage.

The most common cause is nonarteritic anterior ischemic optic neuropathy (NAION), for which the most important risk factor is constitutionally small optic disk ("disk at risk"), and since this usually affects both eyes, there is a risk of

Table 15–1. Types of Fundal Hemorrhage

Type	Location	Source	Shape	Color
Preretinal (subhyaloid)	Between the retina and the vitreous	Superficial disk or retinal vessels usually due to neovascularization	Crescent with gravity-dependent upper border and round lower border determined by the extent of posterior vitreous detachment	Light red to dark red according to density
Superficial retinal	Retinal nerve fiber layer	Radial peripapillary or superficial retinal capillary network	Linear ("flame-shaped") due to orientation of retinal ganglion cell axons	Light red
Intraretinal	Deep retina (inner nuclear layer)	Deep retinal capillary network	Round ("dot" or "blot") aligned perpendicular to the surface of the retina	Medium or dark red
White-centered retinal (Roth spot)	Superficial or deep retina	Superficial or deep retinal capillary network, typically in bacterial endocarditis but more commonly in other conditions including diabetes and leukemia	Round	Red with white or pale center, which is due to partial resolution of hemorrhage, extravasation of white blood cells, or associated cotton-wool spot
Subretinal	Between photoreceptors (neurosensory retina) and retinal pigment epithelium (RPE)	Subretinal neovascularization or optic disk disease	Large with less distinct border than sub-RPE hemorrhage	Light or medium red
Subretinal pigment epithelium (hemorrhagic RPE detachment)	Between retinal pigment epithelium and Bruch's membrane (choroid)	Choroidal network	Large with more distinct border than subretinal hemorrhage	Dark or medium red

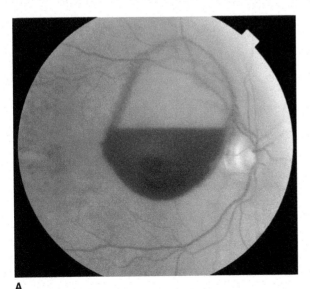
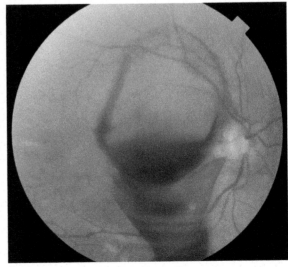

A   B

▲ **Figure 15–1.** Preretinal hemorrhage due to ruptured retinal macroaneurysm. **A:** Large hemorrhage with fluid level lying between the retina and vitreous. **B:** Dispersion into vitreous after disruption of posterior vitreous with YAG laser.

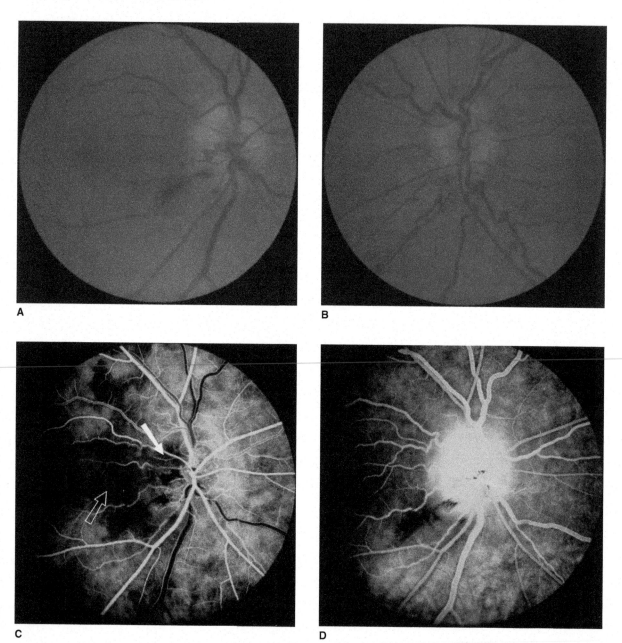

▲ **Figure 15–2.** Anterior ischemic optic neuropathy. Pallid swelling of small optic disk with hemorrhages **(A)** with small optic disk also in the other eye **(B)**. Fluorescein angiogram shows reduced perfusion of a segment of the optic disk **(filled arrow)** and the adjacent choroid **(unfilled arrow)** in the early phase **(C)** and leakage in the late phase **(D)**.

subsequent involvement of the other eye. Hypertension and arteriosclerotic disease are the commonly identified additional factors in middle age, although it is uncertain whether vascular occlusion or a reduced arterial pressure is the precipitating event. With increasing likelihood with increasing age over 50 years, optic disk infarction may be caused by giant cell arteritis. Other systemic vasculitides (such as antineutrophil cytoplasmic antibody–associated vasculitis) may also present with anterior ischemic optic neuropathy. The visual loss is usually less severe than in giant cell arteritis, and the disk may not be small as in NAION. Bilateral optic disk infarction can be seen after sudden hypotension following acute blood loss, but posterior (retrobulbar) optic nerve infarction without optic disk changes in the acute stage is more typical.

B. Choroidal Infarction

This is rare, but permanent sequelae include single or multiple areas of chorioretinal pigmentation that may be focal (Elschnig spot), triangular (Amalric sign), or linear (Siegrist streak) (Figure 15–3).

C. Retinal Infarction or Ischemia

The funduscopic appearance of arteriolar occlusion depends on the size of the vessel occluded, the duration of occlusion, and the time course. Occlusion of major arterioles (retinal arteries) produces total, hemispheric, or segmental pallid swelling of the retina, with corresponding visual loss (Figure 15–4) (see Chapter 10). Central retinal artery occlusion is usually due to atherosclerosis but can result from embolic disease. It can also be a manifestation of giant cell arteritis.

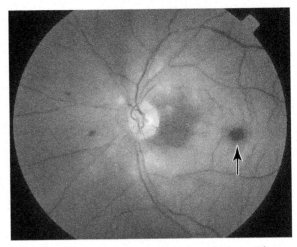

▲ **Figure 15–4.** Central retinal artery occlusion, with pallid retinal swelling and a "cherry red spot" at the fovea **(arrow)** in a patient with hypertension.

Branch retinal artery occlusion is more commonly due to emboli (see later in the chapter).

A cotton-wool spot (Figure 15–5) is caused by interruption of axoplasmic transport in axons of the retinal nerve fiber layer by superficial retinal ischemia that is due usually to occlusion of a precapillary retinal arteriole but occasionally more proximal impairment of retinal blood flow. It consists of pale, slight swelling usually one-fourth to one-half the size of the optic disk. Pathologic examination shows distention

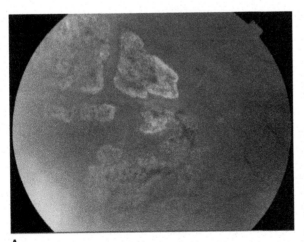

A

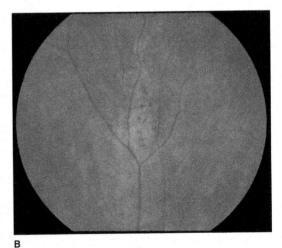

B

▲ **Figure 15–3.** Retinal pigmentation due to choroidal infarction. **A:** Multiple triangular (Almaric sign) in antiphospholipid syndrome. **B:** Single linear (Siegrist streak) in systemic vasculitis.

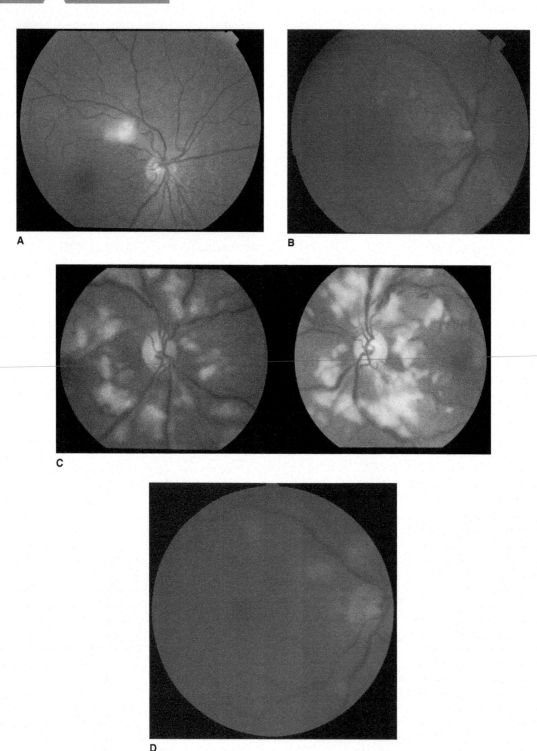

▲ **Figure 15–5.** Cotton-wool spots. **A:** Isolated unexplained cotton-wool spot in a 30-year-old female. **B:** Human immunodeficiency virus infection. **C:** Systemic lupus erythematosus. **D:** Giant cell arteritis.

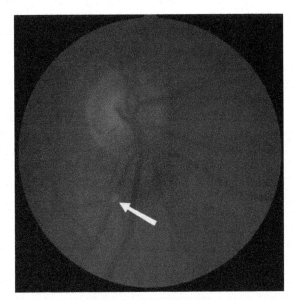

▲ **Figure 15–6.** Retinal embolus **(arrow).**

Table 15–2. Causes of Transient Visual Loss

Retinal embolus (monocular—"amaurosis fugax") **or cerebral embolus** (homonymous hemianopic)
   Carotid artery stenosis, ulceration, or dissection
   Basilar or vertebral artery disease (cerebral not retinal embolus)
   Cardiac dysrhythmia (eg, atrial fibrillation)
   Cardiac valvular disease (eg, infective endocarditis)
   Left ventricular aneurysm with mural thrombus following myocardial infarction

Arterial occlusive disease
   Internal or common carotid artery occlusion
   Basilar or vertebral artery occlusion
   Arteritis (eg, giant cell arteritis)

Systemic disease
   Hematologic
      Anemia
      Polycythemia
      Macroglobulinemia
      Sickle cell disease
   Circulatory failure
      Systemic hypotension
         Blood loss
         Shock
      Cardiac dysrhythmia
      Impaired left ventricular function
      Autonomic dysfunction (eg, diabetes mellitus)
      Endocrine dysfunction (eg, Addison's disease)
      Drugs
   Migraine
      Migraine aura
      Retinal (choroidal) migraine

Ocular disease
   Optic disk swelling
      Papilledema (raised intracranial pressure—"transient visual obscuration")
   Raised intraocular pressure
   Intraocular hemorrhage
      Uveitis-glaucoma-hyphema (UGH) syndrome
   Subluxed lens
   Gaze-evoked amaurosis
      Optic nerve sheath meningioma
      Graves' ophthalmopathy

of neurons, with cytoid bodies; electron microscopy shows accumulation of axoplasm and organelles. Cotton-wool spots resolve over 6 weeks regardless of their cause.

D. Transient Retinal Ischemia due to Emboli (Amaurosis Fugax)

Complete monocular visual loss with full recovery after 5–10 minutes, with the beginning and end often being described as a curtain passing vertically across the vision, is characteristic of transient retinal ischemia due to transit of an embolus through the retinal circulation ("amaurosis fugax") (Figure 15–6). The three main types of retinal emboli are **cholesterol**, from an atheromatous plaque in the great vessels; **platelet-fibrin**, from disease of the great vessels or heart; and **calcific** from a diseased aortic or mitral valve. Overall carotid artery disease is the most common source (see Chapter 14). A cardiac cause such as atrial fibrillation, mitral or aortic valve disease, or infective endocarditis particularly needs to be considered in patients with a history of cardiac disease or age under 40 years. It is important for the ophthalmologist to search the fundus for emboli, although frequently, they are not seen; auscultate for carotid bruits and cardiac murmurs; check the pulse for atrial fibrillation; and arrange investigations for disease of the carotids, including for underlying risk factors and cardiac disease as appropriate. Retinal emboli, whether or not associated with retinal dysfunction, indicate a risk of stroke, and the incidental discovery of usually cholesterol emboli should prompt similar assessment.

Other causes of transient visual loss are listed in Table 15–2.

▶ Chronic Ocular Ischemia

Reduction in the retinal arteriovenous pressure gradient may produce acute signs of ocular ischemia (see preceding pages) or the less frequently recognized chronic changes.

A. Ocular Ischemic Syndrome (Figure 15–7)

Chronic reduction of ocular arterial perfusion pressure sufficient to cause clinical manifestations (ocular ischemic syndrome) usually reflects severe bilateral carotid occlusive disease, of which atherosclerosis is the most common cause.

Retinal ischemia manifests as capillary dilation, micro-aneurysms, predominantly peripheral hemorrhages, cotton-wool spots, optic disk new vessels, and macular edema, but the abnormalities may be mild despite the severity of the carotid disease. The ocular abnormalities mimic and are often ascribed incorrectly to diabetic eye disease or retinal vein occlusion. Anterior segment ischemia, which is less common, manifests as iritis, iris and anterior chamber angle neovascularization, and reduced or increased intraocular pressure.

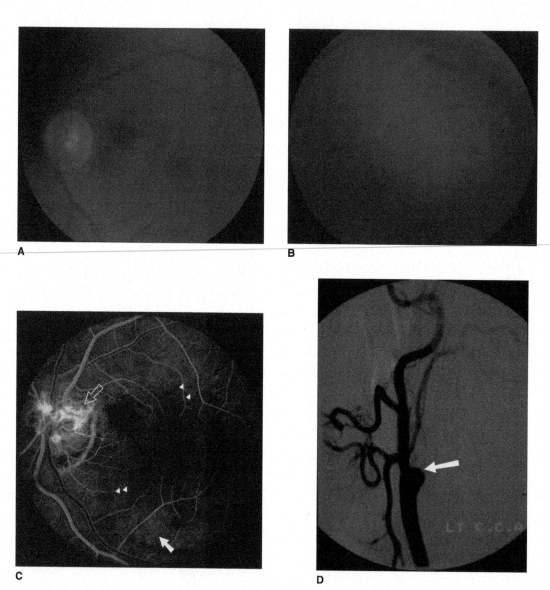

▲ **Figure 15–7.** Ocular ischemic syndrome due to carotid occlusive disease. **A:** Macular hemorrhage. **B:** Peripheral retinal hemorrhages. **C:** Fluorescein angiogram showing capillary dilation **(filled arrow)**, microaneurysms **(arrowheads)**, and optic disk new vessels **(unfilled arrow)**. **D:** Carotid angiogram showing total occlusion of ipsilateral internal carotid artery. **E:** Multiple cotton-wool spots. **F:** Fluorescein angiogram showing macular capillary nonperfusion **(arrows)**. **G:** Fluorescein angiogram in chronic ocular ischemia due to Takayasu's disease with capillary dilation and leakage of dye including from optic disk neovascularization.

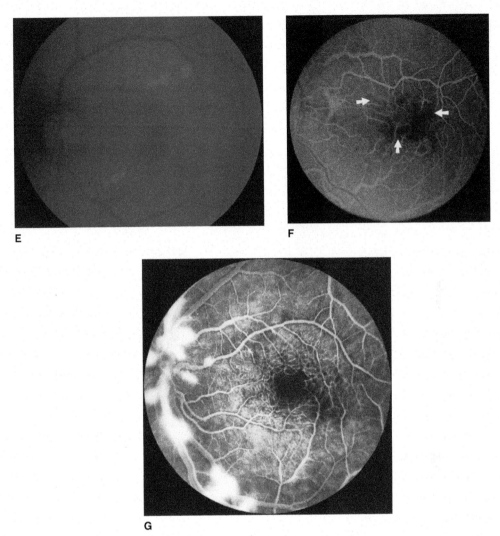

E   F

G

▲ **Figure 15–7.** (*Continued*)

B. Carotid Artery–Cavernous Sinus Fistula (Figure 15–8)

Carotid artery–cavernous sinus fistula results from an abnormal communication between the carotid artery or its branches and the cavernous sinus. Direct fistulas occur as a consequence of rupture of the intracavernous internal carotid artery, due to aneurysm, weakened vessel wall (eg, collagen vascular disease, Ehlers-Danlos syndrome), or trauma. They usually have an acute, florid presentation and commonly require closure. Indirect (dural) fistulas usually are spontaneous, chronic, and often have multiple sites of fistulation but generally are mild. They are associated with diabetes and systemic hypertension and may be a consequence of thrombosis of dural veins. Frequently they resolve

spontaneously. Clinical features of carotid artery–cavernous sinus fistulas include dilated conjunctival and arterialized ("corkscrew") aepiscleral veins, raised intraocular pressure, dilated retinal veins with hemorrhages and fluorescein leakage, ophthalmoplegia (usually lateral rectus), and bruit. Computed tomography (CT) and magnetic resonance imaging (MRI) show thickened ocular muscles and a dilated superior ophthalmic vein, the latter being a differentiating feature from Graves' ophthalmopathy. Reversal of flow ("arterialization") of the superior ophthalmic vein is a characteristic finding on orbital ultrasound blood flow studies. When required, closure of carotid artery–cavernous sinus fistulas is usually achieved by interventional radiologic techniques.

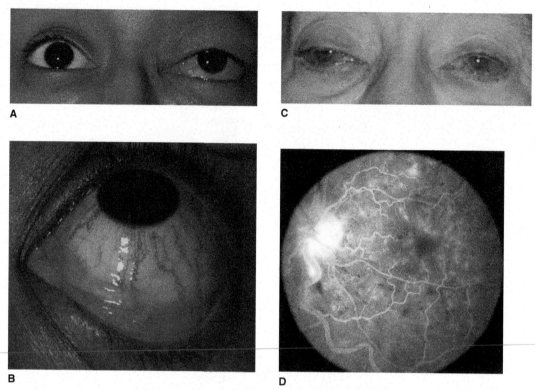

▲ **Figure 15–8.** Carotid artery–cavernous sinus fistula. Traumatic direct **(A)** with arterialized episcleral vessels **(B)**. **C:** Spontaneous indirect. **D:** Fluorescein angiogram showing dilated retinal veins, optic disk neovascularization, and macular edema.

▶ Retinal Vein Occlusion

A. Central Retinal Vein Occlusion (Figure 15–9)

Central retinal vein occlusion is an important cause of visual morbidity in older people, particularly those with systemic hypertension or glaucoma.

Fundus examination shows dilated tortuous veins with retinal and macular edema, linear and round hemorrhages in all four quadrants of the retina, and sometimes cotton-wool spots. The arterioles are usually attenuated, indicating generalized microvascular disease.

Fluorescein angiography demonstrates two types of response: a nonischemic type, with dilation of retinal vessels and edema; and an ischemic type, with large areas of capillary nonperfusion or evidence of retinal or anterior segment neovascularization. In less than 10% of ischemic but over 80% of nonischemic central retinal vein occlusions, the ultimate visual acuity is better than 20/200. Table 15–3 lists risk factors associated with retinal vein occlusion and the appropriate investigations.

Treatment of central retinal vein occlusion is focused on management of neovascularization and macular edema (see Chapter 10). In ischemic central retinal vein occlusion, panretinal laser photocoagulation is effective in preventing and treating anterior segment (iris and/or anterior chamber angle) and secondary neovascular glaucoma; however, the latter may require additional treatment. Macular edema is treated with intravitreal injection of an anti–vascular endothelial growth factor (VEGF) agent or possibly intravitreal steroid.

B. Branch Retinal Vein Occlusion (Figure 15–10)

Branch retinal vein occlusion should be viewed as part of the spectrum of central retinal vein occlusion. Investigations are similar in the two conditions, but vascular risk factors, particularly systemic hypertension, are more common and raised intraocular pressure is less common. Branch retinal vein occlusion occurs more frequently in the superotemporal and inferotemporal regions and particularly at sites where arteries cross over veins.

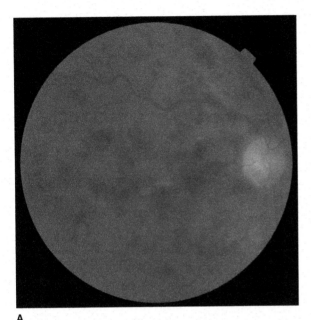

A

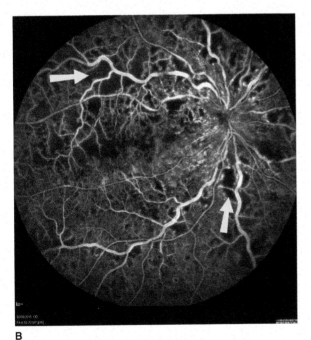

B

▲ **Figure 15–9.** Central retinal vein occlusion. **A:** Linear and round retinal hemorrhages in all four quadrants with a few cotton-wool spots. **B:** Fluorescein angiogram showing areas of capillary nonperfusion **(arrows).**

Table 15–3. Retinal Vein Occlusion

Risk Factors
Age
Raised intraocular pressure
Systemic hypertension
Smoking
Diabetes mellitus
Hyperlipidemia
Collagen vascular diseases
Chronic renal failure
Hyperviscosity syndromes (eg, myeloma, Waldenström's
    macroglobulinemia)

Investigations
Full blood count and hematocrit
Erythrocyte sedimentation rate (ESR)
Renal profile with urine microscopy and renal ultrasound if
    abnormal
Serum lipids
Plasma proteins and protein electrophoresis with 24-hour urinary
    protein for Bence-Jones protein if abnormal or raised ESR
Plasma glucose and glycosylated hemoglobin (HbA1c)
Thrombophilia screen (young patients)
    Lupus anticoagulant
    Cardiolipin antibodies
    Protein C
    Protein S
    Activated protein C resistance (APCR)/factor V Leiden mutation
    Antithrombin III
    Homocysteine

The roles of intravitreal anti-VEGF agents or steroid and laser treatment in the management of branch retinal vein occlusion are discussed in Chapters 10 and 23.

HYPERTENSIVE RETINOCHOROIDOPATHY

The severity of hypertensive retinochoroidopathy is determined by the degree of elevation of the blood pressure and the state of the retinal arterioles. It is predictive of risk for cerebrovascular disease, coronary artery disease, and mortality (Table 15–4).

In young patients with accelerated (malignant) hypertension, an extensive retinopathy is seen, with hemorrhages, cotton-wool spots, choroidal infarcts, and occasionally exudative detachment of the retina. Severe disk edema is a prominent feature and may be accompanied by a macular star of exudates (Figure 15–11). Vision may be impaired and may deteriorate further if blood pressure is reduced too quickly.

In contrast, elderly patients with arteriosclerotic vessels are unable to respond in this manner, and their vessels are thus protected by the arteriosclerosis, so they seldom exhibit florid hypertensive retinochoroidopathy (Figure 15–12).

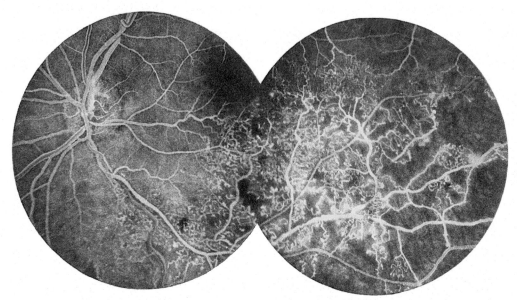

▲ **Figure 15–10.** Branch retinal vein occlusion. Fluorescein angiogram showing within the affected segment irregularity of arterioles and veins, areas of capillary closure, and dilated capillaries with microaneurysms.

IDIOPATHIC (BENIGN) INTRACRANIAL HYPERTENSION

Idiopathic intracranial hypertension is characterized by raised intracranial pressure with no identifiable cause including normal cerebrospinal fluid constituents; normal radiologic studies, particularly no evidence of cerebral venous sinus occlusion; and no causative drug therapy (usually tetracyclines or retinoids). Usually patients are young, overweight women and present with headache. Transient visual obscurations, blurred vision, and diplopia are the ophthalmologic features. Idiopathic intracranial hypertension is rare in adult men except in association with sleep apnea syndrome.

Initially visual fields are normal apart from enlarged blind spots due to papilledema. Generalized field constriction and inferonasal and arcuate defects may occur. CT or

Table 15–4. Mitchell-Wong Classification of Hypertensive Retinopathy

Grade	Classification	Systemic Associations
No retinopathy	No detectable retinal signs	None
Mild retinopathy	One or more of the following arteriolar signs: • Generalized arteriolar narrowing • Focal arteriolar narrowing • Arteriovenous nicking • Arteriolar wall opacity ("silver wiring")	Modest[1] association with risk of stroke, subclinical stroke, coronary artery disease, and mortality
Moderate retinopathy	One or more of the following retinal signs: • Hemorrhage (blot, dot, or flame shaped) • Microaneurysm • Cotton-wool spot • Exudate	Strong[2] association with risk of stroke, cognitive decline, and cardiovascular mortality
Malignant retinopathy	Moderate retinopathy plus optic disk swelling[3]	Strong association with mortality

[1]Modest: risk and odds ratios of > 1 but < 2.
[2]Strong: risks and odds ratio of > 2.
[3]Anterior ischemic optic neuropathy, characterized by unilateral optic disk swelling, visual loss, and sectoral visual field loss, should be excluded.
Source: Adapted from Wong TY, Mitchell P: Hypertensive retinopathy. N Engl J Med 2004;351:2310. [PMID: 15564546]

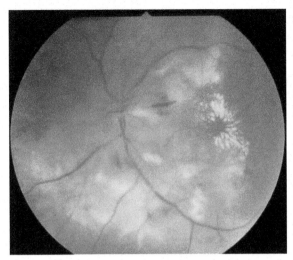

▲ **Figure 15–11.** Accelerated hypertension in a young woman manifesting as marked optic disk edema, macular star of exudates, exudative retinal detachment, retinal hemorrhages, and cotton-wool spots.

MRI usually shows distended optic nerve sheaths, flattened globes, and an empty pituitary sella. The aims of treatment are to minimize permanent visual loss, which occurs in up to 50% of patients, and relieve symptoms. Treatment options include weight loss, oral acetazolamide or other diuretics,

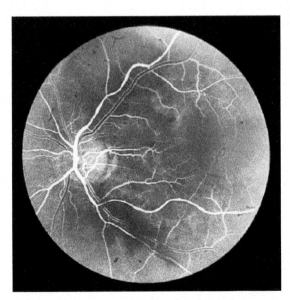

▲ **Figure 15–12.** Accelerated hypertension. Fluorescein angiogram in an elderly woman showing marked arteriolar constriction and irregularity but few signs of florid retinopathy.

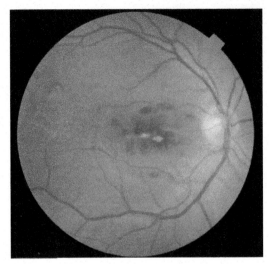

▲ **Figure 15–13.** Infective endocarditis: white-centered retinal hemorrhages (Roth spots).

cerebrospinal fluid shunt, and optic nerve sheath fenestration (see Chapter 14).

INFECTIVE ENDOCARDITIS

Infection of cardiac endothelial surfaces usually on the cardiac valves may produce multiple septic emboli with frequent ocular manifestations that include white centered retinal hemorrhages (Figure 15–13), retinal and choroidal infarction, and mild infective vitritis.

HEMATOLOGIC DISORDERS

Ocular changes in **leukemia** are most common in acute disease. They predominantly affect structures with a good blood supply, including the retina, choroid, and optic disk, and manifest as hemorrhages and infiltrates (Figure 15–14).

In **hyperviscosity syndromes**, reduced blood flow results in dilation of retinal arteries and veins, hemorrhages, microaneurysms, and areas of capillary closure (Figure 15–15). The main causes are polycythemia, either primary or secondary, macroglobulinemia, and multiple myeloma. Treatment of the hyperviscosity can reverse the retinal changes.

Sickle cell hemoglobinopathies are heritable disorders in which normal adult hemoglobin is replaced by sickle hemoglobin resulting in "sickle-shaped" deformity of red blood cells when there is relative deoxygenation. Ocular abnormalities, which are more common in SC and S-thal disease than in SS or AS disease, include conjunctival "comma-shaped" capillaries and retinal changes, comprising hemorrhage with subsequent chorioretinal scarring ("black sunburst"), hemorrhagic arterial occlusion ("salmon patch"),

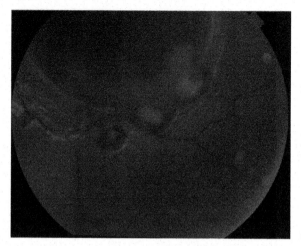

▲ **Figure 15–14.** Acute myeloid leukemia: retinal infiltrates.

and peripheral capillary closure that may lead to new vessel formation, characteristically in a "sea-fan" pattern. Retinal detachment may develop. Laser therapy is rarely needed because the complexes fibrose and reperfusion can occur.

NEOPLASTIC DISEASE

Neoplastic disease may involve the eye and optic pathways by direct spread, metastases, or immunologic mechanisms. The most frequent primary tumors metastasizing to the eye

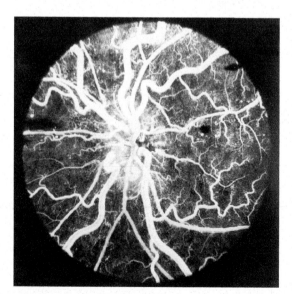

▲ **Figure 15–15.** Hyperviscosity syndrome. Fluorescein angiogram showing dilated arteries and veins, with hemorrhages and microaneurysms.

are carcinoma of the breast in women and bronchial carcinoma in men (see Chapters 7 and 10). Most patients have a known history of cancer, but in a third of patients presenting with ocular metastasis, the primary tumor has yet to be diagnosed. Visual loss also may occur from nonmetastatic disease, due to **cancer-associated retinopathy (CAR)** or **melanoma-associated retinopathy (MAR)**, each of which is associated with specific retinal autoantibodies and characteristic clinical and electrophysiologic abnormalities, or **diffuse uveal melanocytic proliferation**.

METABOLIC DISORDERS

DIABETES MELLITUS

The global prevalence of diabetes mellitus among adults is 8.5%, with a fourfold increase in people with diabetes between 1980 and 2014. It is a complex metabolic disorder that can lead to widespread vascular disease. The risk of ocular complications is increased by poor control of diabetes and systemic hypertension, but they still occur despite seemingly good control. The lengthened life span of diabetics has resulted in a marked increase in the prevalence of ocular complications, of which the prognosis is generally better for type 2 than for type 1 diabetics.

The possibility of diabetes should be considered in all patients with unexplained retinopathy, cataract, extraocular muscle palsy, optic neuropathy, or sudden changes in refractive error.

▶ Diabetic Retinopathy (Figure 15–16)

Diabetic retinopathy is a common cause of blindness. In the Western world, it accounts for almost one-fourth of blind registrations and is the most common cause of new blindness in the working-age population. In the United States, 40–45% of diabetics have retinopathy.

Type 1 diabetics develop a severe form of retinopathy within 20 years in 60–75% of cases even with good diabetic control. The retinopathy is usually proliferative. In the usually older type 2 diabetic patients, retinopathy is more often nonproliferative, with the risk of severe central visual loss from maculopathy.

The clinical features and treatment of diabetic retinopathy are detailed in Chapter 10.

▶ Lens Changes

A. True Diabetic Cataract (Rare)

Bilateral cataracts occasionally occur with a rapid onset in severe juvenile diabetes. The lens may become completely opaque in several weeks.

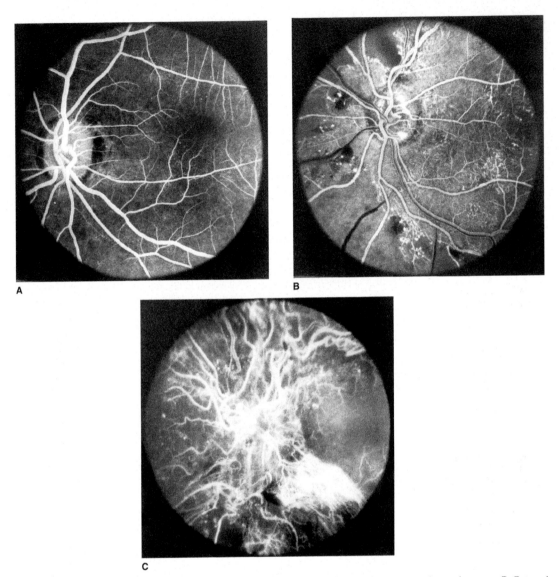

A

B

C

▲ **Figure 15–16.** Fluorescein angiography in diabetic retinopathy. **A:** Microaneurysms in the early stage. **B:** Extensive areas of capillary closure, dilated capillaries with microaneurysms, and early new vessel formation at the optic disk. **C:** Extensive growth of vessels into the vitreous with marked leakage.

B. Age-Related Cataract in the Diabetic (Common)

Nuclear sclerosis, posterior subcapsular changes, and cortical lens opacities occur earlier and more frequently in diabetics (see Chapter 8).

C. Sudden Changes in the Refraction of the Lens

Especially when diabetes is not well controlled, changes in blood glucose levels may cause changes in refractive power by as much as 3 or 4 diopters of hyperopia or myopia.

▶ Iris Changes

Glycogen infiltration of the pigment epithelium and sphincter and dilator muscles of the iris may cause diminished pupillary responses. The reflexes may also be altered by the autonomic neuropathy of diabetes.

Rubeosis iridis is a serious complication of the retinal ischemia that is also the stimulus to retinal neovascularization in severe diabetic retinopathy. Numerous small intertwining blood vessels develop on the anterior surface of the iris.

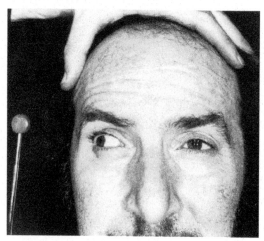

▲ **Figure 15–17.** Pupil-sparing third nerve palsy in diabetes mellitus. Sudden painful ophthalmoplegia, left ptosis, failure of adduction, and normal pupillary responses.

Spontaneous hyphema may occur. Formation of peripheral anterior synechiae blocks aqueous outflow, resulting in secondary (rubeotic) glaucoma.

Extraocular Muscle Palsy (Figure 15–17)

This common occurrence in diabetes is manifested by a sudden onset of diplopia, caused by paresis of one or more extraocular muscles due to infarction of one of the ocular motor nerves. It may be the first manifestation of diabetes. When the third nerve is involved, pain may be a prominent symptom. Differentiation from a posterior communicating aneurysm is important; in diabetic third nerve palsy, the pupil is usually spared (see Chapter 14). Recovery of ocular motor function begins within 3 months after onset and usually is complete. The fourth and sixth nerves may be similarly involved.

Optic Neuropathy (see Chapter 14)

Visual loss is usually due to infarction of the optic disk (nonarteritic anterior ischemic optic neuropathy). Diabetic papillopathy manifests as chronic optic disk swelling, usually with mild visual impairment.

ENDOCRINE DISEASES

THYROID GLAND

1. GRAVES' OPHTHALMOPATHY

Graves' disease is hyperthyroidism (thyrotoxicosis) due to autoimmune thyroid gland disease. In a small proportion of cases, there are eye signs known as Graves' ophthalmopathy

(thyroid eye disease) (Figure 15–18) (see also Chapter 13), which is made more likely and exacerbated by radioiodine therapy for Graves' disease, especially if the resulting hypothyroidism is inadequately treated, and by tobacco smoking. It may develop before any manifestation of hyperthyroidism. It also may occur in autoimmune hypothyroidism (Hashimoto's thyroiditis); thyroid dysfunction due to amiodarone (see later in the chapter); in association with thyroid antibodies without thyroid dysfunction; and occasionally, in the absence of thyroid antibodies and clinical and laboratory evidence of thyroid dysfunction.

Graves' ophthalmopathy is also an autoimmune disorder. Patients usually have serum antibodies to thyroid microsomes (thyroperoxidase), thyroglobulin, and/or thyrotropin (thyroid-stimulating hormone [TSH]) receptors including thyroid-stimulating immunoglobulins. The main target antigen is likely to be the thyrotropin receptor expressed on orbital fibroblasts. The disease process affects the orbital fat and interstitial connective tissue, extraocular muscles, and lacrimal gland. The extraocular muscles may become grossly distended, due to inflammation and intercellular edema secondary to increased concentrations of mucopolysaccharides, and subsequently may become fibrosed.

Clinical Findings (Table 15–5)

Patients may present with nonspecific complaints, such as dry eyes and ocular discomfort, or with prominence of the eyes, double vision, or reduction of vision. The most characteristic sign is dynamic lid lag. The Mourits Clinical Activity Score can be used to monitor disease activity with time and in response to therapy (Table 15–6). The NOSPECS classification quantifies severity of disease (Table 15–7).

Treatment

A. All Cases

1. Prompt restoration and maintenance of euthyroidism
2. Cessation of smoking

B. Mild Disease

1. Lubricants eye drops and/or ointment for ocular surface discomfort
2. Oral selenium 100 μg twice daily

C. Moderate and Severe Disease

1. Optic nerve compression

   • Urgent treatment with high-dose corticosteroid therapy either intravenously (eg, methylprednisolone 1 g daily for 3 days) or orally (eg, prednisolone 100 mg daily)

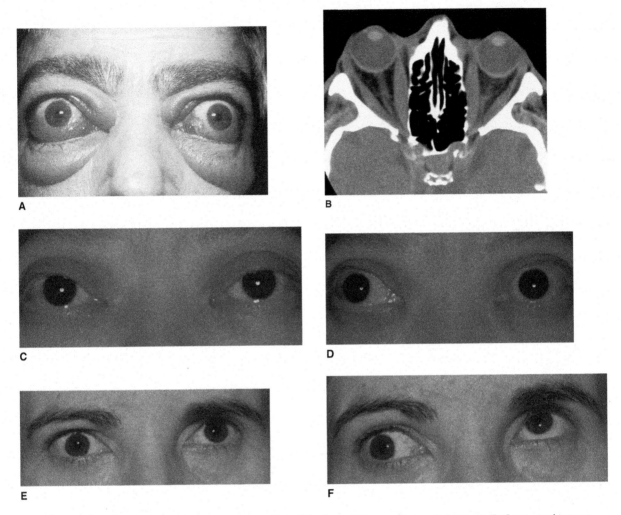

▲ **Figure 15–18.** Graves' ophthalmopathy. **A:** Proptosis, lid edema, lid retraction, and chemosis. **B:** Computed tomography scan showing thickening of the extraocular muscles with optic nerve compression at the orbital apex. Ptosis due to coexistent myasthenia before **(C)** and after **(D)** intravenous edrophonium. Inferior rectus fibrosis causing downward deviation **(E)** and limitation of elevation of right eye **(F)**.

- Options if ongoing treatment required:
  - Orbital decompression (usually achieved by removal of the medial, inferior, and lateral orbital walls via an external or endoscopic approach; decompression of the orbital apex is essential for relief of optic nerve compression)
  - Orbital radiotherapy
  - Long-term corticosteroid therapy
  - Other immunosuppressant therapy (eg, azathioprine) solely or to allow lower maintenance corticosteroid dose
  - Rituximab (anti-CD20 monoclonal antibody) if corticosteroids ineffective
  - Plasmapheresis in refractory cases

2. Corneal exposure
  - Frequent preservative-free lubricants eye drops and/or ointment
  - Topical antibiotics if corneal infection
  - Lateral tarsorrhaphy, other lid surgery, or botulinum toxin–induced ptosis
  - Additional options in severe disease:

Table 15–5. Signs of Graves' Ophthalmopathy

Lid dysfunction
  Lid retraction
    Unilateral or bilateral
    Affects upper and lower lids causing staring expression
    Contributory factors are increased sympathetic nervous
      system activity of hyperthyroidism; fibrosis of the lid
      retractors; widening of the palpebral fissure due to
      exophthalmos; and increased activation of the upper lid
      retractor (levator muscle) when upgaze is restricted due
      to fibrosis of the inferior rectus
  Lid lag
    Unilateral or bilateral
    Affects only the upper lid
    von Graefe sign (dynamic lid lag): elevated upper lid during
      downward movement of the globe (most characteristic sign
      of Graves' ophthalmopathy)
    Lid lag (static lid lag, "hang up"): elevated upper lid on downgaze
  Lagophthalmos
    Incomplete eye closure to which upper and lower lid dysfunction
      and proptosis contribute
  [Ptosis may indicate coexistent myasthenia (Figure 15–18C and D)
  (see Chapter 14).]

Proptosis (often termed exophthalmos in Graves'
  ophthalmopathy) (Figure 15–18A)
  Unilateral or bilateral
  Range from mild (< 24 mm) to severe
  Always axial (see Chapter 13)
  Caused by increase in bulk of ocular muscles and orbital fat
  Magnetic resonance imaging/computed tomography useful for analysis

Ophthalmoplegia
  Typically limitation of elevation with downward deviation due to
    fibrosis (tethering) of inferior rectus muscle (may cause
    increased intraocular pressure on upgaze) (Figure 15–18E and F)
  Often mild limitation of ocular movements in all directions of gaze

Retinal and optic nerve changes
  Retinal or choroidal folds due to compression of the globe
  Compressive optic neuropathy predominantly due to enlargement
    of extraocular muscles at the orbital apex

Corneal changes
  Superior limbic keratoconjunctivitis
  Corneal exposure and ulceration due to lagophthalmos (see above)

- High-dose corticosteroid therapy
- Orbital decompression
- Orbital radiotherapy

3. Double vision (ophthalmoplegia)

- Prisms, either temporary stick-on (Fresnel) or incorporated into spectacles; occlusion of one eye; or possibly extraocular muscle botulinum toxin injections

- Possibly oral corticosteroids and/or other immunosuppressant therapy

Table 15–6. Clinical Activity Score (CAS) of Graves' Ophthalmopathy

Pain
  1. Painful, oppressive feeling on or behind the globe
  2. Pain on attempted eccentric gaze
Redness
  3. Redness of the lids
  4. Diffuse redness of the conjunctiva
Swelling
  5. Chemosis (conjunctival edema)
  6. Swollen caruncle
  7. Edema of the lids
  8. Increase in proptosis of 2 mm or more
Impaired function
  9. Decrease in visual acuity of one or more (Snellen) lines
  10. Decrease of eye movements in any direction equal to or more
    than 5°

One point is given for the presence of each parameter, with the total being the activity score (CAS). Parameters 1–7 provide a score from a single assessment.
Parameters 8–10 are assessed over a period of 1–3 months.
A score of 3 or more indicates likely response to anti-inflammatory therapy.
Increasing score correlates with increasing extraocular muscle enlargement.
Source: Reproduced, with permission, from Mourits MP et al: Clinical criteria for the assessment of disease activity in Graves' ophthalmopathy: A novel approach. Br J Ophthalmol 1989;73:639. [PMID: 2765444]

- Possibly orbital radiotherapy

- Once disease inactive and ophthalmoplegia static for at least 6 months, extraocular muscle surgery for double vision inadequately controlled by prisms

4. Proptosis

- Lid surgery or orbital decompression for permanent problematic or disfiguring proptosis

Table 15–7. NOSPECS Classification of Severity of Graves Ophthalmopathy

Class 0	No symptoms or signs
Class I	Only signs, no symptoms
Class II	Soft tissue involvement
Class III	Proptosis
Class IV	Extraocular muscle involvement
Class V	Corneal involvement
Class VI	Sight loss due to optic nerve compression

Source: Reproduced, with permission, from Werner SC. Modification of the classification of the eye changes of Graves' disease. Am J Ophthalmol 1977;83:725. Copyright © Elsevier. [PMID: 577380]

After treatment of the acute disease, the order of rehabilitative surgery should be orbital decompression if required, extraocular muscle surgery if required, and finally lid surgery if required because orbital decompression may alter the pattern of extraocular muscle abnormality and extraocular muscle surgery may alter the position of the lids.

▼ VITAMIN DEFICIENCIES

VITAMIN A AND VITAMIN E (FIGURE 15–19)

Vitamin A deficiency causes ocular surface disease (see Chapter 6) and retinopathy, predominantly manifesting as rod photoreceptor dysfunction with night blindness (nyctalopia) and peripheral field loss. Peripheral and central retinal degeneration occurs in vitamin E deficiency.

VITAMIN B

Acute **thiamin (vitamin B$_1$) deficiency** causes **Wernicke's encephalopathy**, typically characterized by confusion, ataxia, and nystagmus but also manifesting as ophthalmoplegia, and may result in **Korsakoff's psychosis**. It most commonly occurs in alcoholics. Urgent treatment with parenteral thiamin, initially intravenously, is essential. Chronic thiamin deficiency produces **beriberi**, with ocular disease in 70% of cases. Epithelial changes in the conjunctiva and cornea cause dry eyes. Visual loss may occur as a result of optic atrophy. Treatment is by oral and, if necessary, intramuscular thiamin and correction of dietary deficiency.

Riboflavin (vitamin B$_2$) deficiency has been reported to cause rosacea keratitis, peripheral corneal vascularization, seborrheic blepharitis, and secondary conjunctivitis. **Niacin (nicotinic acid) deficiency (pellagra)** is quite common in alcoholics and is characterized by dermatitis, diarrhea, and dementia. Ocular involvement is rare, but optic neuritis or retinitis may develop. Both riboflavin and niacin deficiency are treated with oral supplementation.

Vitamin B$_{12}$ deficiency (pernicious anemia) is discussed in Chapter 14.

VITAMIN C

In vitamin C (ascorbic acid) deficiency (scurvy), hemorrhages may develop in a variety of sites, for example, skin, mucous membranes, body cavities, the orbits, and subperiosteally in the joints. Hemorrhages may also occur into the lids, subconjunctival space, anterior chamber, vitreous cavity, and retina. Treatment is with oral ascorbic acid and correction of dietary deficiency.

▼ GRANULOMATOUS DISEASES

Many granulomatous diseases cause ophthalmic disease, particularly uveitis (see Chapter 7).

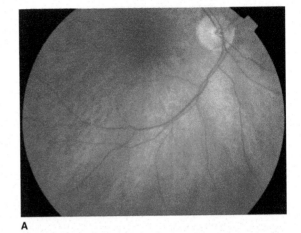

A

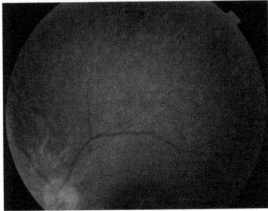

B

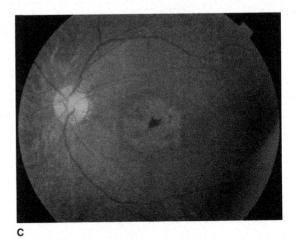

C

▲ **Figure 15–19. A:** Retinal atrophy in vitamin A deficiency. Peripheral **(B)** and central **(C)** retinal degeneration in vitamin E deficiency.

Ocular **tuberculosis** results from endogenous spread from systemic foci. The incidence of eye involvement is less than 1% in known cases of pulmonary tuberculosis. Typically there is a granulomatous panuveitis. Multiple small, discrete, yellowish choroidal nodules may occur especially in miliary tuberculosis (Figure 15–20A). Systemic antituberculosis therapy is required. Anterior uveitis is treated with topical mydriatics and corticosteroids. Posterior uveitis may require systemic corticosteroid therapy. Tuberculosis may also cause ocular motor cranial nerve palsies, papilledema, or damage to the optic nerves or optic chiasm from basal meningitis, vasculitis, or direct infiltration, including a mass lesion (tuberculoma) (Figure 15–20B). There has been a recent increase in the incidence of tuberculosis as a result of human immunodeficiency virus (HIV) infection.

Sarcoidosis (Figure 15–21) is a multisystem disease characterized by noncaseating granulomatous infiltration of affected tissues. The prevalence in North America is 10–80 per 100,000 population, with wide racial and geographic variations: blacks are affected almost 10 times more commonly than whites. Patients may present with pulmonary, ocular, joint, cutaneous, reticuloendothelial system, and exocrine gland manifestations. A granulomatous uveitis may be accompanied by cells in the vitreous, periphlebitis, disk swelling, retinal neovascularization, choroidal disease, and rarely disk granuloma. New vessels may require photocoagulation. Infiltrative optic neuropathy is a rare cause of severe and progressive loss of vision. The ocular and systemic disease may require treatment with corticosteroids and occasionally immunosuppressants.

Eales' disease is characterized by vitreous hemorrhages from areas of retinal neovascularization and was originally reported in young men in poor general health. It is a diagnosis of exclusion; tuberculosis, sarcoidosis, systemic lupus erythematosus, sickle cell disease, and diabetes all need to be excluded. Photocoagulation of the new vessels can reduce the chance of further vitreous hemorrhage.

Leprosy is a chronic granulomatous disorder caused by *Mycobacterium leprae*, an acid-fast bacillus. Three major types are recognized: lepromatous, tuberculoid, and dimorphous. The eye may be affected in any type but is most frequently affected in the lepromatous type. Ocular lesions are due to direct invasion by *M leprae* of the ocular tissues or of the nerves supplying the eye and adnexa. Because the organism grows better at lower temperatures, infection is more apt to involve the anterior than the posterior segment of the eye. Typical features are inadequate eye closure (lagophthalmos) due to facial palsy; loss of the lateral portions of the eyebrows and eyelashes (madarosis); corneal scarring due to corneal exposure, corneal anesthesia, and interstitial keratitis; and granulomatous chronic iritis with pinpoint pupils. Due to widespread availability of multidrug therapy (dapsone, rifampicin, and clofazimine), leprosy is no longer a public health problem (less than 1 case per 10,000 persons).

SYPHILIS

The most common eye lesion in **congenital syphilis** is interstitial keratitis, but it is a late manifestation (discussed in Chapter 6). Chorioretinitis unassociated with interstitial keratitis may occur. Congenital syphilis is treated with large doses of penicillin, although usually it does not influence the interstitial keratitis. In **acquired syphilis**, ocular chancre (primary lesion) occurs rarely on the lid margins and follows

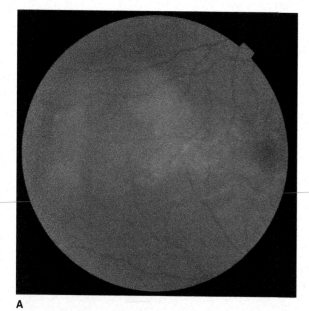

A

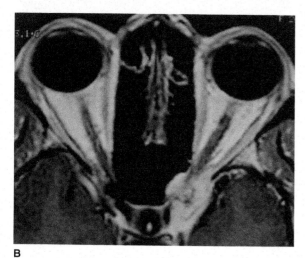

B

▲ **Figure 15–20.** Tuberculosis. **A:** Choroidal nodules. **B:** Orbital apex tuberculoma.

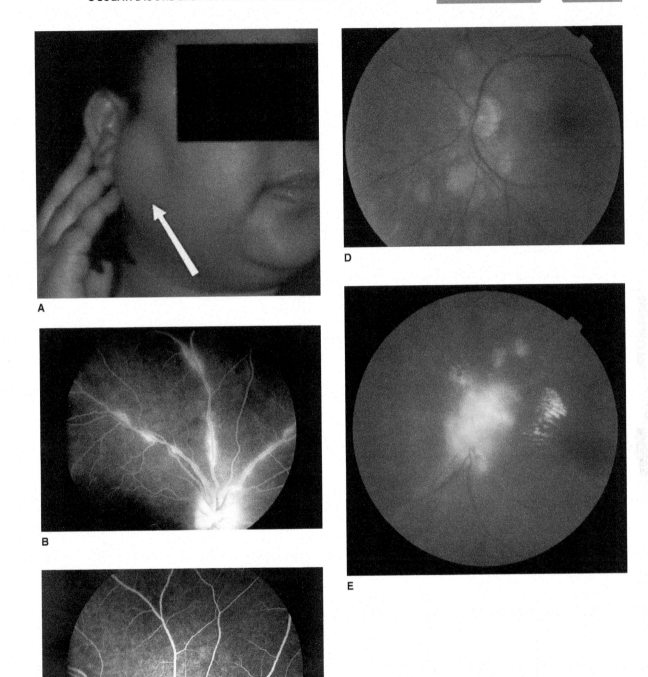

▲ **Figure 15–21.** Sarcoidosis. **A:** Parotitis. Focal periphlebitis and disk leakage may respond dramatically to systemic corticosteroids. **B:** Before treatment. **C:** After 6 weeks of treatment with prednisolone, 30 mg daily. **D:** Choroidal lesions. **E:** Optic disk granuloma.

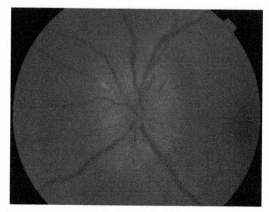

▲ **Figure 15–22.** Secondary syphilis: optic neuritis.

the same course as a genital chancre. In the secondary stage, there may be anterior uveitis, vitritis, various types of retinitis, acute posterior placoid chorioretinitis, and optic neuritis (Figure 15–22). Treatment is parenteral penicillin with the regimen for neurosyphilis.

TOXOPLASMOSIS

Toxoplasma gondii, the protozoal parasite that causes toxoplasmosis infects a great number of animals and birds and has worldwide distribution. Felids are the definitive host. Ocular toxoplasmosis is usually due to reactivation of congenital infection.

▶ Congenital Toxoplasmosis (Figure 15–23)

Infection occurs in utero, and 40% of infants born to mothers who acquired toxoplasmosis during pregnancy—particularly during the third trimester—will be affected (see also Chapter 20).

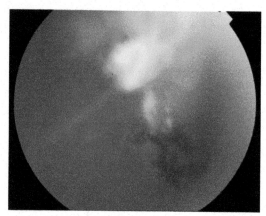

▲ **Figure 15–23.** Toxoplasmosis: active chorioretinitis adjacent to scarring from previous lesion.

There is a posterior uveitis with focal retinochoroiditis, usually in the posterior pole, and an active lesion is often related to an old healed lesion. Panuveitis and optic neuritis may occur but not isolated anterior uveitis. Treatment with antiprotozoal agents, sometimes combined with systemic corticosteroids, reduces inflammation but does not prevent scar formation and is only given for disease that threatens vision (see Chapter 7). Subconjunctival or retrobulbar injection of corticosteroids is contraindicated because it may cause severe exacerbation of disease. Topical corticosteroids and cycloplegics may be useful.

▶ Acquired Toxoplasmosis

Acquired toxoplasmosis affects young adults and is characterized by general malaise, lymphadenopathy, sore throat, and hepatosplenomegaly similar to that seen in infectious mononucleosis. It is endemic in South America and in parts of sub-Saharan Africa. Toxoplasmic retinochoroiditis may rarely follow acquired systemic toxoplasmosis. The diagnosis is confirmed by the finding of both IgG and IgM antibodies.

▼ VIRAL DISEASES

HERPES VIRUSES

▶ Herpes Simplex Virus

There are two morphologic strains of the herpes simplex virus (HSV): type 1 and type 2. Ocular infections are usually produced by type 1, whereas genital infections are caused by type 2. The most common manifestation of herpes simplex is cold sores on the lips. The most common eye lesion is keratitis (see Chapter 6). During primary infection, vesicular skin lesions may occur on the skin of the lids, the lid margins, or the conjunctiva. Uncommon manifestations are iridocyclitis and, more rarely, retinitis (see later in the chapter) and severe encephalitis.

▶ Varicella-Zoster Virus (Chickenpox & Herpes Zoster)

First infection with varicella-zoster virus (VZV) causes chickenpox (varicella). Swollen lids, conjunctivitis, vesicular conjunctival lesions, and (rarely) uveitis and optic neuropathy may occur.

Herpes zoster results from reactivation of latent infection following reduction of immunity, usually due to age, leading to spread of viral infection and associated granulomatous inflammation with vasculitis. It is usually confined to a single dermatome on one side and presents with malaise, headache, and fever followed by burning, itching, and pain in the affected area. Herpes zoster ophthalmicus (HZO) occurs when there is involvement of the first division of the trigeminal nerve. Acutely there may be conjunctivitis, keratitis, episcleritis, scleritis, uveitis when the nasociliary nerve is involved, which is predicted by rash on the tip of the nose (Hutchinson sign), and optic neuropathy (Figure 15–24). Chronic disease that may be recurrent manifests as keratitis, scleritis, and uveitis.

Treatment is not usually required in varicella but should be considered in all cases of ophthalmic zoster. Oral acyclovir, 800 mg five times a day for 7–10 days, started within 72 hours after eruption of the rash, reduces ocular complications, including postherpetic neuralgia. Alternatives are famciclovir, 500 mg three times daily, or valacyclovir, 1 g three times daily. In immunocompromised individuals, both herpes zoster, which may become disseminated, and varicella are likely to be severe and may be fatal. Intravenous acyclovir, 30 mg/kg/d in three divided doses, should be given for at least 7 days. Anterior uveitis requires topical steroids and cycloplegics. A vaccine is available and recommended for older individuals to reduce the risk of herpes zoster.

Acute retinal necrosis has been described following chickenpox and herpes zoster.

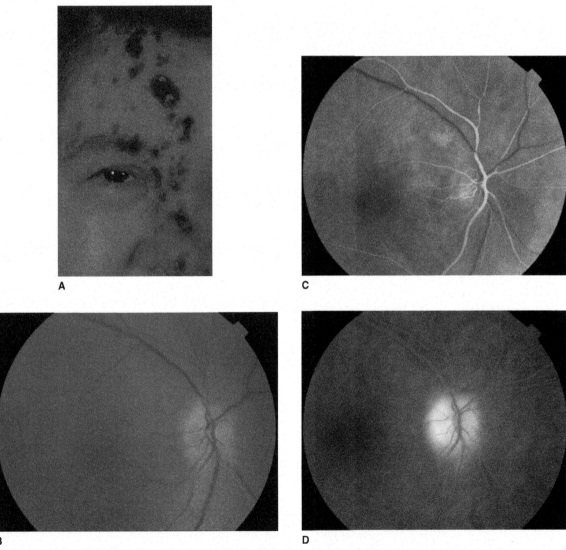

▲ **Figure 15–24.** Herpes zoster ophthalmicus. **A:** Rash involving the tip of the nose (Hutchinson sign). Optic neuropathy with optic disk swelling **(B)**, reduced optic disk and choroidal perfusion in the early phase of fluorescein angiogram **(C)**, and leakage in the late phase **(D)**.

Cytomegalovirus

Infection with cytomegalovirus (CMV) may range from subclinical infection to classic manifestations of cytomegalic inclusion disease. The virus most frequently affects immunocompromised individuals (eg, those with HIV infection, organ transplant recipients). It manifests as a florid necrotizing retinitis with arteriolar occlusion, hemorrhage, and edema. The retinitis itself or secondary retinal detachment can be blinding. In HIV infection, CMV retinitis is more common when CD4 counts are very low.

First-line treatment of CMV retinitis is with intravenous ganciclovir or oral valganciclovir. A standard regimen is a 2-week induction course of intravenous therapy followed by maintenance oral therapy. Alternative treatment can be with a ganciclovir intraocular implant, cidofovir, or foscarnet. Neutropenia is the most important side effect of ganciclovir; renal damage, that of foscarnet. Ocular complications of cidofovir include uveitis, ocular hypotension, and ciliary body necrosis. Maintenance therapy is required unless the immunocompromise can be reversed, such as with highly active antiretroviral therapy (HAART) in HIV infection (see later in the chapter). Congenital CMV infection can cause microphthalmia, cataract, optic atrophy, and optic disk malformation. The differential diagnosis of congenital disease should include toxoplasmosis, rubella, herpes simplex infection, and syphilis. CMV rarely causes retinitis in the newborn.

Epstein-Barr Virus

Infectious mononucleosis (glandular fever) due to Epstein-Barr virus (EBV) can affect the eye directly, causing keratitis, nongranulomatous uveitis, scleritis, conjunctivitis, retinitis, choroiditis, or optic neuritis. Complete recovery is usual, but residual visual loss can result.

Acute Retinal Necrosis

Acute retinal necrosis (ARN) is a disease of healthy individuals, presenting with anterior uveitis with fine keratic precipitates and severe occlusive retinal vasculitis. There is often more than one focus of retinitis, resulting in necrotic areas with discrete borders, which spread circumferentially and posteriorly from the midperipheral retina (Figure 15–25). In most cases, VZV or HSV types 1 or 2 is implicated. CMV and EBV are less commonly responsible. Polymerase chain reaction (PCR) of vitreous samples is helpful to confirm the diagnosis and identify which virus is responsible. Initial treatment is with intravenous acyclovir. Intravenous foscarnet or cidofovir may be effective in infections resistant to acyclovir. Intravitreal ganciclovir or oral valganciclovir may also be used. A 3-month course of oral acyclovir reduces the chances of involvement of the second eye. The disease may result from reactivation of dormant virus, whose antigens

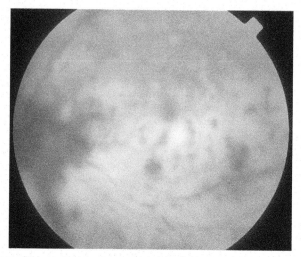

▲ **Figure 15–25.** Acute retinal necrosis due to varicella-zoster virus.

have been found in all layers of the retina, pigment epithelium, and choroid. There may be an immunogenetic predisposition to the disease.

Progressive Outer Retinal Necrosis

Progressive outer retinal necrosis (PORN) is a form of necrotizing retinitis similar to acute retinal necrosis that occurs in immunocompromised patients and is attributed to herpes zoster. There is less inflammation, with multifocal onset in the posterior retina. It has faster progression and a worse outcome when compared with acute retinal necrosis. Retinal detachment may follow the retinal necrosis. Management is the same as for acute retinal necrosis.

OTHER VIRAL DISEASES

Bulbar **poliomyelitis** severe enough to cause lesions of the third, fourth, or sixth cranial nerve is usually fatal. In survivors, any type of internal or external ophthalmoplegia may result. Supranuclear abnormalities ("gaze" palsies, paralysis of convergence or divergence) are rare residual defects. Optic neuritis is uncommon. Treatment is purely symptomatic, although occasionally, a residual extraocular muscle imbalance can be greatly improved by strabismus surgery.

Maternal **rubella** (German measles) during the first trimester of pregnancy causes serious congenital anomalies. The most common eye complication is cataract, which is bilateral in 75% of cases. Other congenital ocular anomalies are frequently associated with the cataracts, for example, uveal colobomas, nystagmus, microphthalmos, strabismus, retinopathy, and infantile glaucoma. Congenital cataract, especially if bilateral, may require surgical removal, but the prognosis is always guarded.

In **measles**, acute conjunctivitis is common early in its course. Koplik's spots may be seen on the conjunctiva, and epithelial keratitis occurs frequently. The treatment of the eye complications of measles is symptomatic unless there is secondary infection, in which case local antibiotic ointment is used.

In **mumps**, the most common ocular complication is dacryoadenitis. A diffuse keratitis with corneal edema resembling the disciform keratitis of herpes simplex occurs rarely.

VACCINATION

Optic neuritis can occur following any vaccination but is most often seen in children following administration of the combined measles-mumps-rubella (MMR) vaccine. Onset is usually within 2 weeks and is bilateral, with visual loss and sometimes pain on eye movements. Examination reveals bilateral disk edema, and MRI shows high signal in the optic nerves. Treatment is with oral corticosteroids, and complete recovery of vision is the anticipated outcome.

FUNGAL DISEASES

CANDIDIASIS

Ocular involvement accompanies systemic candidal infection and candidemia in approximately two-thirds of cases. The initial lesion is a focal necrotizing granulomatous retinitis (Figure 15–26A) with or without choroiditis, characterized by fluffy white exudative lesions associated with cells in the vitreous overlying the lesion. Such lesions may spread to involve the optic nerve and macula. Endophthalmitis, Roth spots, and exudative retinal detachment may occur. Spread into the vitreous cavity may result in formation of vitreous abscesses, sometimes described as "a string of pearls" (Figure 15–26B). Anterior uveitis occurs, and there may be a hypopyon. Treatment consists of intravitreal amphotericin B combined with oral flucytosine and fluconazole, which are synergistic. Early vitrectomy may prevent macular damage.

MUCORMYCOSIS

Mucormycosis is a rare, often fatal infection occurring in debilitated patients, particularly poorly controlled diabetics. The fungi (*Rhizopus*, *Mucor*, and *Absidia*) attack through the upper respiratory tract and invade the arterioles, producing necrotic tissue. Clinical features are the pathognomonic black hemipalate, proptosis, and an ischemic globe with blindness due to ophthalmic artery occlusion. Death occurs from cerebral abscess. Treatment includes removal of the affected tissue, intravenous amphotericin B (preferably liposomal) or possibly posaconazole, and management of the underlying medical condition.

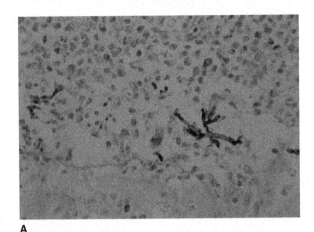

A

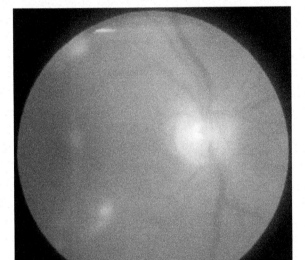

B

▲ **Figure 15–26.** Candidiasis. **A:** Histopathology of retinitis showing fungal elements in the deep retina. **B:** Endophthalmitis with typical "string of pearls" appearance in the vitreous.

ACQUIRED IMMUNODEFICIENCY SYNDROME (AIDS)

AIDS is caused by a retrovirus, HIV, which infects mature T-helper cells, leading to immune suppression, with the severity depending on the balance between the rates of destruction and replacement of T cells. The persistent immunodeficiency results in opportunistic infections.

Transmission of HIV is primarily by exchange of bodily fluids during sexual contact or through the use of contaminated needles by intravenous drug abuse. Transmission may also occur when contaminated blood products are transfused or by needlestick injury.

There may be an acute flu-like illness a few weeks after initial infection, followed months later by weight loss, fever, diarrhea, lymphadenopathy, and encephalopathy. Opportunistic infection with herpes zoster virus, *Candida*, and tuberculosis becomes more frequent as the CD4 count drops below 500 cells/μL. When the CD4 cell count is below 200 cells/μL, infections with protozoa (such as *Pneumocystis* and *Toxoplasma*) and fungi (such as *Cryptococcus*) occur. CMV and *Mycobacterium avium-intracellulare* infections are seen when the CD4 count is below 100 cells/μL.

The eye is involved in 30% of patients with AIDS. The most common abnormalities are retinal microvasculopathy, with cotton-wool spots and hemorrhages, and conjunctival vasculopathy characterized by "comma-shapeda vessels, sludging of the blood, and linear hemorrhages." The cause of these findings is unknown, but they are sometimes associated with increased plasma viscosity and may represent immune complex deposition. An intermediate uveitis may occur when there is a high viral load. Among the opportunistic infections, viral infections of the retina are most common, particularly CMV (Figure 15–27) (see earlier in the chapter). Involvement of the optic nerve by CMV results in gross optic disk edema and severe sudden and irreversible visual loss. Diagnosis is usually based on the clinical picture and confirmation of active viral replication as shown by PCR testing of blood, urine, cerebrospinal fluid, aqueous, or vitreous. Cryptococcal meningitis may cause fulminant optic neuritis as well as optic nerve damage due to raised intracranial pressure.

Treatment of HIV infection is complicated and individualized according to comorbidity and therapeutic response. Initially it involves a combination of at least three drugs (HAART). Usually there is a dramatic drop in the HIV viral load, increase in CD4 count, and improved well-being.

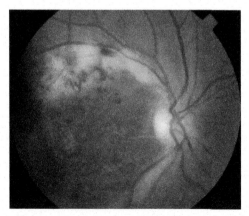

▲ **Figure 15–27.** Retinal changes in human immunodeficiency virus infection: cytomegalovirus retinitis.

Patients with CMV retinitis may develop a "reconstitution uveitis" in which relative immune recovery is followed by panuveitis. It may be possible to stop anti-CMV therapy when the CD4 count has risen above 200/μL for 3 months.

Acute retinal necrosis and progressive outer retinal necrosis (see earlier in the chapter) may occur. If the causative agent of the former is herpes simplex, concurrent encephalitis is common. *Toxoplasma* chorioretinitis is usually bilateral, acquired (congenital infections are rarely reactivated in AIDS), and associated with substantial vitreous reaction. Candidal endophthalmitis is rarely seen except in drug addicts. Less common organisms that typically involve the choroid are *Pneumocystis jiroveci* (formerly *P carinii*), *Cryptococcus neoformans*, and *M avium-intracellulare*. Choroidal infection is blood-borne and portends imminent demise.

Herpes zoster ophthalmicus is a common presenting feature of HIV infection in sub-Saharan Africa and may be very severe, with anterior segment necrosis and ophthalmoplegia. Syphilis in association with HIV infection may produce severe blinding uveitis or optic neuropathy. Herpes simplex, molluscum contagiosum, and Kaposi's sarcoma frequently affect the eyelids and surrounding tissues. The combination of rifabutin and clarithromycin or cidofovir may precipitate symptomatic uveitis.

Neuro-ophthalmologic problems are divided into those related directly to HIV infection of the brain, such as optic neuropathy and supranuclear ophthalmoplegia, and those caused by cerebral abscesses or encephalitis, commonly due to cryptococcal infection, lymphoma, or toxoplasmosis.

MULTISYSTEM IMMUNE-MEDIATED DISEASES AND SYSTEMIC VASCULITIS

SYSTEMIC LUPUS ERYTHEMATOSUS

Systemic lupus erythematosus (SLE) is mediated by autoantibodies (antinuclear, double-stranded DNA, ribonucleoprotein, and antiphospholipid) and immune complexes. Its numerous manifestations include systemic upset with fatigue and malaise, malar ("butterfly") facial rash, musculoskeletal disturbance such as arthralgia and myalgia, hematologic disease particularly anemia, and cardiopulmonary, renal, and neurologic disease. Ocular abnormalities include keratoconjunctivitis sicca in approximately a third of cases, episcleritis, and scleritis. Retinal involvement ranges from microangiopathy, with cotton-wool spots, microaneurysms, exudates, and hemorrhages very similar to diabetic retinopathy, to severe occlusive disease. It may be complicated by hypertensive retinochoroidopathy. Choroidal involvement, with exudative retinal detachment or abnormalities of the retinal pigment epithelium, may occur alone or in association with retinopathy. Retinal and choroidal disease may be accompanied by life-threatening neurologic and renal disease. An optic neuropathy may occur due to an inflammatory or vaso-occlusive disease.

High-dose corticosteroids, cyclophosphamide, and possibly mycophenolate are the most effective treatments for severe disease. Hydroxychloroquine is useful for milder chronic disease but may cause retinopathy with prolonged or high-dose treatment.

ANTIPHOSPHOLIPID ANTIBODY SYNDROME

This diagnosis should be considered in patients with recurrent thromboembolism, recurrent fetal loss, livedo reticularis, thrombocytopenia, and neurologic disease without other features of systemic lupus erythematosus. Visual loss may be due to retinal vein or arterial occlusion or ischemic optic neuropathy. Choroidal infarcts may also occur (Figure 15–3A). The diagnosis is confirmed by the presence of lupus anticoagulant and high-titer IgG and IgM anticardiolipin antibodies.

DERMATOMYOSITIS

In this rare disease, there is characteristically a degenerative subacute inflammation of the muscles, sometimes including the extraocular muscles. The lids are commonly a part of the generalized dermal involvement and may show marked swelling and erythema. Retinopathy with cotton-wool spots and hemorrhages may occur. High doses of systemic corticosteroids will frequently effect a remission that continues even after cessation of therapy. The ultimate prognosis is, however, poor.

SCLERODERMA

This rare chronic disease is characterized by widespread alterations in the collagenous tissues of the mucosa, bones, muscles, skin, and internal organs. Individuals of both sexes between 15 and 45 years of age are affected. The skin in local areas becomes tense and leathery, and the process may spread to involve large areas of the limbs, rendering them virtually immobile. The skin of the eyelids is often involved. Iritis and cataract occur less frequently. Retinopathy, similar to that which occurs in lupus erythematosus and dermatomyositis, may be present. Systemic corticosteroid treatment improves the prognosis.

POLYARTERITIS NODOSA

This collagen disease affects mainly medium-sized arteries, most commonly in men. There is intense inflammation of all the muscle layers of the arteries, with fibrinoid necrosis and a peripheral eosinophilia. The main clinical features include nephritis, hypertension, asthma, peripheral neuropathy, muscle pain with wasting, and peripheral eosinophilia. Cardiac involvement is common, although death is usually caused by renal dysfunction.

Ocular changes are seen in 20% of cases and consist of episcleritis and scleritis (Figure 15–28), which is often painless (see Chapter 7). When the limbal vessels are involved, guttering of the peripheral cornea may occur. A retinal

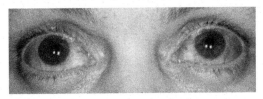

▲ **Figure 15–28.** Polyarteritis nodosa. Bilateral scleritis.

microvasculopathy is common. Sudden dramatic visual loss may be due to an inflammatory steroid-responsive optic neuropathy, ischemic optic neuropathy, or central retinal artery occlusion. Ophthalmoplegia may result from involvement of ocular motor cranial nerves. Systemic corticosteroids and cyclophosphamide are of some value. A few patients have a monophasic disease that resolves completely, but in the remainder, the long-term prognosis is uniformly bad.

GRANULOMATOSIS WITH POLYANGIITIS (WEGENER'S GRANULOMATOSIS)

This granulomatous process shares certain clinical features with polyarteritis nodosa. The three diagnostic criteria are (1) necrotizing granulomatous lesions of the respiratory tract, (2) generalized necrotizing arteritis, and (3) renal involvement with necrotizing glomerulitis.

Ophthalmic manifestations occur in 50% of cases. Proptosis resulting from orbital granulomatous inflammation may lead to extraocular muscle or optic nerve involvement (Figure 15–29A). Nasolacrimal duct obstruction is a rare complication. Involvement of the globe manifests as conjunctivitis, peripheral corneal ulceration (Figure 15–29B), episcleritis, scleritis, uveitis, and retinal vasculitis.

Antineutrophil cytoplasmic antibodies (ANCAs), characteristically C-ANCA, are present in most cases with generalized disease and have both diagnostic and prognostic value, but they are found in only 30% of cases with disease limited to the head and neck. Combined corticosteroids and immunosuppressants (particularly cyclophosphamide) often produce a satisfactory response. Rituximab has been advocated for refractory cases.

RHEUMATOID ARTHRITIS

In rheumatoid arthritis, which is more common in women than in men, scleritis and episcleritis are comparatively common. Scleritis may herald exacerbation of systemic disease, tends to occur with widespread vasculitis, and may lead to scleromalacia perforans (Figure 15–30) (see Chapter 7).

Corticosteroid drops are helpful in episcleritis, but systemic treatment (nonsteroidal anti-inflammatory agents, corticosteroids, and other agents such as methotrexate or tumor necrosis factor inhibitors, albeit the last may exacerbate ocular inflammatory disease) is necessary for scleritis.

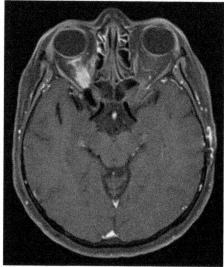

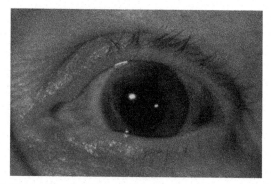

▲ **Figure 15–29.** Granulomatosis with polyangiitis (Wegener's granulomatosis). **A:** Computed tomography scan showing left orbital disease with optic nerve involvement. **B:** Peripheral corneal ulceration.

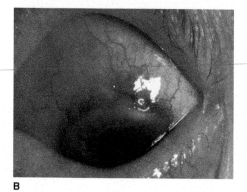

▲ **Figure 15–30.** Rheumatoid arthritis. Scleral thinning due to scleromalacia perforans.

Keratoconjunctivitis sicca is present in 15% of cases (see Chapter 4). Peripheral corneal melting may occur in more severe cases.

JUVENILE IDIOPATHIC ARTHRITIS (JUVENILE CHRONIC ARTHRITIS, JUVENILE RHEUMATOID ARTHRITIS, STILL'S DISEASE)

Ocular complications of juvenile idiopathic arthritis occur most frequently in girls with oligoarticular disease. The systemic disease appears to be disproportionately mild in children with severe visual loss, and diagnosis and treatment may therefore be delayed. Ocular involvement may occur before joint involvement. There is a chronic insidious uveitis with a high incidence of anterior segment complications (eg, posterior synechiae, cataract, secondary glaucoma, band-shaped keratopathy) (see Chapter 7). Whereas antinuclear antibodies are present in 30% of patients with juvenile idiopathic arthritis overall, they are present in 88% who develop uveitis. Most cases are controlled with local corticosteroids and mydriatics, but severe cases require methotrexate and occasionally a short course of high-dose systemic corticosteroids.

SJÖGREN'S SYNDROME

Sjögren's syndrome is a systemic disorder with diverse features but characterized by dry eyes (keratoconjunctivitis sicca) and dry mouth (xerostomia). It may be secondary to a connective tissue disease, usually rheumatoid arthritis. It is more common in females. The onset of ocular symptoms occurs most frequently during the fourth, fifth, and sixth decades. Lymphoid proliferation is a prominent feature and may involve the kidneys, lungs, or liver, causing renal tubular acidosis, pulmonary fibrosis, or cirrhosis. Lymphoreticular malignant disease such as reticulum cell sarcoma may develop after many years.

Histopathologic change in the lacrimal gland is infiltration of lymphocytes, histiocytes, and occasional plasma cells leading to atrophy and destruction of the glandular structures. Because of the relative inaccessibility of the lacrimal gland, labial salivary gland biopsy is the preferred option for diagnosis in patients without serum antibodies to the extractable nuclear antigens Ro (SSA) and La (SSB).

GIANT CELL ARTERITIS (TEMPORAL ARTERITIS)

This is a disease of elderly patients (mostly women over age 60) that causes inflammation and occlusion of medium and large arteries. Clinically branches of the external carotid system are most frequently involved, but pathologic and imaging studies show more widespread involvement, including aortitis. Polymyalgia rheumatica may precede or accompany the disease. Generally patients feel unwell with increasingly severe pain in the region of the superficial temporal and occipital arteries that may be tender, swollen, and pulseless. Increasing jaw pain on chewing (jaw claudication) is almost pathognomonic. Visual loss occurs in 30–60% of cases and is usually due to ischemic optic neuropathy or less commonly central retinal artery occlusion. Involvement of one eye indicates high risk without treatment of involvement of the other eye. Occipital infarction is rare. Other neurologic complications are cranial nerve palsies, although double vision is more likely to be due to orbital ischemia, and brainstem lesions. Usually erythrocyte sedimentation rate (ESR) is markedly raised (80–100 mm in the first hour) and C-reactive protein (CRP) is moderately raised (25–50 mg/dL), but both may be normal. Positive temporal artery biopsy is the most definitive test (see Chapter 14). It is important to make the diagnosis early because immediate high-dose systemic corticosteroids (eg, oral prednisone 1–2 mg/kg/d, possibly preceded by intravenous methylprednisolone 1 g/d for 3 days) produces dramatic relief of pain and prevents further ischemic episodes. Disease activity is monitored by the clinical state aided by the inflammatory markers. In most cases, corticosteroid therapy can be discontinued after 1–2 years, but longer duration therapy is required in up to 30% of cases with the risk of adverse effects including increased mortality.

IDIOPATHIC ARTERITIS OF TAKAYASU (PULSELESS DISEASE)

This disease, found most frequently in young women and occasionally in children, is a polyarteritis of unknown cause with increased predilection for the aorta and its branches. Manifestations include cerebrovascular insufficiency, syncope, absence of pulsations in the upper extremities, and ocular ischemic syndrome (see earlier in the chapter). Thromboendarterectomy, prosthetic graft, and systemic corticosteroid therapy have been reported to be successful.

ANKYLOSING SPONDYLITIS

Ankylosing spondylitis occurs mainly in males 16–40 years of age with HLA-B27 in around 90% of all cases. Anterior uveitis, which is usually acute and painful, occurs in 25–50% of patients and may be complicated by acute angle-closure glaucoma during an acute episode and cataract, glaucoma, or posterior segment complications if there are severe, frequent, or poorly controlled episodes (see Chapter 7).

BEHÇET'S DISEASE

Behçet's disease causes oral and genital ulceration; skin lesions including increased inflammatory reaction to trauma (pathergy test); arthritis; peripheral venous thrombosis and occasional arterial disease; and neurologic disease including cerebral venous sinus thrombosis. Ocular disease occurs in

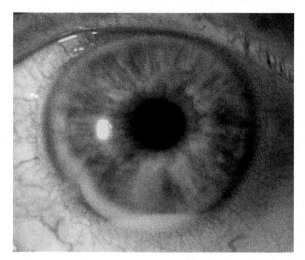

▲ **Figure 15–31.** Behçet's disease: hypopyon.

75% of cases. Uveitis is severe and frequently causes hypopyon (Figure 15–31). Focal retinal infiltrates are typical. Visual loss is usually due to ischemic branch retinal vein occlusions. Treatment often involves multiple immunosuppressants (eg, corticosteroids, anti–tumor necrosis factor-α biologics, cyclosporine, azathioprine, interferon), but visual outcome is still poor in 25% of cases. Ocular involvement is associated with the HLA-B51 haplotype. Tumor necrosis factor gene polymorphisms and possibly the prothrombotic factor V Leiden mutation are associated with more severe ocular disease.

HERITABLE CONNECTIVE TISSUE DISEASES

MARFAN'S SYNDROME

The inherited defect is a mutation in the fibrillin-1 gene located on chromosome 15. Inheritance is autosomal dominant with variable expression, so that mild, incomplete forms of the syndrome are seen, but about 25% of affected individuals have new mutations. The most striking clinical feature is increased length of the long bones, resulting in tall stature, large arm span, and long thin fingers and toes (arachnodactyly). Other characteristics include scanty subcutaneous fat, relaxed ligaments, and, less commonly, developmental anomalies, including congenital heart disease and deformities of the spine and joints. Ocular complications are often seen, particularly superior and nasal lens dislocation (Figure 15–32). Less common are severe refractive errors, megalocornea, cataract, uveal colobomas, and secondary glaucoma. There is a high infant mortality rate. Removal of a dislocated lens may be necessary.

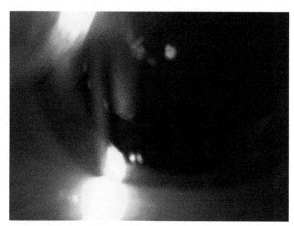

▲ **Figure 15–32.** Marfan'a syndrome with upward dislocation of the lens.

OSTEOGENESIS IMPERFECTA

This rare autosomal dominant syndrome, usually due to a mutation in a type 1 collagen gene, is characterized by multiple fractures, blue scleras, and, less commonly, deafness. The disease usually manifests soon after birth. The long bones are very fragile, fracturing easily and often healing with fibrous bony union. The bones become more fragile with age. The very thin sclera allows the blue color imparted by the underlying uveal tract to show through. There is usually no visual impairment. Occasionally, abnormalities such as keratoconus, megalocornea, and corneal or lenticular opacities are also present. Ophthalmologic treatment is seldom necessary.

HEREDITARY METABOLIC DISORDERS

See Table 15–8 for a list of hereditary metabolic disorders affecting the eye.

MISCELLANEOUS SYSTEMIC DISEASES WITH OCULAR MANIFESTATIONS

VOGT-KOYANAGI-HARADA DISEASE (FIGURE 15–33)

Vogt-Koyanagi disease is characterized by bilateral uveitis, alopecia, poliosis, vitiligo, and hearing defects, usually in young adults. If there is exudative retinal detachment due to exudative choroiditis, the term Harada disease is used. There is a tendency toward recovery of visual function, but this is not always complete. Initial treatment is with local steroids and mydriatics, but systemic steroids in high doses are frequently required to prevent permanent visual loss.

Table 15–8. Hereditary Metabolic Disorders Affecting the Eye

Wilson's disease
  Rare autosomal recessive disease of young adults
  Characterized by abnormal copper metabolism
  Kayser-Fleischer ring (see Chapter 6): peripheral circumferential corneal discoloration due to deposition of copper at Descemet's membrane

Cystinosis
  Rare autosomal recessive derangement of amino acid metabolism
  Cystine crystals deposited throughout the body
  Dwarfism, nephropathy, death in early childhood
  Cystine crystals seen in conjunctiva and cornea

Albinism
  Oculocutaneous (autosomal recessive) or ocular (X-linked recessive)
  Nystagmus, iris transillumination, hypopigmented fundi, hypoplastic foveas
  Increased proportion of decussating axons in optic chiasm can be detected by electrodiagnostic testing

Galactosemia
  Rare autosomal recessive disorder of carbohydrate metabolism
  Cataract (cortical vacuoles)

EPIDERMAL NECROLYSIS (STEVENS-JOHNSON SYNDROME AND TOXIC EPIDERMAL NECROLYSIS)

Epidermal necrolysis, which is characterized by extensive detachment of the epithelium of the skin and mucous membranes, encompasses Stevens-Johnson syndrome (SJS) and toxic epidermal necrolysis (TEN), with the former being less severe. (Erythema multiforme used to be classified with epidermal necrolysis but is now deemed to be a different entity with no or mild involvement of mucous membranes.) Epidermal necrolysis is rare, and the acute phase is self-limiting but associated with severe morbidity, including ocular disease, and mortality (SJS 5–12%, TEN 15–40%). The majority of cases are caused by drugs, most commonly allopurinol and carbamazepine. Prompt discontinuation of the drug is recommended. Whether specific treatment such as corticosteroid therapy is beneficial is uncertain. Supportive treatment is important. The primary ocular abnormality is membranous conjunctivitis, leading to tear deficiency due to occlusion of the lacrimal gland ducts, symblepharon, loss of goblet cells and meibomian glands, and entropion with trichiasis or ectropion. Loss of limbal stem cells exacerbates corneal disease, which may result in corneal ulceration, infection, and perforation, and panophthalmitis. Treatment includes intensive topical preservative-free lubricants and corticosteroids, release of symblepharon, amniotic membrane grafts, lid surgery, and topical antibiotics for secondary infection.

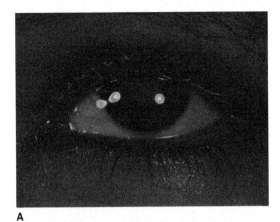

A

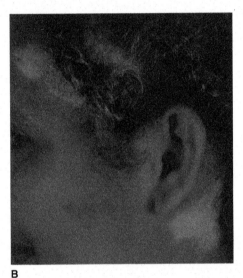

B

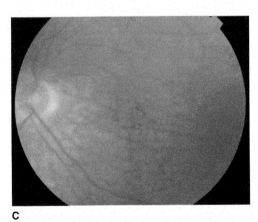

C

▲ **Figure 15–33.** Vogt-Koyanagi-Harada (VKH) disease. **A:** Poliosis of the eyelashes. **B:** Alopecia, vitiligo, and poliosis of the hair. **C:** Late retinal pigment epithelial damage.

ROSACEA (ACNE ROSACEA)

This disease of unknown cause is primarily dermatologic, beginning as hyperemia of the face associated with acneiform lesions and eventually causing hypertrophy of tissues such as rhinophyma (Figure 15–34). Chronic blepharitis is often present. Rosacea keratitis develops in about 5% of cases.

Careful attention to lid hygiene is essential. Topical corticosteroids help in controlling keratitis. Long-term systemic doxycycline or erythromycin therapy is often beneficial.

LYME DISEASE

Lyme disease is a vector-mediated multisystem illness caused by the spirochete *Borrelia burgdorferi*. The usual vectors are small ixodid ticks that have a complex three-host life cycle involving multiple mammalian and avian species.

The disease has three major stages. Initially, in the area of the tick bite, there develops the characteristic skin lesion of erythema chronicum migrans, often accompanied by regional lymphadenopathy, malaise, fever, headache, myalgia, and arthralgia. Several weeks to months later, there is a period of neurologic and cardiac abnormalities. After a few more weeks or even years, rheumatologic abnormalities develop—initially, migratory musculoskeletal discomfort, but later, a frank arthritis that may recur over several years.

Conjunctivitis is a frequent finding in the first stage. Cranial nerve palsies—particularly of the seventh but also of the third, fourth, or sixth cranial nerves—often occur in the neurologic phase. Other ophthalmologic abnormalities that have been reported include uveitis, ischemic optic

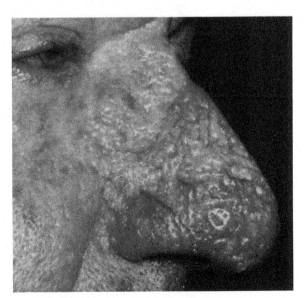

▲ **Figure 15–34.** Acne rosacea: rhinophyma and blepharitis.

neuropathy, optic disk edema and neuroretinitis with macular star, bilateral keratitis, and choroiditis with exudative retinal detachments.

Laboratory diagnosis is by demonstration of specific IgM and IgG antibodies in serum or cerebrospinal fluid. The spirochetes may also be isolated from these sources.

Recommended treatment options include oral doxycycline, amoxicillin, or cefuroxime or intravenous ceftriaxone for 14 days.

IMMUNOSUPPRESSANTS

Immunosuppressants reduce ocular inflammation, but often the treatment is empirical because a specific cause of the inflammation cannot be identified. All patients must undergo medical assessment before treatment is started, including individual susceptibility to adverse effects; be counseled about the benefits and risks of the treatment options; and be monitored throughout the course of treatment. Commonly used drugs are **corticosteroids** (eg, prednisolone), **azathioprine**, **cyclosporine**, **mycophenolate mofetil**, and **cytotoxic agents** such as methotrexate and cyclophosphamide. Biologic agents are being used increasingly, including monoclonal antibodies to cytokines (eg, tumor necrosis factor, interleukin-17A, interferon-2α), cytokine receptors (eg, anti-interleukin-2 receptor, anti-interleukin-6 receptor), T-cell subsets (eg, T-helper cells [Th17]), or other antigens (eg, insulin-like growth factor-1 receptor [IGFR-1R]).

OCULAR COMPLICATIONS OF SYSTEMICALLY ADMINISTERED DRUGS

Adverse ocular effects of systemic drugs are discussed in Chapter 22.

REFERENCES

Aissopou EK et al: The Keith-Wagener-Barker and Mitchell-Wong grading systems for hypertensive retinopathy: Association with target organ damage in individuals below 55 years. J Hypertens 2015;33:2303. [PMID: 26335430]

Amin RM et al: Treatment options for juvenile idiopathic arthritis (JIA) associated uveitis. Ocul Immunol Inflamm 2016;24:81. [PMID: 26652068]

Asoklis R et al: Images in clinical medicine. Ocular rosacea. N Engl J Med 2016;374:771. [PMID: 26933851]

Bakhda RN. Clinical study of fundus findings in pregnancy induced hypertension. J Family Med Prim Care 2016;5:424. [PMID: 27843854]

Bartalena L et al: The 2016 European Thyroid Association/European Group on Graves' Orbitopathy Guidelines for the Management of Graves' Orbitopathy. Eur Thyroid J 2016;5:9. [PMID: 27099835]

Bhatt N et al: Biologic therapies: Anti-tumor necrosis factor-α, anti-interleukins, rituximab and others. Dev Ophthalmol 2016;55:252. [PMID: 26501216]

Borkar DS et al: Incidence of herpes zoster ophthalmicus: Results from the Pacific Ocular Inflammation Study. Ophthalmology 2013;120:451. [PMID: 23207173]

Catt CJ et al: Ocular manifestations of Stevens-Johnson syndrome and toxic epidermal necrolysis in children. Am J Ophthalmol 2016;166:68. [PMID: 27018234]

Chang VS et al: Chronic ocular complications of Stevens-Johnson syndrome and toxic epidermal necrolysis: The role of systemic immunomodulatory therapy. Semin Ophthalmol 2016;31:178. [PMID: 26959145]

Chang YS et al: Risk of nonarteritic anterior ischemic optic neuropathy following end-stage renal disease. Medicine (Baltimore) 2016;95:e3174. [PMID: 27015205]

Chang YS et al: Risk of retinal artery occlusion in patients with end-stage renal disease: A retrospective large-scale cohort study. Medicine (Baltimore) 2016;95:e3281. [PMID: 27057891]

Cohen EJ. Management and prevention of herpes zoster ocular disease. Cornea 2015;34(Suppl 10):S3. [PMID: 26114827]

Correll MH et al: Lyme neuroborreliosis: A treatable cause of acute ocular motor disturbances in children. Br J Ophthalmol 2015;99:1401. [PMID: 25868792]

Cugati S et al: Treatment options for central retinal artery occlusion. Curr Treat Options Neurol 2013;15:63. [PMID: 23070637]

Davies EC et al: Herpes zoster ophthalmicus: Declining age at presentation. Br J Ophthalmol 2016;100:312. [PMID: 26178905]

Gaier ED et al: The enigma of nonarteritic anterior ischemic optic neuropathy: An update for the comprehensive ophthalmologist. Curr Opin Ophthalmol 2016;27:498. [PMID: 27585212]

Generali E et al: Ocular involvement in systemic autoimmune diseases. Clin Rev Allergy Immunol 2015;49:263. [PMID: 26494481]

Govindaraju R et al: Images in clinical medicine. Carotid-cavernous sinus fistula. N Engl J Med 2016;374:e15. [PMID: 27028934]

Gower NJ et al: Drug discovery in ophthalmology: Past success, present challenges, and future opportunities. BMC Ophthalmol 2016;16:11. [PMID: 26774505]

Harrell M et al: Current treatment of toxoplasma retinochoroiditis: An evidence-based review. J Ophthalmol 2014;2014:273506. [PMID: 25197557]

Henderson AD et al: Hypertension-related eye abnormalities and the risk of stroke. Rev Neurol Dis 2011;8:1. [PMID: 21769065]

Henderson AD et al: Grade III or grade IV hypertensive retinopathy with severely elevated blood pressure. West J Emerg Med 2012;13:529. [PMID: 23359839]

Heng YK et al: Epidermal necrolysis: 60 years of errors and advances. Br J Dermatol 2015;173:1250. [PMID: 26769645]

Horie Y et al: HLA-B51 carriers are susceptible to ocular symptoms of Behçet disease and the association between the two becomes stronger towards the East along the Silk Road: A literature survey. Ocul Immunol Inflamm 2016;8:1. [PMID: 26954704]

Hsien YM et al: Why can't I see after my heart is fixed: A case series of ocular complications after cardiac intervention. BMC Ophthalmol 2016;16:32. [PMID: 27013074]

Hsu DY et al: Morbidity and mortality of Stevens-Johnson syndrome and toxic epidermal necrolysis in United States adults. J Invest Dermatol 2016;126:1387. [PMID: 27039263]

Hu LT: Lyme disease. Ann Intern Med 2016;164:ITC65. [PMID: 27136224]

Jain R et al: Stevens-Johnson syndrome: The role of an ophthalmologist. Surv Ophthalmol 2016;61:369. [PMID: 26829569]

Kaniwa N et al: Drugs causing severe ocular surface involvements in Japanese patients with Stevens-Johnson syndrome/toxic epidermal necrolysis. Allergol Int 2015;64:379. [PMID: 26433536]

Karra E et al: Clinical assessment of patients with thyroid eye disease. Br J Hosp Med (Lond) 2016;77:C2. [PMID: 26903467]

Karra E et al: Management of patients with thyroid eye disease. Br J Hosp Med (Lond) 2016;77:C6. [PMID: 26903468]

Katz DM et al: Is there treatment for nonarteritic anterior ischemic optic neuropathy. Curr Opin Ophthalmol 2015;26:458. [PMID: 26367094]

Kim JW et al: Efficacy of combined orbital radiation and systemic steroids in the management of Graves' orbitopathy. Graefes Arch Clin Exp Ophthalmol 2016;254:991. [PMID: 26876240]

Kohanim S et al: Acute and chronic ophthalmic involvement in Stevens-Johnson syndrome/toxic epidermal necrolysis: A comprehensive review and guide to therapy. II. Ophthalmic disease. Ocul Surf 2016;14:168. [PMID: 26882981]

Kolar P. Risk factors for central and branch retinal vein occlusion: A meta-analysis of published clinical data. J Ophthalmol 2014;2014:724780. [PMID: 25009743]

Konstantinidis L et al: Hypertension and the eye. Curr Opin Ophthalmol 2016;27:514. [PMID: 27662019]

Levy-Clarke G et al: Expert panel recommendations for the use of anti-tumor necrosis factor biologic agents in patients with ocular inflammatory disorders. Ophthalmology 2014;121:785. [PMID: 24359625]

Lima GS et al: Current therapy of acquired ocular toxoplasmosis: A review. J Ocul Pharmacol Ther 2015;31:511. [PMID: 26226199]

Marcocci C et al: Selenium and the course of mild Graves' orbitopathy. N Engl J Med 2011;364:1920. [PMID: 21591944]

Moradi A et al: Clinical features and incidence rates of ocular complications in patients with ocular syphilis. Am J Ophthalmol 2015;159:334. [PMID: 25447116]

Northey LC et al: Syphilitic uveitis and optic neuritis in Sydney, Australia. Br J Ophthalmol 2015;99:1215. [PMID: 25788666]

Odouard C et al: Rising trends of endogenous Klebsiella pneumoniae endophthalmitis in Australia. Clin Exp Ophthalmol 2016 Aug 26. [Epub ahead of print] [PMID: 27564396]

Ong YT et al: Hypertensive retinopathy and risk of stroke. Hypertension 2013;62:706. [PMID: 23940194]

Peponis VG et al: Bilateral multifocal chorioretinitis and optic neuritis due to Epstein-Barr virus: A case report. Case Rep Ophthalmol 2012;3:327. [PMID: 23139677]

Pleyer U et al: Ocular toxoplasmosis: Recent aspects of pathophysiology and clinical implications. Ophthalmic Res 2014;52:116. [PMID: 25248050]

Preble JM et al: Ocular involvement in systemic lupus erythematosus. Curr Opin Ophthalmol 2015;26:540. [PMID: 26367085]

Pula JH et al: Update on the evaluation of transient vision loss. Clin Ophthalmol 2016;10:297. [PMID: 26929593]

Raman R et al: Diabetic retinopathy: An epidemic at home and around the world. Indian J Ophthalmol 2016;64:69. [PMID: 26953027]

Saenz-de-Viteri M et al: Optical coherence tomography assessment before and after vitamin supplementation in a patient with vitamin A deficiency: A case report and literature review. Medicine (Baltimore) 2016;95:e2680. [PMID: 26871796]

Sanchez E et al: Diagnosis, treatment, and prevention of Lyme disease, human granulocytic anaplasmosis, and babesiosis: A review. JAMA 2016;315:1767. [PMID: 27115378]

Schaal S et al: Acute retinal necrosis associated with Epstein-Barr virus: Immunohistopathologic confirmation. JAMA Ophthalmol 2014;132:881. [PMID:24743882]

Sharma N et al: Adjuvant role of amniotic membrane transplantation in acute ocular Stevens-Johnson syndrome: A randomized control trial. Ophthalmology 2016;123:484. [PMID: 26686968]

Steeples LR et al: Staphylococcal endogenous endophthalmitis in association with pyogenic vertebral osteomyelitis. Eye 2016;30:152. [PMID: 26449198]

Subramanian PS et al: Progression of asymptomatic optic disc swelling to non-arteritic anterior ischaemic optic neuropathy. Br J Ophthalmol 2016 Aug 26. [Epub ahead of print] [PMID: 27565987]

Suri D et al: Optic nerve involvement in childhood onset systemic lupus erythematosus: Three cases and a review of the literature. Lupus 2016;25:93. [PMID: 26341243]

Tran KD et al: Epidemiology of herpes zoster ophthalmicus: Recurrence and chronicity. Ophthalmology 2016;123:1469. [PMID: 27067924]

Varma DD et al: A review of central retinal artery occlusion: Clinical presentation and management. Eye 2013;27:688. [PMID: 23470793]

Verstraeten A et al: Marfan syndrome and related disorders: 25 years of gene discovery. Hum Mutat 2016;37:524. [PMID: 26919284]

Vodopivec I et al: Management of transient monocular vision loss and retinal artery occlusions. Semin Ophthalmol 2017;32:125. [PMID: 27780399]

Vrcek I et al: Herpes zoster ophthalmicus: A review for the internist. Am J Med 2017;130:21. [PMID: 27644149]

Webster GF et al: Ocular rosacea, psoriasis, and lichen planus. Clin Dermatol 2016;34:146. [PMID: 26903182]

Weinberg DV et al: Amaurosis fugax captured during fluorescein angiography. Retina 2015;35:2669. [PMID: 26049618]

Wong RW et al: Emerging concepts in the management of acute retinal necrosis. Br J Ophthalmol 2013;97:545. [PMID: 23235944]

Woolston SL et al: Ocular syphilis: A clinical review. Curr Infect Dis Rep 2016;18:36. [PMID: 27686678]

Zanaty M et al: Endovascular treatment of carotid-cavernous fistulas. Neurosurg Clin N Am 2014;25:551. [PMID: 24994090]

Zeidan MJ et al: Behçet's disease physiopathology: A contemporary review. Auto Immun Highlights 2016;7:4. [PMID: 26868128]

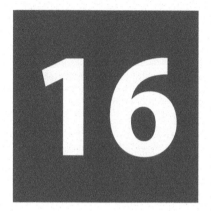

Immunologic Diseases of the Eye

Munir M. Iqbal, MD, and
William G. Hodge, MD, MPH, PhD, FRCSC

Ocular manifestations are a common feature of immunologic diseases even though, paradoxically, the eye is also a site of immune privilege. The propensity for immunologic disease to affect the eye derives from a number of factors, including the highly vascular nature of the uvea, the tendency for immune complexes to be deposited in various ocular tissues, and the exposure of the mucous membrane of the conjunctiva to environmental allergens.

Immunologic diseases of the eye can be grossly divided into two major categories: antibody-mediated and cell-mediated diseases. As is the case in other organs, there is ample opportunity for the interaction of these two systems in the eye.

ANTIBODY-DEPENDENT & ANTIBODY-MEDIATED DISEASES

Before it can be concluded that a disease of the eye is antibody-dependent, the following criteria must be satisfied:

1. There must be evidence of specific antibody in the patient's serum or plasma cells.
2. The antigen must be identified and, if feasible, characterized.
3. The same antigen must be shown to produce an immunologic response in the eye of an experimental animal, and the pathologic changes produced in the experimental animal must be similar to those observed in the human disease.
4. It must be possible to produce similar lesions in animals passively sensitized with serum from an affected animal upon challenge with the specific antigen.

Unless all of the above criteria are satisfied, the disease may be thought of as *possibly* antibody-dependent.

In such circumstances, the disease can be regarded as antibody-mediated if only one of the following criteria is met:

1. If antibody to an antigen is present in higher quantities in the ocular fluids than in the serum (after adjustments have been made for the total amounts of immunoglobulins in each fluid).
2. If abnormal accumulations of plasma cells are present in the ocular lesion.
3. If abnormal accumulations of immunoglobulins are present at the site of the disease.
4. If complement is fixed by immunoglobulins at the site of the disease.
5. If an accumulation of eosinophils is present at the site of the disease.
6. If the ocular disease is associated with an inflammatory disease elsewhere in the body for which antibody dependency has been proved or strongly suggested.

ALLERGIC EYE DISEASE (SEE ALSO CHAPTER 5)

Allergic conjunctivitis (AC) is characterized by conjunctival edema, along with one or more of pruritus, conjunctival hyperemia, chemosis, tearing, and a burning sensation, following exposure to an offending allergen. In severe cases, due to a compromise in the tear film, photophobia and blurred vision can be present. AC is classified as seasonal allergic (hay fever) conjunctivitis (SAC) (usually following exposure to pollen) or perennial allergic conjunctivitis (PAC) (usually following exposure to dust mites, mold, animal dander and occupational allergens).

▶ Pathogenesis

AC is one of the few inflammatory eye disorders for which antibody dependence definitely has been established. It is a form of atopic disease with an implied hereditary susceptibility. Immunoglobulin (Ig) E (reaginic antibody) is attached to mast cells lying beneath the conjunctival epithelium. Binding of the offending antigen to corresponding IgE triggers the release of vasoactive substances, principally leukotrienes and histamine, resulting in vasodilation and chemosis.

Diagnosis

Diagnosis is usually clinical, but it can be confirmed by a high proportion of eosinophils in Giemsa-stained scrapings of conjunctival epithelium. Skin test with a causative allergen produces wheal and flare of an immediate (type 1) hypersensitivity response. Serum and tear fluid can be analyzed for specific IgE, total IgE, and cytokines.

Treatment

In addition to prevention of exposure to relevant allergens and other ocular surface irritants and nonpharmacologic management with lubricants and cold compresses, treatment of AC is quite variable and depends on severity and persistence. For mild cases, topical antihistamines or mast cell stabilizers are recommended. In moderate or persistent cases, dual action topical agents consisting of both antihistamines and mast cell stabilizers are indicated. In severe or particularly persistent cases, topical steroids for short duration and dual action agents are indicated, although steroids are seldom used in practice.

Allergen-specific immunotherapy can produce short- and long-term improvement of symptoms and is indicated in severe, persistent cases, as well as in patients who have simultaneous rhinoconjunctivitis. Patients are dosed either sublingually or subcutaneously with gradually increasing doses of suspected allergens, with attenuation of allergen-specific type 2 T-cell response being the probable mechanism of action.

Other forms of treatment are discussed in Chapter 5.

ATOPIC KERATOCONJUNCTIVITIS AND VERNAL KERATOCONJUNCTIVITIS

Atopic keratoconjunctivitis (AKC) and vernal keratoconjunctivitis (VKC) are manifestations of atopy. Both, but especially AKC, ultimately result in structural modifications of the lids and conjunctiva.

AKC typically begins in the late teens or early twenties, often persisting into the fifth decade of life. It is usually perennial but can have seasonal exacerbations. Symptoms include pruritus, tearing, redness, and burning. There may be severe eczema of the lids and periorbital skin, and the bulbar conjunctiva is hyperemic and thickened. Papillary hypertrophy is often present in the palpebral conjunctiva, particularly inferiorly. Meibomian gland dysfunction and staphylococcal blepharitis are common. Inflammatory mediators and thickening of the lids cause corneal damage including punctate erosions, abrasions, ulcerations, and mucous plaques. There is predisposition to herpes simplex virus keratitis, anterior and posterior subcapsular cataracts, and keratoconus.

VKC characteristically affects children and adolescents and is rare thereafter. It usually occurs in hot, dry climates during the warmer months of the year. Symptoms include severe pruritus, tearing, redness, and frequently photophobia. On examination, there are giant ("cobblestone") papillae of the tarsal conjunctiva (see Figure 5-10). The keratinized epithelium of the papillae may cause punctate corneal erosions and a large abrasion (shield ulcer), over which a fibrin and mucus-containing plaque may form and require surgical removal. At the limbus, there may be gelatinous infiltration, which often is associated with white accumulations of eosinophils and desquamated epithelial cells (Horner-Trantas dots). Compared to AKC, the papillae are larger, and corneal neovascularization and conjunctival scarring are less common.

Pathogenesis

As well as IgE-mediated mast cell degranulation with release of vasoactive amines, non–IgE-mediated disease processes are active in both AKC and VKC. In VKC, there is heavy papillary infiltration by mononuclear cells and T-cell, eosinophil, and cytokine activity, with type 2 helper T cells being the primary driver. In AKC, there is T-cell activity, with type 1 helper T cells being the primary driver.

Diagnosis

There are large numbers of eosinophils in conjunctival scrapings, but they are more numerous and more often degranulated in VKC than in AKC. There is a type 1 hypersensitivity reaction to skin testing with food extracts, pollens, and various other antigens, but the significance of these reactions is not established. Usually the specific inciting antigen is not known.

Treatment

Avoidance or control of known and suspected allergens is beneficial. In AKC, antihistamines and mast cell stabilizers are usually inadequate, and patients often require topical steroid therapy. In VKC, antihistamines and mast cell stabilizers can be quite helpful, with refractory cases requiring topical steroid therapy. In refractory cases, immunomodulators such as cyclosporine and tacrolimus may be beneficial.

Other treatments are discussed in Chapter 5.

JOINT DISEASES AFFECTING THE EYE (SEE ALSO CHAPTERS 5, 7, 15, & 17)

Uveitis and scleritis are the principal ocular manifestations associated with joint diseases. Rheumatoid arthritis may be accompanied by scleritis (see Figures 7–29 to 7–31), peripheral ulcerative keratitis (see Figure 6–9), or episcleritis (see Figures 7–27 and 7–28) as well as dry eyes (secondary Sjögren's syndrome).

Juvenile idiopathic arthritis is associated with uveitis (see Figure 7–7). Unilateral or bilateral chronic anterior uveitis that is often clinically silent is associated particularly with the oligoarticular category, which more commonly affects females with positive antinuclear antibodies, and sometimes the rheumatoid factor–negative polyarticular category. Acute, usually unilateral anterior uveitis occurs particularly in the HLA-B27 enthesitis-related category, which is more common in males. **Ankylosing spondylitis** in adults, which also affects males more frequently than females, may be accompanied by acute anterior uveitis, often with fibrin.

Reactive arthritis affects men more frequently than women. It is triggered by gastrointestinal infection usually with *Shigella*, *Salmonella*, or *Campylobacter* or genitourinary infection particularly with *Chlamydia*. The first attack of ocular inflammation usually consists of a self-limited papillary conjunctivitis. Subsequent attacks consist of acute iridocyclitis of one or both eyes, occasionally with hypopyon.

▶ **Pathogenesis**

Disease activity in rheumatoid arthritis correlates with serum autoantibodies against IgG (rheumatoid factor) and against cyclic citrullinated peptides (CCP) that induce inflammation by several pathways, particularly formation of immune complexes, which is responsible for the occlusive vasculitis that is particularly important in the characteristic necrotizing type of scleritis. Secondary Sjögren's syndrome is caused by antibody-mediated destruction of acinar cells and lymphocytic infiltration of the lacrimal and salivary glands, resulting in dry eyes (keratoconjunctivitis sicca) and dry mouth (xerostomia).

Intraocular inflammation in the seronegative arthropathies is strongly associated with human leukocyte antigen B27 (HLA-B27). Other HLA associations with ophthalmic disease are listed in Table 16–1. Such associations may be causative or coincidental.

Table 16–1. Examples of Human Leukocyte Antigens (HLA) Associated with Ophthalmic Diseases

Acute anterior uveitis	B27
Sympathetic ophthalmia	A11, DRB1
Vogt-Koyanagi-Harada disease	DR4, DRB1
Birdshot chorioretinopathy	A29
Behçet's disease	B51
Giant cell arteritis	DRB1
Mucous membrane pemphigoid	DR4, DQB1
Epidermal necrolysis	
Allopurinol	B58
Carbamazepine	B15
Methazolamide	B59
Cold medicine	A02, B44

▶ **Diagnosis**

Detection of rheumatoid factor and targeted HLA testing may be diagnostic. HLA-B27 is strongly associated with axial spondyloarthritis, including ankylosing spondylitis, and sacroiliitis.

OTHER ANTIBODY-MEDIATED EYE DISEASES (SEE ALSO CHAPTERS 5 & 15)

Systemic lupus erythematosus is a chronic autoimmune disease associated with antinuclear and anti-double-stranded DNA antibodies with inflammatory and vascular consequences that affect a wide variety of organs. There are many ocular manifestations, of which secondary Sjögren's syndrome is most common, and retinal (see Figure 15–5), choroidal, and optic nerve disease are most likely to cause reduction of vision and be associated with nonocular especially cerebrovascular disease. Antiphospholipid antibodies may contribute to pathogenesis.

Mucous membrane (ocular cicatricial) pemphigoid is associated with antibodies to a component of conjunctival basement membrane, provably a protein of hemidesmosomes. It is characterized by subepithelial bullae with chronic conjunctivitis resulting in scarring, symblepharon (see Figure 5–17), contraction of the fornices, and tear deficiency. The end result is bilateral conjunctival and corneal keratinization. Disease control requires systemic immunosuppression. Local treatment includes topical lubricants, lacrimal punctual occlusion, eyelid surgery for trichiasis, and end-stage disease keratoprosthesis.

CELL-MEDIATED DISEASES (SEE ALSO CHAPTERS 7 & 15)

This group of diseases is associated with cell-mediated immunity or delayed hypersensitivity and characterized by infiltration of mononuclear cells, principally lymphocytes and macrophages. The antigenic stimulus may be chronic infection such as tuberculosis, leprosy, toxoplasmosis, and herpes zoster. Such infections are often associated with delayed skin test reactivity following the intradermal injection of an extract of the organism. The granulomatous diseases of the eye are less well understood. They are thought to represent cell-mediated, possibly autoimmune processes, but the antigenic stimuli have not been identified.

SARCOIDOSIS

Ocular sarcoidosis is characterized by a panuveitis with occasional inflammatory involvement of the optic nerve, conjunctiva, choroid, and retinal veins (see Figure 15–21).

Pathogenesis & Diagnosis

Sarcoidosis is an inflammatory disease of unknown etiology. The presence of macrophages and giant cells suggests phagocytosis of particulate matter, which may be the result of mycobacterial infection. Definitive diagnosis requires identification of noncaseating granulomas for which there is no other cause and thus require biopsy, usually lymph node, skin, or pulmonary, including bronchoalveolar lavage. Pulmonary disease, typically bilateral hilar lymphadenopathy, raised serum angiotensin-converting enzyme (SACE), negative tuberculin (Mantoux or Heaf) test, and positive gallium scan are diagnostic pointers.

Treatment

See Chapter 15.

SYMPATHETIC OPHTHALMIA & VOGT-KOYANAGI-HARADA DISEASE

These are uncommon autoimmune diseases affecting pigmented structures of the eye and skin.

Clinical Features

Sympathetic ophthalmia causes bilateral granulomatous uveitis weeks to months (usually within 1 year) following accidental or surgical ocular trauma. Patients usually present with floaters and painless reduction of vision. The typical findings in both the exciting (traumatized) eye and the sympathizing eye are bilateral anterior uveitis with mutton fat keratic precipitates, moderate to severe vitritis, and choroiditis that may manifest as yellow-white nodular lesions under the retinal pigment epithelium (Dalen-Fuchs nodules). Sometimes papillitis and glaucoma occur. There may be vitiligo (depigmentation of the skin) and poliosis (whitening of the hair and eyelashes).

Vogt-Koyanagi-Harada (VKH) disease affects many organs besides the eyes. There is a (meningeal) prodromal stage, during which there may be headache, neck stiffness, encephalopathy, focal neurologic signs and cerebrospinal fluid lymphocytosis, and tinnitus, vertigo, and sensorineural hearing loss. Within a few days, there is bilateral granulomatous panuveitis with choroiditis including Dalen-Fuchs nodules, optic disk edema, and sometimes exudative retinal detachment. Subsequently, there may be vitiligo, poliosis, and alopecia (see Figure 15–33).

Pathogenesis

In both diseases, there is a T-cell–mediated granulomatous inflammation. In sympathetic ophthalmia, the stimulus is exposure of intraocular antigens by the ocular trauma. In VKH, one or more antigens related to melanin are the stimulus, and the disease typically occurs in heavily pigmented individuals such as Hispanics and Japanese. Both conditions are associated with certain HLA types (Table 16–1).

Diagnosis

Both conditions are diagnosed primarily on clinical features. On fundus fluorescein angiography, pinpoint leakage at the level of the retinal pigment epithelium is typical. On ultrasonography, particularly in VKH, there is choroidal thickening. Treatment of both conditions is immunosuppression.

OTHER CELL-MEDIATED EYE DISEASES (SEE ALSO CHAPTER 15)

Giant cell arteritis is a large-vessel vasculitis with a predilection for the branches of the carotid arteries, particularly the (superficial) temporal artery, and for the vertebral arteries. It presents in individuals older than 50 years and typically with temporal headache, scalp tenderness, jaw claudication, malaise, weight loss, and polymyalgia rheumatica. Ocular complications include anterior ischemic optic neuropathy and central retinal artery occlusion and, without prompt treatment, a risk of progression to complete blindness. Initial diagnosis is primarily clinical supplemented by raised erythrocyte sedimentation rate and C-reactive protein. Temporal artery biopsy showing chronic inflammation sometimes with giant cells and typically with fragmentation of the internal elastic lamina is conclusive. Varicella-zoster virus or other infection may be a trigger.

Polyarteritis nodosa is a necrotizing arteritis of medium and small arteries. It can affect both the anterior and posterior segments of the eye and cause neurologic disease with ophthalmic manifestations (see Figure 15–28).

Granulomatosis with polyangiitis (Wegener's granulomatosis) is a systemic vasculitis predominantly affecting small to medium vessels. There is necrotizing granulomatous inflammation, usually involving the respiratory tract and commonly affecting the kidneys. Ophthalmic involvement usually consists of peripheral ulcerative keratitis and scleritis, but retinal vasculitis can occur (see Figure 15–29). The presence of cytoplasmic pattern of antineutrophil cytoplasmic antibodies (C-ANCA) is helpful in making the diagnosis.

Behçet's disease has an uncertain place in the classification of immunologic disorders. It is characterized by recurrent iridocyclitis with hypopyon (see Figure 15–31) and occlusive vasculitis of branch retinal veins. Although it has many of the features of a delayed hypersensitivity disease, dramatic alterations of serum complement levels at the very beginning of an attack suggest an immune complex disorder. Furthermore, high levels of circulating immune complexes have recently been detected in patients with this disease. Most patients with ocular symptoms are positive for HLA-B51 and of eastern Mediterranean or Southeast Asian ancestry.

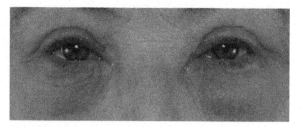

▲ **Figure 16–1.** Periocular contact dermatitis due to delayed hypersensitivity reaction to eye drops.

Contact dermatitis, which may affect the eyelids, represents a significant, although minor, disease caused by delayed hypersensitivity. Topical medications such as brimonidine and atropine, eye drop preservatives, perfumed cosmetics, materials contained in plastic spectacle frames, and other locally applied agents may act as the sensitizing hapten. The lower lid is more extensively involved than the upper lid when the sensitizing agent is applied in drop form (Figure 16–1). There is an erythematous and vesicular rash with pruritus.

Epidermal necrolysis, which encompasses Stevens-Johnson syndrome and toxic epidermal necrolysis, is most commonly incited by drugs such as allopurinol and carbamazepine. It may lead to conjunctival and corneal scarring. Disease manifestations result from keratinocyte apoptosis, which probably is due to immune-mediated cytotoxicity. Certain subtypes are associated with HLA types (Table 16–1).

Phlyctenular keratoconjunctivitis (see Figure 5–14) represents a delayed hypersensitivity response to certain microbial antigens, principally those of *Mycobacterium tuberculosis* and *Staphylococcus aureus* (see also Chapters 5 and 6).

CORNEAL TRANSPLANTATION AND GRAFT REJECTION

Reduction of vision due to central corneal disease may be suitable for a corneal graft that, depending on the extent of disease, may be achieved by penetrating keratoplasty (PKP), in which the full thickness of the cornea is replaced (see Figure 6–13); anterior lamellar keratoplasty, in which part of the anterior portion is replaced; or endothelial keratoplasty, in which only the endothelium is replaced.

Except in the rare instance of exchanging tissue between the two eyes of the same individual (autograft), corneal transplantation is an allograft with the attendant risk of graft rejection. However, due to various factors that limit exposure to the foreign antigens and the immunological response to them, corneal allograft generates a relatively weak immune response. Even though tissue matching for

HLA antigens and systemic immunosuppression are not routinely used, 1-year graft survival for PKP is at least 85%, and in low-risk cases, 5-year survival is over 90%. In contrast, in high-risk cases, such as inflamed or vascularized recipient corneas, 5-year survival is around 55%. The antigens responsible for the vast majority of the immune response are located on the endothelium. Whenever possible, corneal graft surgery is limited to anterior lamellar keratoplasty to minimize the immunogenicity of the graft tissue and the likelihood of rejection.

Both humoral and cellular mechanisms have been implicated in corneal graft rejection. It is likely that early graft rejection (2–4 weeks from surgery) is cell-mediated. Cytotoxic lymphocytes are present at the limbus and in the corneal stroma, and in vivo phase microscopy has shown them attacking donor endothelial cells, but CD8 T-cell knockout mice can mount a vigorous rejection response, with predominance of delayed-type hypersensitivity inflammatory cells, so cytotoxic T cells may not be required. Lymphocytes mediating rejection generally move inward from the periphery of the cornea, forming a "rejection line" that may be seen on the endothelium or the epithelium as they move centrally. The donor cornea becomes edematous as the endothelium becomes increasingly compromised.

Late rejection of a corneal graft may occur weeks to months after surgery and may be antibody-mediated, since cytotoxic antibodies have been isolated from the serum of patients with a history of multiple graft reactions in vascularized corneal beds. These antibody reactions are complement-dependent and attract polymorphonuclear leukocytes, which can form dense rings in the cornea at the sites of maximum deposition of immune complexes.

▶ Treatment

The mainstay of the treatment of corneal graft reactions is intensive topical corticosteroid therapy. Epithelial and stromal damage often is reversible. Due to its lack of regenerative capability, endothelial damage is likely to be irreversible, leading to graft failure such that endothelial rejection requires more aggressive and prolonged treatment. In severe endothelial graft rejections, systemic steroids may be indicated. Systemic and topical cyclosporine or tacrolimus also are effective in preventing and treating graft rejection.

For patients known to be high risk for rejection (eg, corneal neovascularization, prior graft rejection, young age, prior anterior segment surgery, active inflammation, and herpes simplex virus keratitis), especially if the other eye has little or no visual potential, matching for histocompatibility (HLA) and blood group (ABO) antigens and pretreatment with immunosuppressants such as azathioprine, cyclosporine, or mycophenolate mofetil may be undertaken.

RECENT DEVELOPMENTS IN IMMUNOTHERAPY

While in many cases the initiators of ocular inflammatory diseases are still unknown, the components of the inflammatory response are increasingly understood. Of paramount importance in many systemic and ocular inflammatory conditions are T-cell–mediated immune reactions and cytokines.

Immunosuppressants

These include antimetabolites (azathioprine, methotrexate, and mycophenolate mofetil), T-cell inhibitors (cyclosporine and tacrolimus), and alkylating agents (cyclophosphamide and chlorambucil). The treating physician must be familiar with the ocular and systemic side effects of these medications, which are discussed in Chapter 15.

Biologic Response Modifiers

The biologic response modifiers (biologics) most frequently used for ophthalmic disease are the anti–vascular endothelial growth factor (VEGF) agents for choroidal neovascularization, such as in age-related macular degeneration, and for retinal vascular disease, such as diabetic retinopathy. For inflammatory diseases, a wide range of agents have been shown to be beneficial (Table 16–2).

Modes of Delivery

In order to enhance anti-inflammatory effect on the eye and to minimize systemic side effects, alternative modes of delivery of these agents (apart from oral or intravenous) have also been studied. A topical anti–tumor necrosis factor α antibody, ESBA105, is being investigated for its feasibility in treating ocular inflammation. Intraocular methotrexate has shown vision improvement and reduction of macular edema in uveitic patients. Sustained implants of immunosuppressants, as well as intraocular viral and nonviral gene therapies that deliver anticytokine agents, are being investigated in animal studies.

REFERENCES

Abu Samra K et al: Current treatment modalities of JIA-associated uveitis and its complications: Literature review. Ocul Immunol Inflamm 2016;24:431. [PMID: 26765345]

Amouzegar A et al: Alloimmunity and tolerance in corneal transplantation. J Immunol 2016;196:3983. [PMID: 27183635]

Artifoni M et al: Ocular inflammatory diseases associated with rheumatoid arthritis. Nat Rev Rheumatol 2014;10:108. [PMID: 24323074]

Aziz HA et al: Sympathetic ophthalmia: Clinicopathologic correlation in a consecutive case series. Retina 2015;35:1696. [PMID: 25719985]

Broussard KC et al: Autoimmune bullous diseases with skin and eye involvement: Cicatricial pemphigoid, pemphigus vulgaris, and pemphigus paraneoplastica. Clin Dermatol 2016;34:205. [PMID: 26903186]

Cantini F et al: Uveitis in spondyloarthritis: An overview. J Rheumatol Suppl 2015;93:27. [PMID: 26523051]

Catt CJ et al: Ocular manifestations of Stevens-Johnson syndrome and toxic epidermal necrolysis in children. Am J Ophthalmol 2016;166:68. [PMID: 27018234]

Chang VS et al: Chronic ocular complications of Stevens-Johnson syndrome and toxic epidermal necrolysis: The role of systemic immunomodulatory therapy. Semin Ophthalmol 2016;31:178. [PMID: 26959145]

Chen JJ et al: Atopic keratoconjunctivitis: A review. J Am Acad Dermatol 2014;70:569. [PMID: 24342754]

Chu XK et al: Sympathetic ophthalmia: To the twenty-first century and beyond. J Ophthalmic Inflamm Infect 2013;3:49. [PMID: 23724856]

Chuang CT et al: Reversible alopecia in Vogt-Koyanagi-Harada disease and sympathetic ophthalmia. J Ophthalmic Inflamm Infect 2013;3:41. [PMID: 23514340]

Clarke SL et al: Juvenile idiopathic arthritis-associated uveitis. Pediatr Rheumatol Online J 2016;14:27. [PMID: 27121190]

De Smit E et al: Giant cell arteritis: Ophthalmic manifestations of a systemic disease. Graefes Arch Clin Exp Ophthalmol 2016;254:2291. [PMID: 27495301]

Du L et al: Vogt-Koyanagi-Harada disease: Novel insights into pathophysiology, diagnosis and treatment. Prog Retin Eye Res 2016;52:84. [PMID: 26875727]

Ebrahimiadib N et al: Successful treatment strategies in granulomatosis with polyangiitis-associated peripheral ulcerative keratitis. Cornea 2016;35:1459. [PMID: 27362884]

Table 16–2. Examples of Biologic Response Modifiers (Biologics) for Ocular Disease

Anti-VEGF agents	Aflibercept, bevacizumab, pegaptanib, ranibizumab
Anti–tumor necrosis factor (TNF) α agents	Adalimumab, certolizumab, etanercept, golimumab, infliximab
Lymphocyte inhibitors	
T-cells	Abatacept, daclizumab
B cells	Rituximab
Receptor antagonists	
Interleukin-1	Anakinra, gevokizumab
Interleukin-6	Sarilumab, tocilizumab
Interleukin-17	Secukinumab
CD52	Alemtuzumab
CD11a	Efalizumab
Interferons	Alpha-interferon, beta-interferon

El-Shereef RR et al: Ocular manifestation of systemic lupus erythematosus. Rheumatol Int 2013;33:1637. [PMID: 22202921]

Generali E et al: Ocular involvement in systemic autoimmune diseases. Clin Rev Allergy Immunol 2015;49:263. [PMID: 26494481]

Greco A et al: Vogt-Koyanagi-Harada syndrome. Autoimmun Rev 2013;12:1033. [PMID: 23567866]

Hattori T et al: Novel insights into the immunoregulatory function and localization of dendritic cells. Cornea 2016;35:S49. [PMID: 27631349]

Hou S et al: Molecular genetic advances in uveitis. Prog Mol Biol Transl Sci 2015;134:283. [PMID: 26310161]

Kearsley-Fleet L et al: Factors associated with improvement in disease activity following initiation of etanercept in children and young people with juvenile idiopathic arthritis: Results from the British Society for Paediatric and Adolescent Rheumatology Etanercept Cohort Study. Rheumatology (Oxford) 2016;55:840. [PMID: 26721878]

Kharel Sitaula R et al: Role of lupus retinopathy in systemic lupus erythematosus. J Ophthalmic Inflamm Infect 2016;6:15. [PMID: 27174124]

Kolomeyer AM et al: Chronic non-infectious uveitis in patients with juvenile idiopathic arthritis. Ocul Immunol Inflamm 2016;24:377. [PMID: 26902465]

Kubaisi B et al: Granulomatosis with polyangiitis (Wegener's disease): An updated review of ocular disease manifestations. Intractable Rare Dis Res 2016;5:61. [PMID: 27195187]

Lavezzo MM et al: Vogt-Koyanagi-Harada disease: Review of a rare autoimmune disease targeting antigens of melanocytes. Orphanet J Rare Dis 2016;11:29. [PMID: 27008848]

Levitt AE et al: Ocular inflammation in the setting of concomitant systemic autoimmune conditions in an older male population. Cornea 2015;34:762. [PMID: 26053887]

Margo CE et al: Autoimmune disease: Conceptual history and contributions of ocular immunology. Surv Ophthalmol 2016;61:680. [PMID: 27131478]

Minos E et al: Birdshot chorioretinopathy: Current knowledge and new concepts in pathophysiology, diagnosis, monitoring and treatment. Orphanet J Rare Dis 2016;11:61. [PMID: 27175923]

Mitulescu TC et al: Acute anterior uveitis and other extra-articular manifestations of spondyloarthritis. J Med Life 2015;8:319. [PMID: 26351533]

O'Keefe GA et al: Vogt-Koyanagi-Harada disease. Surv Ophthalmol 2017;62:1. [PMID: 27241814]

Oray M et al: Ocular morbidities of juvenile idiopathic arthritis-associated uveitis in adulthood: Results from a tertiary center study. Graefes Arch Clin Exp Ophthalmol 2016;254:1841. [PMID: 27084082]

Papagiannuli E et al: Systemic lupus erythematosus: An update for ophthalmologists. Surv Ophthalmol 2016;61:65. [PMID: 26197421]

Pasadhika S et al: Update on the use of systemic biologic agents in the treatment of noninfectious uveitis. Biologics 2014;8:67. [PMID: 24600203]

Payal AR et al: Long-term drug-free remission and visual outcomes in sympathetic ophthalmia. Ocul Immunol Inflamm 2016 Jan 25. [Epub ahead of print] [PMID: 26808121]

Preble JM et al: Ocular involvement in systemic lupus erythematosus. Curr Opin Ophthalmol 2015;26:540. [PMID: 26367085]

Qazi Y et al: Corneal allograft rejection: Immunopathogenesis to therapeutics. J Clin Cell Immunol 2013;S9:6. [PMID: 26367085]

Queisi MM et al: Update on ocular cicatricial pemphigoid and emerging treatments. Surv Ophthalmol 2016;61:314. [PMID: 26708362]

Sakata VM et al: Diagnosis and classification of Vogt-Koyanagi-Harada disease. Autoimmun Rev 2014;13:550. [PMID: 24440284]

Sánchez-Hernández MC et al: Consensus document on allergic conjunctivitis (DECA). J Invest Allergol Clin Immunol 2015;25(2):94. [PMID: 25997302]

Shaker M et al: An update on ocular allergy. Curr Opin Allergy Clin Immunol 2016;16:505. [PMID: 27490123]

Silpa-archa S et al: Ocular manifestations in systemic lupus erythematosus. Br J Ophthalmol 2016;100:135. [PMID: 25904124]

Smolen JS et al: Rheumatoid arthritis. Lancet 2016;388:2023. [PMID: 27156434]

Stroh IG et al: Occurrence of and risk factors for ocular hypertension and secondary glaucoma in juvenile idiopathic arthritis-associated uveitis. Ocul Immunol Inflamm 2016 Mar 22. [Epub ahead of print] [PMID: 27003850]

Taraborelli M et al: The contribution of antiphospholipid antibodies to organ damage in systemic lupus erythematosus. Lupus 2016;25:1365. [PMID: 26945023]

Tong L et al: The eye: A window of opportunity in rheumatoid arthritis? Nat Rev Rheumatol 2014;10:552. [PMID: 24914693]

Ueta M. Genetic predisposition to Stevens-Johnson syndrome with severe ocular surface complications. Cornea 2015;34:S158. [PMID: 26448174]

Vichyanond P et al: Vernal keratoconjunctivitis: A severe allergic eye disease with remodeling changes. Pediatr Allergy Immunol 2014;25:314. [PMID: 24438133]

Watanabe R et al: Ulcerative keratitis in patients with rheumatoid arthritis in the modern biologic era: a series of eight cases and literature review. Int J Rheum Dis 2015 Jul 14. [Epub ahead of print] [PMID: 26179634]

Yu T et al: High-risk corneal allografts: A therapeutic challenge. World J Transplant 2016;6:10. [PMID: 27011902]

Yücel OE et al: Efficacy and safety of topical cyclosporine A 0.05% in vernal keratoconjunctivitis. Singapore Med J 2016;57:507. [PMID: 26768065]

Special Subjects of Pediatric Interest

17

Paul Riordan-Eva, FRCOphth

Pediatric ophthalmology offers particular challenges to the ophthalmologist, pediatrician, and family physician. Symptoms are often nonspecific, and the usual examination techniques require modification. Development of the visual system is still occurring during the first decade of life, with the potential for amblyopia even in response to relatively mild ocular disease. Because the development of the eye often reflects organ and tissue development of the body as a whole, many congenital somatic defects are mirrored in the eye. Collaboration with pediatricians, neurologists, and other health workers is essential in managing these conditions. Similar collaboration is required in assessing the educational needs of any child with poor vision.

Details of the embryology and the normal postnatal growth and development of the eye are discussed in Chapter 1.

EXAMINATION OF NEONATES

Every newborn's physical examination should include assessment for normal symmetrical external ocular anatomy and normal red reflex in each eye (Table 17–1). If any abnormality is identified, full ophthalmological assessment is required, for which the necessary instruments are hand light, loupe, direct and indirect ophthalmoscopes, and occasionally a portable slitlamp. Any congenital abnormality may be associated with nonocular abnormalities requiring further investigations.

Vision

Assessment of vision of the neonate is limited to observing the following response to a visual target, the most effective being a human face. Visual fixation and following movements can be demonstrated in most neonates; however, during the first 2 months of life, some do not demonstrate consistent fixation behavior and following (smooth pursuit) eye movements may be coarse and jerky.

External Inspection

The eyelids are inspected for growths, deformities, lid notches, and symmetric movement with opening and closing of the eyes. The absolute and relative size of the eyeballs is noted, as well as their position and alignment. The size and luster of the corneas are noted, and the anterior chambers are examined for clarity and iris configuration. The size, position, and light reaction of the pupils are also noted. The pupils are normally relatively dilated until 29 weeks of gestation, at which time the pupillary light response first becomes apparent. The light response is not a reliable test until 32 weeks of gestation. Anisocoria of 0.5 mm can be seen in as many as 20% of neonates. It is important to carefully examine the pupils of any infant with ptosis, looking for anisocoria, as Horner's syndrome, while usually benign, can be due to neuroblastoma.

Ophthalmoscopic Examination

The red reflex is examined with a direct ophthalmoscope. Any abnormality requires direct and/or indirect ophthalmoscopy through dilated pupils. (Phenylephrine 2.5% and cyclopentolate 1% or tropicamide 1% are generally safe in full-term neonates. They may have adverse effects on blood pressure and gastrointestinal function in premature neonates and those with lightly pigmented eyes, for whom combined cyclopentolate 0.2% and phenylephrine 1% [Cyclomydril] should be used.)

Physiologic cupping of the disk is usually not seen in premature infants and is rarely seen at term. In neonates, the optic disk may appear gray, resembling optic nerve atrophy, but if so, there is gradual change to the normal adult pink color by about 2 years of age. Fundal hemorrhages are present in up to 50% of newborns, usually clearing completely within a few weeks and leaving no permanent visual dysfunction. In addition to fundal abnormalities, ophthalmoscopy reveals corneal, lens, and vitreous opacities.

Table 17–1. Pediatric Eye Examination Schedule

Neonatal Examination

External ocular anatomy and red reflex.

In infants requiring examination for retinopathy of prematurity (ROP) or with abnormal red reflex, dilate the pupils with phenylephrine 2.5% and cyclopentolate 1% or tropicamide 1% instilled 1 hour prior to examination. (Cyclopentolate 0.2% and phenylephrine 1% combination [Cyclomydril] is used in babies with lightly pigmented eyes and premature neonates.) Special attention should be paid to the optic disks and maculas; detailed examination of the peripheral retinas is not necessary unless the baby is at risk for ROP.

Age 6 months

Ocular fixation, alignment (looking for strabismus), and movements.

Age 4 years

Visual acuity with Snellen letters, HOTV matching optotypes, or Lea symbols. Visual acuity should be normal (20/20–20/30).

Age 5–16 years

Visual acuity at age 5. If normal, test visual acuity with the Snellen chart every 2 years until age 16. Color vision should be tested at ages 8–12. No other routine eye examination (eg, ophthalmoscopy) is necessary if visual acuity is normal and the eyes appear normal upon inspection.

EXAMINATION OF INFANTS & YOUNG CHILDREN

▶ Vision

Vision should be assessed at each "well child" examination. It is best not to wait until the child is old enough to respond to visual charts, as these may not furnish accurate information until school age. During the first 3–4 years, estimations of vision generally rely on observation and reports about the child's behavior both at play and during interactions with parents and other children. However, seemingly normal visual performance is possible with relatively poor vision. Obviously abnormal performance probably reflects extremely poor vision. The influence of visual impairment on motor and social development must always be borne in mind.

The pupillary responses to light are only a gross test of visual function and are reliable only for ruling out complete dysfunction of the anterior visual or efferent pupillary pathways. The ability to fixate and follow a target is much more informative. The target must be appropriate to the age of the child. Binocular following and convergence are best examined first to establish the child's cooperation. Each eye should then be tested separately, preferably with occlusion of the fellow eye by an adhesive patch. Comparison of the

performance of the two eyes will give useful information about their relative acuities. Resistance to occlusion of one eye suggests that it is the preferred eye and the fellow eye has comparatively poor vision. In nystagmus with a latent component (increased intensity with occlusion of one eye), occlusion of either eye is likely to be resisted because of its adverse effect on visual acuity. Manifest nystagmus may be indicative of an anterior visual pathway disorder or other central nervous system disease (see Chapter 14). After 3 months of age, strabismus, detected by examining the relative position of the corneal light reflections, may be indicative of poor vision in the deviated eye, particularly if this eye does not or is slow to take up fixation of a light upon occlusion of the fellow eye (see Chapter 12).

The developing sensory system can be assessed by the quantitative techniques of optokinetic nystagmus, forced-choice preferential looking methods, and visually evoked responses (see Chapter 2). Although visually evoked potentials have suggested that normal adult visual acuity is attained before 2 years of age, this is probably an overestimate and it is likely that 3–4 years of age is a more accurate estimate (Table 17–2). Forced-choice preferential looking methods provide reliable and relatively easy assessment of visual acuity in preverbal children, even in the very young. However, they tend to overestimate visual acuity in amblyopia.

From about age 4, it is possible to elicit subjective responses with the illiterate "E" chart, child recognition figures, Lea figures, or HOTV cards. Usually, at the first- or second-grade level, the regular Snellen chart may be employed. Stereoacuity can be shown to develop in most infants beginning at 3 months of age, but clinical testing is not generally possible until 3–4 years of age. Absence of stereopsis, as judged with the Random Dot "E" test or the Titmus stereo test, is suggestive of strabismus or amblyopia and should prompt further investigation.

▶ Refraction

Objective refraction is a crucial part of pediatric ophthalmic examination, especially if there is any suggestion of poor vision or strabismus. In young children, this should be performed with cycloplegia to prevent accommodation. In most circumstances, cyclopentolate 1% drops applied twice—separated by an interval of 5 minutes—30 minutes

Table 17–2. Development of Visual Acuity (Approximate)

Age	Visual Acuity
2 months	20/400
6 months	20/100
1 year	20/50
3 years	20/20

prior to examination is sufficient, but atropine may be required if convergent strabismus is present or the eyes are heavily pigmented. Atropine drops can be associated with systemic side effects, so atropine 1% ophthalmic ointment applied once daily for 2 or 3 days prior to examination is recommended. The parents should be warned of the symptoms of atropine toxicity—fever, flushed face, and rapid pulse—and the necessity for discontinuing treatment, cooling the child with sponge bathing, and, in severe cases, seeking urgent medical assistance. Cycloplegic refraction provides the additional advantage of good mydriasis for examination of the fundus.

About 80% of children between the ages of 2 and 6 years are hyperopic, 5% are myopic, and 15% are emmetropic. Since hyperopia can be overcome by accommodation and tends during childhood to decrease with time, only about 10% of children require correction of refractive error before age 7 or 8. Myopia often develops between ages 6 and 9 and increases throughout adolescence, with the greatest change at the time of puberty. Astigmatism is relatively common in babies but decreases in prevalence during the first few years of life. Thereafter, it remains relatively constant in prevalence and degree throughout life. Asymmetric refractive error can lead to (anisometropic) amblyopia, which is detected only by assessing visual acuity.

Anterior & Posterior Segment Examination

Further examination needs to be tailored to each child's age and ability to cooperate. It is generally easier in neonates and babies than in young children because they can be restrained easily by being wrapped in a blanket, and examination is often easily accomplished by allowing the infant to feed or nurse during the examination. Anterior segment examination in the young child may rely on the use of hand light and loupe, but slitlamp examination is often possible in babies with the cooperation of the mother and in young children with appropriate encouragement. Measurement of intraocular pressure and gonioscopy frequently necessitate examination under anesthesia. Fundus examination relies on good mydriasis.

In infants, there is no foveal light reflection. The macula has a bright "mother-of-pearl" appearance with a suggestion of elevation, which is more pronounced in heavily pigmented infants. At 3–4 months of age, the macula becomes slightly concave and the foveal light reflection appears. The peripheral fundus in the infant is gray, in contrast to the orange-red fundus of the adult. In white infants, the pigmentation is more pronounced near the posterior pole and gradually fades at the periphery to almost white, which should not be confused with retinoblastoma. In more heavily pigmented infants, a gray-blue sheen is seen throughout the periphery. During the next several months, pigment continues to be deposited in the retina, and usually at about 2 years of age, the adult color is evident.

CONGENITAL OCULAR ABNORMALITIES

Congenital defects of the ocular structures fall into two main categories: (1) developmental anomalies, of which genetic defects are an important cause; and (2) tissue reactions to intrauterine insults (infections, drugs, etc).

Congenital Abnormalities of the Globe

Failure of formation of the optic vesicle results in **anophthalmos**. Failure of invagination leads to a **congenital cystic eye.** Failure of optic vesicle/fissure closure produces **colobomas of the iris, retina, and/or choroid. Cryptophthalmos** occurs when the eyelids fail to separate.

Abnormally small eyes can be divided into **nanophthalmos**, in which function is normal, and **microphthalmos**, in which function is abnormal and there may be other ocular abnormalities such as cataract, coloboma, or congenital cyst.

Lid Abnormalities

Congenital ptosis is commonly due to dystrophy of the levator muscle of the upper lid (see Chapter 4). Other causes are congenital Horner's syndrome and congenital third nerve palsy. Severe ptosis can lead to unilateral astigmatism or visual deprivation, and thus cause amblyopia.

Palpebral coloboma is a cleft of either the upper or lower eyelid due to incomplete fusion of fetal maxillary processes. Large defects require early repair to avoid corneal ulceration due to exposure. Congenital eyelid colobomas are commonly seen in association with craniofacial disorders such as Goldenhar's syndrome.

Corneal Abnormalities

Partial or complete opacification of the cornea at birth or during childhood may be due to congenital glaucoma, in which case the eye is often larger than normal (buphthalmos); forceps injury at birth, which may cause extensive corneal opacities with edema as a result of rupture of Descemet's membrane that usually clear spontaneously but frequently induce anisometropic amblyopia; faulty development of the corneal endothelium; developmental anterior segment abnormalities with persistent corneal-lens attachments; intrauterine inflammation; interstitial keratitis; and mucopolysaccharide depositions of the cornea as in Hurler's syndrome. Megalocornea is an enlarged cornea with normal clarity and function, usually transmitted as an X-linked recessive trait and an isolated anomaly.

Iris & Pupillary Defects

Displacement of the pupil (**corectopia**) is usually upward and outward. It may be associated with ectopic lens, when it is usually bilateral, congenital glaucoma, or microcornea. **Polycoria** means multiple pupils. **Coloboma of the iris** indicates incomplete closure of the fetal ocular cleft and usually occurs inferiorly and nasally. It may be associated with coloboma of the lens, choroid, and optic nerve, and involvement of these structures can be associated with profound reduction of vision. **Aniridia** (absence of the iris) is a rare abnormality, frequently associated with secondary glaucoma (see Chapter 11) and usually due to an autosomal dominant hereditary pattern. There is a significant association with Wilms' tumor for which the risk can be determined by genetic testing, thus identifying the children who need to undergo screening by renal ultrasound every 3 months until age 8.

The color of the iris is determined largely by heredity. Abnormalities in color include **albinism**, due to the absence of normal pigmentation of the ocular structures and frequently associated with poor visual acuity and nystagmus; and **heterochromia**, which is a difference in color in the two eyes that may be a primary developmental defect with no functional loss, due to congenital Horner's syndrome or secondary to an inflammatory process.

Lens Abnormalities

The lens abnormalities most frequently noted are cataracts (see Chapter 8). Others are faulty development, such as coloboma or subluxation, which occurs in Marfan's syndrome.

Any lens opacity that is present at birth is a congenital cataract, regardless of whether or not it interferes with visual acuity. Congenital cataracts are often associated with other conditions. Maternal rubella during the first trimester of pregnancy is a common cause in emerging countries. Other congenital cataracts have a hereditary background, with autosomal dominant transmission being the most common in developed countries. The time of onset of congenital cataract is often identifiable by its position. The innermost fetal nucleus of the lens forms early in embryonic life and is surrounded by the embryonic nucleus. During adult life, further growth in the lens is peripheral and subcapsular.

If a congenital cataract is too small to occlude the pupil, adequate visual acuity is attained by viewing around it. If the pupil is occluded, normal sight does not develop and visual deprivation may lead to nystagmus and profound irreversible amblyopia. Good visual results have been reported with both unilateral and bilateral cataracts treated by early surgery with prompt correction of aphakia and amblyopia therapy. Aphakic correction is done by using extended-wear contact lenses with the power changed frequently to maintain optimal correction as the globe grows and the refractive status changes or by implantation of an intraocular lens, but determining the appropriate power is difficult.

A common management problem in congenital cataracts is the associated amblyopia. Whether this can be dealt with adequately is the major determinant in deciding whether early surgery for monocular congenital cataract is justified. In the case of bilateral congenital cataracts, the time interval between operating on the two eyes must be as short as possible if amblyopia in the second eye is to be avoided. If early surgery is to be undertaken for congenital cataracts, it is best done within the first 2 months of life, and thus prompt referral to an ophthalmologist is essential.

Developmental Anomalies of the Anterior Segment

Failure of migration or subsequent development of neural crest cells produces abnormalities involving the anterior chamber angle, iris, cornea, and lens. Mutations of the *PAX6* gene cause many of these developmental anomalies of the eye, such as **Axenfeld-Rieger syndrome** and **Peters' anomaly.** Glaucoma is a major clinical problem that often requires surgical intervention, as good control of intraocular pressure is required before considering corneal transplantation.

Congenital Glaucoma

Congenital glaucoma (see Chapter 11) may occur alone or in association with many other congenital lesions. It is often bilateral. Early diagnosis and treatment are essential to preserve useful vision and prevent permanent blindness. The most striking symptom is extreme photophobia. Early signs are corneal haze or opacity, increased corneal diameter, and increased intraocular pressure. Since in childhood the outer coats of the eyeball are not rigid, the increased intraocular pressure expands the cornea and sclera, producing an eye that is larger than normal (buphthalmos). The major differential diagnoses are forceps injuries at birth, developmental anomalies of the cornea or anterior segment, and mucopolysaccharidoses such as Hurler's syndrome, of which none produce enlargement of the globe.

Vitreous Abnormalities

In premature infants, remnants of the tunica vasculosa lentis are frequently visible, in front of and/or behind the lens. Usually they have regressed by term, but rarely, they remain permanently and appear as a complete or partial "cobweb" in the pupil. At other times, remnants of the primitive hyaloid system fail to absorb completely, leaving either a cone on the optic disk that projects into the vitreous (Bergmeister's papilla) or a gliotic tuft on the posterior lens capsule (Mittendorf's dot). Persistent hyperplastic primary vitreous is an important cause of leukocoria that must be differentiated from retinoblastoma, congenital cataract, and retinopathy of prematurity.

Choroid & Retina

Choroidal colobomas, usually in the lower nasal region and sometimes involving the iris and all or part of the optic nerve, are often associated with syndromes such as CHARGE, Aicardi's, in which another feature are focal chorioretinal lesions (lacunae), and Goldenhar's (hemifacial microsomia). Posterior polar chorioretinal scarring is a feature of toxoplasmosis and other maternally acquired intrauterine infections.

Optic Nerve

Congenital anomalies of the optic nerve are relatively common. They are usually benign, such as minor abnormalities of the retinal vessels at the nerve head and tilted disks due to an oblique entrance of the nerve into the globe, but they may be associated with severe visual loss in the case of optic nerve hypoplasia or the rare central coloboma of the disk (morning glory syndrome) (see Chapter 14).

Optic nerve hypoplasia is a nonprogressive congenital abnormality of one or both optic nerves in which the number of axons in the involved nerve is reduced. Previously regarded as rare, it is now recognized to be a major cause of visual loss in children. The degree of visual impairment varies from normal acuity with a wide variety of visual field defects to no perception of light. Clinical diagnosis is hampered by the difficulties of examining young children and the subtlety of the clinical signs. In more marked cases, the optic disk is obviously small and the circumpapillary halo of the normal-sized scleral canal produces the characteristic "double ring sign." In other cases, the hypoplasia may be only segmental and much more difficult to detect.

Optic nerve hypoplasia is frequently associated with midline deformities, including absence of the septum pellucidum, agenesis of the corpus callosum, dysplasia of the third ventricle, pituitary and hypothalamic dysfunction, and midline facial abnormalities. Jaundice and hypoglycemia in the neonatal period and growth retardation, hypothyroidism, and diabetes insipidus during childhood are important consequences. More severe intracranial abnormalities such as anencephaly and porencephaly also occur. Endocrine and neuroradiographic investigations should be undertaken in all patients with optic nerve hypoplasia.

Visual performance in children with optic nerve hypoplasia occasionally may be improved by occlusion therapy. Conversely, optic nerve hypoplasia is an important cause of poor vision that does not normalize with occlusion therapy in children with or without strabismus. A number of patients with optic nerve hypoplasia are not diagnosed until adult life because of the subtlety of the optic nerve abnormality.

Extraocular Dermoids

Congenital rests of surface ectodermal tissues may lead to formation of dermoids that occur frequently in the extraocular structures. They occur most commonly superolaterally, arising from the frontozygomatic suture.

Congenital Nasolacrimal Duct Obstruction

Canalization of the distal nasolacrimal duct normally occurs before birth or during the first month of life, with as many as 30% of infants having epiphora during this time. Approximately 6% have more prolonged symptoms, of which the majority will also resolve aided by lacrimal sac massage and treatment of episodes of conjunctivitis with topical antibiotics. Nasolacrimal probing is usually curative in the remainder and is best deferred until about 1 year of age. In the event of acute dacryocystitis, earlier probing is often indicated. In a few cases, temporary intubation and/or balloon catheter dilation of the lacrimal system or lacrimal surgery is required. The possibility of more extensive congenital nasolacrimal anomalies should be borne in mind in patients with craniofacial anomalies. Epiphora may also be due to inflammatory anterior segment disease, lid abnormalities, and congenital glaucoma.

Orbital Abnormalities

Crouzon's syndrome is a rare autosomal dominant premature fusion of the skull bones (craniosynostosis) characterized by shallow orbits with proptosis, hypoplasia of the maxilla, enlargement of the nasal bones, abnormal increase in the space between the eyes (ocular hypertelorism), and optic atrophy. The palpebral fissures slant downward (in contrast to the upward slant of Down syndrome). Strabismus due to structural anomalies of the muscles and orbit is often present.

INVESTIGATION OF THE BLIND BABY WITH NORMAL OCULAR & NEUROLOGIC EXAMINATION

An important part of pediatric ophthalmology is the investigation of infants with poor visual performance for which clinical examination reveals no ocular or neurologic cause. This presumes that defects such as optic nerve hypoplasia, albinism, and high refractive errors have been excluded. The important conditions to be considered are Leber's congenital amaurosis, cortical blindness, cone dystrophy, ocular motor apraxia, and delayed visual maturation.

Leber's congenital amaurosis and **cone dystrophy** are congenital retinal dystrophies that cause poor vision in infants who present with large-amplitude nystagmus and poor visual fixation. These infants will frequently demonstrate eye poking, pressing, or rubbing (oculodigital sign). Diagnosis is confirmed by electroretinography. **Cerebral (cortical) visual impairment,** a common cause of vision impairment in premature infants and infants who sustained perinatal hypoxic-ischemic encephalopathy, is the leading cause of infantile blindness in developed countries. Diagnosis is confirmed by neuroimaging and clinical history. In **ocular motor apraxia** (infantile-onset saccade initiation delay), a defect in initiation of horizontal saccades gives the impression of visual unresponsiveness, although the visual pathways are normal. Affected children develop characteristic compensatory head movements to overcome the eye movement disorder. **Delayed visual maturation** is a rare condition in which vision does not develop until after 2 months of age. In some cases, there may be associated ocular and neurologic abnormalities that limit final visual performance, but normal vision is attained in those in which it is an isolated condition.

POSTNATAL PROBLEMS

The most common ocular disorders of children are external infections of the conjunctiva and eyelids (bacterial conjunctivitis, hordeola, blepharitis), amblyopia, strabismus, ocular foreign bodies, allergic reactions of the conjunctiva and eyelids, and refractive errors. Since it is more difficult to elicit an accurate history of causative factors and subjective complaints in children, it is not uncommon to overlook significant ocular disorders (especially in very young children).

▶ Ophthalmia Neonatorum (Conjunctivitis of the Newborn)

Conjunctivitis of the newborn may be chemical, bacterial, chlamydial, or viral. Differentiation is sometimes possible according to the timing of presentation, but appropriate smears and cultures are essential. Antenatal diagnosis and treatment of maternal genital infections should prevent many cases of neonatal conjunctivitis. The presence of active maternal genital herpes at the time of delivery may be an indication for elective cesarean section (see Chapter 20). In all cases of chlamydial, gonococcal, and herpes simplex virus neonatal conjunctivitis, the baby must be tested and treated for other sexually transmitted infections, and the mother and her sexual partners should be assessed and treated.

A. Chlamydial Conjunctivitis

Chlamydia is now the most common identifiable infectious cause of neonatal conjunctivitis in the United States. Typically its onset is between 5 and 14 days after birth. Characteristic inclusion bodies are seen in epithelial cells of a conjunctival smear. Direct immunofluorescent antibody staining of conjunctival scrapings is a highly sensitive and specific diagnostic test, and polymerase chain reaction is now clinically available. Systemic therapy with erythromycin is more effective than topical therapy and aids in the eradication of concurrent nasopharyngeal carriage, which may predispose to the development of pneumonitis.

B. Bacterial Conjunctivitis

Bacterial conjunctivitis, usually due to *Staphylococcus aureus, Haemophilus* species, *Streptococcus pneumoniae, Streptococcus faecalis, Neisseria gonorrhoeae,* or *Pseudomonas* species—the last two being the most serious because of potential corneal damage—typically presents between 2 and 5 days after birth. Provisional identification of the causative organism may be made from conjunctival smears. Gonococcal conjunctivitis necessitates parenteral therapy with ceftriaxone, or cefotaxime if there is hyperbilirubinemia. Other types of neonatal bacterial conjunctivitis require topical instillation of antibacterial agents, such as sodium sulfacetamide, bacitracin, or polymyxin-trimethoprim, as soon as results of smears are known.

C. Viral Conjunctivitis

Herpes simplex virus produces characteristic giant cells and viral inclusions on cytologic examination. Herpetic keratitis occurring in children younger than 6 months necessitates admission to hospital for lumbar puncture with polymerase chain reaction evaluation to determine whether there is central nervous system systemic infection and whether systemic therapy is needed. Herpetic keratoconjunctivitis usually resolves spontaneously but may require antiviral therapy, particularly when associated with disseminated infection that occurs chiefly in atopic individuals.

▶ Uveitis in Childhood

Inflammatory eye disease is relatively uncommon in children, but there are a number of important syndromes. The conditions that are seen in the same form as in adults are acute nongranulomatous anterior uveitis associated with the HLA-B27 spondylarthritides, intermediate uveitis, Fuchs' heterochromic iridocyclitis, and idiopathic anterior uveitis. These are treated in the same way as in adults (see Chapter 7), but with care in the use of systemic steroids because of their effects on growth. Uveitis in association with juvenile idiopathic arthritis is generally asymptomatic in its early stages and, if undetected, may produce severe loss of vision due to glaucoma, cataract, or band keratopathy (see Figure 7–9). Regular ophthalmic screening of children with oligoarticular disease, which generally occurs in girls with positive antinuclear antibodies, is essential. Long-term use of topical steroids and mydriatic/cycloplegic agents is often effective in controlling the uveitis, but some patients will require systemic immunosuppression, possibly with agents other than steroids (see Chapters 7 and 15).

▶ Retinopathy of Prematurity

Retinopathy of prematurity (ROP) (see Chapter 10) has been estimated to result in 550 new cases of infant blindness each year in the United States. The major risk factors for ROP are decreasing gestational age and decreasing birth weight. Although recognition of the causative role of supplemental oxygen and its restriction seems to have reduced the incidence of ROP, other factors contribute to the onset and severity of the disease. They include acidosis, apnea, patent ductus arteriosus, septicemia, blood transfusions, and intraventricular hemorrhage. Improved neonatal care has reduced the percentage of babies affected but has also greatly increased the total number at risk.

A. Pathogenesis and Progression

Retinal vascularization proceeds centrifugally from the optic nerve, beginning at the fourth month of gestation. Retinal vessels normally reach the nasal ora serrata at 8 months and the temporal ora serrata at 9 months. ROP develops if this process is disturbed. It is usually bilateral but often asymmetric. The active phase involves changes at the junction of vascularized and avascular retina, initially as an obvious demarcation line (stage 1; Table 17–3), followed by formation of a distinct ridge (stage 2), then extraretinal fibrovascular proliferation (stage 3). Even among patients with stage 3 disease, there is a high incidence of spontaneous regression. Consideration is also given to the location of the changes with respect to distance from the optic disk (zone I or II), the extent of the disease in clock hours, and the presence of venous dilation and arterial tortuosity in the posterior segment ("plus" disease). The cicatricial phase (stages 4 and 5) is defined by increasingly severe retinal detachment, which results in profound vision impairment even with vitreoretinal surgery.

B. Screening and Treatment

All babies with a birth weight of 1500 g or less or gestational age at birth of 30 weeks or less and some infants with a birth weight between 1500 and 2000 g or gestational age at birth greater than 30 weeks, such as those who receive cardiorespiratory support, should undergo screening by a suitably experienced ophthalmologist. Up to 60% of such babies are affected, if only by the early stages. Onset of serious ROP correlates best with postmenstrual age. If gestational age at birth is 27 weeks or less, screening should begin at 31 postmenstrual weeks, or possibly earlier if gestational age at birth is less than 25 weeks. If gestational age at birth is 28 weeks or more, screening should begin at 4 weeks chronological age. Screening is repeated until the retina is fully vascularized,

the retinal changes have undergone spontaneous resolution, or appropriate treatment has been given. Cyclomydril (cyclopentolate 0.2% and phenylephrine 1%) is convenient to dilate the pupils. Tropicamide 0.5% can be used instead of cyclopentolate. If only higher concentrations (2.5–5%) of phenylephrine are available, the risk of systemic adverse effects must be borne in mind.

Laser ablation of the immature retina delivered by a head-mounted indirect ophthalmoscope diode or argon laser is the recommended treatment and should be undertaken once there is any stage disease close to the optic disk (zone I) with plus disease, stage 3 disease in zone I, or stage 2 or 3 disease with plus disease. Previously cryotherapy was the treatment of choice, but there was a higher incidence of complications. Intravitreal injections of anti–vascular endothelial growth factor (VEGF) agents have been shown to be effective in threshold and prethreshold ROP, with regression of neovascular changes and continued peripheral growth of normal retinal vessels. Any treatment should be carried out with the assistance of an experienced neonatologist and under careful monitoring because of the risks of serious systemic complications, including respiratory and cardiorespiratory arrest. Vitreoretinal surgery may be appropriate for eyes with stage 4 or 5 disease but is only recommended when such disease occurs in the better eye as the visual prognosis continues to be poor.

In a significant number of infants with ROP, there is spontaneous regression. Peripheral retinal changes of regressed ROP include peripheral folds and retinal breaks and changes in the posterior retina include straightening of the temporal vessels, temporal stretching of the macula, and retinal tissue that appears to be dragged over the disk. Other ocular findings of regressed ROP include myopia (which may be asymmetric), strabismus, cataract, and angle-closure glaucoma.

▶ Leukocoria (White Pupil)

Parents will occasionally see, or identify on photographs as absence of the "red-eye" effect, a white spot through the infant's pupil (leukocoria). A rare but important cause is retinoblastoma, a rare malignant tumor of childhood that is fatal if untreated and, in 90% of cases, is diagnosed before the end of the third year (see Chapter 10). Leukocoria is more often due to cataract, retinopathy of prematurity, persistent hyperplastic primary vitreous, or refractive error in the case of absence of the red-eye effect, but any affected child must be seen urgently to ensure that vision and life-threatening conditions are diagnosed and treated promptly.

▶ Strabismus

Strabismus (see Chapter 12) is present in about 2% of children. Its early recognition is often the responsibility of the

Table 17–3. Stages of Retinopathy of Prematurity

Stage	Clinical Findings
1	Demarcation line
2	Intraretinal ridge
3	Ridge with extraretinal fibrovascular proliferation
4	Subtotal retinal detachment
5	Total retinal detachment

pediatrician or the family physician. Occasionally, childhood strabismus has neurologic significance. The idea that a child may outgrow crossed eyes should be discouraged. Any child with evidence of strabismus after 3 months of age must be referred as soon as possible for ophthalmologic assessment. Neglect in the treatment of strabismus may lead to undesirable cosmetic effects, psychic trauma, and amblyopia.

Amblyopia

Amblyopia is decreased visual acuity in the absence of sufficient organic eye disease to explain the level of vision.

Normal development of the visual cortex is determined by postnatal visual experience. Visual deprivation due to any cause, congenital or acquired, during the critical period of development (probably lasting up to age 8 in humans) prevents the establishment of normal vision. Reversal of this effect becomes increasingly difficult with increasing age of the child. Early suspicion and prompt referral for treatment of the underlying condition are important in preventing amblyopia.

The most common causes of amblyopia are strabismus, in which the image from the deviated eye is suppressed to prevent diplopia, and anisometropia, in which an inability to focus the eyes simultaneously causes suppression of the image of one eye. High degrees of hypermetropia or astigmatism may cause bilateral amblyopia. Successful treatment depends on early detection and compliance with treatment, which involves appropriate correction of refractive error and then, if necessary, occlusion therapy (patching) of the sound eye for several hours a day or the use of atropine penalization (pharmacologic blurring of the sound eye) daily for several weeks. No matter what therapy is instituted, visual acuity of both eyes must be monitored.

Since poor visual function in a young child may go unnoticed, routine screening by the age of 4 years is recommended (see Chapter 20).

Child Abuse

Child abuse is an important cause of childhood trauma, and its prompt recognition is essential if affected children are to be appropriately protected, but wrong diagnosis must also be avoided if families are not to be unjustly treated.

In the **shaken baby syndrome**, external signs of head injury are absent, but intraretinal, preretinal, and vitreous hemorrhages are common. They are often accompanied by intracranial hemorrhage and may be indicative of the presence of cerebral injury, even if computed tomography is normal. Retinal hemorrhages in children less than 3 years of age without external evidence of head injury is strongly suggestive of child abuse, as long as other causes such as blood dyscrasia have been excluded.

Blunt trauma to the head and eyes is a more readily recognized form of child abuse. Ocular manifestations include subconjunctival hemorrhage; hyphema; cataract; lens subluxation; glaucoma; retinal, vitreous, intrascleral, and optic nerve hemorrhages; and papilledema.

Victims of child abuse may present initially to ophthalmologists, and the diagnosis must be kept in mind. Ophthalmologists may also provide evidence of injuries to the head and eyes in children presenting with unexplained injuries to other parts of the body. The ophthalmologist should work in close collaboration with the pediatrician to ensure that all other potential causes of hemorrhage have been evaluated and to document all other injuries of the child.

Learning Disabilities & Dyslexia

Ophthalmologists are often asked to evaluate children with suspected learning disabilities in order to rule out ocular disorders. Dyslexia is the most common type of learning disability and is characterized by the inability to develop good reading and writing skills. Affected children are usually of normal intelligence and have no associated physical or visual abnormalities. Parents and educators sometimes attribute learning disabilities to visual perceptual abnormalities, but most of these affected children have no visual or ocular impairment. It is believed that dyslexia is caused by a specific defect of information processing in the central nervous system. The diagnosis of learning disabilities should be made by education specialists. Treatment is often effective in ameliorating this condition. When asked to evaluate a child with a learning disorder, the ophthalmologist should perform a complete examination and treat any refractive error, strabismus, or amblyopia as required. It is important to advise the parents that ocular or visual abnormalities generally do not lead to learning disabilities, and special educational programs may be necessary to treat these children. "Vision training," "visual therapy," and "perceptual training" programs have not been evaluated in a scientifically controlled, randomized, or prospective fashion, and thus their efficacy has not been proved.

REFERENCES

Agrawal Y et al: Retinopathy of prematurity screening leading to cardiopulmonary arrest: Fatal complication of a benign procedure. BMJ Case Rep 2016 Jul 28;2016. [PMID: 27469387]

Alajbegovic-Halimic J et al: Risk factors for retinopathy of prematurity in premature born children. Med Arch 2015;69:409. [PMID: 26843736]

American Academy of Pediatrics et al: Joint statement: Learning disabilities, dyslexia, and vision. Pediatrics 2009;124:837. [PMID: 19651597]

Beharry KD et al: Pharmacologic interventions for the prevention and treatment of retinopathy of prematurity. Semin Perinatol 2016;40:189. [PMID: 26831641]

Binenbaum G et al: The natural history of retinal hemorrhage in pediatric head trauma. J AAPOS 2016;20:131. [PMID: 27079593]

Broxterman EC et al: Retinopathy of prematurity: A review of current screening guidelines and treatment options. Mo Med 2016;113:187. [PMID: 27443043]

Callaway NF et al: Retinal and optic nerve hemorrhages in the newborn infant: One-year results of the Newborn Eye Screen Test Study. Ophthalmology 2016;123:1043. [PMID: 26875004]

Casas-Llera P et al: Validation of a school-based amblyopia screening protocol in a kindergarten population. Eur J Ophthalmol 2016;26:505. [PMID: 26776699]

Ceynowa DJ et al: Morning glory disc anomaly in childhood: A population-based study. Acta Ophthalmol 2015;93:626. [PMID: 26173377]

Chen SN et al: Intravitreal anti-vascular endothelial growth factor treatment for retinopathy of prematurity: Comparison between ranibizumab and bevacizumab. Retina 2015;35:667. [PMID: 25462435]

Chua SY et al: Age of onset of myopia predicts risk of high myopia in later childhood in myopic Singapore children. Ophthalmic Physiol Opt 2016;36:388. [PMID: 27350183]

Creavin AL et al: Ophthalmic abnormalities and reading impairment. Pediatrics 2015;135:1057. [PMID: 26009619]

Fierson WM et al: Screening examination of premature infants for retinopathy of prematurity. Pediatrics 2013;131:189. [PMID: 23277315]

Griffith JF et al: The use of a mobile van for school vision screening: Results of 63 841 evaluations. Am J Ophthalmol 2016;163:108. [PMID: 26621684]

Guo DD et al: Stereoacuity and related factors: The Shandong Children Eye Study. PLoS One 2016;11:e0157829. [PMID: 27391873]

Henderson LM et al: Treating reading difficulties with colour. BMJ 2014;349:g5160. [PMID: 25183692]

Hingorani M et al: Aniridia. In: Pagon RA et al, eds. GeneReviews® [Internet]. Seattle, USA: 1993-2016. 2003 May 20 [updated 2013 Nov 14]. [PMID: 20301534]

Isaac M et al: Involution patterns of retinopathy of prematurity after treatment with intravitreal bevacizumab: Implications for follow-up. Eye (Lond) 2016;30:3332. [PMID: 26869159]

Karibe H et al: Acute subdural hematoma in infants with abusive head trauma: A literature review. Neurol Med Chir (Tokyo) 2016;56:264. [PMID: 26960448]

Kelly KR et al: Amblyopic children read more slowly than controls under natural, binocular reading conditions. J AAPOS 2015;19:515. [PMID: 26610788]

Lambert SR et al: Factors associated with stereopsis and a good visual acuity outcome among children in the Infant Aphakia Treatment Study. Eye (Lond) 2016;30:1221. [PMID: 27472216]

Lee HJ et al: A review of the clinical and genetic aspects of aniridia. Semin Ophthalmol 2013;28:306. [PMID: 24138039]

Matejcek A et al: Treatment and prevention of ophthalmia neonatorum. Can Fam Physician 2013;59:1187. [PMID: 24235191]

McGregor ML: Convergence insufficiency and vision therapy. Pediatr Clin North Am 2014;61:621. [PMID: 24852157]

Mehravaran S et al: The UCLA preschool vision program, 2012-2013. J AAPOS 2016;20:63. [PMID: 26917075]

Mian M et al: Shaken baby syndrome: A review. Fetal Pediatr Pathol 2015;34:169. [PMID: 25616019]

Mintz-Hittner HA et al: Efficacy of intravitreal bevacizumab for stage 3+ retinopathy of prematurity. N Engl J Med 2011;364:603. [PMID: 21323540]

Moganeswari D et al: Test re-test reliability and validity of different visual acuity and stereoacuity charts used in preschool children. J Clin Diagn Res 2015;9:NC01. [PMID: 26675120]

Moore DL et al: Preventing ophthalmia neonatorum. Can J Infect Dis Med Microbiol 2015;26:122. [PMID: 26236350]

Moore DL et al: Preventing ophthalmia neonatorum. Paediatr Child Health 2015;20:93. [PMID: 25838784]

Nagamoto T et al: Clinical characteristics of congenital and developmental cataract undergoing surgical treatment. Jpn J Ophthalmol 2015;59:148. [PMID: 25608682]

Nagamoto T et al: Surgical outcomes of congenital and developmental cataracts in Japan. Jpn J Ophthalmol 2016;60:127. [PMID: 26940344]

Naz S et al: Incidence of environmental and genetic factors causing congenital cataract in children of Lahore. J Pak Med Assoc 2016;66:819. [PMID: 27427129]

Nischal KK: Genetics of congenital corneal opacification: Impact on diagnosis and treatment. Cornea 2015;34(Suppl 10):S24. [PMID: 26352876]

Nischal KK: Visual surveillance in craniosynostoses. Am Orthopt J 2014;64:24. [PMID: 25313108]

Nye C: A child's vision. Pediatr Clin North Am 2014;61:495. [PMID: 24852147]

Park MJ et al: Ocular findings in patients with spastic type cerebral palsy. BMC Ophthalmol 2016;16:195. [PMID: 27821110]

Reis LM et al: Conserved genetic pathways associated with microphthalmia, anophthalmia, and coloboma. Birth Defects Res C Embryo Today 2015;105:96. [PMID: 26046913]

Roos L et al: Congenital microphthalmia, anophthalmia and coloboma among live births in Denmark. Ophthalmic Epidemiol 2016;23:324. [PMID: 27552085]

Salman MS: Infantile-onset saccade initiation delay (congenital ocular motor apraxia). Curr Neurol Neurosci Rep 2015;15:24. [PMID: 25783597]

Shah PK et al: Retinopathy of prematurity: Past, present and future. World J Clin Pediatr 2016;5:35. [PMID: 26862500]

Sheeladevi S et al: Global prevalence of childhood cataract: A systematic review. Eye (Lond) 2016;30:1160. [PMID: 27518543]

Traboulsi EI et al: Associated systemic and ocular disorders in patients with congenital unilateral cataracts: The Infant Aphakia Treatment Study experience. Eye (Lond) 2016;30:1170. [PMID: 27315350]

Wahlberg-Ramsay M et al: Evaluation of aspects of binocular vision in children with dyslexia. Strabismus 2012;20:139. [PMID: 23211137]

Yusuf IH et al: Unilateral persistent hyperplastic primary vitreous: Intensive management approach with excellent outcome beyond visual maturation. BMJ Case Rep 2015 Jan 6;2015. [PMID: 25564632]

Ophthalmic Genetics

James J. Augsburger, MD, and Zélia M. Corrêa, MD, PhD

Ophthalmic genetics is concerned with pathogenesis, pattern of transmission, prognosis, and treatment of ophthalmic conditions due to genetic defects. Information on specific conditions, including the availability of genetic testing, is available online (eg, www.ncbi.nlm.nih.gov [National Center for Biotechnology Information] and www.genetest.org).

GENETIC DIAGNOSIS

A great number of ophthalmic conditions are transmitted through families in characteristic hereditary patterns. Others clearly have a genetic (chromosomal) basis but are rarely transmitted through more than one generation. Multigenerational genetic ophthalmic conditions are generally caused by limited deletions, mutations, and/or duplications of small segments of DNA on specific chromosomes, while those affecting only a single individual or a single generation are either due to large chromosomal abnormalities or an autosomal recessive condition.

▶ Principal Patterns of Inheritance

The characteristic features of **autosomal dominant** inheritance are as follows:

1. The genetic abnormality is usually a small mutation in a single gene or small group of adjacent genes on one of the somatic chromosomes. The mutated gene is expressed in almost all individuals who inherit it regardless of the status of the corresponding gene inherited from the unaffected parent.

2. The genetic mutation and its associated condition are present in multiple consecutive generations (unless the condition is fatal before reproductive age).

3. The gene mutation is transmitted on average to half of the children of an affected person.

4. Males and females are affected equally.

Ophthalmic conditions and multisystem disorders with ophthalmic manifestations exhibiting autosomal dominant inheritance and their characteristic ophthalmic features are as follows:

1. Neurofibromatosis type 1: Iris Lisch nodules, multifocal choroidal melanocytic clusters, optic nerve and/or optic chiasm pilocytic astrocytoma (glioma), and periocular plexiform neurofibroma

2. Neurofibromatosis type 2: Combined retinal hamartoma

3. Tuberous sclerosis: Retinal astrocytoma (usually multifocal and bilateral)

4. von Hippel-Lindau disease: Retinal capillary hemangioma (usually multifocal and bilateral)

5. Retinoblastoma (usually multifocal and bilateral)

6. Best's vitelliform macular dystrophy

7. Retinitis pigmentosa (some forms)

8. Gardner's syndrome (familial adenomatous polyposis–carcinoma syndrome): Atypical nonclustered multifocal congenital hypertrophy of retinal pigment epithelium in both eyes

An isolated unilateral unifocal ophthalmic condition that is a feature of an autosomal dominantly inherited condition (eg, retinoblastoma, retinal capillary hemangioma, retinal astrocytoma, and optic nerve or optic chiasm glioma) is not always transmittable, because mutation of the relevant gene can develop in a normal chromosome after conception. If a mutation develops after conception and is present in the gamete (spermatozoa or ova), it can be transmitted to future generations as a novel mutation. Many conditions with an autosomal dominant pattern of inheritance are now known to be due to recessive mutations at the molecular level. The mutation is transmitted from one parent to his or her child but does not manifest unless the same or similar mutation is inherited from the other parent. Thus the clinical disorder develops only when there is a mutation on both chromosomes (recessive trait), but the inheritance pattern is autosomal dominant.

The characteristic features of **autosomal recessive** inheritance are as follows:

1. The genetic abnormality is usually a small mutation in a single gene or small number of adjacent genes on one of the somatic chromosomes and is expressed only when an individual has inherited it from both parents.
2. The condition due to the genetic mutation is usually present in a single generation (unless there is a high level of consanguinity in the mating pool).
3. On average, one in four of the children of parents who both carry the mutated gene manifests the condition and two in four are carriers.
4. Males and females are affected equally.

Ophthalmic conditions exhibiting autosomal recessive inheritance include the following:

1. Retinitis pigmentosa (some forms)
2. Gyrate atrophy
3. Xeroderma pigmentosum

The characteristic features of **X-linked recessive** inheritance are as follows:

1. The genetic abnormality is usually a small mutation in a single gene or small number of adjacent genes on the sex (X) chromosome. This gene is expressed only when it is not balanced by a normal X chromosome inherited from the unaffected parent.
2. The genetic mutation and the associated condition are present in multiple consecutive generations.
3. The mutated X chromosome is transmitted, on average, to half of the children of both affected males and carrier females.
4. Only males are affected by the complete condition, but female carriers may have a limited manifestation.

Ophthalmic conditions exhibiting X-linked recessive inheritance include the following:

1. X-linked retinoschisis
2. Ocular albinism
3. Retinitis pigmentosa (some forms)
4. Norrie's disease
5. Choroideremia (most cases)

The characteristic features of **mitochondrial inheritance** are as follows:

1. The genetic abnormality is a mutation in a single or small group of adjacent genes of mitochondrial DNA, such as the point mutations of the cytoplasmic mitochondria that cause Leber's hereditary optic neuropathy.

2. The genetic abnormality is transmitted from a carrier mother to all her children.
3. Only carrier mothers transmit the condition to their children.
4. Both males and females are affected.

Examples of ophthalmic disorders transmitted by mitochondrial inheritance are as follows:

1. Leber's hereditary optic neuropathy
2. Kearns-Sayre syndrome: Principal ophthalmic features are chronic progressive external ophthalmoplegia and pigmentary retinopathy

Some ophthalmic diseases, including age-related macular degeneration and primary open-angle glaucoma, have a **polygenic and multifactorial pattern** of inheritance, occurring in family members substantially more frequently than expected on the basis of chance alone but without a simple pattern of inheritance. Mutations of multiple different genes have been associated with these conditions, and interactions between them and environmental conditions affect the characteristics of the conditions, such as age at clinical onset, severity at initial detection, rapidity of progression, and ultimate outcome.

▶ Chromosomal Abnormalities

Some ophthalmic conditions are due to a genetic defect but are rarely transmitted through more than one generation. In most of them, there is a major or complete loss or duplication of one or more chromosomes involving numerous genes. Due to absence of half the normal complement of genes associated with a particular chromosome in cases with complete chromosomal deletions and to the presence of 50% more than the normal complement of genes associated with a particular chromosome in cases with complete chromosomal duplications, affected individuals characteristically have multiple morphological abnormalities that frequently prompt chromosomal analysis during infancy or early childhood. Affected individuals frequently are sterile or unsuccessful in reproducing or do not reach reproductive age, thus accounting for the lack of multigenerational transmission. In most cases, the abnormal complement of chromosomes can be identified by karyotyping. The main chromosomal disorders and their common ophthalmic manifestations are as follows:

1. **Trisomy syndromes**
   - Trisomy 13 (Patau's syndrome): Microphthalmia, uveal colobomas, congenital cataract
   - Trisomy 18 (Edward's syndrome): Hypertelorism, hypoplastic supraorbital ridges, eyelid anomalies
   - Trisomy 21 (Down's syndrome): Epicanthal folds, iris hypoplasia, keratoconus
   - XXY trisomy (Klinefelter's syndrome): Epicanthal folds, hypertelorism, upward slant of palpebral fissures

2. **Monosomy syndrome**
   - Monosomy X (Turner's syndrome): Congenital ptosis, strabismus, cataract
3. **Partial chromosomal deletion or duplication syndromes**
   - Chromosome 13q deletion syndrome: Hypertelorism, epicanthal folds, retinoblastoma
   - Chromosome 11p deletion syndrome: Congenital aniridia

PRINCIPAL USES OF GENETIC DIAGNOSIS IN OPHTHALMOLOGY

The principal uses of ophthalmic genetic diagnosis are as follows:

1. Identification of clinically unaffected carriers of a familial disease, for the purposes of familial genetic counseling and risk prognostication
2. Identification of individuals in a family who are predisposed genetically to develop a familial disease but have not yet done so (for the purpose of justifying periodic screening evaluations)

In practice, the clinician first must recognize a familial inheritance pattern in more than one generation or branch of a family or diagnose in one or more members of the same generation of a family an ophthalmic condition that is known to be transmitted genetically in at least some families. In the former situation, a genetic counselor:

1. Investigates the family pedigree, identifies the likely inheritance pattern of the disease, and suggests and arranges for genetic testing of the family.
2. Determines which family members are affected or predisposed to develop the disease and/or determines unaffected carriers who can transmit the disease to their offspring, and advises the family as a whole, affected individuals, and carriers about the genetic findings and their implications.

In diseases for which effective treatment is available if it is detected when limited in extent, genetic differentiation between individuals who are and those who are not predisposed to develop the disease assists targeting of screening programs. For instance, in familial retinoblastoma that is potentially fatal, identification of at-risk individuals justifies frequent ophthalmic examinations under anesthesia to detect newly emerging retinal tumors in infants at risk, and such examinations should be avoided in infants shown not to be at risk. Familial genetic testing allows detection of carrier status of clinically unaffected individuals who have the potential to pass the disease on to their offspring. Such information can be used in family planning or to justify early genetic and clinical evaluation of any future offspring for evidence of the disease or genetic susceptibility to it.

For diagnosis in one or more members of the same generation of a family of an ophthalmic condition known to be transmitted genetically in at least some families and for which genetic testing is currently available (eg, Norrie's disease and Leber's hereditary optic neuropathy), testing of the affected individual(s) and their parents and siblings can be performed to determine the presence of the genetic abnormality. If a relevant genetic abnormality is identified in an affected family member but not in any other family members, it is likely to be due to a new mutation. In contrast, if neither the affected individual nor any first-degree relative has a relevant genetic abnormality, either the clinical diagnosis is incorrect or an unknown genetic abnormality is responsible.

Family pedigrees can be used to support or, in some cases, refute clinical diagnosis of a condition transmitted in at least some families according to a particular genetic pattern. For example, in ophthalmic conditions with maternal inheritance via mitochondrial DNA (eg, Leber's hereditary optic neuropathy, Kearns-Sayre syndrome), affected mothers transmit the disease to their offspring of either sex, but affected fathers do not transmit the disease. Thus, if a child and father are affected, the clinical diagnosis is unlikely to be correct. Similarly, if the inheritance is X-linked recessive (eg, X-linked retinoschisis), the mother of an affected individual is likely to be an unaffected carrier; 50% of sons of a carrier mother manifest the condition; 50% of daughters of a carrier mother are carriers; sons of affected males are unaffected; and daughters of affected males are carriers. Thus, if a son and father are affected, the clinical diagnosis is unlikely to be correct.

GENETIC PROGNOSTICATION

Genetic prognostication refers to the use of genetic information to predict a patient's prognosis.

Retinitis pigmentosa is caused by a variety of mutations with several patterns of inheritance (autosomal dominant, autosomal recessive, or X-linked recessive). Individuals from a particular family, thus having the same genotype, are likely to have the same clinical manifestations (phenotype) (eg, age when visual symptoms are first recognized, severity of visual field loss at initial detection, rate of progression following initial symptoms, and ultimate level of visual loss), whereas individuals from different families will tend to have different clinical manifestations. Such genotype-phenotype correlations have been defined for several genetic subtypes of retinitis pigmentosa. Similarly in von Hippel-Lindau disease, which has an autosomal dominant pattern of inheritance, there are genetic subgroups with substantially different risk of developing renal cell carcinoma.

Many cases of retinoblastoma occur as a familial disease with an autosomal dominant inheritance pattern, but the defect in the retinoblastoma gene in the tumor cells does not seem to influence disease severity or ultimate survival outcome. In contrast, although there is not a strong familial tendency, most primary uveal melanomas that ultimately metastasize have deletion of one chromosome 3 (monosomy 3) or a characteristic gene expression profile (class 2) within the tumor cells. If either abnormality is detected, such as in a biopsy, enucleation, or resection specimen, the patient is at high risk of metastatic disease and should be encouraged to participate in an adjuvant therapy clinical trial to identify interventions that prevent or delay the onset of metastasis (see www.clinicaltrials.gov).

GENE THERAPY

Gene therapy is the attempted elimination or amelioration of disease, due to loss (deletion) or functional inactivation of one or a few adjacent genes, by inserting, incorporating, and activating replacement segments of DNA corresponding to the deleted or nonfunctional gene, so as to achieve normal gene function. In ophthalmology, only a few trials are in progress (eg, retinitis pigmentosa, Leber's hereditary optic neuropathy, and some corneal disease) but with good safety profile of viral vector gene transfer and as-yet limited recovery of function (see www.clinicaltrials.gov).

REFERENCES

Allen KF et al: Genetics of primary inherited disorders of the optic nerve: Clinical applications. Cold Spring Harb Perspect Med 2015;5:a017277. [PMID: 26134840]

Bainbridge JWB et al: Long-term effect of gene therapy on Leber's congenital amaurosis. N Engl J Med 2015;372:1887. [PMID: 25938638]

Benjaminy S et al: Communicating the promise for ocular gene therapies: Challenges and recommendations. Am J Ophthalmol 2015;160:408. [PMID: 26032192]

Branham K et al: Providing comprehensive genetic-based ophthalmic care. Clin Genet 2013;84:183. [PMID: 23662791]

Chan S et al: Advances in the genetics of eye diseases. Curr Opin Pediatr 2013;25:645. [PMID: 24126856]

Comander J et al: Visual function in carriers of X-linked retinitis pigmentosa. Ophthalmology 2015;122:1899. [PMID: 26143542]

Daiger SP et al: Genes and mutations causing retinitis pigmentosa. Clin Genet 2013;84:132. [PMID: 23701314]

Dalkara D et al: Let there be light: Gene and cell therapy for blindness. Hum Gene Ther 2016;27:134. [PMID: 26751519]

Edwards TL et al: Visual acuity after retinal gene therapy for choroideremia. N Engl J Med 2016;374:1996. [PMID: 27120491]

Findeis-Hosey JJ et al: Von Hippel-Lindau disease. J Pediatr Genet 2016;5:116. [PMID: 27617152]

Helgadottir H et al: The genetics of uveal melanoma: Current insights. Appl Clin Genet 2016;9:147. [PMID: 27660484]

Jacobson SG et al: Improvement and decline in vision with gene therapy in childhood blindness. N Engl J Med 2015;372:1920. [PMID: 25936984]

Kaliki S et al: Uveal melanoma: Estimating prognosis. Indian J Ophthalmol 2015;63:93. [PMID: 25827538]

Kersten HM et al: Ophthalmic manifestations of inherited neurodegenerative disorders. Nat Rev Neurol 2014;10:349. [PMID: 24840976]

MacLaren RE et al: Retinal gene therapy in patients with choroideremia: Initial findings from a phase 1/2 clinical trial. Lancet 2014;383:1129. [PMID: 24439297]

Meyerson C et al: Leber hereditary optic neuropathy: Current perspectives. Clin Ophthalmol 2015;9:1165. [PMID: 26170609]

Nash BM et al: Retinal dystrophies, genomic applications in diagnosis and prospects for therapy. Transl Pediatr 2015;4:139. [PMID: 26835369]

Nichols EE et al: Tumor characteristics, genetics, management, and the risk of metastasis in uveal melanoma. Semin Ophthalmol 2016;31:304. [PMID: 27128983]

Riaz M et al: Genetics in retinal diseases. Dev Ophthalmol 2016;55:57. [PMID: 26501365]

Scanga HL et al: Genetics and ocular disorders: A focused review. Pediatr Clin North Am 2014;61:555. [PMID: 24852152]

Soliman SE et al: Knowledge of genetics in familial retinoblastoma. Ophthalmic Genet 2016 Jul 18:1. [Epub ahead of print] [PMID: 27427836]

Sorrentino FS et al: A challenge to the striking genotypic heterogeneity of retinitis pigmentosa: A better understanding of the pathophysiology using the newest genetic strategies. Eye (Lond) 2016;30:1542. [PMID: 27564722]

Wiley LA et al: Stem cells as tools for studying the genetics of inherited retinal degenerations. Cold Spring Harb Perspect Med 2014;5:a017160. [PMID: 25502747]

Zinkernagel MS et al: Recent advances and future prospects in choroideremia. Clin Ophthalmol 2015;9:2195. [PMID: 26648685]

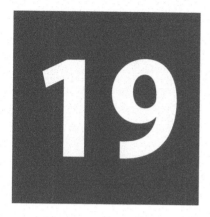

19

Ophthalmic Trauma

Jonathan Pargament, MD, Zélia M. Corrêa, MD, PhD, and James J. Augsburger, MD

The eye and periorbital region are subject to a range of injuries with a wide spectrum of severity and sequelae.

INITIAL EVALUATION

Initial evaluation of ophthalmic trauma, whether by a first responder or an emergency department provider, starts with an assessment of the patient's overall condition to identify and manage any life-threatening problems. Then the circumstances of the injury must be established. The patient's level of consciousness may be altered due to substance abuse, psychiatric disease or brain injury, so family members or bystanders may provide crucial collateral information. Specific questions should include whether a blunt or sharp object inflicted the injury; whether the injury occurred at high or low velocity; whether the patient has any prior history of ocular disease or surgery; and when and what the patient last ate and drank.

The next step is ophthalmic examination, of which the extent will depend on the patient's level of cooperation. The first part does not require significant cooperation and begins with an inspection of the eyes and periorbital tissues for any obvious abnormalities such as lacerations, ecchymosis (Figure 19–1), proptosis, corneal clouding, or gross hyphema. In severe ophthalmic trauma, it is critical to examine the eye as atraumatically as possible to avoid exacerbating the damage. The pupils are examined to determine their absolute and relative sizes and shapes and their responses to direct and consensual illumination. If the patient is conscious and cooperative, visual acuity and confrontation visual fields are tested. Keep in mind that the patient may have broken or lost his or her glasses during the trauma. A pinhole for distance acuity and/or near vision chart and presbyopic reading glasses may be crucial.

If the initial evaluation reveals an injury that warrants further evaluation, ophthalmology consultation is essential. In addition to reviewing the history, the ophthalmologist will perform an external examination, reassess visual acuity and pupillary responses to light, assess ocular position in each orbit, evaluate ocular alignment and motility, if possible perform slitlamp examination of the anterior segment and measure intraocular pressure, and perform indirect ophthalmoscopy of the fundus.

OCULAR INJURIES

Rapid recognition by emergency care providers of chemical and open globe injuries is particularly important because of the need for emergency intervention to minimize their severity.

▶ Chemical Injuries

In adults, ocular chemical injury is usually due to splash or spray of industrial or agricultural chemical, cleaning solution, automotive fluid, or cement or plaster in the work or home environment or assault with alkali or acid. In children, it is frequently caused by a cleaning solution or detergent.

Regardless of the type of chemical or circumstance of the injury, the most important first step is copious eye irrigation as soon as possible. Tap water will suffice until the patient has been transported to the emergency department, where sterile isotonic saline is preferred. Topical anesthetic drops and the use of an eyelid speculum facilitate effective irrigation and removal of particulate matter in the case of cement or plaster. Irrigation should continue until a neutral pH has been achieved or definitive care by an ophthalmologist has been provided.

The next step is to determine the nature of the chemical involved in the injury, which may be indicated by the reaction of a pH strip prior to irrigation. Acid such as from a car battery precipitates necrotic tissue that acts as a barrier to its deeper penetration. Alkali such as in industrial cleaning solutions, household bleach, cement, and plaster causes more severe damage because it does not form such a barrier and penetrates further. Important signs of severe chemical injury are corneal clouding, limbal whitening, and significant conjunctival chemosis. The lack of redness mistakenly may be interpreted to indicate mild injury.

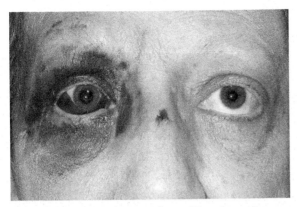

▲ **Figure 19–1.** Prominent right eyelid ecchymosis and subconjunctival hemorrhage due to blunt trauma suffered in a fall.

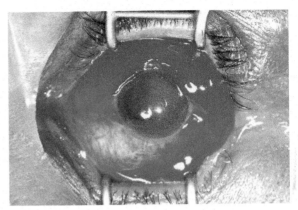

▲ **Figure 19–3.** Massive hemorrhagic chemosis following severe blunt ocular trauma. A globe rupture in the superonasal quadrant was confirmed by surgical exploration.

Further management includes topical antibiotic while there is a corneal epithelial defect; topical cycloplegic to reduce discomfort; topical steroid to reduce inflammation; topical and oral ascorbate (vitamin C) to prevent collagen lysis; topical potassium citrate to chelate calcium to reduce inflammation; oral doxycycline to reduce inflammation and prevent corneal melting; topical lubricants; and oral acetazolamide to treat raised intraocular pressure.

Open Globe Injuries

Open globe injury is an ocular injury that results in a full-thickness defect in the cornea and/or sclera, exposing the intraocular compartments to the external environment. Signs of an open globe injury that can be identified by basic examination include pupillary distortion (usually toward the wound), flat anterior chamber, and extraocular protrusion of uveal tissue (Figure 19–2). Other findings that should arouse

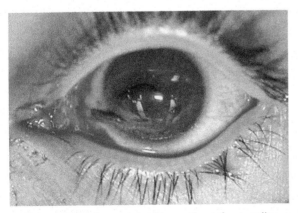

▲ **Figure 19–2.** Corneoscleral laceration inferonasally with pupil displaced toward the laceration and iris incarcerated in wound.

suspicion of an open globe injury are massive hemorrhagic chemosis (Figure 19–3), profoundly soft eye, deep eyelid laceration (Figure 19–4), and intraocular blood (hyphema, vitreous hemorrhage). Open globe injuries are categorized as (1) full-thickness eye wall lacerations and (2) globe ruptures.

A **full-thickness eye wall laceration** is an ocular injury caused by a sharp object or high-velocity projectile that has cut completely through the cornea, sclera, or both. In some cases, the object that caused the cut is not retained at the site but is withdrawn or extruded prior to emergency evaluation (Figures 19–1 and 19–5). In other cases, the object is retained in the wound (Figure 19–6) or inside the eye (Figure 19–7). In still other cases, the object passes completely through the eye, causing both entry and exit wounds (double perforating injury).

In full-thickness eye wall lacerations, the lens capsule may be cut at the time of the injury. When the capsule is disrupted, the lens becomes hydrated, swollen, and opaque. Fragments of the lens may also extrude into the anterior chamber and cause severe inflammation. A lensectomy procedure is required but typically is not performed at the time of the globe repair. It may be delayed for treatment of hyphema and/or inflammation and to more accurately measure and plan for intraocular lens placement.

Intraocular foreign bodies retained in the posterior segment can be very challenging to remove without additional injury to ocular structures. Therefore, they should be left alone during the initial globe repair and a vitreoretinal subspecialist consulted about subsequent removal.

Globe rupture is splitting or tearing of the cornea and/or sclera at a relatively weak point by severe blunt ocular trauma. Relatively common sites are posterior to the extraocular muscles (especially in the superonasal quadrant), along incisions from prior intraocular surgery, and at the

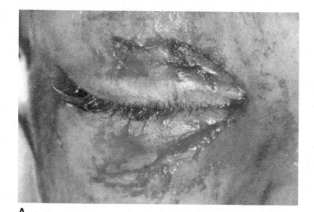

A

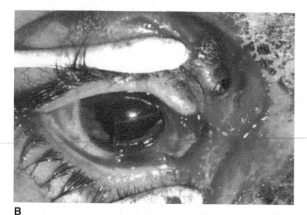

B

▲ **Figure 19–4.** Eyelid laceration with concurrent open globe injury. **A:** Rather innocuous-appearing V-shaped eyelid laceration involving the upper and lower lids and medial canthal skin. **B:** Total dark red hyphema and hemorrhagic chemosis are evident when the lids are separated. Note also that laceration extends through both lacrimal canaliculi.

lamina cribrosa. Globe rupture should be suspected in the setting of any blunt trauma resulting in massive hemorrhagic chemosis or a profoundly soft eye (Figure 19–3).

If an open globe injury is identified or suspected, straightaway a protective shield should be taped over the injured eye and urgent ophthalmology consultation arranged. Analgesic and antiemetic medications should be administered to keep the patient reasonably comfortable and avoid vomiting. Tetanus toxoid vaccine should be administered. In full-thickness eye wall laceration, a computed tomography (CT) scan may be required to identify or rule out a retained intraocular or intraorbital foreign body.

Once an ophthalmologist has confirmed an open globe injury, surgical repair should be undertaken as soon as reasonably possible. General anesthesia should be induced

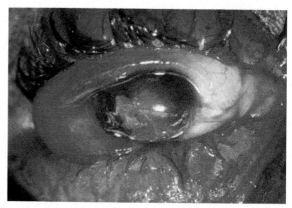

▲ **Figure 19–5.** Pellet gun injury to the right eye resulting in open globe injury. Note massive hemorrhagic chemosis, irregular corneal shape, distorted pupil, and dark brown iris tissue incarcerated into limbal wound.

without the use of depolarizing agents (eg, succinylcholine) as this can lead to increased intraocular pressure and extrusion of intraocular contents. The ophthalmologist explores the wound to determine its full extent and plan the surgical repair. In most cases, corneal lacerations and ruptures are closed using 10-0 nylon sutures with buried knots, and scleral discontinuities are closed using 8-0 or 9-0 nylon sutures. Iris and/or ciliary body tissue incarcerated in the wound may be replaced inside the eye (reposited) if it is not necrotic or grossly contaminated. Precise realignment of the wound edges and release of incarcerated corneal and conjunctival epithelium are important. The sutured wound needs to be watertight. If the conjunctiva was lacerated or incised to facilitate exposure of a scleral wound, it is closed with absorbable 7-0 or 8-0 sutures. Antibiotics

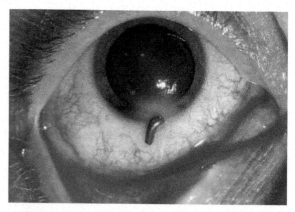

▲ **Figure 19–6.** Ocular laceration with retained foreign body. The tip of a metallic foreign body protrudes from the eye at the limbus inferiorly.

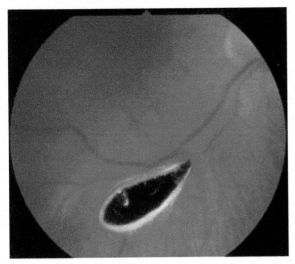

▲ Figure 19–7. Metallic intraocular foreign body lying on the surface of the retina.

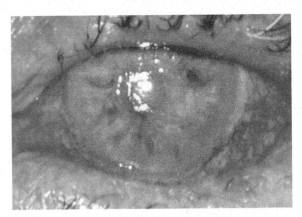

▲ Figure 19–8. Corneal abrasion stained with fluorescein.

and corticosteroids are often injected subconjunctivally at the conclusion of the operation and continued as eye drops postoperatively. The patient should be examined frequently in the postoperative period for wound leaks, infection, recurrent intraocular bleeding, hypotony, and ocular hypertension that may require additional treatment.

Intraocular or Intraorbital Foreign Body

A history of explosion, gunshot wound, or striking of metal upon metal should raise suspicion of an intraocular or intraorbital foreign body. If the optical media are still relatively clear, it may be possible for an ophthalmologist to detect or exclude an intraocular foreign body. Otherwise if an open globe injury is suspected or there is massive orbital swelling, CT scan of the eyes and orbits will detect most foreign bodies and determine their general locations (eg, inside the eyeball, in the wall of the globe, in the orbit). Magnetic resonance imaging (MRI) is contraindicated if a magnetic foreign body is suspected.

Closed Globe Injuries

Corneal abrasion, a scratching or scraping away of some of the corneal epithelium (Figure 19–8), is one of the most common ophthalmic injuries encountered in an emergent care setting. Commonly there is a history of an injury, such as from a finger nail or during manipulation of a contact lens. Typically there is severe foreign body sensation, tearing, light sensitivity, and blurred vision. Administration of a topical anesthetic drop usually improves the patient's symptoms dramatically. Slitlamp examination with fluorescein, which stains the exposed basement membrane, will reveal the extent of the corneal abrasion. Treatment for corneal

abrasion should always include topical broad-spectrum antibacterial agents. Eye patching may decrease pain. The patient should be examined periodically, especially if there are increased symptoms, to ensure that the cornea is healing and there is no associated corneal infection. Under no circumstance should topical anesthetic drops be given to the patient for self-administration as they delay corneal epithelial healing, mask the subjective findings of a worsening course, and if used for a prolonged period, can cause a chronic neurotrophic corneal ulcer.

Corneal or conjunctival foreign body occurs when an object with too little momentum to pass completely through the eye wall becomes embedded in the cornea or conjunctiva. The patient will frequently have a recent history of grinding or striking metal. Symptoms are quite similar to a corneal abrasion including foreign body sensation, light sensitivity, and excessive tearing. Larger corneal foreign bodies may be visible on diffuse light examination. Smaller foreign bodies may be evident only on slitlamp examination (Figure 19–9).

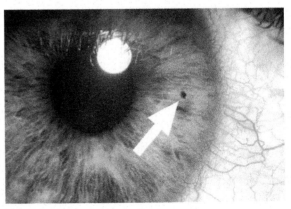

▲ Figure 19–9. Tiny metallic corneal foreign body appearing as dark brown speck on the cornea (**arrow**).

Linear vertical corneal epithelial defects are often indicative of a foreign body embedded in the tarsal conjunctiva of the upper eyelid and should prompt eversion of the eyelid to examine its conjunctival surface and to remove the foreign body with a sterile cotton-tipped applicator stick.

Removal of a corneal foreign body requires proficiency with the slitlamp. Depending on the emergency room provider's training and experience, removal may be attempted. The cornea should first be anesthetized with a topical anesthetic drop. While viewing with the slitlamp, the foreign body is dislodged with a sterile 27-gauge or larger caliber needle. If the foreign body is composed of iron or copper, there may be an associated "rust ring," which can be removed with a battery-operated drill with a burr tip. A broad-spectrum antibacterial should be administered and treatment continued for a corneal abrasion. If there is any question about whether the foreign body has passed completely through the cornea, an ophthalmologist should be consulted immediately.

Subconjunctival hemorrhage results from cutting or tearing of one or more conjunctival or anterior orbital blood vessels leading to accumulation of blood in the substantia propria of the conjunctiva. If greater than 270 degrees or associated with prominent chemosis, it is suspicious of open globe injury (Figure 19–3) and warrants urgent surgical exploration.

Trauma may cause **superficial ocular laceration** of the conjunctiva with or without partial thickness laceration of the sclera and/or cornea. Slitlamp biomicroscopy must be used to ascertain the depth of the laceration and assure that it does not extend completely through the eye wall. Most partial-thickness lacerations can be managed as if they were corneal abrasions with an antibacterial and patching. Extensive superficial laceration may warrant suturing by an ophthalmologist.

Ocular trauma can cause posttraumatic inflammatory reaction involving the iris (**traumatic iritis**) or the iris and ciliary body (**traumatic iridocyclitis**). Typically, symptom onset is 24–48 hours after the injury with increasing eye pain, photophobia, and blurred vision. On slitlamp examination, there are inflammatory cells and flare in the anterior chamber, finely dispersed keratic precipitates on the cornea, and Vossius ring of dark brown pigment on the anterior lens capsule. Adhesions between the pupillary margin of the iris and the anterior lens capsule (posterior synechiae) and adhesions between the peripheral iris and cornea (peripheral anterior synechiae) may occur. Treatment consists of topical cycloplegic drops (eg, atropine 1%) and frequent corticosteroid drops (eg, prednisolone acetate), which should be prescribed by an ophthalmologist, until the intraocular inflammation subsides. Ophthalmological follow-up is required.

Many ocular injuries damage blood vessels of the iris causing hemorrhage into the anterior chamber (**traumatic hyphema**). If the amount of intraocular bleeding is not too severe, the blood becomes layered out gravitationally (Figure 19–10). Symptoms are similar to those of a traumatic

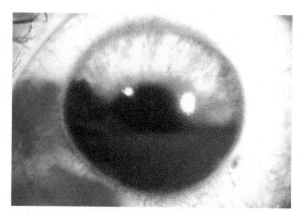

▲ **Figure 19–10.** Traumatic hyphema and associated subconjunctival hemorrhage.

iritis and include blurred vision, eye pain, and light sensitivity. Gross hyphema will be visible on external diffuse light examination, but slitlamp examination is required to detect limited red blood cells in the anterior chamber. Hyphema can be a sign of an open globe injury, so a comprehensive ophthalmic examination is required. Potential complications of hyphema include raised intraocular pressure and corneal blood staining. Treatment of hyphema includes bed rest, ocular antihypertensive drops, frequent topical corticosteroid, and cycloplegic drops. Oral aminocaproic acid reduces breakdown of clot and reduces the risk of re-bleeding.

The concussive shock wave from blunt ocular trauma can damage the iris, ciliary body, and trabecular meshwork. There may be small radial tears through the iris sphincter muscle at the pupillary margin (**traumatic iris sphincter tears**). **Iridodialysis** is more extensive circumferential tear of the iris at the iridociliary junction. **Cyclodialysis** is circumferential separation of the peripheral iris and ciliary body from the sclera at the scleral spur. **Angle recession** is circumferential tear through the trabecular meshwork and is identified as widening of the anterior chamber angle on gonioscopy. These abnormalities typically are accompanied by hyphema and may not be evident until the blood clears. Impairment of the trabecular meshwork function from hyphema and angle recession leads to secondary glaucoma in many cases. Low intraocular pressure (hypotony) can occur with cyclodialysis because the aqueous fluid has direct access to the suprachoroidal space. Ultrasound biomicroscopy is useful for identifying angle recession as well as cyclodialysis with associated ciliochoroidal effusion. These conditions can resolve spontaneously, but surgical intervention may be required for large iridodialysis, cyclodialysis with hypotony, and angle recession glaucoma. Open globe injury with displacement of intraocular contents or blunt ocular injury may cause displacement of the (crystalline) lens (**traumatic lens dislocation**). It is more likely if there is pre-existing weakness of the zonules, such as in Marfan's syndrome and homocystinuria. On slitlamp examination, there may be abnormal movements of the lens with eye movements (**phakodensis**), abnormal position (**subluxation**) of the lens, or complete dislocation of the lens into the anterior chamber or vitreous. Depending on the extent of the dislocation, nonurgent surgery may be required.

Severe ocular contusion may cause focal or geographic retinal whitening (**commotio retinae**) that usually is located opposite the site of impact. Typically it develops within 24 hours after the injury and gradually fades over several days to weeks. If the macula is affected, the visual acuity may be profoundly reduced. There is no active treatment.

Blunt or sharp trauma to the periorbital region can damage the optic nerve (**traumatic optic neuropathy**). Severe blunt trauma to the head, particularly the frontal region, or to the face, particularly if there is a fracture at the orbital apex, may injure the optic nerve as it passes through the optic canal. Penetrating orbital injuries, periocular soft tissue lacerations, and eye gouging can damage the optic nerve without necessarily causing an open globe injury. Depending on the severity of the injury, the visual acuity ranges from normal to no light perception. Treatment with systemic corticosteroids is controversial, and prognosis is variable.

Severe ocular contusion can cause tearing of the retinal pigment epithelium (**choroidal rupture**) in a crescentic or curvilinear pattern that is typically concentric to the optic disk margin (Figure 19–11). Involvement of the central macula can cause permanent profound reduction of visual acuity. Choroidal neovascularization arising from the edge of the choroidal rupture may also cause reduction of visual acuity, but treatments are available.

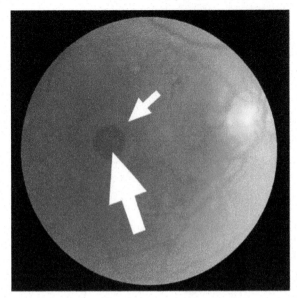

▲ **Figure 19–12.** Traumatic macular hole (**larger arrow**) with surrounding exudative subretinal fluid (**smaller arrow**).

Ocular contusion injury in which the shock wave impacts directly on the fovea can cause a full-thickness retinal hole (**traumatic macular hole**) (Figure 19–12). Vitreoretinal surgery may be indicated, but visual acuity frequently does not improve.

Mechanical ocular injuries often tear superficial retinal blood vessels, leading to traumatic **vitreous hemorrhage**, which can range from mild to severe. Typically, there is an associated partial or complete posterior vitreous detachment. As long as the retina is not torn, the intravitreal blood usually clears spontaneously within a few weeks to months. If the retina is torn, retinal detachment frequently develops, requiring surgery.

ORBITAL INJURIES

Trauma to the periorbital region can result in a variety of injuries including contusions, abrasions, avulsions, and lacerations. The initial evaluation should include a thorough examination of the eyelid margin, nasolacrimal system, and canthi. Contusions and abrasions can be treated conservatively with topical antibacterial ointment. Superficial eyelid lacerations not involving the eyelid margin may be closed as with any skin laceration. Injuries involving the full thickness of the eyelid margin or the nasolacrimal system (Figure 19–13) require an ophthalmology or oculoplastic consultation. Surgery is usually required to achieve precise alignment of the tarsal plate, mucocutaneous junction, lash line, and canaliculus so as to prevent a lid notch and reduced

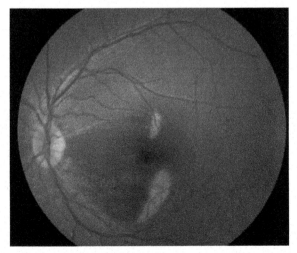

▲ **Figure 19–11.** Traumatic choroidal ruptures with associated subretinal blood.

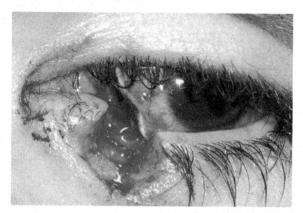

▲ **Figure 19–13.** Full-thickness laceration of left lower eyelid involving its medial margin with underlying eye wall laceration and uveal prolapse.

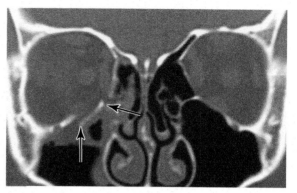

▲ **Figure 19–14.** Coronal computed tomography scan of orbits showing right orbital floor fracture (**arrows**).

the risk of epiphora. All periorbital lacerations should receive a thorough examination to rule out associated ocular injury.

Blunt and penetrating injuries to the periorbital region are frequently associated with **orbital fractures**, either from direct impact with transmission of force through the bones or indirectly by injury to the thin bone of the orbital walls from elevation of intraorbital pressure ("**blowout fracture**"), which most commonly affects the orbital floor and may result in entrapment of orbital tissue sometimes including an extraocular muscle. Clinical signs of an orbital fracture include step defect of the orbital rim, enophthalmos or exophthalmos, paresthesias and numbness in the distribution of the first or second division of the trigeminal nerve, diplopia, and orbital crepitus. Entrapment of an extraocular muscle may cause severe pain and autonomic disturbance with bradycardia and vomiting on attempted eye movement. Particularly in children, blowout fracture with extraocular muscle entrapment may not be accompanied by orbital soft tissue signs ("white-eyed blowout"). CT scan of head and orbits, preferably reviewed by a neuroradiologist, will identify most orbital fractures (Figure 19–14), whether there is entrapment of orbital soft tissues, and whether there are facial or skull fractures requiring maxillofacial or neurosurgical assessment.

Not all orbital fractures need to be repaired, and in many cases, surgery can be delayed by 1–2 weeks to allow resolution of orbital swelling and reduction of the risk of dangerously high intraorbital pressure during surgery. Blowout fractures with severe pain and/or autonomic disturbance require urgent surgical intervention. Blowout fractures with troublesome double vision or risk of persistent enophthalmos benefit from surgery, with optimal timing being determined by individual circumstances. Whether orbital fractures with displaced bony fragments impinging on the optic nerve should be repaired is debatable because existing optic nerve damage is unlikely to be improved and surgery entails a risk of further optic nerve injury.

A wide variety of injuries including from firearms and explosions may result in **intraorbital foreign bodies**. Depending on their composition and location, surgical removal may be attempted, but often it is better avoided unless necessitated by infection or inflammation. CT shows metals well. MRI is contraindicated if the foreign body is known to be or could be magnetic. Copper may cause an inflammatory reaction and, along with iron, may cause retinal toxicity (see below). Lead is relatively inert. Organic foreign bodies including wood may be difficult to appreciate with CT scan and more apparent on MRI. They predispose to orbital infection and should be removed if possible.

Blunt or sharp trauma can cause **retrobulbar hemorrhage**, especially in patients on anticoagulants. Symptoms include marked orbital swelling with lid ecchymosis and subconjunctival hemorrhage, decreased vision, and double vision. On examination, the orbit is tense to retropulsion with increased intraocular pressure and decreased movements of the globe. Markedly increased intraocular pressure and a relative afferent pupillary defect require emergent lateral canthotomy and cantholysis. Ophthalmology consultation should occur without delay.

THERMAL BURNS

Thermal burns of the periocular region occur most commonly from fires and explosions. Mild cases may present with redness and pain. Severe thermal burns will present with severe swelling, redness or whitening, blistering, and charring of the involved tissues. Initial treatment consists of topical antibiotic ointment to keep the tissues lubricated and prevent secondary infection. Full-thickness burns can cause ectropion and lid retraction within a few days, necessitating tarsorrhaphies or skin grafts to prevent corneal exposure. Repeat procedures are frequently required over the ensuing weeks to months in such patients.

Thermal burns to the ocular surface are much less frequent than thermal burns to the eyelids. However, full-thickness eyelid burns frequently result in necrosis and retraction of eyelid tissues, which can lead to ocular surface exposure, fusion of the eyelids to the surface of the eye (symblepharon), microbial keratitis, corneal perforation, intraocular infection, and blindness.

The most common electromagnetic injury to the eye is **ultraviolet radiation–induced superficial keratoconjunctivitis** due to absorption of ultraviolet radiation energy by the corneal and conjunctival epithelium during activities such as arc welding, prolonged exposure to reflected light off of snow, water or white sand, and use of tanning beds. Typically, patients will report a painful red eye with foreign body sensation and tearing several hours after the exposure. Topical anesthetic drops may be required to provide temporary relief sufficient to allow slitlamp examination. Treatment is similar to that described earlier for corneal abrasions.

LATE SEQUELAE OF OPHTHALMIC TRAUMA

Corneal full-thickness lacerations and ruptures frequently heal with sufficient irregular warping to cause profound impairment of visual acuity. Rigid contact lens, corneal laser treatment, or corneal grafting (usually delayed until at least 6 months after the injury) may be required.

Following severe chemical injuries and some thermal injuries, the corneal stroma becomes partially or completely opaque. Also most or all of the limbal stem cells that normally repopulate the corneal epithelium are lost, which results in progressive conjunctivalization of the corneal surface. Limbal stem cell transplantation followed by penetrating keratoplasty or implantation of a prosthetic cornea may restore some vision.

Ocular hypotony means low intraocular pressure, typically defined as less than 6 mm Hg. It leads to corneal folds, diffuse corneal and uveal congestion, and macular edema, which can cause mild to profound visual impairment. It may be caused by exudative ciliochoroidal effusion, cyclodialysis, retinal detachment, unrecognized globe rupture, and posttraumatic intraocular inflammation. If hypotony is not effectively treated, the eye may become shrunken and blind (phthisis bulbi).

Microbial infection is a serious and potentially blinding complication of many ocular injuries. It may be limited to the specific site of injury (eg, cornea, lid) or may extend throughout the eye (endophthalmitis) or orbit (panophthalmitis). It is much more likely after trauma involving a contaminated object and in open globe injuries.

Corneal blood staining complicates ophthalmic trauma associated with major hyphema and concomitant substantial elevation of intraocular pressure. Red blood cells are forced into the stroma of the cornea by the high intraocular pressure. As the red blood cells break down, reddish brown hemosiderin pigment is deposited in the corneal stroma. Typically, the staining is most pronounced centrally and inferiorly and least pronounced peripherally and superiorly. If the blood eventually clears from the anterior chamber and intraocular pressure returns to normal, the corneal blood staining will resolve slowly over many months. While this is a tolerable problem for most adults, it is a potential cause of amblyopia in young children. Therefore, sustained raised intraocular pressure in a child with hyphema should be treated aggressively, possibly including anterior chamber washout.

Iron and copper are toxic to intraocular structures. Iron released from a retained foreign body is absorbed by many intraocular tissues including the cornea, lens, and retina, leading to greenish discoloration (**siderosis oculi**). Copper (**chalcosis oculi**) is deposited particularly in the Descemet's membrane, lens capsule, and retina. In either case, permanent vision loss can occur due to retinal toxicity. Thus intraocular foreign bodies containing iron or copper should be removed whenever possible.

After external exposure of uveal tissue, an autoimmune granulomatous inflammation may develop in both the injured and uninjured eye (**sympathetic ophthalmia**) (see Chapter 7). It is most commonly associated with extensive corneoscleral laceration. Symptoms may begin as early as 1–2 weeks after the trauma but may not develop for several years. Untreated, the inflammation can lead to profound loss of vision in both eyes. Local and systemic immunosuppression with steroids and other agents is required to preserve vision. Removal of a severely traumatized eye within 7–10 days of the injury reduces the likelihood of sympathetic ophthalmia.

Traumatic diplopia can be monocular or binocular. Monocular double vision persists with closure of the fellow eye, whereas binocular double vision resolves when either eye is closed. Significant injury to the cornea will frequently cause substantial corneal warping (irregular astigmatism) leading to monocular diplopia. Binocular diplopia can be caused by injury to the third, fourth, or sixth cranial nerves or to the extraocular muscles. Orbital fractures are a common cause. After surgical repair and release of extraocular muscle entrapment, diplopia may persist because of neuromuscular damage, and extraocular muscle surgery may be required.

Injuries to the nasolacrimal system can occur anywhere from the punctum to the nasolacrimal duct. Obstruction of any component of the nasolacrimal system leads to chronic overflow of tears (**epiphora**). Isolated obstruction of the nasolacrimal duct can also lead to infection of the lacrimal sac (dacryocystitis). Stenosis of the punctum can be treated easily with punctoplasty. Obstruction of the canaliculus or nasolacrimal duct may require dacryocystorhinostomy or a Jones tube.

MANAGEMENT OF ASSOCIATED NONOPHTHALMIC INJURIES

Ophthalmic traumas are rarely isolated injuries. Mechanisms of injury capable of causing ocular and periorbital injury are often sufficient to cause severe facial and brain injury

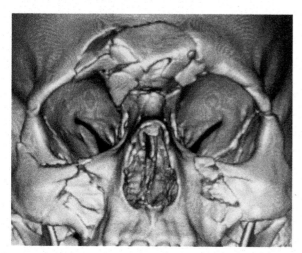

▲ **Figure 19-15.** Three-dimensional reconstructed computed tomography scan of unhelmeted motorcycle accident victim with bilateral panorbital fractures, frontal sinus fractures, and mandibular fracture.

(Figure 19–15). A team-based approach, often with maxillofacial surgeons, plastic surgeons, and neurosurgeons, is necessary to provide the best possible cosmetic and functional outcome for the patient.

REFERENCES

Al Wadeai EA et al: Epidemiological features of pediatric ocular trauma in Egypt. J Ophthalmol 2016;2016:7874084. [PMID: 27800177]

Baharestani S et al: Eyelid reconstruction techniques. In: Ichpujani P et al (eds): *Expert Techniques in Ophthalmic Surgery*. Jaypee Brothers Medical Publishers, 2015.

Bansal S et al: Controversies in the pathophysiology and management of hyphema. Surv Ophthalmol 2016;61:297. [PMID: 26632664]

Baradaran-Rafii A et al: Current and upcoming therapies for ocular surface chemical injuries. Ocul Surf 2017;15:48. [PMID: 27650263]

Batur M et al: Epidemiology of adult open globe injury. J Craniofac Surg 2016;27:1636. [PMID: 27526252]

Bossert RP et al: Blindness following facial fracture: Treatment modalities and outcomes. Craniomaxillofac Trauma Reconstr 2009;2:117. [PMID: 22110805]

Damgaard OE et al: Surgical timing of the orbital "blowout" fracture: A systematic review and meta-analysis. Otolaryngol Head Neck Surg 2016;155:387. [PMID: 27165680]

Eslani M et al: The ocular surface chemical burns. J Ophthalmol 2014;2014:196827. [PMID: 25105018]

Gharaibeh A et al: Medical interventions for traumatic hyphema. Cochrane Database Syst Rev 2013;12:CD005431. [PMID: 24302299]

Guzman-Salas PJ et al: Characteristics of sympathetic ophthalmia in a single international center. Open Ophthalmol J 2016;10:154. [PMID: 27651849]

Haring RS et al: Epidemiologic trends of chemical ocular burns in the United States. JAMA Ophthalmol 2016;134:1119. [PMID: 27490908]

Jung H et al: Prognostic CT findings of diplopia after surgical repair of pure orbital blowout fracture. J Craniomaxillofac Surg 2016;44:1479. [PMID: 27427337]

Kalin-Hajdu E et al: Controversies of the lacrimal system. Surv Ophthalmol 2016;61:309. [PMID: 26700821]

Kim SM et al: Prediction of the development of late enophthalmos in pure blowout fractures: Delayed orbital tissue atrophy plays a major role. Eur J Ophthalmol 2017;27:104. [PMID: 27198642]

Kong Y et al: Six-year clinical study of firework-related eye injuries in North China. Postgrad Med J 2015;91:26. [PMID: 25583736]

Leonard R: *Statistics on Vision Impairment: A Resource Manual, 2000.* Lighthouse International, 2000.

Loporchio D et al: Intraocular foreign bodies: A review. Surv Ophthalmol 2016;61:582. [PMID: 26994871]

Messman AM: Ocular injuries: New strategies in emergency department management. Emerg Med Pract 2015;17:1. [PMID: 26466300]

Movahedan A et al: Long-term management of severe ocular surface injury due to methamphetamine production accidents. Cornea 2015;34:433. [PMID: 25642642]

Nam SM: Microscope-assisted reconstruction of canalicular laceration using Mini-Monoka. J Craniofac Surg 2013;24:2056. [PMID: 24220405]

Neovius E et al: Persistent diplopia after fractures involving the orbit related to nerve injury. J Plast Reconstr Aesthet Surg 2015;68:219. [PMID: 25488468]

Page RD et al: Risk factors for poor outcomes in patients with open-globe injuries. Clin Ophthalmol 2016;10:1461. [PMID: 27536059]

Pargament JM et al: Physical and chemical injuries to eyes and eyelids. Clin Dermatol 2015;33:234-237. [PMID: 25704943]

Rajkumar GC et al: Ocular injuries associated with midface fractures: A 5 year survey. J Maxillofac Oral Surg 2015;14:925. [PMID: 26604465]

Read SP et al: Traumatic open globe injury in young pediatric patients: Characterization of a novel prognostic score. J AAPOS 2016;20:141. [PMID: 27079595]

Rodman RE et al: Controversies in the management of the trauma patient. Facial Plast Surg Clin North Am 2016;24:299. [PMID: 27400843]

Rudnisky CJ et al: Visual acuity outcomes of the Boston keratoprosthesis type 1: Multicenter study results. Am J Ophthalmol 2016;162:89. [PMID: 26550696]

Sadiq MA et al: Eyelid lacerations due to dog bite in children. J Pediatr Ophthalmol Strabismus 2015;52:360. [PMID: 26371465]

Scruggs D et al: Ocular injuries in trauma patients: An analysis of 28,340 trauma admissions in the 2003-2007 National Trauma Data Bank National Sample Program. J Trauma Acute Care Surg 2012;73:1308. [PMID: 22914085]

Septa D et al: Etiology, incidence and patterns of mid-face fractures and associated ocular injuries. J Maxillofac Oral Surg 2014;13:115. [PMID: 24822001]

SooHoo JR et al: Pediatric traumatic hyphema: A review of 138 consecutive cases. J AAPOS 2013;17:565. [PMID: 24215806]

Sosin M et al: Treatment outcomes following traumatic optic neuropathy. Plast Reconstr Surg 2016;137:231. [PMID: 26710028]

Su Y et al: Predictive factors for residual diplopia after surgical repair in pediatric patients with orbital blowout fracture. J Craniomaxillofac Surg 2016;44:1463. [PMID: 27530668]

Sung EK et al: Injuries of the globe: What can the radiologist offer? Radiographics 2014;34:764. [PMID: 24819794]

Tabatabaei SA et al: Systemic oral antibiotics as a prophylactic measure to prevent endophthalmitis in patients with open globe injuries in comparison with intravenous antibiotics. Retina 2016;36:360. [PMID: 26815932]

Toride A et al: Visual outcome after emergency surgery for open globe eye injury in Japan. Clin Ophthalmol 2016;10:1731. [PMID: 27660410]

Vaca EE et al: Facial fractures with concomitant open globe injury: Mechanisms and fracture patterns associated with blindness. Plast Reconstr Surg 2013;131:1317. [PMID: 23416437]

Voss JO et al: The "tight orbit": Incidence and management of the orbital compartment syndrome. J Craniomaxillofac Surg 2016;44:1008. [PMID: 27259677]

Westekemper H et al: Clinical outcomes of amniotic membrane transplantation in the management of acute ocular chemical injury. Br J Ophthalmol 2017;101:103. [PMID: 27150827]

Yardley AE et al: Paediatric ocular and adnexal injuries requiring hospitalisation in Western Australia. Clin Exp Optom 2016 Oct 20. [Epub ahead of print] [PMID: 27762442]

Yildiz M et al: An important cause of blindness in children: Open globe injuries. J Ophthalmol 2016;2016:7173515. [PMID: 27247799]

Yucel OE et al: Clinical characteristics and prognostic factors of scleral rupture due to blunt ocular trauma. Eye (Lond) 2016;30:1606. [PMID: 27589050]

Zhu L et al: Ocular trauma score in siderosis bulbi with retained intraocular foreign body. Medicine (Baltimore) 2015;94:e1533. [PMID: 26426616]

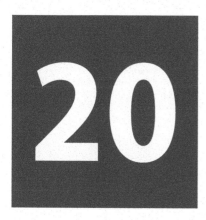

Causes and Prevention of Vision Loss

Dustin Curts, MD, and William G. Hodge, MD, PhD, FRCSC

This chapter addresses vision loss as a worldwide health problem, providing information on causes, with data on prevalence, and measures to prevent it. All of the disorders that may cause vision loss are discussed more fully in other chapters.

Causes of Vision Loss

DEFINITIONS

Reduction of vision has significant consequences. Differentiating between different degrees of reduction of vision is important because the demands for medical, social, and rehabilitative interventions vary.

Reduction of vision has been defined in many different ways, resulting in multiple terms that may not be consistent with one another. Whereas to the lay person it implies complete loss of vision, the term "blindness" is often used for individuals who have significant and useful residual vision, an extreme example being the use of the term "color blindness" for individuals with mild color vision deficiency. "Legal blindness" is used in the United States for those who meet various legal requirements for benefits.

An important challenge is categorizing the broad range of reduction of vision. The World Health Organization (WHO) and almost all population surveys now use the International Classification of Diseases, 10th Revision (ICD-10), of which the 2015 version categorizes reduction of vision according to the presenting (using whatever refractive correction the subject has) distant visual acuity of the better eye as mild or no visual impairment, moderate visual impairment, severe visual impairment, and blindness, but other categorizations are used (Table 20–1). (Confusingly, the term "visual impairment" may be used to encompass the moderate and severe visual impairment and blindness categories of ICD-10, ie, not including

mild visual impairment. In this chapter, the term "vision loss" is used instead.) Maximum diameter of visual field of 20° or less in the better eye is also categorized as blindness by the ICD and as legal blindness in the United States. The *AMA Guides to the Evaluation of Permanent Impairment* provides a graduated categorization of visual field impairment, as it does for impairment of visual acuity. The differences between the various categorizations and the variable terminology emphasize the importance of knowing which definitions are used whenever statistics about reduction of vision are compared.

Presenting visual acuity, rather than best-corrected visual acuity, acknowledges the importance of uncorrected (or undercorrected) refractive error as a cause of vision loss worldwide and almost doubles its overall prevalence. For legal blindness in the United States and eligibility for certification as severely sight impaired (blind registration) or sight impaired (partially sighted registration) across Europe, which are relevant to eligibility for financial and other support, best-corrected visual acuity is still used.

▶ Driving Privileges

In the United States, the visual requirements for driving vary from state to state for both private and commercial drivers. For private drivers, 20/40 best-corrected visual acuity with both eyes is the most common requirement, but some accept less. These requirements set a safety margin between letter

Table 20–1. Categorizations of Reduction of Vision

Snellen Visual Acuity						LogMAR	EDTRS Letters	WHO (ICD-10 2015)[1]	AMA[2]	United States	United Kingdom
20 ft	6 m	4 m	3 m	1 m	Decimal						
				NLP					Total blindness		
20/2000	6/600	4/400	3/300	1/100	0.010	2.00	0	Blindness	Near-blindness	Legal blindness	Severely sight impaired (blind)
20/1600	6/480	4/320	3/240	1/80	0.013	1.90					
20/1250	6/375	4/250	3/188	1/63	0.016	1.80					
20/1200	6/360	4/240	3/180	1/60	0.017	1.78					
20/1000	6/300	4/200	3/150	1/50	0.020	1.70					
20/800	6/240	4/160	3/120	1/40	0.025	1.60	5		Profound low vision		
20/640	6/192	4/128	3/96	1/32	0.031	1.50	10				
20/500	6/150	4/100	3/75	1/25	0.040	1.40	15				
20/400	6/120	4/80	3/60	1/20	0.050	1.30	20	Severe visual impairment	Severe low vision		Sight impaired (partially sighted)
20/320	6/96	4/64	3/48	1/16	0.063	1.20	25				
20/300	6/90	4/60	3/45	1/15	0.067	1.18	26				
20/250	6/75	4/50	3/38	1/13	0.080	1.10	30				
20/200	6/60	4/40	3/30	1/10	0.100	1.00	35				
20/160	6/48	4/32	3/24	1/8	0.125	0.90	40	Moderate visual impairment	Moderate low vision		
20/125	6/38	4/25	3/19	1/9	0.160	0.80	45				
20/120	6/36	4/24	3/18	1/6	0.167	0.78	46				
20/100	6/30	4/20	3/15	1/5	0.200	0.70	50				
20/80	6/24	4/16	3/12	1/4	0.250	0.60	55				
20/70	6/21	4/14	3/11	1/3.5	0.286	0.54	58				
20/63	6/19	4/13	3/10	1/3.2	0.317	0.50	60	Mild or no visual impairment	Near-normal vision (mild loss)		
20/60	6/18	4/12	3/9.0	1/3.0	0.333	0.48	61				
20/50	6/15	4/10	3/7.5	1/2.5	0.400	0.40	65				
20/40	6/12	4/8.0	3/6.0	1/2.0	0.500	0.30	70				
20/32	6/10	4/6.4	3/4.8	1/1.6	0.625	0.20	75				
20/30	6/9.0	4/6.0	3/4.5	1/1.5	0.667	0.18	76		Range of normal vision		
20/25	6/7.5	4/5.0	3/3.8	1/1.3	0.800	0.10	80				
20/20	6/6.0	4/4.0	3/3.0	1/1.0	1.000	0	85				
20/16	6/4.8	4/3.2	3/2.4	1/0.8	1.250	-0.10	90				
20/12.5	6/3.8	4/2.5	3/1.9	1/0.63	1.600	-0.20	95				
20/10	6/3.0	4/2.0	3/1.5	1/0.50	2.000	-0.30	100				

AMA, American Medical Association; ETDRS, Early Treatment Diabetic Retinopathy Study; ICD-10, International Classification of Diseases, 10th Revision; LogMAR, Logarithm of the Minimum Angle of Resolution; WHO, World Health Organization.
[1]Available at: http://apps.who.int/classifications/icd10/browse/2015/en#/H53-H54.
[2]Rondinelli RD et al: *Guides to the Evaluation of Permanent Impairment*, 6th ed. American Medical Association, 2008.

chart performance in the office and on-the-road performance under adverse conditions. The requirements for commercial drivers are often more stringent, not because they drive in a different visual environment, but because a wider safety margin is deemed desirable. In Canada, the legal limit for driving for private drivers is best-corrected visual acuity with both eyes of 20/50 (6/15) or better and a continuous field of vision horizontally no less than 120° and vertically 15° above and below central fixation, and with no evidence of diplopia within the central 40° of fixation. Other countries have similar but varying requirement for visual acuity, visual field, and absence of diplopia. Health professionals, particularly ophthalmologists, are obligated to ensure that patients failing the relevant requirements do not drive, if necessary by informing the licensing body. There are published vision standards for various occupations.

PREVALENCE

Historically, prevalence studies on vision loss were varied and inconsistent, making it difficult to compare reports from different parts of the world. The availability of comparable data from nearly every WHO member state has facilitated more accurate comparison of worldwide statistics. The WHO has estimated that, in 2010, worldwide there were 285 million people with vision loss, of whom 39 million were blind. The prevalence of vision loss was estimated to be 0.3–0.35% in Europe and the Americas; 0.53–6.1% in China and the Western Pacific region; 0.68–0.73% in India, Southeast Asia, and Africa; and 0.85% in the Eastern Mediterranean region.

Population-based studies indicate that the global prevalence of vision loss has been declining since the early 1990s, with less vision loss from infectious diseases such as trachoma but increasing vision loss from conditions related to aging, such as cataract and age-related macular degeneration. Accordingly, the majority of individuals with vision loss are older (82% over the age of 50) but also poor, with close to 90% living in low- and middle-income countries. Vision loss is additionally clustered in disadvantaged communities in rural areas and urban slums, where the risk of blindness is 10–40 times higher than in the industrially developed regions of Europe and America. Women are at much higher risk of vision loss, with population-based surveys estimating that 64% of those with vision loss worldwide are women. There are approximately 19 million children with vision loss, of whom 1.4 million are irreversibly blind with the need for rehabilitation for the rest of their lives.

CAUSES

Uncorrected refractive error is responsible for 42% of worldwide vision loss (Table 20–2). It is estimated that over 12 million children (between the ages of 5 and 15) with impaired vision could have normal vision with correction of refractive error alone. The leading causes of blindness are cataract, glaucoma, age-related macular degeneration, and corneal opacities. Vision loss caused by infectious diseases such as trachoma is decreasing due to improvements in public health. Most recent WHO figures estimate that trachoma affects 1.8 million people visually.

Causes of vision loss around the world are influenced by the level of social development and local geography. In developing countries, besides refractive error, cataract is the leading cause, with glaucoma, trachoma, leprosy, onchocerciasis, and xerophthalmia also being important. Corneal scarring is a significant cause of monocular vision loss in the developing

Table 20–2. Causes of Worldwide Vision Loss and Blindness

Cause	Vision Loss	Blindness
Refractive error	42%	3%
Cataract	33%	51%
Glaucoma	2%	8%
Age-related macular degeneration	1%	5%
Corneal opacity	1%	4%
Childhood	1%	4%
Trachoma	1%	3%
Diabetic retinopathy	1%	1%
Undetermined	18%	1%

Source: Data taken from Pascolini D et al: Global estimates of visual impairment: 2010. Br J Ophthalmol 2012;96:614 [PMID: 22133988].

world, accounting for 850,000 cases of blindness per year in India alone. In more developed countries, vision loss is to a great extent related to the aging process. Although cataract is still an important cause of vision loss, the leading causes of blindness in North America and other developed countries are age-related macular degeneration, diabetic retinopathy, and glaucoma. Other causes are herpes simplex keratitis, retinal detachment, retinal vascular disorders, and inherited retinal degenerative disorders.

In children, retinal diseases such as retinopathy of prematurity (ROP) account for 29% of worldwide vision loss; corneal scarring, predominantly due to xerophthalmia, rubella, and infection, accounts for 21%; and congenital disorders (including cataract, glaucoma, and structural abnormalities of the globe) account for 14%. Differences again exist when comparing the relative causes in developed and developing countries. In developed countries, the major causes are ROP, cataract, hereditary disease of the retina, diseases of the central nervous system (including hypoxic injury to the visual pathway), congenital malformations of the globe (microphthalmos, anopthalmos, and optic nerve hypoplasia), and nystagmus. The major causes in developing countries are corneal scarring, trachoma, genetic diseases, and cataract.

▶ Cataract

Fifty-one percent of blindness worldwide is due to cataract. In many parts of the developing world, the facilities available for treating cataract are grossly inadequate, being hardly sufficient to cope with new cases and completely inadequate for dealing with the backlog of existing cases, currently estimated to be 10 million.

It is not fully understood why the frequency of cataract varies so greatly in different geographic areas, although exposure to ultraviolet radiation and recurrent episodes of dehydration, often occurring in severe diarrheal diseases, are thought to be important. With decreasing mortality rates and changing demographics, age-related causes of vision loss, including cataract, are expected to continue to rise. Worldwide, approximately 20 million people are blind from cataract. By 2020, this number is expected to reach 40 million. Although no current medical treatments exist to delay the development of cataract, it is estimated that a 10-year delay in cataract formation would reduce the number of individuals requiring surgery by 45%. Until an effective treatment that can prevent or delay cataract formation is devised, it will remain a leading cause of vision loss and will become an increasingly important global public health concern.

Uncorrected Refractive Error

Uncorrected refractive error is clearly avoidable through the provision of corrective lenses; however, this remains a major cause of vision loss throughout the world, even in developed countries such as the United States, but particularly in developing countries where limited access to eye care professionals, low prevalence of eye health-seeking behavior, and low affordability of corrective lenses remain major problems. In children, ineffective screening is also a contributing factor.

Glaucoma

The incidence of vision loss due to glaucoma has decreased in recent years as a result of earlier detection, improved medical and surgical treatment, and a greater awareness and understanding of the disorder. However, in many developing countries, glaucoma remains a common cause of vision loss. This is especially the case in West Africa, where untreated open-angle glaucoma is extremely common. In China and Southeast Asia, there appears to be a preponderance of narrow-angle glaucoma. Approximately 3 million individuals worldwide are blind due to glaucoma, and a simple easy method of detecting patients at risk still does not exist. Treatment is also a major problem because of the poor compliance of most patients for taking daily eye drops. A simple but safe surgical procedure may ultimately be the only solution for reducing the needless burden of vision loss from this disease. More research in this area is essential.

Trachoma

Trachoma causes bilateral keratoconjunctivitis, generally in childhood, which leads in adulthood to corneal scarring that, when severe, causes vision loss. About 40 million people have trachoma, most of them in Africa, the Middle East, and Asia. It can be treated with various antibiotics, including tetracyclines and erythromycin, but azithromycin is proving to be the drug of choice. The number of individuals who are blind from trachoma has dropped from 6 million to 1.8 million, which is a testament to current WHO-supervised treatment programs

and the effectiveness of azithromycin. Prevention of spread of infection will require provision of proper sanitary facilities, including clean water for drinking and washing, waste disposal, fly control, and behavioral change in hygiene.

Onchocerciasis

Onchocerciasis is transmitted by bites of the blackfly, which breeds in clear running streams. It is endemic in the greater part of tropical Africa and Central and South America. The most heavily infested zone is the Volta River basin, which extends over parts of Dahomey, Ghana, Ivory Coast, Mali, Niger, Togo, and Upper Volta. Worldwide, 15–20 million people are affected by onchocerciasis, with half a million individuals in hyperendemic areas blinded by the disease.

The major ophthalmic manifestations of onchocerciasis are keratitis, uveitis, retinochoroiditis, and optic atrophy. The disease is prevented by insect eradication and personal protection by screening. Treatment with ivermectin is extremely effective in killing the microfilaria and sterilizing the adult females residing in nodules in the body. The effect of the mass distribution of ivermectin in areas where onchocerciasis is endemic is a public health success story. Like leprosy, onchocerciasis is definitely decreasing in its importance as a worldwide cause of vision loss because of successful treatment programs.

Other Causes

Age-related macular degeneration, diabetic retinopathy, and corneal disorders are discussed elsewhere (see Chapters 6, 10, and 15). Table 20–3 addresses leprosy, xerophthalmia, and hereditary disease.

Table 20–3. Leprosy, Xerophthalmia, and Hereditary Disease

Disease	Notes
Leprosy	Affects 14 million people High ocular involvement 10% become blind Effective triple-drug therapy (dapsone, clofazimine, and rifampin)
Xerophthalmia	Due to vitamin A deficiency Affects 5 million children each year 500,000 develop corneal involvement, 50% of whom develop profound vision loss Symptoms include xerosis, Bitot's spots, and keratomalacia Exacerbated by protein malnutrition Prevented by vitamin A supplementation
Hereditary disease	Burden reduced with genetic counseling

Prevention of Vision Loss

Preventive medicine is increasingly important in attempts to fulfill society's expectations of modern medicine with the resources available. Although prevention is a logical approach to the solution of many problems in all branches of medicine, in practice, there are a number of hurdles to overcome. For any particular condition, it is essential that individuals at risk be easily identified. If their identification requires population screening, the process should be easy to perform, accurate, and reliable. Preventive measures must be both effective and acceptable to the target population. Unwarranted interference with the at-risk individual's lifestyle only leads to poor compliance. Legislation may be required for certain measures but may engender resentment when it is felt to infringe on personal liberty. For preventive medicine to be successful, there must be cooperation among all segments of society—not just the medical community—in identifying problem areas, establishing workable solutions, and disseminating information. The successes that have been achieved in occupational health are an example of what can be accomplished if a consensus of opinion is established.

In ophthalmology, the major avenues for preventive medicine are ocular injuries and infections, genetic and systemic diseases with ocular involvement, and ocular diseases in which the early treatable stages are often unrecognized or ignored.

PREVENTION OF OCULAR INJURIES

Ocular injuries are a very preventable cause of vision loss because simple preventive measures are often available. Injuries can vary from closed globe (blunt trauma or chemical injuries) to open globe injuries including rupture, perforation, and penetration (see Chapter 19). WHO statistics show that over 55 million eye injuries occur each year; 1.6 million people are rendered blind, 2.3 million develop bilateral low vision, and 19 million have monocular blindness or low vision. The US Eye Injury Register (USEIR) statistics show that over 57% of injuries occur in people under 30 years of age, with the percentage being even higher in work-related injuries.

▶ Occupational Injuries

Eye injuries remain a significant risk to worker health, especially among individuals in jobs requiring intensive manual labor. Many manufacturing processes pose a particular threat to the eye. Grinding or drilling commonly propels small fragments of metal into the environment at high velocity, and these projectiles can easily lodge on the cornea or penetrate the globe through the cornea or sclera. Tools with sharp ends are also commonly involved in producing penetrating ocular injuries. Welding arcs produce ultraviolet radiation that may cause epithelial keratitis ("arc eye"). Industrial chemicals—particularly those containing high concentrations of alkali or acid—can rapidly produce severe ocular damage that is often bilateral and associated with a poor visual outcome.

New legislation, increased worker training, particularly targeting groups most at risk, provision of effective eye protection equipment, and development of a culture of safety in the workplace have led to a decline in eye injuries. Workers must be properly trained in the use of tools, machinery, and chemicals. Safety guards must be fitted to all machinery, and safety goggles must be worn whenever the worker is doing hazardous work or is in the workplace area where such hazards exist. It is surprising how many workers assume that they are no longer at risk of injury when they are not themselves performing hazardous tasks even though they are in the vicinity of work being performed by others.

The growing interest in "do-it-yourself" projects in the home exposes many more individuals to the risks of ocular injury from machinery, tools, and chemicals. Education of the public to recognize and minimize such risks, which may not be obvious to the ordinary householder or hobbyist, is particularly important.

Early recognition and urgent expert ophthalmologic assessment of any injuries sustained are essential. In the case of chemical injuries, immediate copious lavage of the eyes with sterile water, saline if available, or tap water for at least 5 minutes is the most important method of limiting the damage incurred. Neglect of penetrating injuries or corneal foreign bodies markedly increases the potential for long-term morbidity. Obtaining an accurate history is crucial in identifying the possibility of a penetrating injury. This is particularly true when medical help is sought some time after the injury and the patient may not realize the importance of a seemingly minor episode of trauma. Any worker who presents with unexplained visual loss or intraocular inflammation must be carefully questioned about the possibility of recent ocular injuries, and the possibility of an occult intraocular foreign body must be borne in mind.

Chronic exposure to ultraviolet light or ionizing radiation, such as from improperly screened nuclear materials or in radiology departments, can lead to early and rapid cataract, and care must be taken to monitor and decrease exposure. In one study, the prevalence of cataract was 64% in radiology technicians, 16% in radiologists, 10% in respiratory physicians, and 2% in nuclear medicine department staff, with an overall relative risk of 5 compared to unexposed health care workers.

Table 20–4. Sports and Other Activities Predisposing to Ocular Injuries and the Types of Such Injuries

Activities	Injuries
Sports	Hyphema
Racquetball	Raised intraocular pressure
Squash	Blowout fracture
Baseball	Commotio retinae
Hockey	Vitreous hemorrhage
	Retinal break
	Macular hole
	Corneal laceration
	Globe rupture
Objects	
Champagne Corks	
Pressurized containers	
Sharp objects (scissors, pencils, darts)	
Firearms and explosives	
BB/pellet guns	
Fireworks	
Assault	

Nonoccupational Injuries

The marked reduction in the incidence of severe ocular and facial damage associated with car windshield injuries as a result of legislation requiring the wearing of seatbelts demonstrates the effectiveness of such regulations. Similar attempts to reduce the incidence of injuries from fireworks by limiting their availability have not yet been as successful.

Various sports and other activities are notorious for the high incidence of severe injuries to the eye (Table 20–4). Protective, toughened plastic glasses with refractive correction are available to lower risk in certain situations.

Acute keratitis from **ultraviolet irradiation,** such as seen after exposure to a welding arc, may also occur during skiing if protective goggles are not worn. People wearing contact lenses and with previous history of eye diseases are more vulnerable. Prevention of the keratitis is best achieved with sunglasses with sidepieces and goggles with polarized or photochromic lenses. The role of long-term exposure to ultraviolet light in the etiology of age-related macular degeneration is still debated. There is substantial evidence linking ultraviolet exposure to the development of cataract. However, since ultraviolet exposure occurs from the time of birth, the benefit of regular use of ultraviolet filters in spectacle lenses or sunglasses as a preventive measure has not been demonstrated. The role of ultraviolet light exposure in the etiology of certain corneal disorders—particularly pterygium—and of basal cell carcinoma and melanoma of the eyelids is widely accepted. Education of the public about the dangers of skin cancer following prolonged sun exposure is

very important. Ultraviolet-blocking skin creams should not be used around the eyes, and for that reason, reliance must be placed on avoiding unnecessary exposure to the sun or the use of sunglasses. In patients with xeroderma pigmentosum, the eyelids and bulbar conjunctiva frequently develop carcinomas and melanomas, and their development can be minimized, if not prevented entirely, by protective lenses.

Solar retinitis (eclipse retinopathy) is a specific type of radiation injury that usually occurs after solar eclipses as a result of direct observation of the sun without an adequate filter. Under normal circumstances, sun-gazing is difficult because of the glare, but cases have been reported in young people who have suffered self-inflicted macular damage by deliberate sun-gazing, perhaps while under the influence of drugs. The optical system of the eye behaves as a strong magnifying lens, focusing the light onto a small spot on the macula, usually in one eye only, and producing a thermal burn. The resulting edema of the retinal tissue may clear with minimal loss of function, or it may cause significant atrophy of the tissue and produce a defect that is visible ophthalmoscopically. A permanent central scotoma then results. Eclipse retinopathy can easily be prevented by the use of adequate filters when observing eclipses.

Similar to eclipse retinopathy is the iatrogenic retinal damage that may occur from use of the operating microscope, indirect ophthalmoscope (photic retinopathy), and misdirected recreational laser. The risk of damage from the operating microscope can be reduced by the use of filters to block both ultraviolet light and the blue portion of the visible spectrum, light barriers such as an opaque disk placed on the cornea, or air injected into the anterior chamber.

PREVENTION OF ACQUIRED OCULAR INFECTION

Infections are a major cause of preventable ocular morbidity. Preventive measures are based on maintenance of the integrity of the normal barriers to infection and avoidance of inoculation with pathogenic organisms. The pathogenicity of various organisms and the size of the inoculum required to establish infection vary enormously according to the state of the eye. Most organisms enter the eye through a defect in the ocular surface or via the bloodstream, but some organisms are able to penetrate intact corneal epithelium (Table 20–5). A compromised eye is highly susceptible to infection.

Table 20–5. Organisms Able to Penetrate Intact Corneal Epithelium

Acanthamoeba species	*Neisseria gonorrhea*
Corynebacterium diphtheria	*Neisseria meningitides*
Haemophilus aegyptius	*Shigella* species
Listeria monocytogenes	*Serratia marcescens*

The major barrier to exogenous ocular infection is the epithelium of the cornea and conjunctiva. This can be damaged directly by trauma, including surgical trauma and contact lens wear, or by the secondary effects of other abnormalities of the outer eye, such as lid abnormalities or tear deficiency. In all such situations, particular care must be taken to avoid or recognize secondary infection in its earliest stages.

In the presence of a corneal or conjunctival epithelial defect, particularly when there is an associated full-thickness wound of the cornea or sclera, it is essential to use prophylactic antibiotic therapy and most importantly to make certain that any drops or ointments are sterile. Accidental epithelial injury should be avoided whenever possible, particularly in compromised eyes, such as in exophthalmic eyes with exposure, abnormal eyelid function from facial palsy, or eyes with corneal anesthesia. The classic situation is the combination of fifth and seventh nerve dysfunction such as occurs after surgery for cerebellopontine angle tumor, producing a dry, anesthetic eye with poor eyelid closure. Any comatose patient is also at risk of corneal exposure, and prophylactic ocular lubrication and possibly eyelid taping should be undertaken.

Any unnecessary exposure of the eye to pathogenic organisms should be avoided, but it becomes critical in certain situations. During intraocular surgery, the normal barriers to infection are circumvented, and meticulous attention must be paid to avoiding contamination of the eye with organisms. The ocular environment must be assessed preoperatively to identify and treat any sources of pathogenic organisms. These include colonization or infection of the lacrimal sac; the lid margins, which are frequently colonized by *Staphylococcus epidermidis*—a major cause of endophthalmitis after cataract surgery; the conjunctiva; and the cornea. Considerations may need to be given to other sites of bacterial colonization or infection, such as the bladder, throat, nose, and skin. In emergency situations, it may only be possible to identify such sources and use prophylactic antibiotic therapy to reduce the chances of subsequent infection, whereas for elective surgery, more definitive therapy to eradicate or minimize the pathogenic organisms should be possible. In patients with no identifiable external ocular disease, immediate preoperative instillation of povidone iodine into the conjunctival sac has been shown to be beneficial, and postoperative antibiotics are presumed to be important. Intraocular injection of cefuroxime at the conclusion of cataract surgery reduces the risk of postoperative endophthalmitis, but the correct formulation must be used to avoid corneal damage. Whether inclusion of antibiotic, such as vancomycin, in the infusion fluid during cataract surgery is appropriate continues to be debated. Sterility of the operative field, instruments, intraocular and topical medications, and other fluids introduced into the eye must be ensured. During the postoperative period, sterile medications must be used and contact with other patients with established ocular infections avoided.

Contact lens wear is strongly associated with suppurative keratitis due to the combination of an abnormal load of pathogenic organisms and probable recurrent minor trauma to the corneal epithelium. The incidence of suppurative keratitis is particularly high with soft lenses, especially with extended wear. Overnight wear increases the risk five-fold compared to daily wear with regular replacement. It is apparent that many people wearing contact lenses for cosmetic reasons are not aware of the risks involved. Whereas it may be reasonable to face the risks of infection with extended-wear soft lenses in elderly aphakes who are dependent on contact lenses for refractive correction and cannot cope with daily wear lenses, or in patients with highly compromised eyes that are symptomatic from bullous keratopathy, the arguments in favor of extended-wear soft lenses for refractive correction in patients with low refractive errors are less strong. A number of patients in this latter group start off their contact lens career using extended-wear disposable lenses, which is of course an attractive arrangement because it dispenses with the need for lens cleaning and the associated paraphernalia, but this practice is likely to require an unwelcome sacrifice of safety for convenience. The use of preservative-free solutions, multipurpose solutions, and no rub formulas may have increased the chances of suppurative keratitis by providing less antimicrobial activity. Epidemics of *Fusarium* and *Acanthamoeba* keratitis have been related to particular contact lens solutions.

All contact lens wearers must be apprised of the relative risk of suppurative keratitis and the need for meticulous contact lens hygiene and avoidance of overnight wear or continuing to use lenses beyond their disposal time. Many do not realize that many ocular infections are contracted in swimming pools and hot tubs, with chlorine levels not being adequate to kill protozoa like *Acanthamoeba*; thus, contact lenses should be removed in these situations. All contact lens wearers should be advised to keep a pair of spectacles available so that contact lens wear can be discontinued immediately whenever an eye becomes uncomfortable or inflamed. If ocular discomfort or inflammation persists, the wearer should seek ophthalmologic advice without delay.

In developing countries where contact lens wear is uncommon, the greatest risk factor for corneal ulceration is trauma, usually experienced in the course of everyday agricultural activities. These undocumented abrasions are now recognized as the cause of a "silent epidemic" of corneal ulceration that is a major cause of monocular vision loss in those regions. Studies in India have shown that both bacterial and fungal ulcers that occur after corneal abrasion can be prevented by the application of an antibiotic ointment three times a day for 3 days in the injured eye. The biological mechanism for fungal ulcer prevention by an antibiotic is not readily understood.

Neonatal conjunctivitis (see Chapter 17) is a good example of exposure to a heavy load of pathogenic organisms with the added inherent susceptibility of the poorly developed immune mechanisms of the neonatal eye. The major organisms that may produce neonatal conjunctivitis are *Neisseria gonorrhoeae,* chlamydiae, herpes simplex, *Staphylococcus aureus, Haemophilus* species, and *Streptococcus pneumoniae.* Exposure to these organisms occurs during passage down the birth canal. It should be possible to prevent neonatal conjunctivitis by treating mothers harboring these organisms prior to delivery, and this has been achieved for the bacteria, including *Chlamydia.* The alternative approach is the routine ocular prophylaxis of neonates. This started with the silver nitrate prophylaxis of Credé and has been superseded in a number of centers by topical erythromycin in view of the predominance of chlamydial neonatal conjunctivitis. Neonatal gonococcal infection can rapidly lead to corneal perforation such that urgent treatment with intravenous ceftriaxone is important.

PREVENTION OF IATROGENIC OCULAR AND NONOCULAR INFECTION

Ophthalmologists have been clearly implicated in the transmission of infectious eye disease. Outbreaks of **epidemic keratoconjunctivitis** have been traced to contamination within the hospital or ophthalmologist's office. The adenovirus is transmitted via hands, a tonometer, or solutions contaminated by droppers accidentally rubbed against the infected conjunctiva or lid margin of a patient. Contaminated ophthalmic solutions have also been the source of infection in bacterial corneal ulcers and endophthalmitis following intraocular surgery. Spread of infection can be reduced by infection control policies. A study from the United Kingdom demonstrated a reduction in the proportion of adenovirus infections that were hospital acquired from 48.4% to 22.7% at 12 months and 3.4% at 24 months after new infection control policy, including separate waiting and examination areas and expediting examination of suspected cases. *Pseudomonas aeruginosa* used to be a common contaminant of ophthalmic solutions, particularly fluorescein. Instillation of contaminated fluorescein solution to delineate corneal epithelial defects (eg, after removal of a corneal foreign body) may result in severe keratitis and, frequently, loss of the eye.

The ophthalmologist should be alert to the possibility of transmission by ophthalmic instruments or, in donor cornea or sclera, of agents responsible for nonocular infection, including hepatitis B virus, human immunodeficiency virus (HIV), and prions. Applanation tonometer tips may be adequately sterilized with respect to many infectious agents, including hepatitis B virus, HIV, herpes simplex virus, and adenovirus, by wiping with 70% isopropyl alcohol swabs and then allowing the instrument to dry by evaporation. It is imperative that the tonometer tip be completely dry before use on the next patient or corneal epithelial damage

will result. However, this method of sterilization is probably not effective against prions, for which immersion in hypochlorite, which is less practical and more likely to damage the tonometer tip, resulting in corneal injury, is required. In this case, the tonometer tip should be rinsed in tap water and dried before use. Immersion in hypochlorite at the end of each working day and after examination of high-risk patients is a possible compromise. Many ophthalmologists have changed to routine or as-required use of disposable tonometer tips, which provide reliable results. The noncontact tonometer is recommended for reducing the risks of disease transmission, but it may generate an aerosol spray that endangers the individual operating the tonometer. Goldmann three-mirror and similar contact lenses used for patient examination are also susceptible to damage from immersion in hypochlorite, and use of disposables is not always feasible. Ophthalmologists must maintain the highest level of personal hygiene at all times and must use standard sterile technique when appropriate, keeping in mind the possibility of contamination of any solution brought into contact with the eye.

Hands play a major role in the transmission of infection. They should be washed or disinfected (eg, with isopropyl alcohol) before and after the examination of every patient, especially if an ocular infection is thought to be present.

PREVENTION OF OCULAR DAMAGE DUE TO CONGENITAL INFECTIONS

Viral disease of the mother with resultant embryopathy may lead in the offspring to many damaging ocular conditions (eg, microphthalmos, retinopathy, infantile glaucoma, iridocyclitis, cataract), and in some cases, prevention may be possible. Two viruses, rubella and cytomegalovirus, can be extremely damaging to the infant; however, rubella virus can be prevented by vaccination. Once a common childhood disease, universal vaccination in developed countries has rendered rubella essentially eradicated in this part of the world. However, it still poses a risk in the developing world and areas where vaccination is refused. If a mother contracts rubella during early pregnancy, she should be informed of the likelihood of ocular and other abnormalities in her baby, and the arguments for and against abortion should be presented. Unfortunately, cytomegalovirus continues to be a serious and unsolved threat, potentially causing life- and sight-threatening complications. No protective vaccine is available, although one is under study. At present, early diagnosis and treatment with intravenous and intravitreal ganciclovir is the best way to prevent complications.

Toxoplasmosis is another important cause of congenital infection, leading to (1) chorioretinitis; (2) cerebral or cerebellar calcification; (3) hydrocephalus; and, occasionally, (4) more severe central nervous system abnormalities. Unless the mother is immunocompromised, fetal infection occurs only if she acquires primary infection during pregnancy, with a 40% risk of transmission to the fetus. Maternal infection can be prevented by eating only meat that is well cooked, by washing vegetables and fruits, and by wearing gloves when disposing of cat litter or working in the garden so that contact with viable oocysts and tissue cysts is avoided. It has been shown that if acute maternal infection during pregnancy is identified with serologic testing, appropriate antibiotic treatment as early as the 15th week of gestation reduces the incidence of congenital infection and improves the clinical outcome in fetuses that are infected.

Herpes simplex virus 2 (HSV-2) infection is a sexually transmitted disease, with a 50% risk of transmission to the neonate if the mother has active genital infection at the time of delivery. Women who acquire HSV-2 as a primary infection in the second half of pregnancy, rather than prior to pregnancy, are at greatest risk of transmitting the virus. An additional risk factor for neonatal HSV infection is the use of a fetal-scalp electrode. HSV-2 infection causes not only ocular disease (vesicular eyelid lesions, conjunctivitis, keratitis, cataract, or retinochoroiditis), but also disseminated infection, which has 75% mortality.

If primary genital infection is acquired during the first two trimesters, repeated viral cultures of genital secretions should be carried out from the 32nd week of gestation. If two consecutive cultures are negative and there are no active herpetic genital lesions at the time of delivery, it is safe to perform a vaginal delivery. If primary genital infection is acquired during the third trimester of pregnancy, guidelines are unclear, but the current recommendation is to perform elective cesarean section.

Pregnant women with a first clinical episode or recurrent infection, particularly within a few weeks of delivery, may be treated with acyclovir or valacyclovir. Neither drug is approved for treatment of pregnant women. No increase in fetal abnormalities has been attributed so far to such treatment.

PREVENTION OF GENETIC DISEASE WITH OCULAR INVOLVEMENT

The genetic nature of many disorders that affect the eye is now recognized and their transmission better understood. Diseases such as retinitis pigmentosa, retinoblastoma, or neurofibromatosis and their genetic predisposition are of crucial importance when parents are considering conception.

Prenatal diagnosis, with the option of abortion if the diagnosis is made sufficiently early, is available for an increasing number of conditions. Postnatal screening to facilitate early diagnosis is also important when there is a relevant family history. For example, children at risk of retinoblastoma should be examined every 6 months until the age of 5 or 6 or until genetic testing has been performed.

PREVENTION OF OCULAR DAMAGE DUE TO SYSTEMIC DISEASES

It is important for nonophthalmologic practitioners, particularly internists, general practitioners, and pediatricians, to be aware of the systemic diseases that have avoidable ophthalmic consequences.

Diabetic retinopathy is the most common cause of blindness developing between ages 20 and 64 in developed countries. Treatment is available to prevent such vision loss, but for best effect, it must be administered before visual loss has occurred; that is, diabetics must undergo regular fundal examination and be referred whenever treatment is indicated. Even more important is prevention of development of diabetic retinopathy, which is dependent on optimization of blood sugar, blood pressure, serum lipids, and renal function.

Occasional cases of **vitamin A deficiency**, potentially leading to visual loss due to photoreceptor dysfunction or due to xerophthalmia with associated corneal disease (keratomalacia), still occur. In developing countries, where nutrition is often poor, xerophthalmia is still common. Worldwide, the usual cause of vitamin deficiency is poor diet associated with poverty (see earlier in the chapter). Other causes are poor absorption from the gastrointestinal tract due to gastrointestinal disease, bowel resection, or bariatric surgery, weight-reducing diets, dietary management of food allergy, and chronic alcoholism. Because of the ocular manifestations (night blindness, Bitot's spots, and a lackluster corneal epithelium), the ophthalmologist may be the first to recognize vitamin A deficiency. Early recognition and treatment can prevent loss of vision. Treatment of the acute condition may require large intramuscular doses of vitamin A followed by corrective diet and careful analysis of all possible causes. Individuals at risk of deficiency, such as due to severe gastrointestinal disease or following bowel resection or bariatric surgery, should be prescribed prophylactic vitamin A supplementation.

PREVENTION OF VISUAL LOSS DUE TO DRUGS

It is the ophthalmologist's responsibility to prevent visual loss or major ocular disability from drugs used to treat eye diseases. Topical **corticosteroids** predispose to bacterial keratitis and exacerbate herpes simplex keratitis. Long-term use of topical, oral, or inhaled corticosteroids may lead to open-angle glaucoma and posterior subcapsular cataract. **Topical anesthetics** should never be prescribed or made available for long-term use because severe corneal ulceration and scarring may result. **Preservatives** in eye drops are commonly the cause of allergic reactions and, with long-term use, may cause a cicatrizing conjunctivitis similar to cicatricial pemphigoid (see Chapter 5).

Many drugs used **systemically** have serious ocular side effects and may cause conditions such as Stevens-Johnson syndrome (erythema multiforme), angle-closure glaucoma, optic neuropathy, and retinopathy (see Chapter 22). For this reason, the ophthalmologist must take a careful history of the patient's use of drugs as part of the initial examination.

EARLY DETECTION OF TREATABLE OCULAR DISEASE

Early diagnosis and treatment markedly improve the visual outcome of many ophthalmic conditions. For some, such as suppurative keratitis, acute angle-closure glaucoma, neovascular age-related macular degeneration, retinal detachment, and giant cell arteritis, the crucial factor is the recognition by health care workers and advice to patients of the importance of seeking ophthalmological assessment as soon as visual symptoms occur. Other conditions may have minimal symptoms or findings in the early stages. Unfortunately, this may be when treatment might be most effective, and routine screening may be indicated. It needs to be established, however, that screening is effective both in terms of cost and its impact on the course of disease.

▶ Primary Open-Angle Glaucoma

Primary open-angle glaucoma is a major cause of preventable vision loss worldwide, particularly among individuals of African or Caribbean racial origin. About 2 million Americans have the disease, although half are undiagnosed. The prevalence of primary open-angle glaucoma increases from 0.1% for those age 40–49 to 5% for those over age 75. Symptoms do not usually occur until there is advanced visual field loss. For treatment to be effective, the disease must be detected at a much earlier stage. Screening programs are hampered by the high prevalence of raised intraocular pressure in the absence of glaucomatous visual field loss (ocular hypertension), which is 10 times more common than primary open-angle glaucoma; the high frequency of normal intraocular pressure on a single reading in untreated open-angle glaucoma; and the complexities of screening for optic disk or visual field abnormalities. Nevertheless, the best means of detecting primary open-angle glaucoma early is annual tonometry and optic disk assessment of adults and first-degree relatives of affected individuals with referral to an ophthalmologist of all those with relevant abnormalities. Examination of all individuals over age 50 every 3–5 years may also be worthwhile, particularly in high-risk populations.

▶ Diabetic Retinopathy

As already discussed (see earlier in the chapter), in developed countries, diabetic retinopathy is the leading cause of new blindness among adults age 20–65 years. It is present in about 40% of diagnosed diabetic patients, and its prevalence is particularly increasing in individuals age 65 years or older. Retinopathy increases in prevalence and severity with increasing duration and poorer glycemic control. In type 1 diabetes, retinopathy is not detectable for at least 3 years after diagnosis. In type 2 diabetes, retinopathy is present in up to 20% of patients at diagnosis and may be the presenting feature. Diabetic retinopathy is broadly classified as **nonproliferative** or **proliferative** with or without maculopathy. To reduce the risk of permanent visual loss, the main abnormalities to which screening programs are directed are new vessel formation, particularly on the optic disk, and exudates around the macula. Screening programs generally rely on review of at least annual fundal photographs following pupil dilation, with referral to an ophthalmologist when vision-threatening abnormalities are detected. More frequent screening is needed during pregnancy. Any diabetic developing visual loss should be referred for ophthalmic assessment. (See Chapters 10 and 15.)

▶ Retinopathy of Prematurity

Retinopathy of prematurity is the consequence of disturbance of the retinal vascularization that normally occurs in utero during the latter half of pregnancy. The main risk factors are decreased gestational age and low birth weight. It has been estimated to result in 400–600 new cases of infant blindness each year in the United States (see Chapter 17). In many cases, retinopathy of prematurity regresses spontaneously, but laser treatment for severe active disease is beneficial. It is recommended that all babies younger than 30 weeks of gestational age, with a birth weight of 1500 g or less, or who receive supplemental oxygen therapy undergo regular screening from 2–4 weeks after birth until the retina is fully vascularized in both eyes, any retinopathy of prematurity has regressed, or any necessary treatment has been completed.

▶ Amblyopia ("Lazy Eye")

Amblyopia literally means poor vision but is generally used to mean reduced visual acuity in excess of that explained by structural, ocular, or visual pathway disease. Central vision develops from birth to age 8, after which time further development is unlikely to occur. The formation of the necessary neural structures and connections for development of central vision is dependent on normal visual experience. The common entities preventing this are **strabismus**, impairing binocular function, and unequal refractive error (**anisometropia**), causing a less well-focused retinal image in one eye. The consequence is preferential development of central vision in the fixing or more focused eye and hindered central vision in the fellow eye. Media opacity, marked refractive error, or severe ptosis can also result in amblyopia.

Amblyopia is treated by correction of the inciting cause and then patching of the dominant eye. A crucial determinant of treatment success is how early the amblyopia is detected and treated.

Routine neonatal examinations should include assessment of red reflex to identify media opacity. This should also include screening for strabismus via the cover-uncover test. Any child observed to have strabismus after the age of 3 months should be seen by an ophthalmologist. All preschool children should have their visual acuity tested. **Photorefraction**, which relies on assessment of the red reflex from each eye, is useful in screening for anisometropia, ametropia, astigmatism, and strabismus in preschool children.

Parents should be made aware of the importance of reporting strabismus, abnormal ocular appearance, or poor visual performance, particularly if there is a relevant family history. Visual acuity testing can be performed at home with the illiterate "E" chart, which is sometimes known as the "Home Eye Test." Abnormalities of the red reflex on photographs may alert parents to ocular abnormalities.

▶ Juvenile Idiopathic Arthritis

Uveitis associated with oligoarticular juvenile idiopathic arthritis, which generally occurs in girls with positive antinuclear antibodies, is typically asymptomatic in its early stages and often remains undetected until severe loss of vision due to glaucoma, cataract, or band keratopathy has already occurred. Regular ophthalmic screening every 6 months should take place.

REFERENCES

Causes of Vision Loss

Abdull MM et al: Causes of blindness and visual impairment in Nigeria: The Nigeria National Blindness and Visual Impairment Survey. Invest Ophthalmol Vis Sci 2009;50:4114. [PMID: 19387071]

Bastawrous A et al: Six-year incidence of blindness and visual impairment in Kenya: The Nakuru Eye Disease Cohort Study. Invest Ophthalmol Vis Sci 2016;57:5974. [PMID: 27820953]

Bourne RR et al: Number of people blind or visually impaired by glaucoma worldwide and in world regions 1990-2010: A meta-analysis. PLoS One 2016;11:e0162229. [PMID: 27764086]

Bowen M et al: The Prevalence of Visual Impairment in People with Dementia (the PrOVIDe study): A cross-sectional study of people aged 60–89 years with dementia and qualitative exploration of individual, carer and professional perspectives. Southampton (UK): NIHR Journals Library 2016 Jul. [PMID: 27489923]

Chong CF et al: A cross-sectional study of prevalence and etiology of childhood visual impairment in Auckland, New Zealand. Asia Pac J Ophthalmol (Phila) 2014;3:337. [PMID: 26107975]

Correia C et al: Global sensory impairment in older adults in the United States. J Am Geriatr Soc 2016;64:306. [PMID: 26889840]

Eckert KA et al: A simple method for estimating the economic cost of productivity loss due to blindness and moderate to severe visual impairment. Ophthalmic Epidemiol 2015;22:349. [PMID: 26395661]

Fenwick EK et al: Association of vision impairment and major eye diseases with mobility and independence in a Chinese population. JAMA Ophthalmol 2016;134:1087. [PMID: 27467140]

Fenwick EK et al: Vision impairment and major eye diseases reduce vision-specific emotional well-being in a Chinese population. Br J Ophthalmol 2016 Aug 26. [Epub ahead of print] [PMID: 27565988]

Frick KD et al: The global burden of potential productivity loss from uncorrected presbyopia. Ophthalmology 2015;122:1706. [PMID: 26190438]

Gain P et al: Global survey of corneal transplantation and eye banking. JAMA Ophthalmol 2016;134:167. [PMID: 26633035]

GBD 2015 Disease and Injury Incidence and Prevalence Collaborators: Global, regional, and national incidence, prevalence, and years lived with disability for 310 diseases and injuries, 1990-2015: A systematic analysis for the Global Burden of Disease Study 2015. Lancet 2016;388:1545. [PMID: 27733282]

Holden BA et al: Nearly 1 billion myopes at risk of myopia-related sight-threatening conditions by 2050: Time to act now. Clin Exp Optom 2015;98:491. [PMID: 26769175]

Khairallah M et al: Number of people blind or visually impaired by cataract worldwide and in world regions, 1990 to 2010. Invest Ophthalmol Vis Sci 2015;56:6762. [PMID: 26567788]

Kyari F et al: Prevalence of blindness and visual impairment in Nigeria: The National Blindness and Visual Impairment Study. Invest Ophthalmol Vis Sci 2009;50:2033. [PMID: 19117917]

Leasher JL et al: Global estimates on the number of people blind or visually impaired by diabetic retinopathy: A meta-analysis from 1990 to 2010. Diabetes Care 2016;39:1643. [PMID: 27555623]

Lee CM et al: The global state of cataract blindness. Curr Opin Ophthalmol 2017;28:98-103. [PMID: 27820750]

Lindfield R et al: Outcome of cataract surgery at one year in Kenya, the Philippines and Bangladesh. Br J Ophthalmol 2009;93:875. [PMID: 19211611]

Mariotti SP et al: Trachoma: Global magnitude of a preventable cause of blindness. Br J Ophthalmol 2009;94:563. [PMID: 19098034]

Mohammadpour M et al: Trachoma: Past, present and future. J Curr Ophthalmol 2016;28:165. [PMID: 27830198]

Naidoo KS et al: Global vision impairment and blindness due to uncorrected refractive error, 1990-2010. Optom Vis Sci 2016;93:227. [PMID: 26905537]

Ozturk T et al: Changing trends over the last decade in the aetiology of childhood blindness: A study from a tertiary referral centre. Br J Ophthalmol 2016;100:166. [PMID: 26159454]

Pan CW et al: Visual impairment among older adults in a rural community in Eastern China. J Ophthalmol 2016;2016:9620542. [PMID: 27777793]

Park SJ et al: Burden of visual impairment and chronic diseases. JAMA Ophthalmol 2016;134:778. [PMID: 27196876]

Pascolini D et al: Global estimates of visual impairment: 2010. Br J Ophthalmol 2012;96:614. [PMID: 22133988] (Also available at: http://www.who.int/blindness/GLOBALDATAFINALforweb.pdf)

Paul P et al: Prevalence and visual outcomes of cataract surgery in rural South India: A cross-sectional study. Ophthalmic Epidemiol 2016;23:309. [PMID: 27552313]

Rondinelli RD et al (eds): *Guides to the Evaluation of Permanent Impairment*, 6th ed. American Medical Association, 2008.

Senjam SS et al: Prevalence of visual impairment due to uncorrected refractive error: Results from Delhi-Rapid Assessment of Visual Impairment Study. Indian J Ophthalmol 2016;64:387. [PMID: 27380979]

Taylor HR: The global issue of vision loss and what we can do about it: José Rizal Medal 2015. Asia Pac J Ophthalmol (Phila) 2016;5:95. [PMID: 26939111]

Ting DS et al: Diabetic retinopathy: Global prevalence, major risk factors, screening practices and public health challenges: a review. Clin Exp Ophthalmol 2016;44:260. [PMID: 26716602]

Varma R et al: Visual impairment and blindness in adults in the United States: Demographic and geographic variations from 2015 to 2050. JAMA Ophthalmol 2016;134:802. [PMID: 27197072]

Varma R et al: Prevalence and causes of visual impairment and blindness in Chinese American adults: The Chinese American Eye Study. JAMA Ophthalmol 2016;134:785. [PMID: 27196952]

World Health Organization: Change to the definition of blindness. Available at http://www.who.int/blindness/Change%20 the%20Definition%20of%20Blindness.pdf. Accessed February 19, 2010.

Zhu RR et al: Prevalences and causes of vision impairment in elderly Chinese: A socioeconomic perspective of a comparative report nested in Jiangsu Eye Study. Int J Ophthalmol 2016;9:1051. [PMID: 27500116]

Prevention of Visual Loss

Allen UD et al: Prevention and management of neonatal herpes simplex virus infections. Paediatr Child Health 2014;19:201. [PMID: 24855418]

American Academy of Pediatrics; Section on Ophthalmology; American Association for Pediatric Ophthalmology and Strabismus; American Academy of Ophthalmology; American Association of Certified Orthoptists: Red reflex examination in neonates, infants, and children. Paediatrics 2008;122:1401. [PMID: 19047263]

Andersen N et al: The Danish Registry of Diabetic Retinopathy. Clin Epidemiol 2016;8:613. [PMID: 27822108]

Au CP et al: Efficacy and cost-effectiveness of intracameral vancomycin in reducing postoperative endophthalmitis incidence in Australia. Clin Exp Ophthalmol 2016;44:803. [PMID: 27311743]

Blanchet K et al: A need for more equity in prevention of blindness. Ophthalmic Epidemiol 2015;22:293. [PMID: 26395655]

Boodhna T et al: More frequent, more costly? Health economic modelling aspects of monitoring glaucoma patients in England. BMC Health Serv Res 2016;16:611. [PMID: 27770792]

Carnt N et al: Strategies for the prevention of contact lens-related Acanthamoeba keratitis: A review. Ophthalmic Physiol Opt 2016;36:77. [PMID: 26691018]

Committee on Public Health Approaches to Reduce Vision Impairment and Promote Eye Health (US): Making eye health a population health imperative: Vision for tomorrow. National Academies Press (US); 2016. [PMID: 27656731]

Cope JR et al: Acanthamoeba keratitis among rigid gas permeable contact lens wearers in the United States, 2005 through 2011. Ophthalmology 2016;123:1435. [PMID: 27117780]

Cope JR et al: Contact lens-related corneal infections: United States, 2005-2015. MMWR Morb Mortal Wkly Rep 2016;65:817. [PMID: 27538244]

DeBuc DC: The role of retinal imaging and portable screening devices in tele-ophthalmology applications for diabetic retinopathy management. Curr Diab Rep 2016;16:132. [PMID: 27841014]

Du Toit N et al: Randomised controlled trial of prophylactic antibiotic treatment for the prevention of endophthalmitis after open globe injury at Groote Schuur Hospital. Br J Ophthalmol 2016 Oct 28. [Epub ahead of print] [PMID: 27793818]

Ellerton JA et al: Eye problems in mountain and remote areas: Prevention and onsite treatment—Official recommendations of the International Commission for Mountain Emergency Medicine ICAR MEDCOM. Wilderness Environ Med 2009;20:169. [PMID: 19594215]

Haring RS et al: Epidemiologic trends of chemical ocular burns in the United States. JAMA Ophthalmol 2016;134:1119. [PMID: 27490908]

Haring RS et al: Epidemiology of sports-related eye injuries in the United States. JAMA Ophthalmol 2016;134:1382. [PMID: 27812702]

Haugen OH et al: Visual impairment in children and adolescents in Norway. Tidsskr Nor Laegeforen 2016;136:996. [PMID: 27325032]

Healy SA et al: Primary maternal herpes simplex virus-1 gingivostomatitis during pregnancy and neonatal herpes: Case series and literature review. J Pediatric Infect Dis Soc 2012;1:299. [PMID: 26619423]

Hendler K et al: Refractive errors and amblyopia in the UCLA Preschool Vision Program: First year results. Am J Ophthalmol 2016;172:80. [PMID: 27640004]

Hoskin AK et al: Eye injury prevention for the pediatric population. Asia Pac J Ophthalmol (Phila) 2016;5:202. [PMID: 27183290]

Jabbarvand M et al: Endophthalmitis occurring after cataract surgery: Outcomes of more than 480 000 cataract surgeries, epidemiologic features, and risk factors. Ophthalmology 2016;123:295. [PMID: 26704882]

Jovanovic N et al: Prevalence and risk factors associated with work-related eye injuries in Bosnia and Herzegovina. Int J Occup Environ Health 2016;22:325. [PMID: 27813453]

Karim-Zade K et al: Pediatric eye trauma in the Republic of Tajikistan: More than meets the eye. Ophthalmic Epidemiol 2016;23:331. [PMID: 27340930]

Massey J et al: Notes from the field: Health care-associated outbreak of epidemic keratoconjunctivitis–West Virginia, 2015. MMWR Morb Mortal Wkly Rep 2016;65:382. [PMID: 27078721]

Mehravaran S et al: The UCLA preschool vision program, 2012-2013. J AAPOS 2016;20:63. [PMID: 26917075]

Moon S et al: Analysis on sports and recreation activity-related eye injuries presenting to the Emergency Department. Int J Ophthalmol 2016;9:1499. [PMID: 27803871]

Mu Y et al: Performance of spot photoscreener in detecting amblyopia risk factors in Chinese pre-school and school age children attending an eye clinic. PLoS One 2016;11:e0149561. [PMID: 26882106]

Pawiroredjo JC et al: The cataract situation in Suriname: An effective intervention programme to increase the cataract surgical rate in a developing country. Br J Ophthalmol 2017;101:89. [PMID: 27836828]

Pineda R: Corneal transplantation in the developing world: Lessons learned and meeting the challenge. Cornea 2015;34:S35. [PMID: 26266438]

Pinninti SG et al: Preventing herpes simplex virus in the newborn. Clin Perinatol 2014;41:945. [PMID: 25459782]

Pratt B et al: Occupational injuries in Canadian youth: An analysis of 22 years of surveillance data collected from the Canadian Hospitals Injury Reporting and Prevention Program. Health Promot Chronic Dis Prev Can 2016;36:89. [PMID: 27172126]

Ramke J et al: Equity and blindness: Closing evidence gaps to support universal eye health. Ophthalmic Epidemiol 2015;22:297. [PMID: 26395657]

Ruão M et al: Photoscreening for amblyogenic risk factors in 1-year-olds: Results from a single center in Portugal over a 9-year period. J AAPOS 2016;20:435. [PMID: 27647116]

Sanchez I et al: Advantages, limitations, and diagnostic accuracy of photoscreeners in early detection of amblyopia: A review. Clin Ophthalmol 2016;10:1365. [PMID: 27555744]

Scheetz J et al: Accuracy and efficiency of orthoptists in comprehensive pediatric eye examinations. Am Orthopt J 2016;66:98. [PMID: 27799583]

Schmier JK et al: An updated estimate of costs of endophthalmitis following cataract surgery among Medicare patients: 2010-2014. Clin Ophthalmol 2016;10:2121. [PMID: 27822008]

Tailor V et al: Childhood amblyopia: Current management and new trends. Br Med Bull 2016;119:75. [PMID: 27543498]

Tang Y et al: Prevalence of age-related cataract and cataract surgery in a Chinese adult population: The Taizhou Eye Study. Invest Ophthalmol Vis Sci 2016;57:1193. [PMID: 26975031]

Tranos P et al: Current perspectives of prophylaxis and management of acute infective endophthalmitis. Adv Ther 2016;33:727. [PMID: 26935830]

Yardley AE et al: Paediatric ocular and adnexal injuries requiring hospitalisation in Western Australia. Clin Exp Optom 2016 Oct 20. [Epub ahead of print] [PMID: 27762442]

Zhu Z et al: Cataract-related visual impairment corrected by cataract surgery and 10-year mortality: The Liwan Eye Study. Invest Ophthalmol Vis Sci 2016;57:2290. [PMID: 27127927]

Optics & Refraction

21

Paul Riordan-Eva, FRCOphth

GEOMETRIC OPTICS

▶ Speed, Frequency, & Wavelength of Light

Speed, frequency, and wavelength of light are related by the following expression:

$$\text{Frequency} = \frac{\text{Speed}}{\text{Wavelength}}$$

In different optical media, speed and wavelength of light change, but frequency is constant. Color depends on frequency, so that the color of a ray of light is not altered as it passes through optical media except by selective non-transmittance or fluorescence. The optical characteristics of a substance can only be defined with respect to clearly specified frequencies of light. A substance to be used for lenses to refract visible light is usually tested with the yellow sodium light (D line) and the blue (F line) and the red (C line) of a rarefied hydrogen discharge tube.

In a vacuum, the speed of all frequencies of light is the same (approximately 3×10^8 meters per second). Since the frequency of the yellow D line is approximately 5×10^{14} Hz, the wavelength of this line in a vacuum is approximately 6×10^{-7} m (0.6 μm). Similarly, the wavelengths in a vacuum of the blue F and red C lines are approximately 5 and 7×10^{-7} m, respectively.

▶ Index of Refraction

If the speed of a light ray is altered by a change in the optical medium, refraction of the ray will also occur (Figure 21–1). The effect of an optical substance on the speed of light is expressed as its index of refraction, n; the higher the index, the slower the speed and the greater the effect on refraction.

In a vacuum, n has the value 1.00000. The **absolute index of refraction** of a substance is the ratio of the speed of light in a vacuum to the speed of light in the substance. The **relative index of refraction** of a substance is calculated with reference to the speed of light in air. The absolute index of refraction of air is about 1.0003. In optics, n is assumed to be relative to air unless specified as absolute.

▶ Thermal Coefficient of Index of Refraction

The index of refraction increases with increasing temperature of the medium, but the rate of change varies from one medium to another, being approximately 150 times greater for plastic and aqueous than for glass. This makes plastic undesirable for precision optical devices. In the human eye, the problem is overcome by the maintenance of a steady temperature.

▶ Dispersion of Light

In all media besides a vacuum, the index of refraction is different for each color (frequency), being larger at the blue end and smaller at the red end of the spectrum. This difference can be quantified as the dispersion value, V:

$$V = \frac{n_D - 1}{n_F - n_C},$$

where n_D, n_F, and n_C are the indices of refraction for the yellow sodium line and the blue and the red hydrogen lines.

The higher the value of V, the lesser is the dispersion of colors. Table 21–1 gives the indices of refraction and some dispersion values for substances of ophthalmologic interest.

▶ Transmittance of Light

Optical materials vary in their transmittance or transparency to different frequencies. Some "transparent" materials such as glass are almost opaque to ultraviolet light. Red glass would be almost opaque to the green frequency. Optical media must

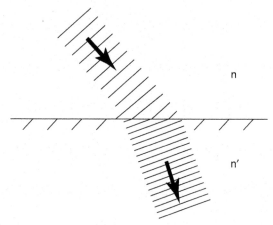

▲ **Figure 21-1.** Refraction of light as it enters a transparent medium of higher refractive index n′.

be selected according to the specific wavelength of light with which they are to be used.

Laws of Reflection & Refraction (Figure 21–2)

1. Incident, reflected, and refracted rays all reside in a plane known as the plane of incidence, which is normal (at a right angle) to the interface.

2. For reflection, relative to the normal, the angles of reflection and incidence are equal.

3. For refraction, the product of the index of refraction of the medium of the incident ray and the sine of the angle of incidence of the incident ray is equal to the product of the same terms of the refracted ray (designated by a prime): $n \sin I = n' \sin I'$ (Snell's law).

4. A ray of light passing from one point to another follows the path that takes the least time to negotiate (Fermat's principle). Optical path length is the index of refraction times the actual path length.

▶ Critical Angle & Total Reflection

In the example of refraction in Figure 21–2, the arriving ray is in the less-dense medium (air) and is refracted toward the normal within the denser medium (glass). Conversely, if the arriving ray were in the denser medium, it would be refracted away from the normal. In this situation, as the angle of incidence is increased, the critical angle is reached when the light is totally reflected (total internal reflection) and the sine of the incident ray in the denser medium reaches the value n′/ n. Total internal reflection obeys the laws of regular reflection, allowing perfect reflection without coatings and being used extensively in fiberoptics.

For aqueous ($n = 1.34$), the critical angle is 48° [$\sin 48° = 1/1.34$]. In Figure 21–3, the shaded area is not directly visible from the surface, explaining why visualization of the anterior chamber angle of the eye requires a gonioscopy lens (see Chapter 2). (The index of refraction of the aqueous, not the index of refraction of the tears or cornea, is the determining factor in this context.)

Table 21–1. Indices of Refraction and Dispersion Values of Some Substances of Ophthalmologic Interest

Substance (20°C unless noted)	Indices of Refraction (n_D)	Dispersion Values (V)
Water	1.333	
Water 37°C	1.331	56
Sea water	1.34	
Sea water, 11,000 m depth	1.36	
Polymethylmethacrylate	1.492	57
Polymethylmethacrylate 37°C	1.489	
Acrylonitrile styrene copolymer	1.57	35
Polystyrene	1.59	31
Fluorite	1.43	95
Spectacle crown glass	1.52	59
Flint glass	1.62	37
Aqueous and vitreous 37°C	1.34	56
Hydroxyethylmethacrylate (HEMA)	1.43	
Cellulose acetate butyrate (CAB)	1.47	
Silicone	1.44	

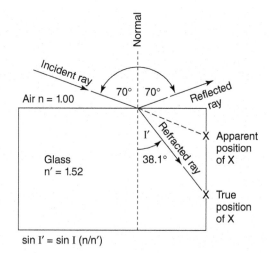

$\sin I' = \sin I \ (n/n')$

▲ **Figure 21-2.** Examples of the laws of reflection and refraction.

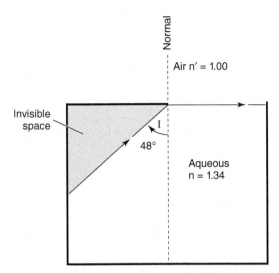

▲ **Figure 21–3.** Example of the critical angle.

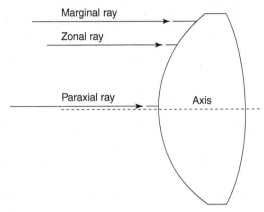

▲ **Figure 21–4.** Illustration of three rays traced in the trigonometric method.

CALCULATIONS USED IN OPTICS

There are two approaches to the application of the principles of geometric optics to single lenses and compound lens systems. The **trigonometric method** is more valid and exact, as it makes no assumptions other than those already determined by the laws of refraction. The **algebraic method** is based on a number of assumptions that greatly simplify calculation of the effects of various lenses but also limit accuracy to an ever-increasing extent as the lens systems become more complex. The algebraic method cannot be relied on for accurate results, particularly in the assessment of the optical effects of contact lenses, intraocular lenses, and keratorefractive procedures.

Certain considerations are universal whichever method is used. For any optical system, the object and its image are said to lie in **conjugate planes.** If the object were to be placed in the plane of its own image, the optical system would produce its new image in the original object plane. Thus, the effects of any optical system will be the same for whichever direction light travels through the system. Each optical system has an infinite number of pairs of conjugate planes. Corresponding points on conjugate planes are known as **conjugate points.**

▶ Trigonometric Method

The trigonometric method mathematically plots the course of certain specified rays through the lens systems. The three rays most frequently plotted are shown in Figure 21–4. The zonal ray represents the average luminous flux of light passing through the lens. At each refracting surface, the change in direction of each of these rays is calculated according to the principles of Snell's law.

The trigonometric method provides an exact determination of the point of focus and information on the quality of the image formed by a lens system. The difference between the back focal lengths (distance along the optical axis from the last refracting surface to the point of focus) of the marginal and paraxial rays is a measure of the "spread of focus," thus indicating the degree of **spherical aberration** (see later in the chapter). Similarly, if rays of different color (frequency), with their different indices of refraction in each medium, are plotted through the system, the degree of **chromatic aberration** (see later in the chapter) will be determined. The optical pathway is the sum of the actual distance a ray passes through the substances multiplied by the index of refraction in the various substances through which it passes. The brightness and contrast of the final image are determined by how closely the optical pathways of the marginal and paraxial rays match.

▶ Algebraic Method

The algebraic method generally assumes that lenses are "infinitely thin," placed close together, and of small diameter, such that any angle will be so small that the size of the angle measured in radians will have the same value as the sine of the angle and that the sine and the tangent of the angle can be assumed to be the same. The results are the **thin lens equations** used by opticians to calculate curves for lenses. "Fudge factors" derived from experience are then necessary to correct for the inaccuracies of these equations.

Use of the algebraic method depends on certain definitions. The position of the lens, reduced to a single line, is the **principal plane,** which intersects the optical axis at the **nodal point** (optical center). The **primary focal point (F)** is that point along the optical axis where an object must be placed to form an image at infinity. The **secondary focal point (F′)** is that point along the optical axis where parallel incident rays

$$\text{Lens power} \cong \frac{1}{\text{Focal length}} \cong \frac{1}{\text{Distance of image}} - \frac{1}{\text{Distance of object}}$$

$$\text{Lens power} \cong (n-1)\ \frac{1}{\text{Front surface radius}} - \frac{1}{\text{Back surface radius}}$$

$$\frac{\text{Size of image}}{\text{Distance of image}} \cong \frac{\text{Size of object}}{\text{Distance of object}}$$

$$\text{Magnification} = \frac{\text{Size of image}}{\text{Size of object}} \cong \frac{\text{Distance of image}}{\text{Distance of object}}$$

Power for Several Lenses Combined

$$\text{Total power} \cong \text{Power}_1 + \text{Power}_2 + \text{Power}_3,\ \text{etc}$$

▲ **Figure 21–5.** Algebraic thin lens approximations. All lengths in meters.

are brought to a focus. If the medium on either side of the lens is of the same refractive index, the distance between the nodal point and each of the focal points, the **focal length,** is the same.

Figure 21–5 shows some of the important thin lens equations.

The **diopter (D)** is a measure of lens power derived from the algebraic method. It is defined as the reciprocal of the focal length of a lens in air measured in meters. Diopters are additive, but only for low-power lenses. The result of combining lenses of high power varies greatly with their thickness and the separation distance. High-power lenses must be described by three values: (1) radii of curvature, (2) index of refraction, and (3) thickness.

The algebraic method treats a high-power lens as if there are two nodal points and two principal planes (n and n′ and H and H′ in Figure 21–6). The nodal points lie on the principal planes only if the refractive medium is the same on either side of the lens. The true focal lengths are measured from the principal planes to the focal points, but the front and back focal lengths—essential to the prescription of corrective lenses—are measured from the respective surfaces of the lens to the focal points. The reciprocal of the back focal length corresponds to the back vertex power as measured with a lensometer.

For contact lenses, a derivation of the thin lens equations (using 1.34 for the index of refraction as it is determined by the aqueous) provides an approximate relationship between power (diopters) and radius of curvature (meters):

$$\text{Power} \approx \frac{(n-1)}{r} = \frac{1.34-1}{r} = \frac{0.34}{r}$$

$$\text{and r (in millimeters)} \approx \frac{340}{\text{Power}}$$

For making high plus contact lenses or thick-spectacle lenses, according to the algebraic method, the equation for lens power (diopters) is:

$$\text{Power} \cong \frac{1}{F} \cong (n-1)\left[\frac{1}{r_1} - \frac{1}{r_2} - \frac{(n-d)d}{nr_1r_2}\right]$$

where F = focal length, r_1 = front surface radius, r_2 = back surface radius, and d = thickness of lens, all measured in meters, and n = refractive index.

The ray tracing method commonly described in ophthalmic optics texts is a graphic representation of the algebraic method (in contrast to true graphic ray tracing, which is a graphic representation of the trigonometric method). Rays are traced through the optical system to connect conjugate points. The positions of the conjugate planes are derived mathematically from the thin lens equations. The size and orientation of the object are then determined by tracing the central ray, which passes straight through the tip of the image, the nodal point of the lens (without being refracted), and the tip of the object. The rays that traverse the focal points of the lens are derived by extrapolation (Figure 21–7).

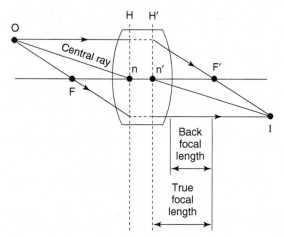

▲ **Figure 21–6.** Description of a high-power lens in the algebraic method.

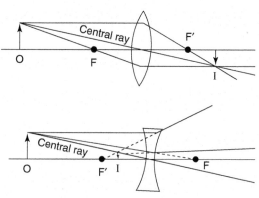

▲ **Figure 21–7.** Ray tracing through plus and minus lenses.

For multiple lens systems, the conjugate planes and the path of the central ray are determined for each lens in succession, producing an image that becomes the object for the next lens until the size and orientation of the final image is located. In the case of a thick lens, refraction occurs at the principal planes of the lens, the position of rays being translated from one principal plane to another without any change in their vertical separation from the optical axis (Figure 21–6). The central ray passes from the tip of the object to the first nodal point and then emerges from the second nodal point parallel to its original direction to reach the tip of the image. When the media on either side of the lens have different refractive indices, the nodal points do not coincide with the principal planes.

Magnification

Linear magnification is the ratio of the height of the image to the height of the object. For an infinitely thin lens in air—as assumed by the algebraic method—this ratio is equal to the ratio of the distance of the image to the distance of the object. For real lens systems, such as those of the eye, a more complex equation including the index of refraction of the initial and final media must be used. The trigonometric method quickly provides other information necessary for the calculation.

Change of Vertex Distance

If the vertex distance (the distance from the eye) of a lens of given power is altered, the effective power of the lens will also change. To calculate a new lens that will have the same effect at the new distance, a derivation of the thin lens equations can be used:

$$Power_2 \approx \frac{1}{\dfrac{1}{Power_1} - (D_1 - D_2)}$$

where $Power_1$ and $Power_2$ are the old and new lens powers (diopters) and D_1 and D_2 are the old and new vertex distances (meters), respectively.

Example 1: A + 13 diopter lens at 11 mm (0.011 m) is to be replaced by a lens at 9 mm (0.009 m).

$$Power_2 \cong \frac{1}{\dfrac{1}{13} - (0.011 - 0.009)} \cong 13.4 \text{ diopters}$$

Example 2: Same lens to be replaced by a contact lens ($D_2 = 0$).

$$Power_2 \cong \frac{1}{\dfrac{1}{13} - (0.011)} \cong 15.2 \text{ diopters}$$

This vertex equation is also an approximation and should not be used for intraocular lens calculations, but it is useful for conversion from spectacle to contact lens powers.

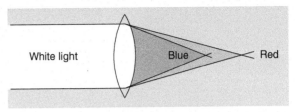

Figure 21–8. Chromatic aberration of lenses.

Aberrations of Spherical Lenses

Spherical lenses are subject to a number of aberrations that reduce the quality of image produced. The variation of refractive index with frequency of light (dispersion) results in greater refraction of blue than red light (**chromatic aberration**) (Figure 21–8). Marginal rays are refracted more than paraxial rays, producing **spherical aberration** (Figure 21–9). **Coma,** a characteristic comet-shaped blur, is the result of spherical aberration of light originating away from the optical axis of the lens. When light traverses a spherical lens obliquely, there is an additional cylindrical lens effect—**astigmatism of oblique incidence. Curvature of field** is the production of a curved image from a flat object. Prismatic effects of the lens periphery also cause image distortion. Achromatic lenses may be made by cementing together plus and minus lenses of different refractive indices. The nonchromatic aberrations are overcome by combining or shaping lenses to reduce the power of the lens periphery, by restricting the area of the lens used to the paraxial zones, and by use of meniscus lenses.

Cylindrical Lenses

A **planocylindrical lens** (Figure 21–10) has one flat surface and one cylindrical surface, resulting in no optical power in the meridian of its axis and maximum power 90° away and forming a line image, parallel to the axis of the lens, from a point object. The ophthalmic convention for specifying the orientation of the meridian of the axis of a cylindrical lens is shown in Figure 21–11.

In a **spherocylindrical** lens, the cylindrical surface is curved in two meridians but not to the same extent. In ophthalmic lenses, these principal meridians are at 90° to each other. The effect of a spherocylindrical lens on a point object is to produce a geometric figure known as the **conoid of Sturm** (Figure 21–12), consisting of two focal lines separated by the interval of Sturm. The position of the focal lines relative to the lens is determined by the power of the two meridians and their orientation by the angle between the meridians. Cross-sections through the conoid of Sturm reveal lines at the focal lines and generally ellipses elsewhere. In one position, the cross-section will be a circle that represents the **circle of least confusion.**

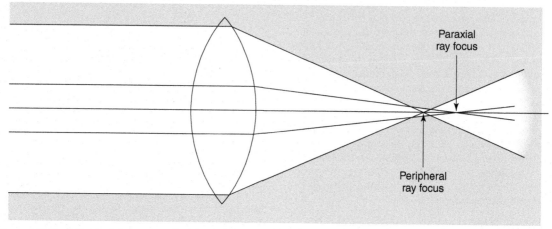

▲ **Figure 21–9.** Spherical aberration of a biconvex lens.

A spherocylindrical lens can be thought of as a combination of a spherical lens and a planocylindrical lens. It can then be specified by the orientation of principal meridians and the power acting in each (Figure 21–13). In a cross diagram, the arms are drawn parallel to the principal meridians and labeled with the relevant power. In longhand notation, the cylinder is specified by the orientation of its axis, which is 90° away from the meridian of maximum power.

Writing prescriptions for spherocylindrical lenses uses longhand notation, and the lens can be specified in either plus or minus cylinder form (Figure 21–13). To transpose between these forms: (1) algebraically sum the original sphere and cylinder; (2) reverse the sign of the cylinder; and (3) change the axis of the cylinder by 90°.

If their principal meridians correspond, combinations of spherocylindrical lenses can be summed mathematically. Otherwise, trigonometric formulas are required. Alternatively, the power of such combinations can be determined by placing them together in a lensometer. The principal meridians of any such combination will be 90° apart.

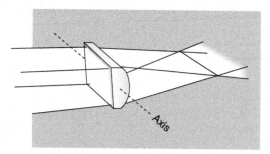

▲ **Figure 21–10.** A planocylindrical lens with axis in the horizontal meridian.

▶ Prisms

A prism consists of a transparent material with nonparallel flat surfaces. In cross-section, it has an apex and a base. The prism is specified by its power and the orientation of its base.

A prism refracts light toward its base, whereas an object seen through a prism appears deviated toward the apex of the prism. The amount of deviation varies according to the tilt of the prism, that is, the angle of incidence of the light. For glass prisms, calibration is performed in the **Prentice position,** in which the incident light is perpendicular to the face of the prism (Figure 21–14). For plastic prisms and in general optics, a prism is calibrated in the **position of minimum deviation,** in which the amount of refraction at the two surfaces of the prisms is equal (Figure 21–14). When prisms are used in clinical practice, these orientations must be adhered to for accurate results.

For a glass prism in the Prentice position, the incident rays are not refracted at the first surface because they are perpendicular to one another (Figure 21–15). At the second surface, the angle of incidence is the same as the apex angle of the prism (A). If I′ is the angle of the final refracted ray, from Snell's law, sin I′ = (n/n′) sin A, with n being the refractive index of the prism and n′ the refractive index of the surrounding medium. For example, if the prism is of glass with n = 1.523 and A = 30°, then sin I′ is 1.523 × 0.5, or 0.7615. I′ is 49.6°. The angle of deviation is I′ – A, or 19.6°.

The power of a prism is measured in prism diopters (PD). One prism diopter deviates an image 1 cm at 1 m (Figure 21–16). The arc tangent of 1/100 is 0.57°. Therefore, 1 PD produces an angle of deviation of almost one-half degree. The "rule of thumb" is that a prism of 2 PD produces an angle of deviation of 1°, but this cannot be applied to prisms of more than 100 PD.

Prisms are used in ophthalmology both to measure and to treat heterotropia and heterophoria. The orientation of

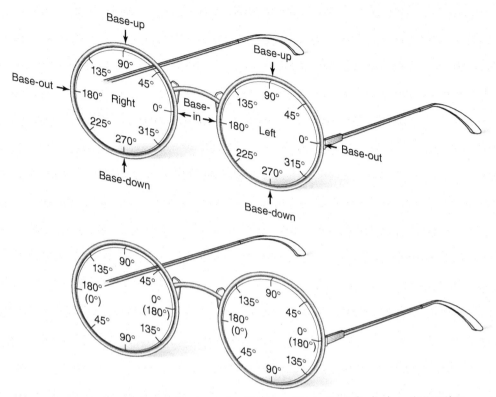

▲ **Figure 21–11. Top:** Illustration of prism base notation. **Bottom:** Illustration of cylinder axis notation.

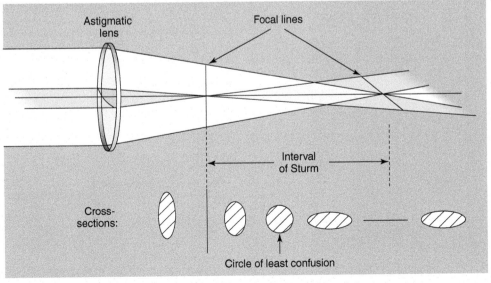

▲ **Figure 21–12.** The conoid of Sturm, formed by light refracted by an astigmatic lens.

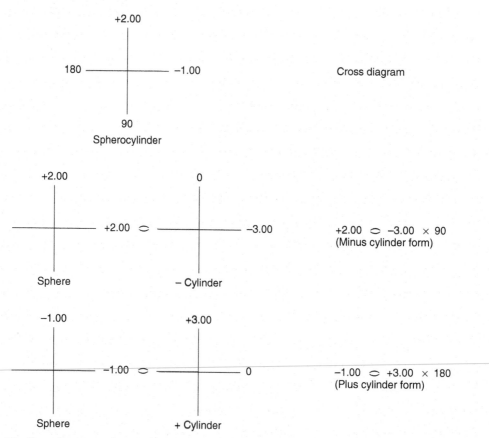

▲ **Figure 21–13.** Cross diagram and equivalent combinations, including longhand notations, for a spherocylindrical lens.

a prism's base is indicated by its direction, usually descriptively, that is, "base-up right eye," "base-down left eye," "base-in" or "base-out," or occasionally by a mathematical system (Figure 21–11).

Fresnel prisms are lightweight plastic prisms consisting of narrow, parallel strips of prism with the same apex angle as the desired single prism (Figure 21–17). They are available as press-on prisms for attachment to the back of spectacle lenses, providing an easily adjusted temporary prismatic correction that is less heavy than conventional glass prisms. Their disadvantages are the image degradation due to light scatter and dirt within the grooves.

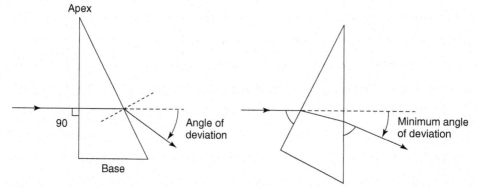

▲ **Figure 21–14.** Calibration of prisms. Glass prisms and spectacle prisms are calibrated according to the Prentice position, whereas plastic prisms are calibrated according to the position of minimum deviation.

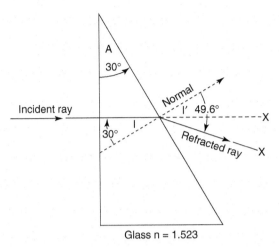

▲ **Figure 21–15.** Example of the prism as used in ophthalmology.

Prismatic Effect of Spherical Lenses

Spherical lenses have increasing prismatic power as the light path moves away from the optical center of the lens. The amount of prism power can be calculated from Prentice's rule, which states that the prism power in prism diopters is equal to the dioptric power of the lens in diopters multiplied by the displacement from the optical center in centimeters. For example, at 0.5 cm away from the optical center of a 6-diopter lens, the prismatic power is 3 PD. Plus lenses produce prism power with the base oriented toward the optical center of the lens, and minus lenses produce prism power with the base oriented away from their optical center.

The prismatic effect of spherical lenses is an important consideration in the correction of anisometropia. Appropriate spectacle lenses may produce significant vertical prismatic deviation when the peripheral portions of the lenses are used. This occurs mainly when the patient attempts to read. The prismatic effect can be overcome by adopting a chin-down position, thus using the optical centers of the lenses once again, by grinding of a compensatory prism into the reading segment of the glasses (**slab-off prism**) or by changing to contact lenses.

If a prism needs to be incorporated into a patient's spectacle correction, such as in the control of hypertropia, it may be achieved by decentration of the spherical lens rather than by addition of a prism to the spherical component.

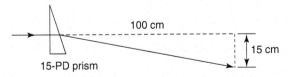

▲ **Figure 21–16.** Power of a prism in prism diopters.

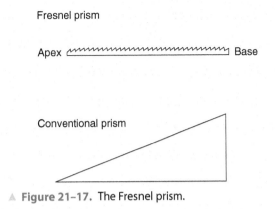

▲ **Figure 21–17.** The Fresnel prism.

Rapid Detection of Lens Characteristics

The nature of a spherical lens may be rapidly detected by looking through it 0.5 m (20 in) or so from the eye and moving the lens at right angles to the visual axis. The image seen through a minus (concave) lens will tend to move *with* the lens. The same test with a plus (convex) lens causes the image to tend to move *away from* the direction of motion. This effect is due to the prismatic effect of the periphery of the lens. The power of the lens can be approximated by neutralization of these movements by lenses of known power. A cylindrical lens shows changing distortion of the image when the lens is rotated about the visual axis. (Spherical lenses do not.) The orientations of the lens in which the image is clearest indicate the principal meridians. The power in each of the principal meridians can then be determined by the method described above for spherical lenses. A prism is recognized by deviation of the image as the static lens is viewed through its center.

OPTICS & THE EYE

Many attempts have been made to simplify the optical system of the human eye, particularly using the thick lens equations of the algebraic method of optical calculations. Much has been made of the concept that the image on the retina is formed by two lens elements, the cornea contributing about 43 D and the lens the remaining 19 D, but this is a gross oversimplification. The **schematic eye of Gullstrand** and its reduced form (Figure 21–18) are models from which mathematical values for the optical characteristics of the eye were derived. For instance, in the reduced schematic eye, the cornea is assumed to be the only refracting surface, the principal plane (H) being placed at its apex and a single nodal point (n) at its center of curvature. The globe has an axial length of 22.5 mm, and the refractive index of the eye is said to be 1.33. Unfortunately, these numbers have become accepted by many as true physiologic values rather than as the convenient mathematically derived values they really are. The refractive index of aqueous is about 1.3337 (for the sodium D line at 37°C).

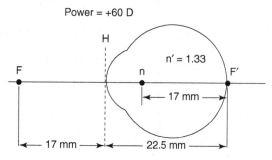

Power = +60 D

▲ **Figure 21–18.** The reduced schematic eye.

Trigonometric ray tracing demonstrates that the optical system of the human eye is more accurately conceptualized as a three-lens system: the aqueous lens, the crystalline lens, and the vitreous lens (Figure 21–19). Contrary to popular belief, the cornea itself has almost no power of refraction in the optical system but is important only in shaping the anterior curve of the aqueous lens. The crystalline lens is an interesting optical component because its index of refraction varies throughout its thickness rather than being constant, as assumed in most optical calculations. The vitreous lens is particularly important because of its major effect on magnification.

Reassessment of models for the optical system of the human eye is essential now that much of ophthalmic surgery, whether it is cataract surgery, keratorefractive procedures, or vitreous surgery, produces profound effects on individual

components of the system. Gullstrand's models, in which the system is assumed to function as an integrated unit, cannot be applied under such circumstances.

▶ **Accommodation**

The eye changes refractive power to focus on near objects by a process called accommodation. Study of Purkinje images, which are reflections from various optical surfaces in the eye, has shown that accommodation results from changes in the crystalline lens. Contraction of the ciliary muscle results in thickening and increased curvature of the lens, probably due to relaxation of the lens capsule.

▶ **Visual Acuity**

Assessment of visual acuity with the Snellen chart is described in Chapter 2. The average resolving power of the normal human eye is 1 minute of arc. Since the Snellen letters are made from squares of 5×5 units (Figure 21–20), the 20/20-size letter has a visual angle of 5 minutes of arc at 20 ft. This is equivalent to 8.7 mm (0.35 in) width and height. The eye minifies an image at 20 ft by about 350 times. Therefore, the size of the 20/20 letter on the retina is 0.025-mm high and wide. This is equivalent to a resolution capacity of 100 lines per millimeter. For a 6-mm pupil and light of wavelength 0.56 μm (in air), the absolute theoretic limit would be 345 lines per millimeter.

REFRACTIVE ERRORS

Emmetropia is absence of refractive error, and **ametropia** is the presence of refractive error.

▶ **Presbyopia**

The loss of accommodation that comes with aging to all people is called **presbyopia** (Table 21–2). A person with

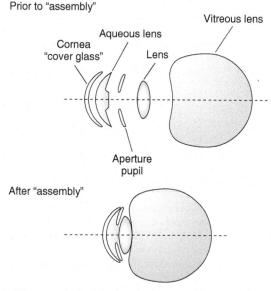

▲ **Figure 21–19.** The optical system of the eye, illustrating the three-lens concept.

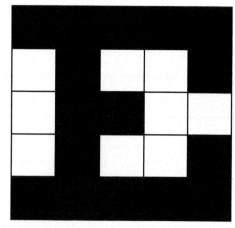

▲ **Figure 21–20.** Snellen block E.

Table 21–2. Table of Accommodation

Age (years)	Mean Accommodation (diopters)
8	13.8
25	9.9
35	7.3
40	5.8
45	3.6
50	1.9
55	1.3

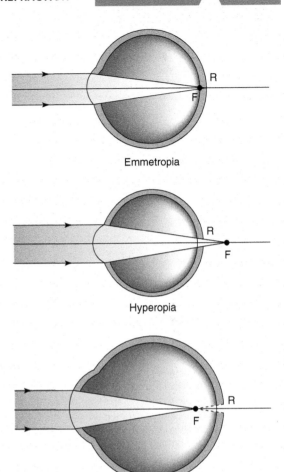

▲ **Figure 21–21.** Spherical refractive errors as determined by the position of the secondary focal point with respect to the retina.

emmetropic eyes (no refractive error) will begin to notice inability to read small print or discriminate fine close objects at about age 44–46. This is worse in dim light and usually worse early in the morning or when the subject is fatigued. These symptoms increase until about age 55, when they stabilize but persist.

Presbyopia is corrected by use of a plus lens to make up for the lost automatic focusing power of the lens. The plus lens may be used in several ways. Reading glasses have the near correction in the entire aperture of the glasses, making them fine for reading but blurred for distant objects. Half-glasses can be worn to abate this nuisance by leaving the top open and uncorrected for distance vision. Bifocals do the same but allow correction of other refractive errors. Trifocals correct for distance vision by the top segment, the middle distance by the middle section, and the near distance by the lower segment. Progressive power (varifocal) lenses similarly correct for far, middle, and near distances but by progressive change in lens power rather than stepped changes.

▶ **Myopia**

When the image of distant objects focuses in front of the retina in the unaccommodated eye, the eye is myopic, or nearsighted (Figure 21–21). If the eye is longer than average, the error is called axial myopia. (For each additional millimeter of axial length, the eye is approximately 3 diopters more myopic.) If the refractive elements are more refractive than average, the error is called curvature myopia or refractive myopia. As the object is brought closer than 6 m, the image moves closer to the retina and comes into sharper focus. The point reached where the image is most sharply focused on the retina is called the "far point." One may estimate the extent of myopia by calculating the reciprocal of the far point. Thus, a far point of 0.25 m would suggest a 4-diopter minus lens correction for distance. The myopic person has the advantage of being able to read at the far point without glasses even at the age of presbyopia. A high degree

of myopia results in greater susceptibility to degenerative retinal changes, including retinal detachment.

Concave spherical (minus) lenses are used to correct the image in myopia. These lenses move the image back to the retina.

▶ **Hyperopia**

Hyperopia (hypermetropia, farsightedness) is the state in which the unaccommodated eye would focus the image behind the retina (Figure 21–21). It may be due to reduced axial length (axial hyperopia), as occurs in certain congenital disorders, or reduced refractive error (refractive hyperopia), as exemplified by aphakia.

Hyperopia is a more difficult concept to explain than myopia. The term "farsighted" contributes to the difficulty, as does the prevalent misconception among laymen that presbyopia is farsightedness and that one who sees well far away is farsighted. If hyperopia is not too great, a young person may obtain a sharp distant image by accommodating, as a normal eye would to read. The young hyperopic person may also make a sharp near image by accommodating more—or much more than one without hyperopia. This extra effort may result in eye fatigue that is more severe for near work. The degree of hyperopia a person may have without symptoms is variable. However, the amount decreases with age as presbyopia (decrease in ability to accommodate) increases. Three diopters of hyperopia might be tolerated in a teenager but will require glasses later, even though the hyperopia has not increased. If the hyperopia is too high, the eye may be unable to correct the image by accommodation. The hyperopia that cannot be corrected by accommodation is termed manifest hyperopia. This is one of the causes of deprivation amblyopia in children and can be bilateral. There is a reflex correlation between accommodation and convergence of the two eyes. Hyperopia is therefore a frequent cause of esotropia (crossed eyes) and monocular amblyopia (see Chapter 12).

▶ Latent Hyperopia

As explained above, a prepresbyopic person with hyperopia may obtain a clear retinal image by accommodation. The degree of hyperopia overcome by accommodation is known as latent hyperopia. It is detected by refraction after instillation of cycloplegic drops, which determines the sum of both manifest and latent hyperopia. Refraction with a cycloplegic is very important in young patients who complain of eyestrain when reading and is vital in esotropia, where full correction of hyperopia may achieve a cure.

Remember that a moderately "farsighted" person may see well for near or far when young. However, as presbyopia comes on, the hyperope first has trouble with close work—and at an earlier age than the nonhyperope. Finally, the hyperope has blurred vision for near *and far* and requires glasses for both near and far.

▶ Astigmatism

In **astigmatism**, the eye produces an image with multiple focal points or lines. In **regular astigmatism,** there are two principal meridians, with constant power and orientation across the pupillary aperture, resulting in two focal lines. The astigmatism is then further defined according to the position of these focal lines with respect to the retina (Figure 21–22). When the principal meridians are at right angles and their axes lie within 20° of the horizontal and vertical, the astigmatism is subdivided into **astigmatism with the rule,** in which the greater refractive power is in the vertical meridian, and **astigmatism against the rule,** in which the greater refractive power is in the horizontal meridian. Astigmatism with the rule is more commonly found in younger patients,

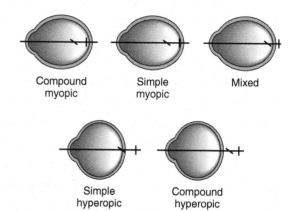

▲ **Figure 21–22.** Types of regular astigmatism as determined by the positions of the two local lines with respect to the retina.

and astigmatism against the rule is found more commonly in older patients (Figure 21–23). **Oblique astigmatism** is regular astigmatism in which the principal meridians do not lie within 20° of the horizontal and vertical. In **irregular astigmatism,** the power or orientation of the principal meridians changes across the pupillary aperture.

The usual cause of astigmatism, particularly irregular astigmatism, is abnormalities of corneal shape. The crystalline lens may also contribute. In contact lens terminology, lenticular astigmatism is called residual astigmatism because it is not corrected by a spherical hard contact lens, which does correct corneal astigmatism.

Regular astigmatism often can be corrected with cylindrical lenses, frequently in combination with spherical lenses, or sometimes more effectively by altering corneal shape with rigid contact lenses, which are usually the only optical means of managing irregular astigmatism. Because the brain is capable of adapting to the visual distortion of an uncorrected astigmatic error, new glasses that do correct the error may cause temporary disorientation, particularly an apparent slanting of images.

▶ Natural History of Refractive Errors

Most babies are slightly hyperopic, with mean refractive error at birth being 0.5 D. The hyperopia slowly decreases, with a slight acceleration in the teens, to approach emmetropia. The corneal curvature is much steeper (6.59-mm radius) at birth and flattens to nearly the adult curvature (7.71 mm) by about 1 year. The lens is much more spherical at birth and reaches adult conformation at about 6 years. The mean axial length is short at birth (16.6 mm), lengthens rapidly in the first 2 or 3 years (to 21.8 mm), then moderately (0.4 mm per year) until age 6, and then slowly (about 1 mm total) to stability (24 mm) at about 10 or 15 years. Presbyopia becomes manifest in the fifth decade.

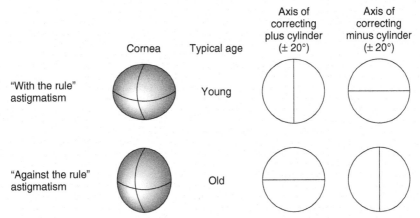

▲ **Figure 21–23.** Types of astigmatism as determined by the orientation of the principal meridians and the orientation of the correcting cylinder axis.

Refractive errors are inherited. The mode of inheritance is complex, as it involves so many variables. Refractive error, although inherited, need not be present at birth any more than tallness, which is also inherited, need be present at birth. For example, a child who reaches emmetropia at age 10 years will probably soon become myopic. Myopia usually increases during the teens. Factors influencing progression of myopia are poorly defined but probably include close work. Optical and pharmacological treatments to retard progression of myopia in children have not yet been shown to have long-term benefit.

▶ Anisometropia

Anisometropia is a difference in refractive error between the two eyes. It is a major cause of amblyopia because the eyes cannot accommodate independently and the more hyperopic eye is chronically blurred. Refractive correction of anisometropia is complicated by differences in size of the retinal images (**aniseikonia**) and oculomotor imbalance due to the different degree of prismatic power of the periphery of the two corrective lenses. Aniseikonia is predominantly a problem of monocular aphakia. Spectacle correction produces a difference in retinal image size of approximately 25%, which is rarely tolerable. Contact lens correction reduces the difference in image size to approximately 6%, which can be tolerated. Intraocular lenses produce a difference of less than 1%.

▶ Correction of Refractive Errors

A. Spectacle Lenses

Spectacles continue to be the safest method of refractive correction. To reduce nonchromatic aberrations, the lenses are made in meniscus form (corrected curves) and tilted forward (pantascopic tilt).

B. Contact Lenses

The first contact lenses were glass fluid-filled scleral lenses. These were difficult to wear for extended periods and caused corneal edema and much ocular discomfort. Hard corneal lenses, made of polymethylmethacrylate, were the first really successful contact lenses and gained wide acceptance for cosmetic replacement of glasses. Subsequent developments include gas-permeable lenses, made of cellulose acetate butyrate, silicone, or various silicone and plastic polymers, and soft contact lenses, made of various hydrogel plastics, all of which provide increased comfort but greater risk of serious complications.

Rigid (hard and gas-permeable) lenses correct refractive errors by changing the curvature of the anterior surface of the eye. The total refractive power consists of the power induced by the back curvature of the lens, the base curve, together with the actual power of the lens due to the difference between its front and back curvatures. Only the second is dependent on the refractive index of the contact lens material. Rigid lenses overcome corneal astigmatism, including irregular astigmatism, by modifying the anterior surface of the eye into a truly spherical shape.

Soft contact lenses, particularly the more flexible forms, adopt the shape of the patient's cornea. Thus, their refractive power resides only in the difference between their front and back curvature, and they correct little corneal astigmatism unless a cylindrical correction is incorporated to make a toric lens.

Contact lens base curves are selected according to corneal curvature, as determined by keratometry or trial fittings. The front curvature is then calculated from the results of overrefraction with a trial contact lens, or from the patient's spectacle refraction as corrected for the corneal plane.

Rigid contact lenses are specifically indicated for the correction of irregular astigmatism, such as in keratoconus. Soft contact lenses are used for the treatment of corneal surface disorders, but for control of symptoms rather than for refractive reasons. All forms of contact lenses are used in the refractive correction of aphakia, particularly in overcoming the aniseikonia of monocular aphakia, and the correction of high myopia, in which they produce a much better visual image than spectacles. However, the vast majority of contact lenses worn are for cosmetic correction of low refractive errors. This has important implications for the risks that can be reasonably accepted in the use of contact lenses. (Further discussion of therapeutic and cosmetic contact lens use, and the associated complications, is given in Chapter 6.)

C. Keratorefractive Surgery

Keratorefractive surgery encompasses a range of methods for changing the curvature of the anterior surface of the eye. The expected refractive effect is generally derived from empirical results of similar procedures in other patients and not based on mathematical optical calculations. Further discussion of the methods and outcome of keratorefractive procedures is included in Chapter 6.

D. Intraocular Lenses

Implantation of an intraocular lens has become the preferred method of refractive correction for aphakia, usually being undertaken at the time of cataract surgery but sometimes deferred in complicated cases. A large number of designs are available, with foldable lenses, made of silicone or hydrogel plastics, which can be inserted into the eye through a small incision, generally being preferred when available and applicable, but rigid lenses, most commonly consisting of an optic made of polymethylmethacrylate and loops (haptics) made of the same material or polypropylene, also still being used. The safest position for an intraocular lens is within an intact capsular bag following extracapsular surgery.

Intraocular lens power was usually determined by the empirical regression method of analyzing experience with lenses of one style in many patients, from which was derived a mathematical formula based on a constant for the particular lens (A), average keratometer readings (K), and axial length in millimeters (L). A simple example is the **SRK (Sanders–Retzlaff–Kraff) equation:**

$$\text{Power IOL} = A - 2.5L - 0.9K$$

A derivation is the SRK II formula. However, regression formulas are now rarely used. Theoretic formulas using a lens constant, keratometer readings, and axial length, together with estimated anterior chamber depth following surgery, include the SRK/T, Haigis, Holladay, and Hoffer Q formulas. Unfortunately, none of these formulas are based on trigonometric ray tracing methods, which do accurately predict the correct power of intraocular lens for an individual patient. However, satisfactory results are generally obtained with selection of the most reliable formula for the particular axial length. Hoffer Q is indicated for short eyes (axial length less than 22 mm), Holladay for relatively long eyes (axial length 24.6–26 mm), and Haigis or SRK/T for especially long eyes (axial length greater than 26 mm). Because there is a tendency to underestimate the required power in eyes that have previously undergone keratorefractive surgery, calculation of the correct intraocular lens is much more difficult in such cases but is assisted by knowledge of refractive error and keratometer readings prior to the refractive surgery.

An additional (piggyback) intraocular lens is sometimes implanted to correct residual refractive error. Intraocular lenses are occasionally inserted without removal of the crystalline lens (phakic intraocular lens) for treatment of refractive error in young individuals without cataract and prior to onset of presbyopia.

E. Clear Lens Extraction for Myopia

Extraction of noncataractous lenses may be undertaken for the refractive correction of moderate to high myopia, with reported outcomes comparable to those achieved with laser keratorefractive surgery. The operative and postoperative complications of intraocular surgery, particularly in high myopia, need to be borne in mind.

METHODS OF REFRACTION

Determination of a patient's refractive correction can be achieved by objective or subjective means and is best accomplished by a combination of the two methods where possible.

▶ Objective Refraction

Objective refraction is performed by retinoscopy, in which a streak of light, known as the **intercept,** is projected into the patient's eye to produce a similarly shaped reflex, the **retinoscopic reflex,** in the pupil (Figure 21–24).

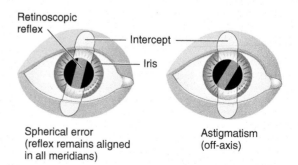

Retinoscopic reflex — Intercept — Iris

Spherical error (reflex remains aligned in all meridians)

Astigmatism (off-axis)

▲ **Figure 21–24.** The retinoscopic reflex.

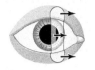 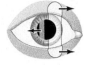

"With"
movement

"Against"
movement

Neutralization

▲ **Figure 21–25.** Movement of the retinoscopic reflex.

Parallel alignment of the intercept and the retinoscopic reflex indicates the presence of only a spherical error, or an additional cylindrical error in which the intercept coincides with one of the principal meridians. Rotation of the projected streak will determine which of these applies and the location of the other principal meridian in the case of a cylindrical error.

The intercept is then swept across the patient's pupil, and the effect on the retinoscopic reflex is noted (Figure 21–25). If it moves in the same direction (**with movement**), plus lenses are placed before the patient's eye; and if it moves in the opposite direction (**against movement**), minus lenses are added—until the pupillary reflex fills the whole pupillary aperture and no movement is detected (**point of neutralization**). When the point of neutralization has been reached, the patient's refractive error has been corrected with an additional correction related to the distance between the patient and examiner (**working distance**). Spherical power equal to the reciprocal of the working distance (measured in meters) is subtracted to compensate for this additional correction and obtain the patient's refractive correction. The working distance is usually 2/3 m, and the correction to be subtracted for the working distance thus is usually 1.5 D.

Automated refractors are available to rapidly determine the objective refraction, but they are not useful in young children or in adults with significant anterior segment disease.

Subjective Refraction

In cooperative patients, subjective refraction produces more accurate results than objective refraction. It relies on the patient's response to alterations in lens power and orientation, using objective refraction or the patient's current refractive correction as the starting point.

The spherical correction is checked by small changes, initially increasing the plus power so as to overcome any accommodative effort, until the clearest image is obtained. The duochrome test of black letters on red and green backgrounds uses the normal chromatic aberration of the eye to refine spherical correction. When the black letters of the two halves of the chart are equally clear, the end point has been reached.

A **cross cylinder** consists of two planocylindrical lenses of equal power but opposite sign superimposed such that their axes of refractive power lie at right angles to one another. This is equivalent to a spherocylindrical lens in which the power of the cylinder is twice the power of the sphere and of the opposite sign. The cross cylinder allows rapid small changes in the axis and power of a cylindrical correction.

Cycloplegic Refraction

In the determination of full hyperopic refractive correction, either in the management of childhood esotropia or the assessment of eyestrain in adult hyperopes, it is necessary to overcome accommodation. This can usually be achieved in adults by fogging techniques in which plus lenses are used to overcome accommodative effort. But otherwise—and always in children—accommodation has to be relaxed by cycloplegic drugs. Cyclopentolate 1%, 1 drop instilled twice 30 minutes prior to refraction, may be sufficient, but atropine 0.5% or 1% ointment, applied twice a day for 3 days, may be necessary in children with dark irides and in the initial assessment of accommodative esotropia. Parents should be warned of the symptoms of atropine toxicity (fever, flushed face, and rapid pulse) and the necessity for discontinuing treatment, cooling the child with sponge bathing, and—in severe cases—seeking urgent medical assistance.

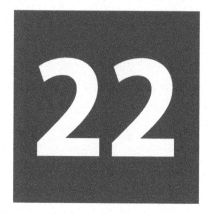

Ophthalmic Therapeutics

Paul Riordan-Eva, FRCOphth, Frederick W. Fraunfelder, MD, MBA, and Lindsey M. McDaniel, MD

22.1 Commonly Used Eye Medications
Paul Riordan-Eva, FRCOphth

The following is a concise formulary of commonly used ophthalmic drugs. Product leaflets, package inserts, and standard pharmacology and toxicology texts should be consulted for more detailed information.

TOPICAL ANESTHETICS

Topical anesthetics are useful for diagnostic and therapeutic procedures, including tonometry, removal of foreign bodies or sutures, gonioscopy, corneal or conjunctival scraping, and minor surgical operations on the cornea and conjunctiva. Cataract (phacoemulsification) surgery is increasingly being carried out under topical anesthesia, supplemented if necessary by (intracameral) injection of local anesthetic into the anterior chamber (see later in the chapter) or oral or intravenous sedation. One or two instillations of topical anesthetic are usually sufficient, but the dosage may be repeated during the procedure.

Proparacaine, tetracaine, and benoxinate are the most commonly used topical anesthetics. For practical purposes, they can be said to have equivalent anesthetic potency. Lidocaine 3.5% gel (Akten) and cocaine 1–4% solution are also used for topical anesthesia.

Note: *Topical anesthetics should never be prescribed for home use, since prolonged application may cause corneal complications and mask serious ocular disease.*

Benoxinate Hydrochloride

Preparation: Solution, 0.4% combined with 0.25% fluorescein sodium (Flurate, Fluress).

Dosage: 1 drop and repeat as necessary.

Onset and duration of action: Anesthesia begins within 1 or 2 minutes and lasts for 10–15 minutes.

Proparacaine Hydrochloride (Proxymetacaine)

Preparations: Solution, 0.5% (Alcaine, Ophthaine, Ophthetic); 0.5% combined with 0.25% fluorescein (Fluoracaine).

Dosage: 1 drop and repeat as necessary.

Onset and duration of action: Anesthesia begins within 20 seconds and lasts 10–15 minutes.

Comment: Least irritating of the topical anesthetics and most suitable for corneal scraping for microbiological cultures.

Tetracaine Hydrochloride (Pontocaine)

Preparation: Solution, 0.5% (Altacaine, Opticaine).

Dosage: 1 drop and repeat as necessary.

Onset and duration of action: Anesthesia occurs within 1 minute and lasts for 15–20 minutes.

Comment: Stings considerably on instillation.

LOCAL ANESTHETICS FOR INJECTION

Lidocaine, mepivacaine, and ropivacaine are shorter-acting local anesthetics for eye surgery. Longer-acting agents are bupivacaine and levobupivacaine. A combination of drugs from the two groups may be used. Local anesthetics are extremely safe when used with discretion, but the physician must be aware of the potential systemic toxic action when rapid absorption occurs from the site of the injection, with excessive dosage, or following inadvertent intravascular injection. When combined with a local anesthetic to prolong the duration of effect, the concentration of epinephrine (adrenaline) should not exceed 1:200,000, particularly in older patients, due to the risk of cardiac arrhythmia. The addition of hyaluronidase encourages spread of local anesthetic and shortens the onset to as little as 1 minute. It is commonly used in peribulbar injections prior to intraocular surgery. For peribulbar and sub-Tenon's injections, 5–10 mL of local anesthetic is usually sufficient, and 15 mL is the maximum volume.

Cataract surgery is commonly performed under topical anesthesia, supplemented by (intracameral) injection of local anesthetic into the anterior chamber, but it is essential that the anesthetic injected into the eye does not contain preservative.

Bupivacaine Hydrochloride

Preparations: Solution, 0.25%, 0.5%, and 0.75% (Marcaine, Sensorcaine); solution, 0.25% with 1 in 200,000 epinephrine, 0.5% with 1 in 200,000 epinephrine.

Dosage: The 0.75% solution is used most frequently. The maximum safe dose for local infiltration in an adult is 150 mg (20 mL of 0.75% solution). Bupivacaine is frequently mixed with an equal amount of lidocaine.

Onset and duration of action: The onset of action is slower than that of lidocaine, but it persists much longer (up to 6–10 hours).

Levobupivacaine Hydrochloride

Preparation: Solution, 0.25%, 0.5%, and 0.75% (Chirocaine)

Dosage: The maximum safe dose for local infiltration in an adult is 150 mg.

Comment: Longer duration of action than bupivacaine.

Lidocaine (Lignocaine) Hydrochloride

Preparations: Solution, 0.5%, 1%, 2%, and 4% (Xylocaine); solution, 0.5% with 1 in 200,000 epinephrine, 1% with 1 in 100,000 epinephrine, 1% with 1 in 200,000 epinephrine, 1.5% with 1 in 200,000 epinephrine, 2% with 1 in 100,000 epinephrine, and 2% with 1 in 200,000 epinephrine (Xylocaine with epinephrine); preservative-free solution, 0.5%, 1%, and 2%.

Dosage: Up to 30 mL of 1% solution, without epinephrine, may be used safely for local anesthesia. The maximum safe dose is 4.5 mg/kg without epinephrine and 7 mg/kg with epinephrine. Intracameral injection requires preservative-free solution.

Comment: Due to its rapid onset and longer action (1–2 hours), lidocaine has become the most commonly used local anesthetic.

Mepivacaine Hydrochloride

Preparations: Solution, 1%, 1.5%, and 2% (Carbocaine, Polocaine).

Dosage: Infiltration and nerve block, up to 20 mL of 1% or 2% solution. The maximum safe dose is 7 mg/kg.

Duration of action: Approximately 2 hours.

Comment: Carbocaine is similar to lidocaine in potency. It is usually used in patients who are allergic to lidocaine.

Ropivacaine Hydrochloride

Preparations: Solution, 0.2%, 0.5%, 0.75%, and 1% (Naropin)

Dosage: Infiltration and nerve block, up to 20 mL of 0.5% or 0.75% solution.

Duration of action: Approximately 2 hours.

MYDRIATICS & CYCLOPLEGICS

Mydriatics dilate the pupil. Cycloplegics paralyze accommodation. They are commonly used singly and in combination, primarily to (1) dilate the pupil to facilitate ophthalmoscopy and intraocular surgery; (2) dilate the pupil and paralyze accommodation, particularly in young patients, as an aid in refraction; and (3) dilate the pupil and paralyze accommodation in uveitis to prevent synechia formation and relieve pain and photophobia. Mydriatics should be used with extreme caution in eyes with narrow anterior chamber angles as they can cause angle-closure glaucoma. Pupil dilation for cataract surgery can be achieved by intracameral injection of mydriatic at the commencement of surgery.

1. MYDRIATICS

Sympathomimetics are mydriatic with no cycloplegic effect.

Phenylephrine Hydrochloride

Preparations: Solution, 0.12%, 2.5%, and 10% (several including Neo-Synephrine).

Dosage: 1 drop and repeat in 5–10 minutes.

Onset and duration of action: The effect usually occurs within 30 minutes after instillation and lasts 2–3 hours.

Comment: Phenylephrine is used both singly and with cycloplegics to facilitate ophthalmoscopy and to dilate the pupil prior to cataract surgery. The 10% solution should not be used in newborn infants, in cardiac patients, or in patients receiving reserpine, guanethidine, or tricyclic antidepressants, because of increased susceptibility to the vasopressor effects.

2. CYCLOPLEGICS

Anticholinergics are mydriatic and cycloplegic.

Atropine Sulfate

Preparations: Solution, 0.5–3%; ointment, 0.5% and 1%.

Dosage: For refraction in children, instill 1 drop of 0.25–0.5% solution in each eye twice a day for 1 or 2 days before the examination and then 1 hour before the examination; ointment, 0.5-cm ribbon twice a day for 2 days prior to examination.

Onset and duration of action: Onset of action is within 30–40 minutes. Maximum effect is reached in about 2 hours. The effect lasts for up to 2 weeks in a normal eye, but in the presence of acute inflammation, the drug must be instilled 2 or 3 times daily to maintain its effect.

Toxicity: Atropine drops must be used with caution to avoid toxic reactions resulting from systemic absorption. Restlessness and excited behavior with dryness and flushing of the skin of the face, dry mouth, fever, inhibition of sweating, and tachycardia are prominent toxic symptoms, particularly in young children.

Comment: Atropine is an effective and long-acting cycloplegic. In addition to its use for cycloplegia in children, atropine is applied topically 2 or 3 times daily in the treatment of iritis. It is also used to maintain a dilated pupil after intraocular surgical procedures.

Scopolamine Hydrobromide

Preparation: Solution, 0.25%.

Dosage: 1 drop 2 or 3 times daily.

Onset and duration of action: Cycloplegia occurs in about 40 minutes and lasts for 3–5 days in normal eyes. The duration of action is much shorter in inflamed eyes.

Toxicity: Scopolamine occasionally causes dizziness and disorientation, mainly in older people.

Comment: Scopolamine is an effective cycloplegic. It is used in the treatment of uveitis, in refraction of children, and postoperatively.

Homatropine Hydrobromide

Preparations: Solution, 2% and 5%.

Dosage: For refraction, 1 drop in each eye and repeat 2 or 3 times at intervals of 10–15 minutes.

Onset and duration of action: Maximum cycloplegic effect lasts for about 3 hours, but complete recovery time is about 36–48 hours. In certain cases, the shorter action is an advantage over scopolamine and atropine.

Toxicity: Sensitivity and side effects associated with the topical instillation of homatropine are rare.

Comment: Homatropine is an effective cycloplegic often used in the treatment of uveitis.

Cyclopentolate Hydrochloride

Preparations: Solution, 0.5%, 1%, and 2% (several including Cyclogyl).

Dosage: For ophthalmoscopy or refraction, 1 drop in each eye and repeat after 10 minutes.

Onset and duration of action: The onset of dilatation and cycloplegia is within 30–60 minutes. The duration of action is less than 24 hours.

Comment: Cyclopentolate is more popular than homatropine and scopolamine for examinations because of its shorter duration of action. Occasionally, neurotoxicity may occur, manifested by incoherence, visual hallucinations, slurred speech, and ataxia. These reactions are more common in children.

Tropicamide

Preparations: Solution, 0.5% and 1% (several including Mydriacyl); 0.25% with 1% hydroxyamphetamine hydrobromide (Paremyd).

Dosage: 1 drop of 1% solution 2 or 3 times at 5-minute intervals.

Onset and duration of action: The time required to reach the maximum cycloplegic effect is usually 20–25 minutes, and the duration of this effect is only 15–20 minutes; therefore, the timing of the examination after instilling tropicamide is important. Complete recovery requires 5–6 hours.

Comment: Tropicamide is an effective mydriatic with weak cycloplegic action and is therefore most useful for ophthalmoscopy.

3. COMBINATION PREPARATIONS

Cyclopentolate Hydrochloride-Phenylephrine Hydrochloride

Preparations: Solution, 0.2% cyclopentolate hydrochloride and 1% phenylephrine hydrochloride (Cyclomydril).

Dosage: 1 drop every 5–10 minutes for 2 or 3 doses.

Onset and duration of action: Mydriasis and some cycloplegia occur within the first 3–6 minutes. The duration of action is usually less than 24 hours. This drug combination is of particular value for pupillary dilation in examination of premature and small infants.

Phenylephrine Hydrochloride-Tropicamide

Preparation: Ophthalmic insert, 5.4 mg phenylephrine and 0.28 mg tropicamide (Mydrasert)

Dosage: Inserted prior to ocular examination or intraocular surgery.

Phenylephrine Hydrochloride-Tropicamide-Lidocaine Hydrochloride

Preparations: Solution for intracameral injection, 0.31% phenylephrine hydrochloride, 0.02% tropicamide, and 1% lidocaine (Mydrane).

Dosage: 0.2 mL injected into the anterior chamber at the commenced of cataract surgery.

DRUGS USED IN THE TREATMENT OF GLAUCOMA

The dose, frequency of administration, and number of drugs should be minimized to achieve adequate control of intra-ocular pressure for the individual patient.

1. TOPICAL PROSTAGLANDIN ANALOGS

The prostaglandin analogs reduce intraocular pressure by increasing outflow of aqueous, mainly via the uveoscleral pathway. Each agent may be used alone or in combination with other types of glaucoma medication, but additive effect is more likely when used in conjunction with agents that reduce aqueous production.

Toxicity: All preparations are associated with increased brown pigmentation of the iris, eyelash growth, hyper-pigmentation of periorbital skin, conjunctival hyperemia, punctate epithelial keratopathy, and foreign body sensation. In addition, they may aggravate ocular inflammation, have been associated with the development of macular edema, and may cause structural changes of the orbital soft tissues.

Bimatoprost

Preparation: Solution, 0.03% (Lumigan).

Dosage: 1 drop once daily at night.

Latanoprost

Preparation: Solution, 0.005% (Xalatan, Monopost [preservative-free]).

Dosage: 1 drop once daily at night.

Tafluprost

Preparation: Solution, 0.0015% (Taflotan, Saflutan [preservative-free] [not available in United States], Zioptan [preservative-free])

Dosage: 1 drop once daily at night.

Travoprost

Preparation: Solution, 0.004% (Travatan, Travatan Z [ben-zalkonium chloride-free]).

Dosage: 1 drop once daily at night.

Unoprostone Isopropyl

Preparation: Solution, 0.15% (Rescula).

Dosage: 1 drop twice daily.

2. TOPICAL BETA-ADRENERGIC RECEPTOR ANTAGONISTS

Beta-adrenergic blocking agents reduce intraocular pressure by suppressing aqueous production. The nonselective β-blockers have similar potency.

Toxicity: All preparations, particularly the nonselective agents, have the potential to cause adverse systemic effects (see discussion in separate section), especially bronchocon-striction and bradycardia but also depression, confusion, and fatigue. They are contraindicated in patients with obstructive airways disease, either asthma or chronic obstructive pul-monary disease (COPD), although betaxolol with its relative β_1-receptor selectivity is safer in this context, and in patients with cardiac conduction defects.

Betaxolol Hydrochloride (Betoptic, Betoptic S)

Preparations: Solution, 0.5% (Betoptic); suspension, 0.25% (Betoptic S).

Dosage: 1 drop twice daily.

Comment: Betaxolol is less potent than the nonselective β-blockers.

Carteolol Hydrochloride

Preparations: Solution, 1% and 2% (Ocupress, Teoptic [not available in United States]).

Dosage: 1 drop twice daily.

Comment: Nonselective β-blocker.

Levobunolol Hydrochloride

Preparations: Solution, 0.25% and 0.5% (Betagan).

Dosage: 1 drop once or twice daily.

Comment: Nonselective β-blocker.

Metipranolol Hydrochloride

Preparation: Solution, 0.3% (OptiPranolol).

Dosage: 1 drop twice daily.

Comment: Non-selective beta-blocker.

Timolol/Timolol Maleate

Preparations: Solution, 0.25% and 0.5%; gel, 0.25% and 0.5% (Betimol, Istalol, Ocudose [preservative-free], Timoptic, Timoptic XE, Timoptic GFS).

Dosage: 1 drop once or twice daily. Gel once daily.

Comment: Nonselective β-blocker.

3. TOPICAL ADRENERGIC RECEPTOR AGONISTS (SYMPATHOMIMETICS)

The α_2-adrenergic agonists apraclonidine and brimoni-dine reduce intraocular pressure primarily by decreasing production of aqueous but possibly also by increasing its drainage through the uveoscleral pathway.

Apraclonidine Hydrochloride

Preparations: Solution, 0.5% and 1% (Iopidine).

Dosage: 1 drop of 1% solution before anterior segment laser treatment and a second drop upon completion of the procedure. One drop of 0.5% solution 2 or 3 times a day as short-term adjunctive treatment in glaucoma uncontrolled by other medications.

Comment: Apraclonidine is specifically indicated for prevention and management of intraocular pressure elevations after anterior segment laser procedures and as adjunctive therapy in patients on maximally tolerated medical therapy who need further reduction of intraocular pressure. Systemic side effects include decreased diastolic blood pressure, bradycardia, and central nervous system symptoms of insomnia, irritability, and decreased libido. Ocular side effects include conjunctival blanching, upper lid elevation, mydriasis, and burning.

Brimonidine Tartrate

Preparation: Solution, 0.2% (Alphagan, Alphagan P [benzalkonium chloride-free]).

Dosage: 1 drop 2 or 3 times daily.

Comment: May be used as monotherapy or in combination with other glaucoma medications. Frequently used as a replacement drug in patients unable to tolerate β-blockers.

Toxicity: Brimonidine has only minimal effect on heart rate and blood pressure. Stinging on instillation, conjunctival hyperemia, and dry mouth are common side effects.

4. TOPICAL CARBONIC ANHYDRASE INHIBITORS

Inhibition of carbonic anhydrase in the secretory epithelium of the ciliary body reduces production of aqueous. Dorzolamide and brinzolamide can be used topically because they have sufficient corneal penetration to reach the ciliary body. They may be used as monotherapy but most frequently are used in combination with other glaucoma medications except for oral carbonic anhydrase inhibitors (see later in the chapter).

Toxicity: Local reactions include burning and stinging, superficial punctate keratopathy, and allergic reactions of the conjunctiva. Bitter aftertaste is common. The systemic side effects associated with oral carbonic anhydrase agents are rare. Both drugs are sulfonamide derivatives but probably do not cross-react with sulfonamides with respect to hypersensitivity reactions.

Brinzolamide

Preparation: Suspension, 1% (Azopt).

Dosage: 1 drop 3 times daily when used alone or twice daily if being used in combination with other topical glaucoma treatment.

Dorzolamide Hydrochloride

Preparation: Solution, 2% (Trusopt).

Dosage: 1 drop 3 times daily when used alone or twice daily if being used in combination with other topical glaucoma treatment.

5. TOPICAL DIRECT-ACTING CHOLINERGIC AGONISTS

All cholinergics decrease intraocular pressure by increasing the outflow of aqueous through the trabecular meshwork.

Carbachol

Preparations: Solution, 1.5% and 3% (Isopto Carbachol).

Dosage: 1 drop in each eye 3 or 4 times a day.

Comment: Carbachol is poorly absorbed through the cornea and usually is used if pilocarpine is ineffective. Its duration of action is 4–6 hours. If benzalkonium chloride is used as the vehicle, the penetration of carbachol is significantly increased. The pharmacodynamics of carbachol also include indirect activity. [Carbachol (Miostat) 0.01% solution can be injected into the anterior chamber (intracameral injection) during intraocular surgery to cause pupillary constriction. Acetylcholine (Miochol-E) 1:100 solution is an alternative.]

Pilocarpine Hydrochloride & Nitrate

Preparations: Solution, 1–4%, 6%, 8%, and 10% (Isopto Carpine); gel, 4% (Pilopine HS).

Dosage: 1 drop up to 4 times a day; 1-cm ribbon of gel in lower conjunctival cul-de-sac at bedtime.

Comment: Pilocarpine should be avoided in eyes with active uveitis.

6. TOPICAL COMBINATION PREPARATIONS

Increasing numbers of topical preparations combining pharmacologically different agents are being developed, mainly advocated to improve compliance but not necessarily resulting in as large a reduction in intraocular pressure as expected from summation of the effects of the individual agents administered separately.

Azarga (brinzolamide 1% and timolol 0.5%), 1 drop twice daily (not available in United States).

Betoptic Pilo (betaxolol 0.25% and pilocarpine 1.75%), 1 or 2 drops 3 times daily.

Combigan (brimonidine 0.2% and timolol 0.5%), 1 drop twice daily.

Cosopt, Cosopt PF [preservative-free] (dorzolamide 2% and timolol 0.5%), 1 drop twice daily.

Duotrav (travoprost 0.004% and timolol 0.5%), 1 drop once daily (not available in United States).

Ganfort (bimatoprost 0.03% and timolol 0.5%), 1 drop once daily (not available in United States).

Simbrinza (brinzolamide 1% and brimonidine 0.2%), 1 drop three times daily.

Taptiqom [preservative-free] (tafluprost 0.0015% and timolol 0.5%), 1 drop once daily (not available in United States).

Xalacom (latanoprost 0.005% and timolol 0.5%), 1 drop once daily in the morning (not available in United States).

7. SYSTEMIC CARBONIC ANHYDRASE INHIBITORS

Systemic administration of carbonic anhydrase inhibitors increases their efficacy, being able to reduce aqueous production by 40–60%. It is used mainly when intraocular pressure cannot be controlled with topical therapy and in acute situations, including management of acute angle closure when parenteral therapy may be necessitated by vomiting as well as the urgency of the situation. The maximum effect occurs approximately 2 hours after oral administration, lasting 4–6 hours, and 20 minutes after intravenous administration.

Systemic administration is associated with several adverse effects including potassium depletion, particularly if the patient is also on diuretic therapy, acidosis, gastric distress, diarrhea, epidermal necrolysis, renal stone formation, shortness of breath, fatigue, and tingling of the extremities. Acetazolamide and methazolamide are sulfonamide derivatives but probably do not cross-react with sulfonamides with respect to hypersensitivity reactions. In Han Chinese individuals, certain human leukocyte antigen (HLA) alleles predispose to cutaneous adverse drug reactions with methazolamide.

Developments in topical medications and laser therapy for glaucoma have reduced the use of systemic carbonic anhydrase inhibitors.

Acetazolamide

Preparations and dosages: Tablets, 125 mg and 250 mg; give 125–250 mg 2 to 4 times a day (dosage not to exceed 1 g in 24 h) (Diamox). Sustained-release capsules, 250 mg and 500 mg; give 1 capsule once or twice a day (Diamox SR, Diamox Sequels, Eytazox). (In idiopathic intracranial hypertension, dosage up to 4 g per day has been used.) 500 mg for injection intravenously or intramuscularly (dosage not to exceed 1 g in 24 h) (Diamox).

Methazolamide

Preparation: Tablets, 25 and 50 mg (Neptazane).

Dosage: 50–100 mg 2 or 3 times daily (total not to exceed 600 mg/d).

8. SYSTEMIC OSMOTIC AGENTS

Hyperosmotic agents such as urea, mannitol, and glycerin are used to reduce intraocular pressure by making the plasma hypertonic to aqueous. They are generally used in the management of acute (angle-closure) glaucoma unresponsive to other treatments and occasionally preoperatively.

Glycerin

Preparations and dosage: Glycerin is given orally usually as 50% solution with water, orange juice, or flavored normal saline solution over ice (1 mL of glycerin weighs 1.25 g) (Osmoglyn). Dose is 1–1.5 g/kg.

Onset and duration of action: Maximum hypotensive effect occurs in 1 hour and lasts 4–5 hours.

Toxicity: Nausea, vomiting, and headache occasionally occur.

Comment: Oral administration and the absence of diuretic effect are significant advantages of glycerin over the other hyperosmotic agents.

Isosorbide

Preparation: 45% solution (Ismotic).

Dosage: 1.5 g/kg orally.

Onset and duration of action: Similar to glycerin.

Comment: Unlike glycerin, isosorbide does not produce calories or elevate blood sugar. Other side effects are similar to glycerin. Each 220 mL of isosorbide contains 4.6 meq of sodium.

Mannitol

Preparation: 5–25% solution for injection (Osmitrol).

Dosage: 1.5–2 g/kg intravenously, usually in 20% concentration.

Onset and duration of action: Maximum hypotensive effect occurs in about 1 hour and lasts 5–6 hours.

Comment: Problems with cardiovascular overload and pulmonary edema are more common with this agent because of the large fluid volumes required.

Urea

Preparation: 30% solution of lyophilized urea in invert sugar (Ureaphil).

Dosage: 1–1.5 g/kg intravenously.

Onset and duration of action: Maximum hypotensive effect occurs in about 1 hour and lasts 5–6 hours.

Toxicity: Accidental extravasation at the injection site may cause local reactions ranging from mild irritation to tissue necrosis.

TOPICAL CORTICOSTEROIDS

Topical corticosteroid therapy is indicated for inflammatory conditions of the anterior segment of the globe. Corticosteroids and their derivatives vary in their anti-inflammatory activity. The potency relative to hydrocortisone is 4 times for prednisolone and 25 times for dexamethasone and betamethasone. Adverse effects are not decreased with the higher-potency drugs even though the therapeutic dosage is lower.

The duration of treatment will vary according to the underlying disease process and may extend from a few days to several months. Initial therapy for a severely inflamed eye consists of instilling drops every 1 or 2 hours while awake. When a favorable response is observed, gradually reduce the dosage and discontinue as soon as possible.

Caution: Adverse effects of topical corticosteroid therapy are exacerbation or development of microbial keratitis, including reactivation of herpes simplex keratitis; ocular hypertension, including the risk of development of open-angle glaucoma; and rarely cataract formation. (These effects occur also with periocular corticosteroid therapy and to a lesser degree with systemic corticosteroid therapy, except for development of cataract that is typically posterior subcapsular.) Any patient receiving topical corticosteroid therapy should be under the care of an ophthalmologist.

Prednisolone acetate suspension, 0.12% and 1%.

Prednisolone sodium phosphate solution, 0.125% and 1%.

Dexamethasone sodium phosphate suspension 0.1%; ointment, 0.05%.

Medrysone suspension, 1%.

Fluorometholone suspension, 0.1% and 0.25%; ointment, 0.1%.

Rimexolone suspension, 1%.

Loteprednol etabonate suspension, 0.5%.

TOPICAL COMBINATION CORTICOSTEROID & ANTI-INFECTIVE AGENTS

There are numerous commercial products containing fixed-dose combinations of corticosteroid and one or more anti-infective agents. They are used for conditions that require both agents (eg, marginal keratitis due to a combined staphylococcal infection and allergic reaction, blepharoconjunctivitis, and phlyctenular keratoconjunctivitis) and postoperatively for the anti-inflammatory effect and prophylactic antibacterial cover.

These mixtures should not be used to treat conjunctivitis or blepharitis due to unknown causes. They should not be used as substitutes solely for anti-infective agents but only when a clear indication for corticosteroids exists as well.

Mixtures of corticosteroid and anti-infective agents may cause all of the same complications that occur with the topical steroid preparations alone.

NONSTEROIDAL ANTI-INFLAMMATORY AGENTS (NSAIDs)

Oral NSAIDs—indomethacin 75 mg daily, flurbiprofen 150 mg daily, or ibuprofen 600 mg daily—are the first-line treatment for nonnecrotizing scleritis. Gastric irritation and hemorrhage are risks. Topical ophthalmic preparations of several NSAIDs provide ocular bioavailability with little toxicity. These agents act primarily by blocking prostaglandin synthesis through inhibition of cyclooxygenase, the enzyme catalyzing the conversion of arachidonic acid to prostaglandins.

▷ Bromfenac

Preparation: Solution 0.09% (BromSite, Prolensa).

Dosage: 1 drop twice daily.

Comment: 2-week course to reduce inflammation following cataract surgery.

▷ Diclofenac Sodium

Preparation: Solution 0.1% (Voltaren Ophthalmic, Voltarol Ophtha [preservative-free] [not available in United States]).

Dosage: 1 drop every half hour for 2 hours prior to cataract surgery and 1 drop up to 4 times daily after surgery.

Comment: Inhibition of intraoperative miosis during cataract surgery and reduction of inflammation following cataract, corneal laser, or strabismus surgery or after glaucoma laser surgery.

▷ Flurbiprofen Sodium

Preparation: Solution 0.03% (Ocufen).

Dosage: 1 drop every half hour for 2 hours prior to surgery and 4 times daily postoperatively.

Comment: Inhibition of intraoperative miosis during cataract surgery and postoperative reduction of inflammation and treatment of cystoid macular edema.

▷ Indomethacin

Preparation: Solution 1% (Indocid [not available in United States]).

Dosage: 1 drop 4 times daily.

Comment: Treatment of allergic eye disease and 2-week course to reduce inflammation following cataract surgery and corneal laser surgery.

▷ Ketorolac Tromethamine

Preparation: Solution 0.5% (Acular, Acular LS, Acuvail); solution concentrate, 4 mL of 0.3% with 1% phenylephrine for intraocular infusion during intraocular surgery (Omidria).

Dosage: Solution, 1 drop 4 times daily; solution concentrate diluted in 500 mL of irrigating solution.

Comment: Treatment of allergic eye disease and 2-week course to reduce inflammation following cataract or corneal laser surgery, and intraocular infusion to maintain pupil dilation during intraocular surgery and reduce postoperative pain.

▷ Nepafenac

Preparation: Solution 0.1% (Nevanac, Ilevro).

Dosage: 1 drop 3 times daily

Comment: 2-week course to reduce inflammation following cataract surgery.

OTHER AGENTS USED IN THE TREATMENT OF ALLERGIC CONJUNCTIVITIS

1. ANTIHISTAMINES

▷ Emedastine Difumarate

Preparation: Solution, 0.05% (Emadine).

Dosage: 1 drop 4 times daily.

▷ Levocabastine Hydrochloride

Preparation: Suspension, 0.05% (Livostin [not available in United States]).

Dosage: 1 drop 4 times daily (up to 2 weeks).

Comment: Selective, potent histamine H1-receptor antagonist with relief of symptoms within minutes and lasting up to 2 hours.

2. MAST CELL STABILIZERS

▷ Cromolyn Sodium

Preparation: Solution, 4% (Crolom, Opticrom).

Dosage: 1 drop 4–6 times daily.

Comment: Response to therapy usually occurs within a few days but sometimes not until treatment is continued for several weeks. It is not useful in the treatment of acute symptoms.

▷ Lodoxamide Tromethamine

Preparation: Solution, 0.1% (Alomide).

Dosage: 1 drop 4 times a day.

Comment: Indicated for allergic eye disease, including vernal conjunctivitis and vernal keratitis. Therapeutic response does not usually occur until after a few days of treatment.

▷ Nedocromil Sodium

Preparation: Solution, 2% (Alocril).

Dosage: Twice daily.

Comment: Rapid onset similar to mast cell stabilizers.

▷ Pemirolast Potassium

Preparation: Solution, 0.1% (Alamast [not available in United States], Alegysal [not available in United States]).

Dosage: Twice daily.

3. COMBINATION ANTIHISTAMINE & MAST CELL STABILIZERS

▷ Alcaftadine

Preparation: Solution, 0.25% (Lastacaft).

Dosage: 1 drop once daily (up to 6 weeks).

▷ Azelastine Hydrochloride

Preparation: Solution, 0.5% (Optivar).

Dosage: 1 drop 2–4 times daily (up to 6 weeks).

▷ Bepotastine Besilate

Preparation: Solution, 1.5% (Bepreve).

Dosage: 1 drop twice daily.

Comment: Bepotastine is a histamine H1-receptor antagonist with mast cell–stabilizing and eosinophil-modulating/inhibiting activity.

▷ Epinastine Hydrochloride

Preparation: Solution, 0.05% (Elestat, Relestat [not available in United States]).

Dosage: 1 drop twice daily (up to 8 weeks).

▷ Ketotifen Fumarate

Preparation: Solution, 0.025% (Alaway, Zaditor, Zyrtec Itchy Eye Drops).

Dosage: Twice daily.

▷ Olopatadine Hydrochloride

Preparations and dosages: Solution, 0.1% (Patanol) twice a day at intervals of 6–8 hours, 0.2% (Pataday) once daily, 0.7% (Pazeo) once daily.

4. VASOCONSTRICTORS & DECONGESTANTS

There are many commercially available over-the-counter (OTC) ophthalmic vasoconstrictive agents that constrict the superficial vessels of the conjunctiva to relieve redness and relieve minor surface irritation and itching of the conjunctiva, which can represent a response to noxious or irritating agents such as smog or swimming pool chlorine. The active ingredients in these agents usually are ephedrine 0.123%, naphazoline 0.012–0.1%, phenylephrine 0.12%, or tetrahydrozoline 0.05–0.15%. Products also are available that contain an antihistamine, antazoline phosphate 0.25–0.5%, or pheniramine maleate 0.3%.

TOPICAL IMMUNOMODULATOR

Cyclosporine

Preparation: Emulsion, 0.05% (Restasis).

Dosage: 1 drop twice daily.

Comment: Cyclosporine suppresses T-cell activation by inhibiting calcineurin and is an effective systemic immunosuppressant, particularly used in transplant medicine. The topical ophthalmic formulation is approved by the US Food and Drug Administration (FDA) to treat dry eye disease, an inflammatory component to the underlying pathogenesis having been established, and increasingly is being tried for other ocular inflammatory diseases, including severe allergic disease, posterior blepharitis, and herpetic stromal keratitis, as well as in high-risk corneal graft patients. Few adverse effects have been reported in individuals treated for up to 4 years.

Tacrolimus

Preparation: Ointment, 0.1% (not available in United States).

Dosage: 1-cm ribbon 2–3 times daily.

Comment: Being tested in severe allergic eye disease.

DRUGS USED IN THE TREATMENT OF OCULAR INFECTIONS

1. TOPICAL SULFONAMIDES

The advantages of the sulfonamides include (1) activity against both gram-positive and gram-negative organisms, (2) relatively low cost, (3) low allergenicity, and (4) the fact that their use is not complicated by secondary fungal infections, as sometimes occurs following prolonged use of antibiotics. The most commonly employed are as follows.

Sulfacetamide Sodium

Preparations: Ophthalmic solution, 10%, 15%, and 30%; ointment, 10% (multiple brand names).

Dosage: Instill 1 drop frequently, depending on the severity of the conjunctivitis.

Sulfisoxazole

Preparations: Ophthalmic solution, 4%; ointment, 4% (Gantrisin).

Dosage: As for sulfacetamide sodium (above).

2. TOPICAL ANTIBIOTICS

Several antibiotics for ophthalmic use are available commercially as solutions or ointments. Higher concentration (fortified) preparations of gentamicin (1.5%) and tobramycin (1.5%), various cephalosporins (eg, cefuroxime [5%], cefazolin [5% and 10%], and ceftazidime [5%]), and amikacin (2.5%) can be obtained from compounding pharmacies (off-label use).

As a general principle, topical use of antibiotics commonly used systemically should be avoided to reduce the risk of development of resistant organisms and because sensitization of the patient may interfere with future systemic use. However, clinical circumstances may necessitate their use. The availability for ophthalmic use of fluoroquinolones (ciprofloxacin, gatifloxacin, moxifloxacin, norfloxacin, and ofloxacin), with their efficacy against a wide variety of gram-positive and gram-negative ocular pathogens, including *Pseudomonas aeruginosa,* has made them the first choice for treatment of corneal ulcers and resistant bacterial conjunctivitis.

Azithromycin

Preparation: Solution, 1% (Azasite).

Dosage: For treatment of conjunctivitis, 1 drop 2 times daily for 2 days, then once daily for 5 days.

Bacitracin (also see Polymyxin B)

Preparation: Ointment, 500 U/g (AK-Tracin, Ocu-Tracin).

Dosage: For treatment of conjunctivitis or blepharitis, apply ointment every 3–4 hours.

Comment: Most gram-positive organisms are sensitive to bacitracin. It is not used systemically because of its nephrotoxicity.

Besifloxacin

Preparation: Suspension, 0.6% (Besivance).

Dosage: For treatment of conjunctivitis, 1 drop every 2–4 hours. For treatment of keratitis, 1 drop every hour during the day and every 2 hours during the night for 48 hours, then gradually reducing.

Chloramphenicol

Preparations: Solution, 0.5%; ointment, 1% (Chloromycetin, Chloroptic) (not available in United States except from compounding pharmacy [off-label use]).

Dosage: For treatment of conjunctivitis or blepharitis, apply ointment or drops every 3–4 hours.

Comment: Chloramphenicol is effective against a wide variety of gram-positive and gram-negative organisms. It rarely causes local sensitization, but cases of aplastic anemia have been associated with long-term therapy.

Ciprofloxacin

Preparation: Solution and ointment, 0.3% (Ciloxan).

Dosage: For treatment of conjunctivitis, 1 drop every 2–4 hours. For treatment of keratitis, 1 drop every hour during the day and every 2 hours during the night for 48 hours, then gradually reducing.

Erythromycin

Preparation: Ointment, 0.5%.

Dosage: For treatment of conjunctivitis, apply ointment every 3–4 hours.

Comment: Particularly effective in staphylococcal conjunctivitis. It may be used instead of silver nitrate in prophylaxis of ophthalmia neonatorum.

Fusidic Acid

Preparation: Gel, 1% (Fucithalmic) (not available in United States).

Dosage: For treatment of conjunctivitis, apply twice daily.

Comment: Popular for treatment of bacterial conjunctivitis because of twice-daily dosage.

Gatifloxacin

Preparation: Solution, 0.3% and 0.5% (Zymar, Zymaxid).

Dosage: For treatment of conjunctivitis, 1 drop every 2–4 hours. For treatment of keratitis, 1 drop every hour during the day and every 2 hours during the night for 48 hours, then gradually reducing.

Comment: This fourth-generation fluoroquinolone is more effective against a broader spectrum of gram-positive bacteria and atypical mycobacteria than earlier fluoroquinolones.

Gentamicin

Preparations: Solution, 0.3% and 1.5% (fortified preparation from compounding pharmacy [off-label use]); ointment, 0.3% (Garamycin, Genoptic, Gentacidin, Gentak).

Dosage: For treatment of conjunctivitis, apply drops (3 mg/mL) or ointment every 2–4 hours. For treatment of keratitis, 1 drop (15 mg/mL) every hour during the day and every 2 hours during the night for 48 hours, then gradually reducing.

Comment: Gentamicin is widely accepted for use in serious ocular infections, especially keratitis caused by gram-negative organisms. It is also effective against many gram-positive staphylococci but is not effective against streptococci. Many strains of bacteria resistant to gentamicin have developed.

Levofloxacin

Preparation: Solution, 0.5% and 1.5% (Iquix, Oftaquix, Quixin).

Dosage: For treatment of conjunctivitis (0.5%), 1 drop every 2–4 hours. For treatment of keratitis (1.5%), 1 drop every hour during the day and every 2 hours during the night for 48 hours, then gradually reducing.

Comment: Comparable to ciprofloxacin.

Moxifloxacin

Preparation: Solution, 0.5% (Vigamox).

Dosage: For treatment of conjunctivitis, 1 drop every 2–4 hours. For treatment of keratitis, 1 drop every hour during the day and every 2 hours during the night for 48 hours, then gradually reducing.

Comment: This fourth-generation fluoroquinolone is more effective against a broader spectrum of gram-positive bacteria and atypical mycobacteria than earlier fluoroquinolones.

Neomycin

Preparations: Solution, 0.25% and 0.5%; ointment, 0.35–0.5%. Commercially available in combinations with bacitracin, polymyxin B, and gramicidin (Neocidin, Neocin-PG, Neosporin).

Dosage: Apply ointment or drops 3 or 4 times daily; 5–10% solutions (from compounding pharmacy [off-label use]) have been used for keratitis.

Comment: Effective against gram-negative and gram-positive organisms. Neomycin is usually combined with some other drug to widen its spectrum of activity. Contact skin sensitivity develops in 5% of patients if the drug is continued for longer than a week.

Norfloxacin

Preparation: Solution, 0.3% (Chibroxin, compounding pharmacy in United States [off-label use]).

Dosage: For treatment of conjunctivitis, 1 drop every 2–4 hours. For treatment of keratitis, 1 drop every hour during the day and every 2 hours during the night for 48 hours, then gradually reducing.

Comment: Comparable to ciprofloxacin.

Ofloxacin

Preparation: Solution, 0.3% (Ocuflox).

Dosage: For treatment of conjunctivitis, 1 drop every 2–4 hours. For treatment of keratitis, 1 drop every hour during the day and every 2 hours during the night for 48 hours, then gradually reducing.

Comment: Comparable to ciprofloxacin.

Polymyxin B

Preparations: Ointment, 10,000 U/g, in combination with bacitracin (Duospore, Polysporin) or bacitracin and neomycin (Neocidin, Neo-Polycin); solution, 10,000 U/mL, in combination with trimethoprim (Polytrim).

Dosage: For treatment of conjunctivitis or blepharitis, apply ointment or drops every 3–4 hours.

Comment: Polymyxin B is effective against many gram-negative organisms but not gram-positive, hence the need for combination with other drugs.

Propamidine Isethionate

Preparations: Solution, 0.1%; ointment, 0.1% (Brolene) (not available in United States).

Dosage: For treatment of conjunctivitis, apply ointment or drops every 3–4 hours. For treatment of keratitis, initially 1 drop every hour during the day and every 2 hours during the night, then gradually reducing.

Comment: Particularly indicated for *Acanthamoeba* keratitis.

Tetracyclines

Preparations: Suspension, 1%; ointment, 1% (Achromycin [not available in United States], Aureomycin [not available in United States], Ocudox Convenience Kit).

Dosage: For treatment of conjunctivitis or blepharitis, apply ointment or drops every 3–4 hours.

Comment: Use generally limited to treatment of chlamydial conjunctivitis and for prophylaxis of ophthalmia neonatorum.

Tobramycin

Preparations: Solution, 0.3% and 1.5% (fortified preparation from compounding pharmacy [off-label use]); ointment, 0.3% (Tobrex, AK-Tob).

Dosage: For treatment of conjunctivitis, apply drop (0.3%) or ointment every 2–4 hours. For treatment of keratitis, 1 drop (1.5%) every hour during the day and every 2 hours during the night for 48 hours, then gradually reducing.

Comment: Similar antimicrobial activity to gentamicin but more effective against streptococci. Best reserved for treatment of *Pseudomonas keratitis,* for which it is more effective.

3. INTRAOCULAR ANTIBIOTICS

The adult doses of agents for bacterial intraocular infections (exogenous or endogenous endophthalmitis) are detailed in Table 22–1.

Cefuroxime

Preparation: Powder for solution, 50 mg (Aprokam [not available in United States]).

Dosage: 1 mg (0.1 mL of 50 mg/5 mL solution) injected into the anterior chamber at the completion of cataract surgery.

Comment: Prophylaxis against postoperative infection.

4. TOPICAL ANTIFUNGAL AGENTS

POLYENES

Amphotericin B

Preparation: 0.1–0.5% solution (compounding pharmacy [off-label use]).

Natamycin

Preparation: Suspension, 5% (Natacyn).

Dosage: Instill 1 drop every 1–2 hours.

Comment: Effective against filamentary and yeast forms. Initial drug of choice for fungal keratitis.

AZOLES

Voriconazole (0.2–1%), **fluconazole** (0.2%), **miconazole** (1%), **ketoconazole** (1%), and **econazole** (2%) as parenteral or compounding pharmacy preparations (off-label use).

The adult doses of agents for fungal intraocular infections are detailed in Table 22–1.

5. ANTIVIRAL AGENTS

Acyclovir

Preparations: Tablets, 200, 400, and 800 mg; ophthalmic ointment, 3% (not available in United States) (Zovirax).

Dosage: Tablets 800 mg 5 times daily for 7–10 days for herpes zoster ophthalmicus; 400–800 mg 3–5 times daily for 7–21 days for herpes simplex keratitis (off-label use in United States). Ointment 5 times daily for 1 week then 3 times daily for 1 week for herpes simplex keratitis.

Comment: Selective activity against herpes simplex virus (HSV) types 1 and 2, varicella-zoster virus, Epstein-Barr virus, and cytomegalovirus.

Famciclovir

Preparation: Tablets, 125, 250, and 500 mg (Famvir).

Dosage: 500 mg 3 times daily for 7–10 days for herpes zoster ophthalmicus; 250–500 mg twice daily for 7–21 days for HSV keratitis (off-label use in United States).

Ganciclovir

Preparation: Gel, 0.15% (Zirgan); intravitreal implant, 4.5 mg (Vitrasert).

Table 22–1. Usual Adult Dose of Selected Antimicrobials for Intraocular Infection

	Intravitreal Dose (0.1 mL)[1,2]	Subconjunctival Dose (0.5 mL)[3]	Oral or Intravenous Dose[3]
Acyclovir (Zovirax)			5–10 mg/kg IV every 8 h[3]
Amikacin (Amikin)	0.4 mg	25 mg	6 mg/kg IV every 12 h
Amphotericin B (Fungizone)	0.005–0.01 mg	1–2 mg	Determined on case-by-case basis
Cefamandole (Mandol)	1–2 mg	75 mg	1 g IV every 6–8 h[4]
Cefazolin (Ancef, Ketzol)	2.25 mg	100 mg	1–1.5 g IV every 6–8 h
Ceftazidime (Fortraz, others)	2.25 mg	100 mg	2 g IV every 12 h
Ceftriaxone (Rocephin)	1 mg		1–2 g IV once or twice a day
Cidofovir (Vistid)			5 mg/kg IV once weekly for 2 wk for induction therapy[5]
Ciprofloxacin (Cipro)			750 mg orally twice a day
Clindamycin (Cleocin)	0.5–1 mg	30 mg	600–900 mg IV every 8 h
Foscarnet (Foscavir)	1.2–2.4 mg		90 mg/kg IV every 12 h for induction therapy
Ganciclovir (Cytovene)	0.2–2 mg or 4.5 mg implant		5 mg/kg IV every 12 h for induction therapy[3]
Gentamicin (Garamycin, Jenamycin)	0.1–0.2 mg	20 mg	1 mg/kg IV every 8 h[4]
Methicillin (Staphcillin)	2 mg	100 mg	1–2 g IV every 6 h
Miconazole (Monistat)	0.025 mg	5 mg	200–600 mg IV every 8 h
Moxifloxacin (Avelox)	0.4 mg		400 mg orally or IV every 24 h
Tobramycin (Nebcin)	0.5 mg	20 mg	1 mg/kg IV every 8 h[4]
Valacyclovir (Valtrex)			1–2 g orally 3 times daily[3]
Valganciclovir (Valcyte)			900 mg orally twice a day for induction therapy[3]
Vancomycin (Vancocin, others)	1 mg	25 mg	1 g IV every 12 h
Voriconazole (Vfend)	0.1 mg		6 mg/kg IV every 12 h for 2 doses then 4 mg/kg IV every 12 h

[1] Principal theory for microbial endophthalmitis is intravitreal, supplemented by subconjunctival and topical therapy especially if primary ocular surface infection. Systemic therapy does not appear to be of additional advantage in exogenous endophthalmitis following primary intraocular surgery but is indicated in endogenous endophthalmitis and for the treatment and prophylaxis of endophthalmitis complicating ocular trauma.
[2] Intravitreal antibiotic preparations should not contain preservatives.
[3] Renal excretion. Dose adjusted according to creatinine clearance.
[4] Nephrotoxic. Dose adjusted according to creatinine clearance and body weight.
[5] Nephrotoxic. Pretreatment with probenecid and adequate hydration required.

Dosage: 5 times daily for 1 week, then 3 times daily for 1 week; intravitreal implant every 5–8 months as required.

Comment: Active against all human herpes viruses (cytomegalovirus, HSV types 1 and 2, varicella-zoster virus, and Epstein-Barr virus) and adenovirus. The ganciclovir intravitreal insert allows treatment of cytomegalovirus retinitis without the adverse effects of systemic therapy.

▷ **Trifluridine**

Preparation: Solution, 1% (Viroptic).
Dosage: 1 drop 9 times daily for 7 days, then 5 times daily.
Comment: Effective in herpes simplex keratitis.

▷ **Valacyclovir**

Preparation: Tablets, 500, 1000 mg (Valtrex).

Dosage: 1000 mg 3 times daily for 7–10 days for herpes zoster ophthalmicus; 1000–2000 mg 3 times daily for acute retinal necrosis; 500–1000 mg twice daily for 7–21 days for herpes simplex keratitis (off-label use in United States).

Valganciclovir

Preparation: Tablet, 450 mg (Valcyte).

Dosage: 900 mg twice daily for 21 days of induction therapy, then once-daily maintenance therapy for cytomegalovirus retinitis.

The adult doses of agents for viral retinitis are detailed in Table 22–1.

DIAGNOSTIC DYE SOLUTIONS

Fluorescein Sodium

Preparations: Solution, 1% and 2%, in single-use disposable units (Minims); solution, 0.25% with 4% lidocaine in single-use disposable units (Minims); sterile paper strips, 0.6 and 1 mg (BioGlo, Fluorets, Ful-Glo, Fluorescein GloStrips); 10% sterile solution for intravenous use.

Dosage: 1 drop.

Comment: Used topically for detection of corneal epithelial defects, in applanation tonometry, and in fitting contact lenses and intravenously for fluorescein angiography.

Indocyanine Green

Preparation: Powder for solution, 25 mg for dilution in 10 mL (IC-Green).

Comment: Administered intravenously for indocyanine green angiography.

Lissamine Green

Preparation: Strip, 1.5 mg (GreenGlo [off-label use in United States]).

Dosage: Moistened with sterile saline and applied.

Comment: For detection of ocular surface disease, better tolerated than rose bengal.

Rose Bengal

Preparation: Strip, 1.5 mg (Rose Bengal GloStrips).

Dosage: Moistened with sterile saline and applied.

Comment: For detection of ocular surface disease.

TEAR REPLACEMENT & LUBRICATING AGENTS

Hydroxypropyl methylcellulose (HPMC) and related chemicals such as carboxymethylcellulose (camellose), hydroxypropyl guar, sodium hyaluronate, polyvinyl alcohol and related chemicals, carbomers (polymers of acrylic acid), castor oil, soft paraffin, and gelatin are used in the formulation of artificial tears, ophthalmic lubricants, contact lens solutions, and gonioscopic lens solutions. These agents are particularly useful in the treatment of keratoconjunctivitis sicca (see Chapter 5). They may be combined with an active agent such as vitamin A (VitA-POS ointment [not available in United States]).

To increase viscosity and prolong corneal contact time, methylcellulose is sometimes added to eye solutions (eg, pilocarpine). Preservative-free preparations are available for use in patients with sensitivities to these substances.

CORNEAL DEHYDRATING AGENTS

Dehydrating solutions and ointments applied topically to the eye reduce corneal edema by creating an osmotic gradient in which the tear film is made hypertonic to the corneal tissues.

Preparations: Anhydrous glycerin solution (Ophthalgan); hypertonic sodium chloride 2% and 5% ointment and solution (Adsorbonac, AkNaCl, Muro-128).

Dosage: 1 drop of solution or ¼-in strip of ointment to clear cornea. May be repeated every 3–4 hours.

VASCULAR ENDOTHELIAL GROWTH FACTOR INHIBITORS

There are several vascular endothelial growth factor (VEGF) inhibitors, initially developed for wet age-related macular degeneration but now used for many retinal diseases, with a wide variety of treatment protocols.

Aflibercept

Preparation: Intravitreal injection, 2 mg (0.05 mL) (Eylea).

Bevacizumab

Preparation: Intravitreal injection, 1.25 mg in 0.05 mL (Avastin [off-label use]).

Pegaptanib Sodium

Preparation: Intravitreal injection, 0.3 mg (0.1 mL) (Macugen).

Ranibizumab

Preparation: Intravitreal injection, 0.5mg (0.05 mL) (Lucentis).

22.2 Ocular & Systemic Side Effects of Drugs

Frederick W. Fraunfelder, MD, and Lindsey M. McDaniel, MD

Ocular medications, often the preservative rather than the drug itself, can cause ocular side effects, and the drugs can cause systemic side effects. Conversely, systemic medications can cause ocular side effects. Tables 22–2 to 22–4 list commonly used ocular and systemic drugs and some of their possible ocular and systemic side effects. Three points in particular bear mentioning as far as side effects of ocular medications: the significance of the risk of systemic effects from topical β-adrenergic blockers, such as timolol, used to reduce intraocular pressure; the importance of teaching patients the correct method for self-administration of eye drops or ointment, and the value of reporting cases of drug-associated ocular side effects to the National Registry of Drug-Induced Ocular Side Effects (www.eyedrugregistry.com).

SYSTEMIC SIDE EFFECTS OF TOPICAL BETA-BLOCKERS

While all topical ocular drugs, merit similar consideration in regard to the risk of systemic side effects, ocular β-adrenoceptor blocking drugs (β-blockers), such as timolol, are particularly known to cause systemic side effects, including severe and sometimes fatal reactions. Plasma drug concentrations sufficient to cause systemic adrenoceptor-blocking effects can occasionally result from ocular administration of these agents. When ocular timolol is administered in infants, blood levels are often more than six times the minimum therapeutic levels achieved when the drug is given orally. If the lacrimal outflow system is functioning, an estimated 80% of a timolol eye drop is absorbed from the nasal mucosa and passes almost directly into the vascular system. This first-order pass effect happens with all drugs that are easily absorbed through mucosal tissue in the head. Drugs absorbed through the nasal mucosa "drain" to the right atrium (first pass), with the blood containing this drug pumped back to various target organs before returning to the left atrium. The second pass occurs through the liver, where primary detoxification occurs before the blood is returned to the right heart. A small amount applied to the nasal mucosa can therefore result in therapeutic blood levels. When timolol is given orally, its first pass includes absorption via the gastrointestinal tract and then the liver, where 80–90% is detoxified before reaching the right atrium. In the United States, approximately 8% of the white population, 24% of the black population, and 1% of the Far Eastern population (Japanese, Chinese) lack the cytochrome P450 enzyme that

metabolizes timolol, placing such individuals at increased risk of systemic side effects from the drug.

A cardiopulmonary history should be obtained before initiating β-blocker glaucoma therapy. Pulmonary function studies should be considered in patients with bronchoconstrictive disease, and electrocardiogram should be ordered on selected patients with cardiac disease. Specifically, the precautions set forth in the package insert should be heeded carefully. Patients with known bronchial asthma, chronic respiratory disease, cardiovascular disease, or sinus bradycardia may need screening before implementing topical β-blocker therapy. These drugs should be used with caution in patients receiving other systemic β-blocking agents. Although the β_1 receptor selectivity of betaxolol reduces the risk of pulmonary side effects, this property is counterbalanced by betaxolol's lesser efficacy at reducing intraocular pressure.

WAYS TO DIMINISH SYSTEMIC SIDE EFFECTS

One important principle for avoiding systemic side effects from topical ocular medications is to prevent overdosing. The lowest therapeutically effective concentration of medication should be prescribed. Only one drop of medication is needed at each dosage, since the volume the conjunctival sac can hold is much less than one drop. Figures 22–1 to 22–4 illustrate the proper method of topical administration of ocular medication. In children, administering cyclopentolate eye drops on a closed eyelid has been shown to provide similar cycloplegia to administration in the inferior cul-de-sac.

NATIONAL REGISTRY OF DRUG-INDUCED OCULAR SIDE EFFECTS

The National Registry of Drug-Induced Ocular Side Effects (NRDIOSE) is a clearinghouse of drug information on ocular toxicology based at the Casey Eye Institute, Oregon Health and Science University. The principle underlying its establishment is the assumption that the suspicions of practicing clinicians regarding possible ocular toxicity of drugs can be pooled to help detect significant adverse ocular side effects from medications. Physicians who wish to report suspected adverse drug reactions should make contact via www.eyedrugregistry.com, or call or fax the Casey Eye Institute, OHSU Foundation, Mailstop 45, PO Box 4000, Portland, OR 97208-9852 (Fax: 503-494-4286).

Table 22–2. Examples of Adverse Ocular Effects Secondary to Systemic Drugs

Drug	Adverse Effects	Drug	Adverse Effects
Acetazolamide	Epidermal necrolysis, myopia, angle-closure glaucoma	Donepezil	Complications during (floppy-iris syndrome) and after cataract surgery
Alfuzosin	Complications during (floppy-iris syndrome) and after cataract surgery	Doxazosin	Complications during (floppy-iris syndrome) and after cataract surgery
Amiodarone	Vortex keratopathy, Graves ophthalmopathy (Figure 15–18), optic neuropathy	Doxycycline	Papilledema, scleral discoloration
Amphetamines	Mydriasis, angle-closure glaucoma, retinal hemorrhage	Ethambutol	Optic neuropathy, color vision defect
Anticholinergics	Angle-closure glaucoma, accommodative paresis, nystagmus, dry eyes	Finasteride	Complications during (floppy-iris syndrome) and after cataract surgery
Anticoagulants	Conjunctival, retinal, and vitreous hemorrhage
Warfarin taken during pregnancy may cause fetal facial deformity with nasolacrimal duct obstruction, microphthalmos, cataract, and optic atrophy	Fluorouracil	Lacrimal obstruction, corneal opacity
		Gold salts	Conjunctival deposits, corneal opacity, nystagmus, pigmentation of lens
		Haloperidol	Cataract, mydriasis
		Hepatitis B vaccine	Uveitis
Barbiturates	Epidermal necrolysis, ptosis, optic atrophy, nystagmus, extraocular muscle paralysis	Indomethacin	Corneal opacity
		Interferon	Optic neuropathy, diplopia, retinopathy
Beta-adrenoceptor agonists	Angle-closure glaucoma	Isoniazid	Optic neuropathy
		Isotretinoin	Conjunctivitis, corneal opacity, papilledema, pseudotumor cerebri
Bisphosphonates	Scleritis, episcleritis, uveitis	Ketamine	Nystagmus
Carbamazepine	Impaired smooth pursuit eye movements, nystagmus (gaze-evoked, downbeat), gaze palsy	Labetalol	Complications during (floppy-iris syndrome) and after cataract surgery
		Levonorgestrel	Pseudotumor cerebri
Chloramphenicol	Color vision defect (yellow tinge), optic neuropathy	Linezolid	Optic neuropathy, retinopathy
Chloroquine, hydroxychloroquine	Vortex keratopathy, retinal degeneration, "bull's eye" maculopathy	Lithium	Impaired smooth pursuit eye movements, nystagmus (gaze-evoked, downbeat), opsoclonus, internuclear ophthalmoplegia, gaze palsy
Chlorpromazine	Complications during (floppy-iris syndrome) and after cataract surgery	Methyldopa	Conjunctivitis
		Mianserin	Complications during (floppy-iris syndrome) and after cataract surgery
Chlorpropamide	Epidermal necrolysis, cataract, color vision defect (red-green)	Minocycline	Papilledema, scleral discoloration
Chlorthalidone	Angle-closure glaucoma	Morphine	Miosis
Cisplatin	Optic neuropathy, color vision defect (yellow-blue axis)	Nalidixic acid	Papilledema
		Naproxen	Corneal opacity
Clofazimine	Crystalline deposits (conjunctiva, cornea, iris)	Oral contraceptives	Retinal artery or vein occlusion, papilledema (cerebral venous sinus thrombosis)
Corticosteroids	Raised intraocular pressure, cataract		
Desferrioxamine	Retinopathy, optic neuropathy, lens opacities	Oxygen	Premature infants who are given supplemental oxygen are at increased risk of developing retinopathy of prematurity
In adults, administration of hyperbaric oxygen (3 atm) can cause constriction of the retinal arterioles
Diazepam	Nystagmus, visual field defects		
Digoxin	Retinal degeneration, changes in color vision, glare		
Disulfiram	Optic neuropathy		
Docetaxel	Optic neuropathy		

(continued)

Table 22–2. Examples of Adverse Ocular Effects Secondary to Systemic Drugs (*Continued*)

Drug	Adverse Effects	Drug	Adverse Effects
Paroxetine	Angle-closure glaucoma	Silodosin	Complications during (floppy-iris syndrome) and after cataract surgery
Penicillamine	Extraocular muscle paralysis, ptosis, optic neuritis	Statins	Diplopia, blepharoptosis, ophthalmoplegia
Phenothiazines	Pigmentation of conjunctiva, cornea and anterior lens capsule, angle-closure glaucoma, retinal degeneration, oculogyric crisis	Sulfonamides	Epidermal necrolysis, myopia, angle-closure glaucoma
Phenytoin	Impaired smooth pursuit eye movements, nystagmus (gaze-evoked, downbeat, periodic alternating), gaze palsy, convergence spasm, opsoclonus (in conjunction with diazepam) Fetal optic nerve hypoplasia if taken during pregnancy	Tacrolimus	Optic neuropathy, cortical blindness
		Tamoxifen	Macular intraretinal deposits with cysts, cataract, optic neuropathy
		Tamsulosin	Complications during (floppy-iris syndrome) and after cataract surgery
Prazosin	Complications during (floppy-iris syndrome) and after cataract surgery	Terazosin	Complications during (floppy-iris syndrome) and after cataract surgery
Quetiapine	Complications during (floppy-iris syndrome) and after cataract surgery	Tetracyclines	Papilledema
Quinacrine	Conjunctival deposits, mydriasis	Thiazides	Angle-closure glaucoma
Quinine	Retinal toxicity with initial thickening of the retinal nerve fiber layer, tonic pupils	Thioridazine	Corneal and lenticular pigmentation, retinal degeneration, oculogyric crisis
Retinoids	Papilledema	Topiramate	Angle-closure glaucoma, myopia
Rifampin	Optic neuritis	Tricyclic antidepressants	Angle-closure glaucoma, accommodative paresis
Risperidone	Complications during (floppy-iris syndrome) and after cataract surgery	Vigabatrin	Visual field constriction (requires monitoring)
Ropinirole	Complications during (floppy-iris syndrome) and after cataract surgery	Vitamin A	Conjunctival deposits, papilledema
Salicylates	Retinal hemorrhage	Vitamin D	Conjunctival deposits, corneal opacity
Sildenafil	Color vision defect (blue-tinge), optic neuropathy	Zonisamide	Angle-closure glaucoma

Table 22–3. Examples of Adverse Systemic Effects of Topical Ocular Medications

Medication	Adverse Effects
Anesthetics, topical local Benoxinate, proparacaine, tetracaine	Allergic reactions, anaphylactic reactions, convulsions, faintness, hypotension, syncope
Antibiotics Chloramphenicol Sulfacetamide, sulfamethizole, sulfisoxazole Tetracycline	Bone marrow depression, including aplastic anemia; gastrointestinal symptoms Photosensitivity, epidermal necrolysis Photosensitivity, skin discoloration
Anticholinergics Atropine, homatropine, scopolamine, cyclopentolate, tropicamide	Confusion, dermatitis, dry mouth, excitement, fever, flushed skin, hallucinations, psychosis, tachycardia, thirst, amnesia, ataxia, convulsions, disorientation dysarthria

(*continued*)

Table 22–3. Examples of Adverse Systemic Effects of Topical Ocular Medications (*Continued*)

Medication	Adverse Effects
Anticholinesterases, long-acting Demecarium, echothiophate, isoflurophate	Abdominal cramps, diarrhea, fatigue, nausea, rhinorrhea, weight loss
Anticholinesterases, short-acting Neostigmine, physostigmine	Abdominal cramps, depigmentation, diarrhea, vomiting
Anti-inflammatory agents Corticosteroids	Exogenous Cushing's syndrome
Beta-adrenoceptor blocker Betaxolol, carteolol, levobunolol, metipranolol, timolol	Asthma, brachycardia, cardiac arrhythmia, confusion, depression, dizziness, dyspnea, hallucinations, impotence, myasthenia, psychosis
Parasympathomimetics Carbachol, pilocarpine	Abdominal cramps, diarrhea, hypotension, increased salivation, muscle tremors, nausea, respiratory distress, rhinorrhea, slurred speech, sweating, vomiting, weakness
Sympathomimetics Ephedrine, epinephrine, hydroxyamphetamine, phenylephrine	Cardiac arrhythmias, hypertension, palpitations, subarachnoid hemorrhage, tachycardia

Table 22–4. Examples of Adverse Ocular Effects of Topical Ocular Medications

Medication	Adverse Effects
Anesthetics, local Benoxinate, proparacaine, tetracaine	Allergic reactions, keratitis, decreased corneal wound healing
Antibiotics Tetracycline Neomycin	Allergic reactions, corneal discoloration Allergic reactions, follicular conjunctivitis, keratitis
Anticholinergics Cyclopentolate, tropicamide	Angle-closure glaucoma, blurred vision, photophobia
Anticholinesterases Demecarium, echothiophate, isoflurophate	Accommodative spasm, cataract, depigmentation of lids, iris cysts, lacrimal outflow obstruction
Anti-inflammatory agents Corticosteroids	Cataracts, corneal infection, decreased corneal wound healing, glaucoma
Antivirals Trifluridine	Cicatricial pseudopemphigoid, keratitis, lacrimal outflow obstruction
Beta-adrenoceptor blockers Betaxolol, carteolol, levobunolol, metipranolol, timolol	Blepharoconjunctivitis, corneal anesthesia, diplopia, dry eyes, keratitis, ptosis
Carbonic anhydrase inhibitors Brinzolamide, dorzolamide	Allergic reactions, keratitis
Parasympathomimetics Pilocarpine	Accommodative spasm, cicatricial pseudopemphigoid, corneal haze (gel), myopia, retinal detachment
Preservatives Benzalkonium chloride, phenyl mercuric nitrate, polyquaternium-1, thimerosal	Allergic reactions, corneal opacity, keratitis
Prostaglandin analogs Bimatoprost, la tanoprost, tafluprost, travoprost, unoprostone	Conjunctival hyperemia, increased iris pigment, increased length and darkening of eyelashes, new lashes, keratitis, anterior uveitis, macular edema, orbitopathy
Sympathomimetics Apraclonidine, brimonidine	Conjunctival hyperemia, allergic reactions, follicular conjunctivitis

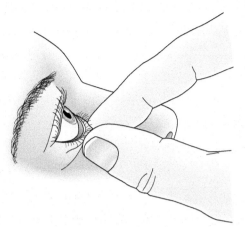

▲ **Figure 22–1.** With the head tilted back, lower eyelid is grasped below the lashes and gently pulled away from the eye to enlarge the inferior cul-de-sac.

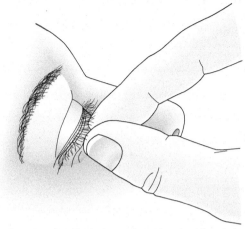

▲ **Figure 22–3.** With the patient then looking downward, the lower eyelid is gently lifted to make contact with the upper lid so as to deepen the inferior cul-de-sac.

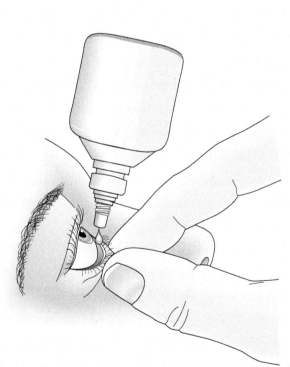

▲ **Figure 22–2.** While the patient looks up, to prevent the medication from first "hitting" the cornea, which would stimulate tearing and dilute the medication, one drop of solution or 1-cm ribbon of ointment is instilled in the inferior cul-de-sac, taking care not to touch the lashes or eyelids, thus avoiding contamination.

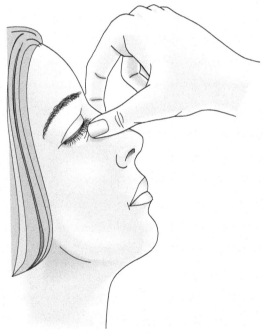

▲ **Figure 22–4.** To decrease systemic absorption, for 2 minutes or more, firm pressure is maintained with the forefinger or thumb over the inner corner of the closed eyelids, which obstructs the lacrimal drainage system and halts the pump function of eyelid movements. Any excess medication is blotted away before pressure is released or the eye is opened. If more than one medication is being administered, 10 minutes should elapse before each administration so that the previously applied medication is not washed away, and ointment should be administered after drops.

REFERENCES

Commonly Used Eye Medications

Abri Aghdam K et al: Comparison of the effect of cycloplegic versus NSAID eye drops on pain after photorefractive keratectomy. J Curr Ophthalmol 2016;27:87. [PMID: 27239584]

Aksoy A et al: Topical proparacaine abuse resulting in evisceration. BMJ Case Rep 2013;22:2013. [PMID: 23608875]

Cheema A et al: Update on the medical treatment of primary open-angle glaucoma. Asia Pac J Ophthalmol 2016;5:51. [PMID: 26886120]

Enright JM et al: Floppy iris syndrome and cataract surgery. Curr Opin Ophthalmol 2017;28:29. [PMID: 27653607]

Erdem E et al: Topical anesthetic eye drops abuse: Are we aware of the danger? Cutan Ocul Toxicol 2013;32:189. [PMID: 23410261]

Ghali AM: The efficacy of 0.75% levobupivacaine versus 0.75% ropivacaine for peribulbar anesthesia in vitreoretinal surgery. Saudi J Anaesth 2012;6:22. [PMID: 22412772]

Giles K et al: Cataract surgery with intraocular lens implantation in children aged 5-15 in local anaesthesia: Visual outcomes and complications. Pan Afr Med J 2016;24:200. [PMID: 27795795]

Guay J et al: Sub-Tenon's anaesthesia versus topical anaesthesia for cataract surgery. Cochrane Database Syst Rev 2015;8:CD006291. [PMID: 26308931]

Guerrier G et al: Bicarbonate-buffered ropivacaine-mepivacaine solution for medial caruncle anaesthesia. Anaesth Crit Care Pain Med 2016 Oct 6. [Epub ahead of print] [PMID: 27720981]

Gupta A et al: Alleviating pain in oculoplastic procedures by reducing the rate of injection of local anaesthetic. Open Ophthalmol 2015;9:156. [PMID: 26862357]

Han JW et al: Prospective, comparative study of the pain of local anesthesia using 2% lidocaine, 2% lidocaine with epinephrine, and 2% lidocaine with epinephrine-bupivicaine mixture for eyelid surgery. Ophthal Plast Reconstr Surg 2017;33:132. [PMID: 26974418]

Hoffman RS et al: Cataract surgery and nonsteroidal antiinflammatory drugs. J Cataract Refract Surg 2016;42:1368. [PMID: 27697257]

Hovanesian JA et al: Intracameral phenylephrine and ketorolac during cataract surgery to maintain intraoperative mydriasis and reduce postoperative ocular pain: Integrated results from 2 pivotal phase 3 studies. J Cataract Refract Surg 2015;41:2060. [PMID: 26703280]

Hoy SM: Tafluprost/timolol: A review in open-angle glaucoma or ocular hypertension. Drugs 2015;75:1807. [PMID: 26431840]

Huang AS et al: Glaucoma-intraocular pressure reduction. Handb Exp Pharmacol 2016 Nov 4. [Epub ahead of print] [PMID: 27812895]

Inoue K: Managing adverse effects of glaucoma medications. Clin Ophthalmol 2014;8:903. [PMID: 24872675]

Joshi RS: Proparacaine hydrochloride topical drop and intracameral 0.5% lignocaine for phacotrabeculectomy in patients with primary open angle glaucoma. Middle East Afr J Ophthalmol 2014;21:210. [PMID: 25100903]

Kim SJ et al: Routine use of nonsteroidal anti-inflammatory drugs with corticosteroids in cataract surgery: Beneficial or redundant? Ophthalmology 2016;123:444. [PMID: 26902558]

Lee RM et al: Severe adverse events associated with local anaesthesia in cataract surgery: 1 year national survey of practice and complications in the UK. Br J Ophthalmol 2016;100:772. [PMID: 26405103]

Lim BX et al: Prophylactic non-steroidal anti-inflammatory drugs for the prevention of macular oedema after cataract surgery. Cochrane Database Syst Rev 2016;11:CD006683. [PMID: 27801522]

M K: Present and new treatment strategies in the management of glaucoma. Open Ophthalmol J 2015;9:89. [PMID: 26069521]

Mäenpää J et al: Cardiac safety of ophthalmic timolol. Expert Opin Drug Saf 2016;15:1549. [PMID: 27534869]

Novack GD et al: Ocular pharmacology. J Clin Pharmacol 2016;56:517. [PMID: 26360129]

Özcan KS et al: Management and outcome of topical beta-blocker-induced atrioventricular block. Cardiovasc J Afr 2015;26:210. [PMID: 26659434]

Palte HD: Ophthalmic regional blocks: Management, challenges, and solutions. Local Reg Anesth 2015;8:57. [PMID: 26316814]

Park Y et al: Principles of ocular pharmacology. Handb Exp Pharmacol 2016 Oct 12. [Epub ahead of print] [PMID: 27730396]

Patel M et al: Toxicity of topical ophthalmic anesthetics. Expert Opin Drug Metab Toxicol 2013;9:983. [PMID: 23617273]

Pinnock C et al: Topical beta-blockers and cardiovascular mortality: Systematic review and meta-analysis with data from the EPIC-Norfolk Cohort Study. Ophthalmic Epidemiol 2016;23:277. [PMID: 27551956]

Sarkar S et al: Comparison of preoperative nepafenac (0.1%) and flurbiprofen (0.03%) eye drops in maintaining mydriasis during small incision cataract surgery in patients with senile cataract: A randomized, double-blind study. Indian J Pharmacol 2015;47:491. [PMID: 26600636]

Sharma R et al: Comparison of eye drop instillation before and after use of drop application strips in glaucoma patients on chronic topical therapy. J Glaucoma 2016;25:e438. [PMID: 26550965]

Thevi T et al: Trends and complications of local anaesthesia in cataract surgery: An 8-year analysis of 12 992 patients. Br J Ophthalmol 2016;100:1708. [PMID: 26994109]

Uche NJ et al: Topical-intracameral anesthesia in manual small incision cataract surgery: A pilot study in a tertiary eye care center in Africa. Niger J Clin Pract 2016;19:201. [PMID: 26856281]

van Minderhout HM et al: Adverse reactions following routine anticholinergic eye drops in a paediatric population: An observational cohort study. BMJ Open 2015;5:e008798. [PMID: 26700273]

Westborg I et al: Intracameral anesthesia for cataract surgery: A population-based study on patient satisfaction and outcome. Clin Ophthalmol 2013;7:2063. [PMID: 24204107]

Yu AY et al: Pupil dilation with intracameral epinephrine hydrochloride during phacoemulsification and intraocular lens implantation. J Ophthalmol 2016;2016:4917659. [PMID: 26904274]

Ocular & Systemic Side Effects of Drugs

Achiron A et al: Acute angle closure glaucoma precipitated by olanzapine. Int J Geriatr Psychiatry 2015;30:1101. [PMID: 26376106]

Araújo JR et al: Acute transient myopia with shallowing of the anterior chamber induced by sulfamethoxazole in a patient with pseudoxanthoma elasticum. J Glaucoma 2014;23:415. [PMID: 25075463]

Bouffard MA: Re-treatment with ethambutol after toxic optic neuropathy. J Neuroophthalmol 2017;37:40. [PMID: 27636749]

Chatziralli IP et al: Risk factors for intraoperative floppy iris syndrome: A prospective study. Eye 2016;30:1039. [PMID: 27367744]

Chen SH et al: Bilateral acute angle closure glaucoma associated with hydrochlorothiazide-induced hyponatraemia. BMJ Case Rep 2014 Dec 4;2014. [PMID: 25477363]

Dettoraki M et al: The role of multifocal electroretinography in the assessment of drug-induced retinopathy: A review of the literature. Ophthalmic Res 2016;56:169. [PMID: 27351191]

Fraunfelder FT: *Drug-Induced Ocular Side Effects and Drug Interactions*, 7th ed. Elsevier Saunders, 2015.

Fraunfelder FW et al: Restricting topical ocular chloramphenicol eye drop use in the United States. Did we overreact? Am J Ophthalmol 2013;156:420. [PMID: 23953152]

Grewal DS et al: Bilateral angle closure following use of a weight loss combination agent containing topiramate. J Glaucoma 2015;24:e132. [PMID: 25304279]

Grzybowski A et al: Toxic optic neuropathies: An updated review. Acta Ophthalmol 2015;93:402. [PMID: 25159832]

Karli SZ et al: Optic neuropathy associated with the use of over-the-counter sexual enhancement supplements. Clin Ophthalmol 2014;8:2171. [PMID: 25378904]

Karuppannasamy D et al: Linezolid-induced optic neuropathy. Indian J Ophthalmol 2014;62:497. [PMID: 24088636]

Kim YH et al: Comparison of the efficacy of fluorometholone with and without benzalkonium chloride in ocular surface disease. Cornea 2016;35:234. [PMID: 26619385]

Llovet-Rausell A et al: Severe ocular side effects with acetazolamide: Case report. Arch Soc Esp Oftalmol 2016;91:543. [PMID: 27179669]

Lochhead J: SSRI-associated optic neuropathy. Eye 2015;29:1233. [PMID: 26139049]

Matoba AY et al: Dendritiform keratopathy associated with exposure to polyquarternium-1, a common ophthalmic preservative. Ophthalmology 2016;123:451. [PMID: 26686962]

Moloney TP et al: Toxic optic neuropathy in the setting of docetaxel chemotherapy: A case report. BMC Ophthalmol 2014;14:18. [PMID: 24564293]

Moschos MM et al: Pathophysiology of visual disorders induced by phosphodiesterase inhibitors in the treatment of erectile dysfunction. Drug Des Devel Ther 2016;8:3407. [PMID: 27799745]

Oluleye TS et al: Chloroquine retinopathy: Pattern of presentation in Ibadan, Sub-Sahara Africa. Eye 2016;30:64. [PMID: 26427986]

Park DH et al: Linezolid induced retinopathy. Doc Ophthalmol 2015;131:237. [PMID: 26526593]

Park HS et al: Comparative clinical study of conjunctival toxicities of newer generation fluoroquinolones without the influence of preservatives. Int J Ophthalmol 2015;8:1220. [PMID: 26682177]

Pomeranz HD: The relationship between phosphodiesterase-5 inhibitors and nonarteritic anterior ischemic optic neuropathy. J Neuroophthalmol 2016;36:193. [PMID: 26720519]

Renard D et al: Spectrum of digoxin-induced ocular toxicity: A case report and literature review. BMC Res Notes 2015;8:368. [PMID: 26298392]

Sheppard JD: Topical bromfenac for prevention and treatment of cystoid macular edema following cataract surgery: A review. Clin Ophthalmol 2016;10:2099. [PMID: 27822006]

Singer JR et al: Uveal effusion as a mechanism of bilateral angle-closure glaucoma induced by chlorthalidone. J Glaucoma 2015;24:84. [PMID: 24448565]

Symes RJ et al: Risk of angle-closure glaucoma with bupropion and topiramate. JAMA Ophthalmol 2015;133:1187. [PMID: 26158444]

Wahl M et al: Intraoperative floppy iris syndrome and its association with various concurrent medications, bulbus length, patient age and gender. Graefes Arch Clin Exp Ophthalmol 2017;255:113. [PMID: 27761703]

Weiler DL: Zonisamide-induced angle closure and myopic shift. Optom Vis Sci 2015;92:e46. [PMID: 25525893]

Yang F et al: Research on susceptible genes and immunological pathogenesis of cutaneous adverse drug reactions in Chinese Hans. J Investig Dermatol Symp Proc 2015;17:29. [PMID: 26067314]

Zurevinsky J et al: A clinical randomized trial comparing the cycloplegic effect of cyclopentolate drops applied to closed eyelids versus open eyelids. Am Orthopt J 2016;66:114. [PMID: 27799585]

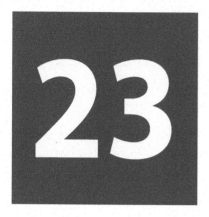

Lasers in Ophthalmology

James McHugh, FRCOphth, and Edward Pringle, MRCP, FRCOphth

LASER TECHNOLOGY

"Laser" is an acronym for light amplification by stimulated emission of radiation. Most light sources radiate energy in all directions, with waves that are out of phase (incoherent), and with multiple wavelengths. By contrast, laser light has a single wavelength (monochromatic) and waves that are in phase (coherent) with very little tendency to spread out (collimated), so they can illuminate with extremely high power (irradiance). A 1-watt laser produces a retinal irradiance approximately 100 million times greater than a 100-watt light bulb.

Laser light is generated from a "gain" medium such as a transparent crystal rod, a semiconductor diode (solid-state laser), a gas, or a liquid dye (Figure 23–1). The gain medium is housed in a resonator cavity with a fully reflective mirror at one end and a partially reflective mirror at the other. An optical or electrical source "pumps" energy into the gain medium, raising the energy level of the atoms to a high and unstable level.

When a high-energy electron returns to a lower energy level, the excess energy is released as a photon of light (Figure 23–2). If this photon encounters another atom in the nonexcited ground state, it will be absorbed, and an electron of the recipient atom will be promoted to a higher energy level. If the photon encounters another atom that is already in a high-energy state, the photon will not be absorbed, but instead will stimulate the release of a second photon. Critically, the new photon will have the same wavelength, phase, and direction as the first photon.

If the gain medium is excited to the point where more atoms are in an excited than a nonexcited (absorbing) state, "population inversion" is said to have occurred. In this unnatural state, photons encountering an atom are more likely to stimulate further photon emission than to be absorbed, resulting in an amplification cascade of exponentially increasing photon release. The presence of mirrors at either end of the resonator cavity, positioned a whole number of wavelengths apart, allows a standing wave of stimulated photon emission in the gain medium between the mirrors. A proportion of photons exits the resonator cavity through the partially reflective mirror, giving an output of laser light.

▶ Pulsed Laser

Laser energy can be emitted continuously or in pulses, which usually have pulse durations of nanoseconds (1 ns = 10^{-9} s) or less.

Q-switching is a method of pulse generation in which the quality (Q) of the resonator is decreased by closing an optical switch between the mirrors of the resonator cavity, preventing the establishment of a standing wave of stimulated emission. Energy losses are limited to spontaneous emission alone, so that pumped energy accumulates in the gain medium. When the optical switch is opened, the stimulated emission of radiation is able to resume, and the energy stored in the gain medium is released in a giant pulse lasting a few nanoseconds.

Mode locking pulse generation relies on the ability of many laser devices to support multiple "axial modes," or slightly different wavelengths of laser light. When the modes are synchronized (locked), constructive interference between their waves results in peaks of very intense amplitude that oscillate within the resonator cavity. Mode locking typically causes extremely brief low-power laser pulses of 1 picosecond or less (1 ps = 10^{-12} s), repeated at several megahertz (MHz). A second gain medium is usually needed to amplify output power while decreasing repetition to manageable rates (hundreds of kHz).

LASER-TISSUE INTERACTIONS

Light of wavelengths of 315 to 1400 nanometers (1 nm = 10^{-9} m) penetrates into the eye, whereas light of other wavelengths is absorbed by the cornea with some transmission to the

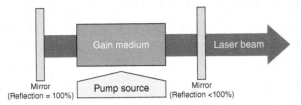

▲ **Figure 23–1.** Laser components.

lens (Table 23–1). Laser light's interaction with tissue can be grouped into categories depending on the intensity and duration of interaction (Figure 23–3).

Photochemical

Exposure of ocular tissue to visible or near ultraviolet (UV) light for durations of 10 seconds or more can cause damage via the creation of oxygen free radicals, which are cytotoxic. Toxicity is increased by the use of a topical or systemic photosensitizing agent, which accumulates in the target tissue and produces free radicals when excited by laser. Treatments based on photochemical interaction include corneal crosslinking and retinal photodynamic therapy (PDT).

Photothermal (Vaporization and Coagulation)

Light energy is converted to heat if its wavelength is within the absorption spectrum of the target and if the exposure is longer than a few microseconds. The absorption spectrums of ocular pigments differ (Figure 23–4). Melanin, which is located in retinal pigment epithelium, absorbs across the spectrum

Table 23–1. Ocular Penetration of Different Wavelengths of Light

Radiation Category	Wavelength	Ocular Absorption
Ultraviolet (UV) light		
UV-C	100–280 nm	Cornea
UV-B	280–315 nm	Cornea
UV-A	315–380 nm	Lens
Visible light	380–780 nm	Retina/retinal pigment epithelium/choroid
Infrared (IR) light		
IR A (near infrared)	780–1400 nm	Retinal pigment epithelium/choroid
IR B	1.4–3.0 μm	Cornea, lens
IR C	3.0 μm–1 mm	Cornea

including infrared light; hemoglobin absorbs blue, green, and yellow and weakly absorbs red and infrared light; oxyhemoglobin absorbs blue, green, and particularly yellow light; and the macular pigment xanthophyll particularly absorbs blue light. The variation between the absorption spectra has led to "tuning" of lasers to a specific wavelength, eg, yellow to target oxyhemoglobin, but the clinical value is uncertain.

A rise of 10–20°C within the retina or choroid will cause photocoagulation (tissue burn). If the temperature reaches 100°C, water vaporizes, causing localized disruption.

The time required for peak heat to be conducted from laser-absorbing tissue to adjacent tissues is known as the thermal relaxation time, typically measured in microseconds for micrometer distances. When laser pulses have a duration that is much shorter than the tissue's thermal relaxation time, they cause thermal damage to laser-absorbing pigmented cells without any significant rise in the temperature of adjacent nonabsorbing tissue (selective thermolysis). Micropulse diode laser and selective laser **trabeculoplasty**, using pulsed FD (frequency doubled) YAG laser, use nanosecond pulses to achieve selective photothermal effects.

Photoablation

Photons of shorter wavelength light have higher energy. Short-wavelength lasers, such as the 193-nm argon-fluoride excimer ("excited dimer") laser, have sufficient energy to break molecular bonds. Biological polymers subjected to excimer laser will degrade to small molecules, while water is explosively evaporated. The duration of photoablative excimer laser pulses is much shorter than the thermal relaxation time of corneal tissue. The superficial cornea is therefore ablated with extreme precision, without any significant thermal collateral damage.

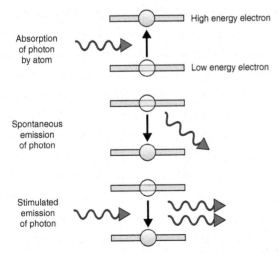

▲ **Figure 23–2.** Photon absorption resulting in spontaneous or stimulated emission according to the level of electron excitation.

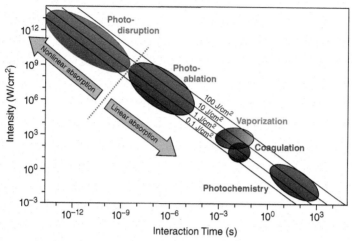

Figure 23–3. Categories of laser tissue interaction.

Photomechanical (Photodisruption/Plasma-Mediated Ablation)

In practice, laser light rays are slightly divergent, and a beam of laser light has points of greater intensity called transverse modes. The point of greatest intensity is called the fundamental mode. Apertures within the laser cavity can be used to eliminate nonfundamental modes, so that a single point of focus of a few micrometers in diameter can be treated with maximum laser irradiance, while tissues outside the target plane are not affected.

High-energy laser causes photomechanical disruption by means of very large temperature gradients at the point

of focus and an intense electrical field that is able to strip electrons from atoms, creating a plasma of ionized atoms and high-energy free electrons ("optical breakdown"). These effects cause a shock wave that expands with supersonic speed and a subsequent microscopic cavitation bubble. The pulse durations of photomechanical lasers are far shorter than the thermal relaxation time of ocular tissues, so there is no significant heat transfer to adjacent tissues.

Photomechanical interactions are the basis of Q-switched Nd:YAG lasers, which are used to perform capsulotomy and iridotomy, and mode-locked femtosecond lasers, which are used for precise computer-controlled cutting of the cornea or lens.

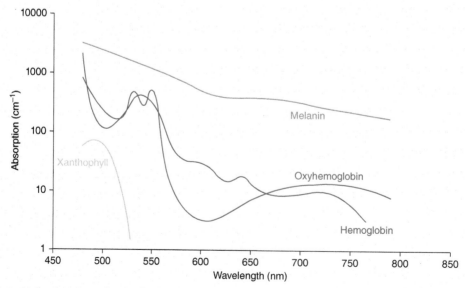

Figure 23–4. Light absorption by ocular pigments.

LASER SAFETY

The International Electrotechnical Commission (IEC) laser classification system (Table 23–2) ranks lasers according to their relative risk; almost all ophthalmic lasers are in class 4, indicating high risk. Rules concerning safe use of lasers vary between jurisdictions. Typically, designated laser safety officers are responsible for the safety of laser equipment, procedure for laser use, and staff training. Laser rooms should have clear warning signs, and doors should be locked during treatment. Interlocks may be used, cutting power to the laser when the door is open. Laser output should be directed away from doorways. Windows and reflective surfaces must be covered.

Slitlamp laser delivery systems use inbuilt filters within the microscope to prevent the surgeon from being harmed by reflected laser light. Surgeons using handheld lasers and observers of all types of laser treatment must wear goggles filtering the wavelength in use. Users must check that the goggles have a high optical density (OD) for the wavelength of the laser to be used (Figure 23–5). OD has a logarithmic scale, so that material with OD1 at a given wavelength would transmit 10% of light, whereas OD2 would transmit 1% and OD3 0.1%. Most laser safety goggles have an OD of 7 for

Table 23–2. International Electrotechnical Commission 60825-1 Laser Safety Categories

Class	Visible (V)/ Nonvisible (NV)	Notes
1: Safe	V/NV	Safe under all foreseeable conditions of operation.
1M: Safe without viewing aids	V/NV	Safe due to divergent or broad beam. May be hazardous if viewed through a lens.
1C: Safe due to mechanical enclosure	V/NV	Device contains higher-powered laser system, but user access to laser controlled by engineering. Safe unless modified.
2: Safe	Visible only	Safe due to blink reflex. Maximum power 1 mW.
2M: Safe without viewing aids	Visible only	Safe due to blink reflex. Divergent or broad beam. Hazardous if viewed through a lens.
3R: Hazardous. Low power	V/NV	Risk of ocular injury. Maximum power 5 mW.
3B: Hazardous. Medium-high power	V/NV	Risk of ocular injury. Specular reflections hazardous. Diffuse reflections usually safe. Maximum continuous wave power 500 mW.
4: Hazardous. High power	V/NV	Risk of ocular and skin injury. Specular and diffuse reflections hazardous. Fire hazard.

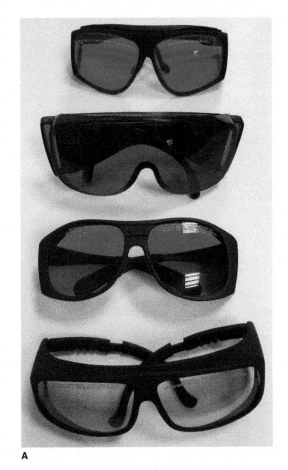

A

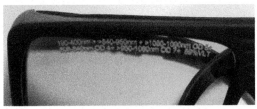

B

▲ **Figure 23–5.** Laser safety glasses **(A)**, each are marked with their optical densities for different wavelengths of light **(B)**.

the wavelength of their intended laser (ie, transmission of 0.00001% of energy at that wavelength).

A wide variety of lasers are used in ophthalmology (Table 23–3).

CORNEAL REFRACTIVE SURGERY

▶ Corneal Surface Ablation

Excimer laser allows extremely precise ablation of ocular surface tissue without significant damage to adjacent tissue. **Photorefractive keratectomy (PRK)** uses excimer laser to treat myopia by ablating the central corneal surface so that it becomes flatter (Figure 23–6), or to treat hypermetropia by ablating the periphery so that the central cornea becomes steeper. PRK is uncomfortable for several days until the epithelium has healed and usually produces subepithelial haze lasting several months.

Laser epithelial keratomileusis (LASEK) is a development of PRK in which the corneal epithelium is loosened with alcohol and detached and then repositioned after excimer laser ablation of the stroma. This causes less pain,

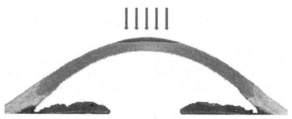

▲ **Figure 23–6.** Diagram of photorefractive keratectomy (PRK).

less haze, and faster visual recovery than PRK. **Epi-LASIK** likewise removes the epithelium prior to laser ablation, using a mechanical microkeratome rather than alcohol.

Phototherapeutic keratectomy (PTK) uses excimer ablation of the anterior corneal stroma to treat conditions such as recurrent corneal erosion syndrome, superficial scarring, some corneal dystrophies, nodular and spheroidal degeneration, and band keratopathy.

▶ Laser In Situ Keratomileusis (LASIK)

Laser in situ keratomileusis (LASIK) is the most widely used laser refractive procedure. A flap of anterior corneal

Table 23–3. Lasers Used in Ophthalmology

Laser Medium	Wavelength	Absorption	Applications
Argon-fluoride (excimer)	193 nm (ultraviolet)	Cornea	Corneal ablation (LASIK, LASEK, PRK, PTK)
Argon	488 nm (blue), 514 nm (green)	Melanin, hemoglobin (blue and green), xanthophyll (blue)	Retinal laser, trabeculoplasty, iridoplasty, iridotomy pretreatment
Frequency-doubled neodymium-YAG (FD-YAG)	532 nm (green)	Melanin, hemoglobin	Single-shot lasers similar to argon laser. Pattern retinal lasers. Q-switched pulses for selective laser trabeculoplasty.
577-nm diode	577 nm (yellow)	Melanin, hemoglobin	Retinal laser (including micropulse). Very low absorption by xanthophyll diminishes collateral thermal damage from macular laser.
Helium-neon	633 nm (red)	Melanin	Used as low-power aiming beam for other lasers.
810-nm diode	810 nm (near infrared)	Melanin; good penetration of sclera and hemoglobin	Retinal laser (including micropulse laser), endoscopic and transscleral cyclophotoablation
Neodymium:glass (femtosecond)	1053 nm (near infrared)	Melanin	Mode-locked femtosecond pulses used to cut corneal incisions for LASIK, corneal grafting, and both corneal and lens incisions for cataract surgery.
Neodymium-YAG (Nd:YAG)	1064 nm (near infrared)	Melanin	Q-switched nanosecond pulses for capsulotomy, iridotomy, and vitreolysis. Continuous wave for transscleral cyclophotocoagulation.

Abbreviations: LASEK, laser epithelial keratomileusis; LASIK, laser in situ keratomileusis; PRK, photorefractive keratectomy; PTK, phototherapeutic keratectomy

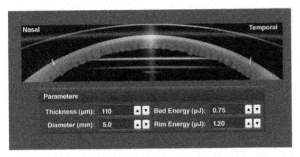

Figure 23–7. Planning of femtosecond laser in situ keratomileusis (LASIK) flap using the Victus system. (Used with permission from Bausch & Lomb Incorporated.)

stroma is cut with a femtosecond laser or an automated keratome (Figures 23–7 and 23–8). The flap is reflected, and the underlying stroma is treated with excimer laser. The corneal flap is then repositioned.

LASIK can be used to treat a broader range of refractive errors than PRK or LASEK. It is essential that at least 250 μm of corneal stroma is left after ablation to avoid iatrogenic corneal ectasia, and occult (forme fruste) keratoconus is a contraindication to LASIK. Wavefront custom ablation improves the accuracy of treatment, reduces spherical aberration, and may cause fewer night-vision problems.

LASIK offers minimal discomfort and very rapid visual recovery, but the use of a corneal flap introduces risks such as epithelial ingrowth, diffuse lamellar keratitis, flap buttonholing, or amputation. Transection of corneal nerves often causes dry eye symptoms after laser refractive surgery and particularly after LASIK.

Small Incision Lenticule Extraction (SMILE)

Femtosecond laser allows extremely precise cutting within the cornea and lens, in which cavitation bubbles separate lamellae without significant thermal or mechanical damage. **Small incision lenticule extraction (SMILE)** uses femtosecond laser to correct myopia by cutting a convex lenticule within the corneal stroma, which is mechanically removed via a laser-cut incision (Figure 23–9). Early studies

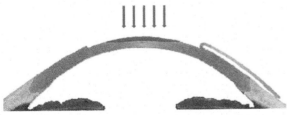

Figure 23–8. Diagram of laser in situ keratomileusis (LASIK). Superficial stromal flap has been reflected (right) allowing ablation of underlying stroma.

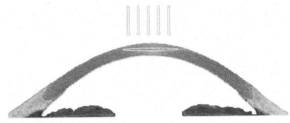

Figure 23–9. Small incision lenticule extraction (SMILE) surgery. Femtosecond laser is used to cut an intrastromal lenticule, as well as an incision for its removal.

have shown that SMILE gives broadly comparable results to LASIK and LASEK, but may be slightly superior in treating higher degrees of myopic astigmatism, with lower spherical aberration postoperatively. SMILE may cause less postoperative dry eye symptoms than excimer refractive procedures.

CATARACT SURGERY

Femtosecond Cataract Surgery

Femtosecond laser has been used to cut clear corneal incisions and limbal relaxing incisions (keratotomies); perform capsulorhexis; and fragment the lens nucleus, reducing the required phacoemulsification energy (Figure 23–10). Femtosecond laser is safe and highly repeatable, in particular allowing optimization of capsulorhexis size. This may be particularly valuable in pediatric cataract surgery. However, at present, there is no evidence of better visual outcomes when compared with conventional cataract surgery performed by an experienced surgeon. A barrier to widespread use is the high cost of femtosecond laser.

Postoperative Capsulotomy

It is common for the posterior lens capsule to opacify after cataract surgery, due to proliferation and metaplasia of lens epithelial cells. Q-switched Nd:YAG laser is used to cut a posterior capsulotomy in either a cross, circular, or inverted U pattern, clearing the opacified capsule from the visual axis (Figure 23–11). An Abraham or Peyman lens helps focusing on the capsule to minimize the power required. Low laser power, starting at 0.8 mJ and increasing until sufficient to breach the capsule, may help to minimize the risk of retinal detachment and postlaser rise of intraocular pressure. Some surgeons advocate routine use of topical antihypertensives (eg, single dose of apraclonidine 1%). Laser applied too anteriorly will pit the lens, and the use of posterior defocus limits this risk. If a circular capsulotomy is cut, any lens pits will be away from the center of the visual axis, but the circular technique may cause a large floater in some patients. The capsulotomy tends to enlarge by 20–30% over the first 3 months after laser due to capsular tension.

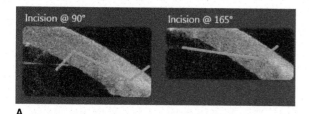

A

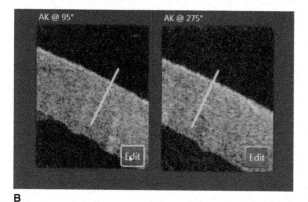

B

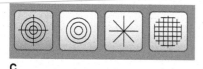

C

▲ **Figure 23–10.** Planning femtosecond laser cataract surgery using the Victus system. **(A)** Main incision and paracentesis. **(B)** Arcuate keratotomy. **(C)** Lens disruption patterns. (Used with permission from Bausch & Lomb Incorporated.)

Anterior capsulotomy is required if phimosis of the anterior capsule encroaches upon the visual axis. Nd:YAG laser is used to make radial incisions in the anterior capsulotomy margin (Figure 23–12), using a capsulotomy lens and anterior defocus to avoid lens pitting. Higher power is generally required for anterior than posterior capsulotomy.

▷ Anterior Vitreolysis

Incomplete clearance of vitreous from the anterior chamber during the management of vitreous loss secondary to trauma or cataract surgery may result in pupillary distortion, chronic uveitis, and cystoid macular edema. The vitreous bands can be cut with the Nd:YAG laser, using a capsulotomy contact lens. Topical pilocarpine constricts the pupil, tightening the vitreous strands to allow easier cutting. Multiple low-power burns limit concussion of the cornea and iris.

GLAUCOMA

▷ Iris Laser Treatment

In primary angle-closure glaucoma, contact between the lens and the iris impedes flow of aqueous through the pupil (pupil block). Increased pressure in the posterior chamber results in forward bowing of the peripheral iris (iris bombé) that occludes the trabecular meshwork leading to increased intraocular pressure (see Chapter 11). Laser iridotomy creates a small hole in the peripheral iris to overcome pupil block. In acute angle-closure glaucoma, it is undertaken to treat and prevent recurrence in the affected eye and for prophylactic treatment of the fellow eye. It is also undertaken in chronic and subacute primary angle-closure glaucoma and in secondary angle-closure glaucoma due to posterior synechiae.

The usual site for laser iridotomy is within an iris crypt between the 10 and 2 o'clock position, so that the upper lid prevents glare from light passing through the iridotomy (Figure 23–13). Following treatment with pilocarpine to constrict the pupil and apraclonidine to reduce any elevation of intraocular pressure due to the laser treatment, with an Abraham or Wise contact lens, the iridotomy is created with a Q-switched Nd:YAG laser, using a few high-power (2.0–8.0 mJ) burns or a greater number of moderate power (0.8–2.0 mJ) burns. In dark irises, the iridotomy site can be pretreated with argon or FD-YAG laser, using 20–40 low-power (120 mW, 50 ms, 50 μm) burns followed by 20 high-power (700 mW, 100 ms, 50 μm) burns to form a crater, which is easier to breach with the Nd:YAG laser. If the view of the iris is obscured by pigmented debris, the treatment is suspended for a few minutes to let it clear. Successful breach of the iris results in a gush of aqueous and pigmented cells through the iridotomy into the anterior chamber. The iridotomy is enlarged to around 200 μm diameter to ensure its patency. Bleeding from iris vessels is arrested by gentle pressure on the contact lens. The intraocular pressure is checked at least 1 hour later, and any pressure spike is treated with topical and/or systemic treatment. A short course of topical steroid is used to reduce intraocular inflammation.

Argon laser peripheral iridoplasty (ALPI) can be used when an acute angle-closure glaucoma does not respond to medical treatment such that laser iridotomy cannot be performed and also for angle closure not due to pupil block, such as in plateau iris. Using an iridotomy lens, a ring of argon or FD-YAG laser burns (1–2 per clock hour, 500 μm diameter, 500 ms duration, power increasing from 200 mW until the iris fibers visibly contract) is applied to the peripheral iris stroma to cause the iris to pull away from the anterior chamber angle, leading to reduction of intraocular pressure and potentially allowing iridotomy. An alternative treatment for acute angle-closure glaucoma unresponsive to medical therapy is surgical peripheral iridectomy (see Chapter 11).

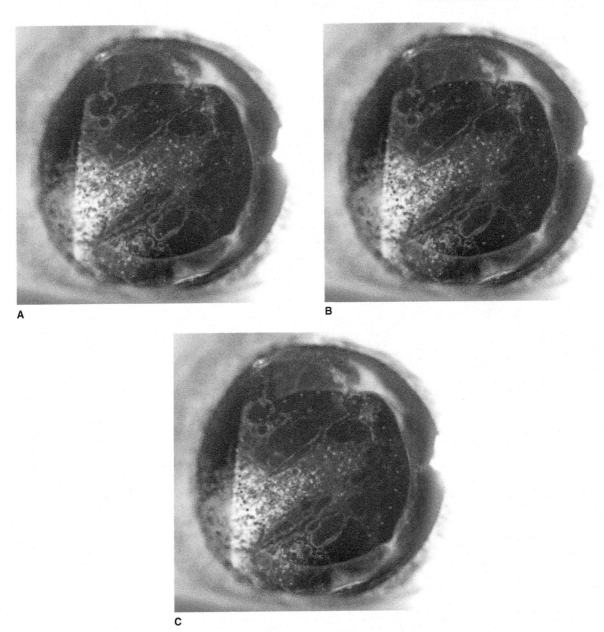

▲ Figure 23–11. Posterior capsule opacification showing outline of laser capsulotomy using (A) cross, (B) circle, and (C) inverted U patterns. Red dots show positions of intended laser burns with closer spacing in the sector of denser opacification.

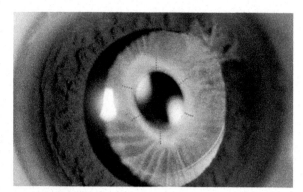

Figure 23–12. YAG laser anterior capsulotomy for capsular phimosis. Red dots show lines of intended laser burns.

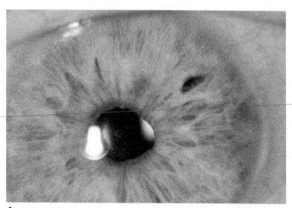

A

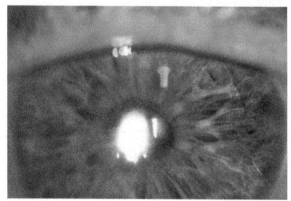

B

Figure 23–13. Patent iridotomy at 2 o'clock position seen by **(A)** direct illumination and **(B)** retroillumination, with the edge of the intraocular lens being visible through the iridotomy. A location of 10 to 2 o'clock is generally preferred for iridotomy because the upper lid then prevents glare.

Trabecular Meshwork Laser Treatment

Laser trabeculoplasty can be used to improve trabecular outflow in open-angle glaucoma. It probably attracts macrophages that clear debris from the trabecular meshwork and may also cause mechanical opening of Schlemm's canal and untreated trabecular spaces.

In argon laser trabeculoplasty (ALT), using a gonioscopy lens, approximately 100 burns (50 μm diameter, 100 ms duration) are placed circumferentially at the junction of the pigmented and nonpigmented trabecular meshwork. The desired end point is transient blanching or a tiny bubble. The effectiveness of ALT declines over time, and most patients will return to baseline pressure within 4 years. ALT causes focal scarring of the trabecular meshwork, so that repeat ALT treatments are much less effective, and may also cause peripheral anterior synechiae.

Selective laser trabeculoplasty (SLT) has largely replaced ALT. It uses the Q-switched FD-YAG laser to apply photothermal treatment to pigmented cells within the trabecular meshwork. The 3-nanosecond pulse duration is much shorter than the thermal relaxation time of pigmented trabecular tissue, preventing damage to nonpigmented trabecular cells. The spot size is 400 μm, significantly larger than ALT, and covers the entire trabecular meshwork. Starting at 0.8 mJ, the power is titrated to 0.1 mJ below the level at which "champagne bubbles" are seen. Either 180° or 360° is treated, with 50 or 100 nonoverlapping burns, respectively.

Histopathologic studies have shown less damage to the trabecular meshwork following SLT than following ALT (Figure 23–14), and peripheral anterior synechiae are much rarer following SLT. Intraocular pressure reduction from initial treatment with ALT and SLT has been shown to be equivalent at 12 months. SLT retreatment is much more effective than ALT retreatment.

Both SLT and ALT may cause a high pressure spike within 1–2 hours of treatment. Prophylactic topical antihypertensives should be used (eg, apraclonidine 1% immediately before laser), and intraocular pressure should be checked at least an hour after laser. A short course of topical steroids is sometimes used following trabeculoplasty.

Ciliary Body Laser Treatment

Aqueous production can be decreased by photothermal laser treatment to the ciliary body (Figure 23–15). Transscleral cyclophotocoagulation (TCP) (cyclodiode) is performed under sub-Tenon's, peribulbar, or general anesthesia. An oblique light source reveals the anterior edge of the ciliary body, which does not transilluminate (Figure 23–16). The laser probe is applied over the ciliary body, and 8–10 burns (1.5 W and 1.5 s for diode laser; 7–9 W and 0.7 s for Nd:YAG) are applied per quadrant around the circumference of the ciliary body, avoiding the 3 and 9 o'clock positions to

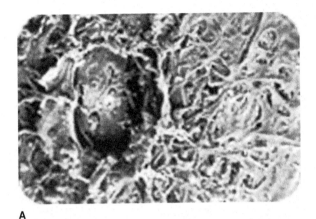

A

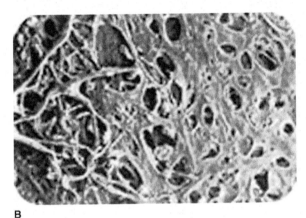

B

▲ **Figure 23–14.** Electron micrographs of trabecular meshwork following **(A)** argon laser trabeculoplasty (ALT) and **(B)** selective laser trabeculoplasty (SLT). (Used with permission from Lumenis.)

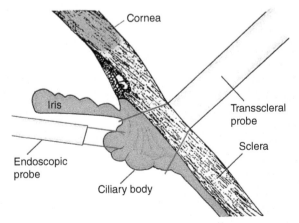

▲ **Figure 23–15.** Diagram of transscleral (cyclodiode) and endoscopic cyclophotocoagulation (ECP) of the ciliary body to reduce aqueous production.

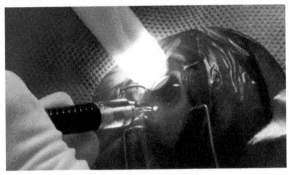

▲ **Figure 23–16.** During cyclodiode, the anterior edge of the ciliary body is silhouetted by oblique illumination. (Used with permission from I. Rodrigues.)

prevent ciliary nerve damage. A "pop" sound indicates tissue vaporization requiring reduction of power.

TCP requires less intensive postoperative management than trabeculectomy or shunt surgery but may hasten phthisis. Intense inflammation is common, and postoperative steroid drops are essential. TCP greatly diminishes aqueous production and has traditionally been reserved for patients with painful blind eyes due to uncontrollable pressure. However, there is evidence that it can be used safely earlier in the natural history of glaucoma.

Laser endocyclophotocoagulation (ECP) uses an endoscopic diode laser probe to visualize and treat the ciliary processes (Figure 23–15). This can be performed via the pars plana during vitrectomy or via corneal incisions at the time of cataract surgery. Laser treatment is applied to each ciliary process for approximately 2 seconds, with power titrated to produce visible blanching and shrinkage (300–900 mW) (Figure 23–17). ECP causes more localized coagulation of

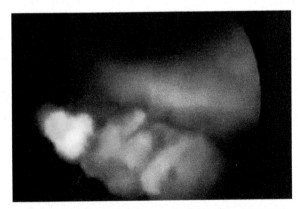

▲ **Figure 23–17.** Endoscopic view of the ciliary processes during endoscopic cyclophotocoagulation (ECP). The laser aiming spot is red. The treated ciliary processes are white. (Used with permission from I. Rodrigues and S. Goyal.)

the ciliary epithelium than TCP, requiring much less laser energy and with lower risks of hypotony, choroidal effusion, and loss of vision.

▶ Laser Suture Lysis

Following trabeculectomy, aqueous drainage into the conjunctival bleb can be increased by the use of laser to break the sutures securing the scleral flap. A Hoskins or Blumenthal suture lysis lens is used to compress the overlying conjunctiva and Tenon's capsule, and argon or FD-YAG laser pulses cut the sutures.

RETINAL LASER TREATMENT

▶ Pan-Retinal Photocoagulation (Scatter Laser)

Retinal ischemia may lead to retinal or iris neovascularization. The most common causes are diabetic retinopathy and retinal vein occlusion. Other causes are sickle cell disease, ocular ischemic syndrome, uveitis, Coats' disease, and retinopathy of prematurity. The definitive treatment for retinal and iris neovascularization is laser pan-retinal photocoagulation (PRP), which decreases the oxygen demand of the peripheral retina and hence the production of vascular endothelial growth factor (VEGF).

PRP may be achieved with argon laser or now, more commonly, with FD-YAG pattern scanning laser. Pattern lasers use briefer laser pulses of higher power. They are less uncomfortable and deliver multiple spots at each activation so that treatment can be performed more quickly. A wide angle contact lens is used to treat the entire retina, apart from the macula and around the disk (Figure 23–18). Burns of 200–500 μm in diameter are placed 0.5–1 burn widths apart. Shot duration is typically 100 milliseconds with a conventional argon or YAG laser or 20 milliseconds with a pattern laser. Power is adjusted to produce a gently blanching burn. It needs to be readjusted during treatment as more peripheral retina requires lower power. Most patients find the procedure uncomfortable but tolerable; peribulbar or sub-Tenon's anesthesia is occasionally required.

PRP is usually split into sessions of approximately 1000–1500 burns 1–2 weeks apart to reduce the incidence of uveitis, macular edema, and exudative retinal detachment. The inferior retina is often treated first as any subsequent vitreous hemorrhage is more likely to obscure this area. At least 2000 and sometimes 6000 or more burns are required to cause regression of new vessels. If retinal ischemia is localized, as in branch retinal vein occlusion, sectoral PRP may be performed, treating only areas shown to be ischemic on fluorescein angiography. If there is significant preexisting macular edema, macular laser treatment is performed before or at the same time as PRP to avoid exacerbating it.

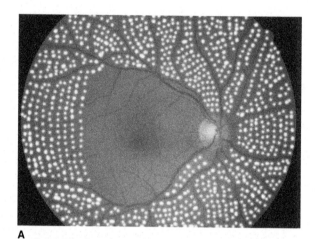

A

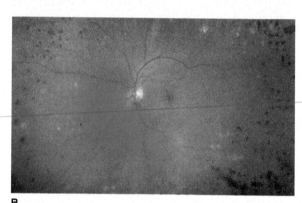

B

▲ **Figure 23–18.** Pan-retinal photocoagulation. **A:** Diagram showing planned distribution of laser burns separated by 0.5–1 burn diameter, avoiding main blood vessels. **B:** Wide angle fundus photograph showing retinal scars.

If there is vitreous hemorrhage dense enough to prevent slitlamp PRP, PRP may be performed during vitrectomy surgery using diode laser delivered via a fiberoptic intraocular probe (**endolaser**). PRP can also be delivered by diode laser using an indirect ophthalmoscope via the pupil (eg, when treating retinopathy of prematurity) or by transscleral diode laser.

In diabetic patients, PRP should be performed urgently if there is high-risk proliferative diabetic retinopathy (see Chapter 10). PRP may also be performed in patients with low-risk proliferative retinopathy, as it reduces the risk of progression to high-risk retinopathy by 50%. Patients with severe nonproliferative diabetic retinopathy are sometimes treated, for example, in an only eye where the first eye was lost to proliferative disease, if patients are difficult to examine, or if patients are at high risk of missing follow-up appointments.

Ischemic central retinal vein occlusion (CRVO) carries a high risk of iris rubeosis, and patients are reviewed frequently to check for its development so that urgent PRP can be performed before rubeotic glaucoma occurs. Intravitreal anti-VEGF agents may be used as an adjunct to laser treatment. Proliferative retinopathy occurs less frequently than rubeosis in CRVO and also is treated with urgent PRP. Areas of retinal hemorrhage should be avoided during PRP unless with a diode laser, which is minimally absorbed by blood. Patients with extensive ischemia sometimes undergo prophylactic PRP in the absence of neovascularization if regular follow-up by an ophthalmologist is not possible.

Laser for Macular Edema

Retinal laser is the standard treatment for macular edema due to retinal vascular disease. Macular laser requires lower power than PRP and is thought to decrease edema by photostimulatory effects on the retinal pigment epithelium. In recent years, it has been supplemented and to some extent replaced by intravitreal corticosteroid and anti-VEGF injections. However, it still has an important role, providing long-lasting treatment at relatively low cost.

Burns of 50–100 μm in diameter are applied as a grid, spaced 1–2 burn widths apart across the superior, temporal, and inferior macula (full grid treatment), or in a modified grid limited to areas of retinal thickening, with additional direct burns to leaking microaneurysms (Figure 23–19). No laser is used within 500 μm of the center of the fovea (foveal avascular zone). The papillomacular bundle, between the disk and fovea, should be treated with caution. Power is titrated to cause faint blanching of the retina close to the vascular arcades or to be just below the threshold for blanching (subthreshold treatment).

Diode micropulse laser uses either 810-nm (infrared) or 577-nm (yellow) light, delivered in very brief bursts— 100 micropulses each 0.1 millisecond in duration during an "on" period of 200 milliseconds, giving a 5% duty cycle. The micropulses are shorter than the thermal relaxation time of retinal tissue, minimizing heat buildup, and the bursts are separated by longer (1800 ms) "off" periods to allow heat to dissipate. Yellow laser has the advantage of low absorption by xanthophyll, minimizing collateral heat damage to the macula. Unlike continuous wave macular laser treatments, micropulse retinal laser is applied in a confluent grid to thickened areas of macula, with power adjusted to half the power needed to cause visible blanching. The lack of a visible end point can make administration difficult, but confluent diode laser is slightly more effective in decreasing edema than conventional macular grid laser, with a lower risk of retinal scarring.

In diabetic macular edema, the Early Treatment Diabetic Retinopathy Study (ETDRS) criteria are used to identify patients likely to benefit from macular laser treatment (see Chapter 10).

If edema is limited to the fovea, intravitreal steroid or anti-VEGF injections may be more appropriate.

Retinal laser is ineffective for macular edema due to central retinal vein occlusion. However, modified grid laser is effective for macular edema due to branch retinal vein occlusion and should be considered if acuity is 20/40 or worse and the edema has persisted for 3 months after the onset of symptoms. Macular laser is avoided in patients with extensive macular hemorrhage due to retinal vein occlusion, because hemorrhage limits laser effectiveness and increases the risk of retinal burns. Intravitreal anti-VEGF injections are better.

Laser for Retinal Tear (Retinopexy)

Peripheral retinal tears, usually due to vitreous traction during posterior vitreous detachment, can lead to retinal detachment. If retinal tears are detected prior to the accumulation of subretinal fluid, they can be encircled by retinal laser to create an adhesion of the adjacent neural retina to the pigment epithelium. Using either pattern or single-shot FD-YAG or argon laser and a wide-angle or three-mirror contact lens, two or three rings of confluent 200–500 μm 100-millisecond burns are placed around the tear. The power is titrated to achieve moderate blanching. Tears in the extreme retinal periphery cannot be treated with a slitlamp laser but can be treated with indirect laser with scleral indentation (Figure 23–20).

Retinopexy is indicated for almost all U-shaped retinal tears and for any retinal breach with a small associated area of subretinal fluid. It is not indicated for fully operculated round holes, except for round holes in lattice in high-risk situations, such as recent symptoms of posterior vitreous detachment or history of retinal detachment in the fellow eye.

Laser for Choroidal Neovascular Membrane

Choroidal neovascular membrane (CNVM) growing through a break in Bruch's membrane is most commonly found in wet macular degeneration, but also occurs in high myopia, traumatic choroidal rupture, and presumed ocular histoplasmosis syndrome (POHS). Photodynamic therapy (PDT) was the treatment of choice for CNVM prior to intravitreal anti-VEGF injections. Verteporfin, a photosensitizing agent, is administered intravenously. The lesion is treated with 689-nm laser (spot size 1000 μm greater than the diameter of the lesion, for 83 seconds). PDT is still useful in patients who are allergic to anti-VEGF treatments and in polypoidal choroidal vasculopathy (PCV). CNVM can also be treated with confluent, strongly blanching argon or FD-YAG laser burns covering the entire lesion. This causes an immediate positive scotoma. Laser is also an option for extra-foveal CNVM threatening vision if repeated anti-VEGF injections are not possible.

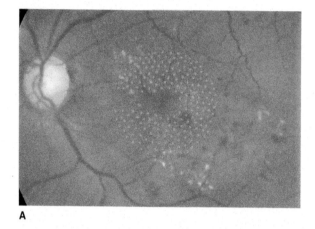

A

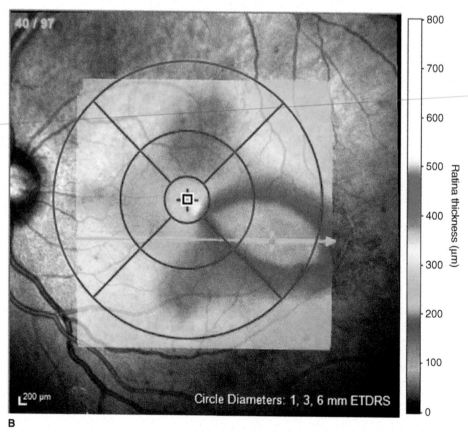

B

▲ **Figure 23–19.** Macular grid laser for diabetic macular edema. **A:** Fundus color photograph showing intended distribution of laser burns for full grid. Modified grid: **B:** Optical coherence tomography (OCT) scan showing retinal thickening inferotemporal and superior to the fovea. **C:** Fluorescein angiogram showing corresponding areas of fluorescein leakage. **D:** Fundus color photograph showing intended distribution of laser burns. (*continued*)

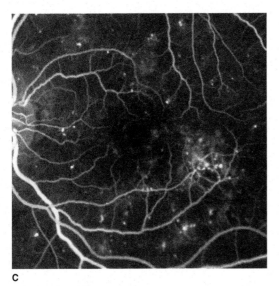

C

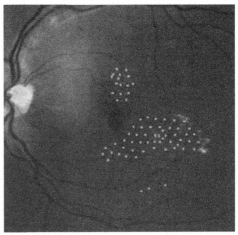

D

▲ **Figure 23–19.** *(Continued)*

▶ Laser for Retinal Macroaneurysm

There is a high rate of spontaneous resolution of retinal artery macroaneurysm, especially following hemorrhage. However, if exudation from the macroaneurysm threatens or involves the central macula, laser treatment may be indicated. A single ring of confluent, lightly blanching, 200-μm diameter FD-YAG or argon laser burns is applied around the aneurysm. Laser may also be applied directly to blanch the aneurysm, but this carries a small risk of occluding the distal arteriole.

REFERENCES

Abouzeid H et al: Femtosecond-laser assisted cataract surgery: A review. Acta Ophthalmol 2014;92:597. [PMID: 24835818]

Agarwal A et al: Current and effective advantages of femto phaco-emulsification. Curr Opin Ophthalmol 2017;28:49. [PMID: 27801688]

Alipour F et al: Hinged capsulotomy: Does it decrease floaters after yttrium aluminum garnet laser capsulotomy? Middle East Afr J Ophthalmol 2015;22:352. [PMID: 26180476]

Amoozgar B et al: Update on ciliary body laser procedures. Curr Opin Ophthalmol 2017;28:181. [PMID: 27898468]

Awan MT et al: Improvement of visual acuity in diabetic and nondiabetic patients after Nd:YAG laser capsulotomy. Clin Ophthalmol 2013;7:2011. [PMID: 24143068]

Bhargava R et al: Neodymium-yttrium aluminium garnet laser capsulotomy energy levels for posterior capsule opacification. J Ophthalmic Vis Res 2015;10:37. [PMID: 26005551]

Blindbaek S et al: Prophylactic treatment of retinal breaks: A systematic review. Acta Ophthalmol 2015;93:3. [PMID: 24853827]

Bloom PA et al: A comparison between tube surgery, ND:YAG laser and diode laser cyclophotocoagulation in the management of refractory glaucoma. Biomed Res Int 2013;2013:371951. [PMID: 24222905]

Cetinkaya S et al: The influence of size and shape of Nd:YAG capsulotomy on visual acuity and refraction. Arq Bras Oftalmol 2015;78:220. [PMID: 26375335]

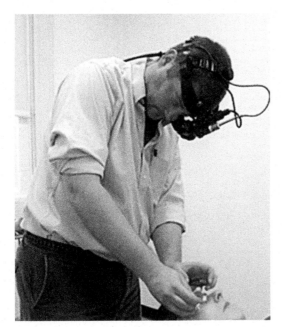

▲ **Figure 23–20.** Indirect retinal diode laser. (Used with permission from G. Bowler.)

Chen G et al: Subthreshold micropulse diode laser versus conventional laser photocoagulation for diabetic macular edema: A meta-analysis of randomized controlled trials. Retina 2016;36:2059. [PMID: 27096529]

Cohen A et al: Endoscopic cyclophotocoagulation for the treatment of glaucoma. Surv Ophthalmol 2016 Oct 5. [Epub ahead of print] [PMID: 27717892]

Day AC et al: Laser-assisted cataract surgery versus standard ultrasound phacoemulsification cataract surgery. Cochrane Database Syst Rev 2016;7:CD010735. [PMID: 27387849]

Ekici F et al: Current and future of laser therapy in the management of glaucoma. Open Ophthalmol J 2016;10:56. [PMID: 27014388]

Evans JR et al: Laser photocoagulation for proliferative diabetic retinopathy. Cochrane Database Syst Rev 2014;11:CD011234. [PMID: 25420029]

Francis BA et al: Endoscopic ophthalmic surgery of the anterior segment. Surv Ophthalmol 2014;59:217. [PMID: 23931901]

Ishida K: Update on results and complications of cyclophotocoagulation. Curr Opin Ophthalmol 2013;24:102. [PMID: 23313903]

Kaplowitz K et al: The use of endoscopic cyclophotocoagulation for moderate to advanced glaucoma. Acta Ophthalmol 2015;93:395. [PMID: 25123160]

Kara N et al: Comparison of two laser capsulotomy techniques: Cruciate versus circular. Semin Ophthalmol 2014;29:151. [PMID: 24475914]

Karahan E et al: An overview of Nd:YAG laser capsulotomy. Med Hypothesis Discov Innov Ophthalmol 2014;3:45. [PMID: 25738159]

Khan AA et al: Retinal detachment following laser retinopexy. Acta Ophthalmol 2016;94:e76. [PMID: 25847400]

Lam FC et al: Macular grid laser photocoagulation for branch retinal vein occlusion. Cochrane Database Syst Rev 2015;5:CD008732. [PMID: 25961835]

Leahy KE et al: Selective laser trabeculoplasty: Current perspectives. Clin Ophthalmol 2015;9:833. [PMID: 26005327]

Liu M et al: Clinical outcomes after SMILE and femtosecond laser-assisted LASIK for myopia and myopic astigmatism: A prospective randomized comparative study. Cornea 2016;35:210. [PMID: 26684046]

Min JK et al: A new technique for Nd:YAG laser posterior capsulotomy. Int J Ophthalmol 2014;7:345. [PMID: 24790883]

Othman IS et al: Subthreshold diode-laser micropulse photocoagulation as a primary and secondary line of treatment in management of diabetic macular edema. Clin Ophthalmol 2014;8:653. [PMID: 24729679]

Patel V et al: Long-term outcomes in patients initially responsive to selective laser trabeculoplasty. Int J Ophthalmol 2015;8:960. [PMID: 26558209]

Pitkänen L et al: Retinal arterial macroaneurysms. Acta Ophthalmol 2014;92:101. [PMID: 23800325]

Popovic M et al: Efficacy and safety of femtosecond laser-assisted cataract surgery compared with manual cataract surgery: A meta-analysis of 14,567 eyes. Ophthalmology 2016;123:2113. [PMID: 27538796]

Qian Y et al: Comparison of femtosecond laser small-incision lenticule extraction and laser-assisted subepithelial keratectomy to correct myopic astigmatism. J Cataract Refract Surg 2015;41:2476. [PMID: 26703499]

Qiao G et al: Sub-threshold micro-pulse diode laser treatment in diabetic macular edema: A meta-analysis of randomized controlled trials. Int J Ophthalmol 2016;9:1020. [PMID: 27500112]

Randleman JB et al: Corneal cross-linking. Surv Ophthalmol 2015;60:509. [PMID: 25980780]

Roberts SJ et al: Efficacy of combined cataract extraction and endoscopic cyclophotocoagulation for the reduction of intraocular pressure and medication burden. Int J Ophthalmol 2016;9:693. [PMID: 27275423]

Saeger M et al: Variability of panretinal photocoagulation lesions across physicians and patients. Quantification of diameter and intensity variation. Graefes Arch Clin Exp Ophthalmol 2017;255:49. [PMID: 27405976]

Sandoval HP et al: Modern laser in situ keratomileusis outcomes. J Cataract Refract Surg 2016;42:1224. [PMID: 27531300]

Santhiago MR et al: Microkeratome versus femtosecond flaps: Accuracy and complications. Curr Opin Ophthalmol 2014;25:270. [PMID: 24837579]

Saxena S et al: In vivo early retinal structural alterations following laser photocoagulation using three-dimensional spectral domain optical coherence tomography. BMJ Case Rep 2016 Jul 11;2016. [PMID: 27402655]

Sayman Muslubaş I et al: Macular burns from nonmedical lasers. Turk J Ophthalmol 2016;46:138. [PMID: 27800276]

Shah DN et al: Complications of femtosecond-assisted laser in-situ keratomileusis flaps. Semin Ophthalmol 2014;29:363. [PMID: 25325862]

Shalchi Z et al: Safety and efficacy of epithelium removal and transepithelial corneal collagen crosslinking for keratoconus. Eye (Lond) 2015;29:15. [PMID: 25277300]

Siegel MJ et al: Combined endoscopic cyclophotocoagulation and phacoemulsification versus phacoemulsification alone in the treatment of mild to moderate glaucoma. Clin Exp Ophthalmol 2015;43:531. [PMID: 25684216]

Singh K et al: Diode laser cyclophotocoagulation in Indian eyes: Efficacy and safety. Int Ophthalmol 2017;37:79. [PMID: 27061905]

Tan JC et al: Endoscopic cyclophotocoagulation and pars plana ablation (ECP-plus) to treat refractory glaucoma. J Glaucoma 2016;25:e117. [PMID: 26020690]

Titiyal JS et al: Comparative evaluation of femtosecond laser-assisted cataract surgery and conventional phacoemulsification in white cataract. Clin Ophthalmol 2016;10:1357. [PMID: 27555743]

Wang L et al: Femtosecond laser penetrating corneal relaxing incisions combined with cataract surgery. J Cataract Refract Surg 2016;42:995. [PMID: 27492097]

Woreta FA et al: LASIK and surface ablation in corneal dystrophies. Surv Ophthalmol 2015;60:115. [PMID: 25307289]

Yang Y et al: Comparison of efficacy between endoscopic cyclophotocoagulation and alternative surgeries in refractory glaucoma: A meta-analysis. Medicine (Baltimore) 2015;94:e1651. [PMID: 26426659]

Yotsukura E et al: Effect of neodymium:YAG laser capsulotomy on visual function in patients with posterior capsule opacification and good visual acuity. Cataract Refract Surg 2016;42:399. [PMID: 27063520]

Yusuf IH: Transscleral cyclophotocoagulation in refractory acute and chronic angle closure glaucoma. BMJ Case Rep 2015 Sep 30;2015. [PMID: 26424819]

Low Vision

24

Gwen K. Sterns, MD

The patient with impaired vision represents a challenge to eye-care professionals. Whether temporary or permanent, low vision is the consequence of an eye disorder, and ophthalmologists and optometrists have a responsibility to manage it. If the outcome of optimal medical and surgical intervention is diminished functional vision, the patient needs vision rehabilitation (see also Chapter 25). No person with low vision should have to search far and wide for low-vision care. Some level of care should be integrated into every ophthalmic practice, either on-site or by referral to a low-vision center.

Low-vision patients typically have impaired visual performance: their visual acuity is not correctable with conventional glasses or contact lenses. They may have cloudy vision, constricted field of vision, large visual field defects (scotomas), glare sensitivity, abnormal color perception, diminished contrast, or diplopia. Patients are often confused by overlapping but dissimilar images from each eye.

The term "low vision" covers a wide range of visual problems, ranging from near-normal vision to severe loss. All low-vision patients have some degree of useful vision even though the loss may be profound. They should not be considered "blind" unless they no longer have useful visual clues. Performance varies with each individual.

In the United States, over 6 million persons are visually impaired but not classified as legally blind.[1] Over 75% of patients seeking treatment are age 65 or older. Age-related macular degeneration accounts for an increasing number of cases. Other common causes of low vision are glaucoma, diabetic retinopathy, cataract, optic atrophy, corneal disease, cerebral damage, degenerative myopia, and retinitis pigmentosa. Approximately 9% of the low-vision population is pediatric, with visual loss from congenital eye disorders or trauma. (See Chapter 20 for discussion of the worldwide prevalence and causes of visual impairment.)

Effective low-vision intervention starts as soon as the patient experiences difficulty performing ordinary tasks. A treatment plan should consider the level of function, realistic goals for intervention, and the varieties of devices that could be helpful. Patients must face the fact that impaired vision is usually progressive. The sooner they adapt to low-vision devices, the sooner they can adjust to the new techniques of using their vision. Low-vision evaluation should never be delayed unless the person is in an active phase of medical or surgical treatment.

Visual performance can be improved by optical and non-optical devices. The general term for corrective devices is "low-vision aids." In this chapter, the emphasis will be on assessment techniques, descriptions of useful devices, and a discussion of some of the functional aspects of common eye diseases.

MANAGEMENT OF THE PATIENT WITH LOW VISION

Comprehensive management includes (1) history of onset of the eye condition and the effect of the loss of vision on daily life; (2) examination for best corrected acuity, visual fields, contrast sensitivity, and color perception (and glare sensitivity if it pertains to the patient's symptoms); (3) evaluation of near vision and reading skills; (4) selection and prescription (or lending) of aids that accomplish task objectives; (5) instruction in correct use and application of devices; and (6) follow-up to reinforce new patterns.

HISTORY TAKING

Specific features of the onset, treatments given, and current medications should be verified. Patients' responses indicate their understanding of their condition. Unrealistic

---

[1]Legal blindness—defined as best corrected visual acuity of 20/200 or less in the better eye or a visual field of 20° or less—affects 1,000,000 individuals in the United States (see Chapter 20). It is an administrative definition that does not mean that the patient is unable to see anything.

Table 24–1. Common Activities That Are Adversely Affected by Visual Impairment with Suggestions for Low-Vision Aids

Activity	Optical Aids	Nonoptical Aids
Shopping	Hand magnifier	Lighting, color cues
Fixing a snack	Spectacle magnifier	Color cues, consistent storage plan
Eating out	Hand magnifier	Flashlight, portable lamp
Identifying money	Spectacle, spectacle-mounted, or hand magnifier	Arrange wallet in compartments, fold banknotes of different denominations differently
Reading print	Spectacle, spectacle-mounted, dome, hand, stand, or portable video magnifier Computer reading system	Lighting, high-contrast print, large print, reading slit
Writing	Hand magnifier	Lighting, bold-tip pen, black ink, line guide
Dialing a telephone	Telescope Hand magnifier	Large-print dial, hand-printed directory
Crossing streets	Telescope	Cane, ask directions
Finding taxis and bus signs	Telescope	
Reading medication labels	Hand magnifier	Color codes, large print
Reading stove dials	Hand magnifier	Color codes
Thermostat adjustment	Hand magnifier	Enlarged-print model
Using a computer	Intermediate add spectacles	High-contrast color, large-print program
Reading signs	Spectacle or spectacle-mounted magnifier Telescope Portable electronic magnifier	Move closer
Watching sporting event	Telescope	Sit in front rows

or unreasonable attitudes need to be documented. Does the person understand the limitations of what can be achieved with low-vision rehabilitation? It is helpful to refer to a list of common daily activities the patient may not be able to perform efficiently (Table 24–1). From this list, it is possible to arrive at realistic treatment objectives for that person.

EXAMINATION

The pupils should not be dilated before a low-vision evaluation. Refractive status should be confirmed to rule out a significant change, particularly after surgical intervention such as cataract or glaucoma surgery. A patient may have become myopic from a nuclear cataract or astigmatic from corneal warping after glaucoma drainage surgery. The most accurate acuity test is the Early Treatment Diabetic Retinopathy Study (ETDRS) chart (Figure 24–1), which has 14 five-letter lines of 0.1 log unit size difference with a LogMAR (logarithm of minimum angle of resolution) scale and a convenient metric or Snellen conversion. Masking of other lines may facilitate letter recognition. An integrated light box standardizes illumination. A 4-meter test distance is used when acuity is 20/20 to 20/200; a 2-meter distance for acuities less than 20/200 but 20/400 or better; and a 1-meter distance for acuities less than 20/400. The ETDRS chart makes obsolete the imprecise expression "finger counting." Alternatively, a Snellen chart can be used, either at the conventional testing distance of 20 feet (6 m) or less (see Chapter 2).

Projector charts are not recommended for testing subnormal vision because of low contrast and insufficient letter choice at low acuities.

The dominant eye and preferred eye should be noted.

The Amsler grid (Figure 2–21) is the traditional test for evaluating the central field. Although relatively insensitive, it can be used to advantage in low vision, particularly to identify the dominant eye. It is viewed at the normal reading distance (28–30 cm). The patient should first look at the chart *binocularly*. ("Can you see the dot?") Observe for eye or head turn. If the dot is seen, the patient is using either a viable macula or an eccentric viewing area. An eye turn or head tilt may confirm this. Ask the patient to report distortion or blank areas seen binocularly. Then check the grid

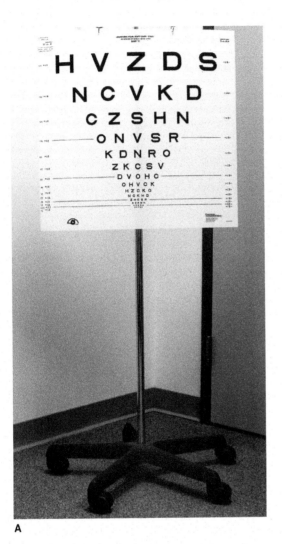

A

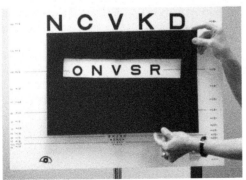

B

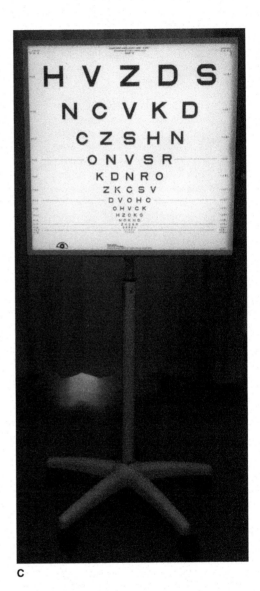

C

▲ **Figure 24–1. A:** Lighthouse modification of the Ferris–Bailey Early Treatment Diabetic Retinopathy Study (ETDRS) chart. **B:** Masking of other lines to facilitate letter recognition. **C:** With integrated light box to standardize illumination.

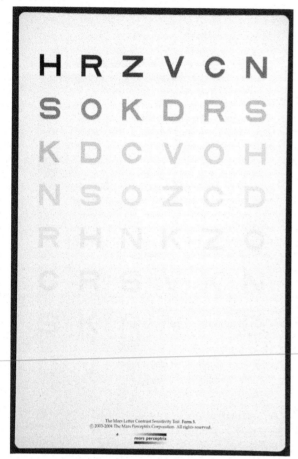

The Mars Letter Contrast Sensitivity Test. Form 3.
© 2003-2004 The Mars Perceptrix Corporation. All rights reserved.

mars perceptrix

▲ **Figure 24–2.** Mars Letter-Contrast Sensitivity Test chart.

The contrast of each letter decreases by a constant factor of 0.04 log unit, which makes it the most sensitive of the clinical contrast tests. Contrast sensitivity is a predictor of the retina's response to magnification. Regardless of acuity, if contrast is subthreshold or in the severe loss category, the patient is less likely to respond to optical magnification.

Simple color identification tests are done if the patient's complaints include difficulty with color cues.

NEAR VISION

Near vision may be evaluated with a combination of single-letter tests, such as with a reduced version of the ETDRS chart, and graded text of short sentences with simple vocabulary (Figure 24–3). Single letters and short words are presented first to establish near acuity. Graded text is then presented to establish reading skills with the selected optical devices.

SELECTION OF DEVICES & PATIENT INSTRUCTION

The dioptric range is selected from the outcome of acuity tests, modified by the results of the Amsler grid and contrast sensitivity tests. A rule of thumb for the starting power is to calculate the reciprocal of visual acuity—for example, an acuity of 20/160 suggests a starting lens of 8 diopters (160/20). Keep in mind that visual acuity is not a particularly sensitive measure of function. Scotomas within the reading field and the contrast sensitivity of the paramacular retina have a greater influence on ability to read magnified print through an optical lens.

After the dioptric range has been agreed upon, the three major categories of devices are presented in sequence in the selected power. Lenses in a spectacle mounting are presented and evaluated first, followed by hand-held magnifiers and, third, stand-mounted magnifiers. Telescopes and television or computer-designed devices are increasingly prescribed as the population becomes more sophisticated in the use of advanced technology.

INSTRUCTION

Part of effective management of every low-vision patient is skilled instruction in using a device. Attention should be paid to daily living activities, which can be complemented by low-vision lenses but may also require referral to an agency for the visually impaired.

The patient uses the various devices under the supervision of an instructor until proficiency is achieved. The patient is allowed ample time to learn correct techniques in one or more sessions and possibly provided a loaner lens for home or job trial. Older patients usually need more

monocularly and again ask the patient to report seeing the center fixation dot and any distortion or scotoma. If the grid is presented in this manner, the patient understands what is expected and the test can provide helpful data. For example, if a large scotoma in the dominant eye overrides the better nondominant eye, the patient probably will require occlusion of the dominant eye. If the dominant eye is the better eye, it will override the poorer nondominant eye, and the patient can benefit from binocular correction.

Tests of contrast express the functional level of retinal sensitivity more accurately than any other test, including acuity. Of the available tests for contrast sensitivity, the Mars test using letters arranged on three 14 × 19 charts in 8 rows of 6 letters each is rapid and accurate (Figure 24–2).[2]

---

[2]MARS Letter Contrast Sensitivity Test. Available from The Mars Perceptrix Corporation, 49 Valley View Road, Chappaqua, NY 10514-2523, www.marsperceptrix.com, Tel: 914-239-3526.

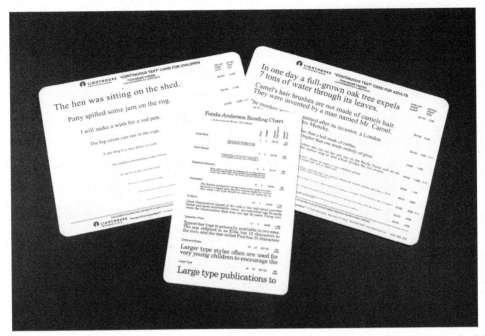

△ **Figure 24–3.** Near-vision test charts, including the Lighthouse Continuous Text Cards for children and adults.

adaptation time and reinforcement than younger or congenitally impaired persons.

Practitioners and staff benefit from training programs to learn how to manage a low-vision patient in the office. Basic setups for incorporating low vision into a practice are reviewed in a number of publications.

FOLLOW-UP

In 2 to 3 weeks, the patient's progress is reviewed, adjustments are made, and prescriptions are finalized. If minor problems arise within the first few days after the appointment, they can usually be resolved by telephone.

▼ LOW-VISION AIDS

There are five types of low-vision aids: (1) convex-lens aids such as spectacle (including bifocal), spectacle-mounted, dome, hand-held, and stand-mounted magnifiers (Figure 24–4); (2) telescopes, either spectacle-mounted or hand-held (Figure 24–5); (3) nonoptical devices (adaptive aids) such as large print, reading stands, marking devices, reading, writing, and signature guides, pill organizers, liquid level indicators, and large numeral and talking clocks, watches, timers, calculators, and scales (Figure 24–6); (4) tints and filters, including antireflective lenses (Figure 24–7), and illumination; and (5) electronic devices such as portable or desktop closed-circuit television (CCTV) reading machines (Figure 24–8), image scanners, and magnification, and voice synthesis and recognition computer software (Figure 24–9).

CONVEX-LENS AIDS (FIGURE 24–4)

Convex-lens aids, such as spectacle, spectacle-mounted, dome, hand, and stand magnifiers, are prescribed for over 90% of patients. The various mountings have inherent advantages and disadvantages.

The main advantage of spectacle (Figure 24–4A) and spectacle-mounted magnifiers (Figure 24–4B) is that both hands remain free to hold the reading material. They require the reading material to be held at the focal distance of the lens, for example, 10 cm for a 10-diopter lens. Increasing lens strength shortens the reading distance and increases the tendency to obstruct light. Lamps with flexible arms may be required for uniform lighting. Patients with binocular function may use 4- to 14-diopter spectacles with base-in prisms to reduce the requirement for convergence (Figure 24–4C). Above 14 diopters, a monocular sphere must be used for the better eye.

Dome magnifiers (Figure 24–4D and E), which are placed directly on the reading material, also allow both hands to be free, always provide a focused image, and maximize

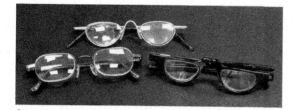

A

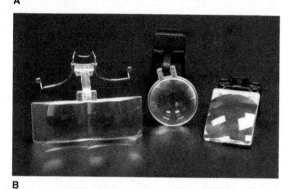

B

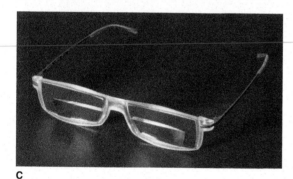

C

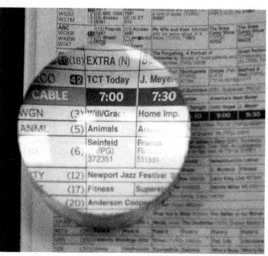

D

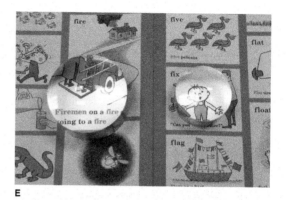

E

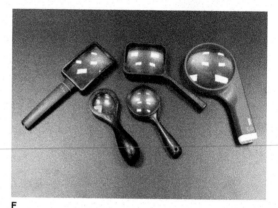

F

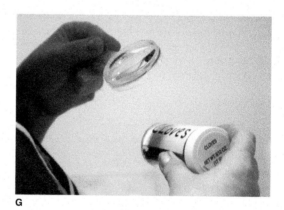

G

▲ **Figure 24–4.** Convex-lens aids. **A:** Spectacle magnifiers. **B:** Spectacle-mounted magnifiers. **C:** High-power reading spectacles with prisms to reduce the requirement for convergence. **D and E:** Dome magnifiers. **F:** Hand magnifiers of various strengths. **G:** Hand magnifier in use. **H:** Hand magnifiers suitable for carrying in a pocket or purse. **I:** Illuminated hand magnifiers of various strengths. **J–L:** Illuminated hand magnifiers with LED blue, green, and yellow light. **M:** Fixed focus stand magnifier, allowing writing on the material being read.

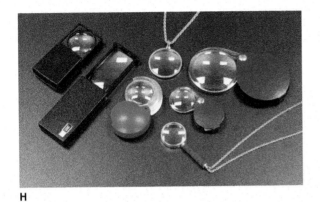

H

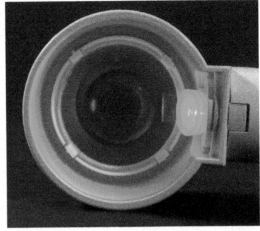

K

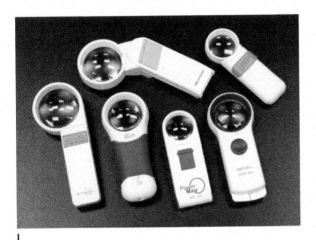

I

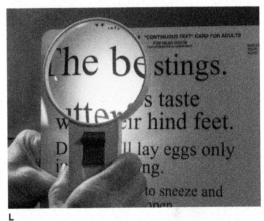

L

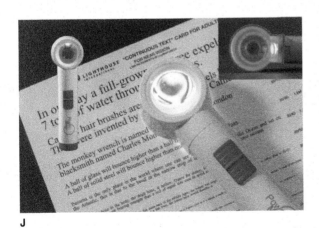

J

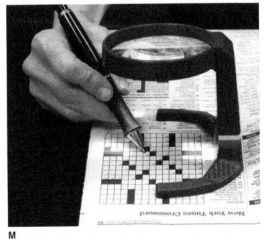

M

▲ **Figure 24–4.** (*Continued*)

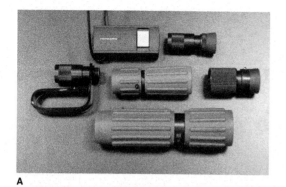

A

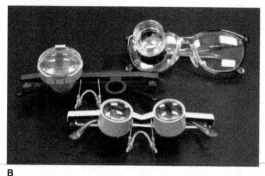

B

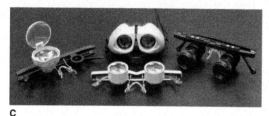

C

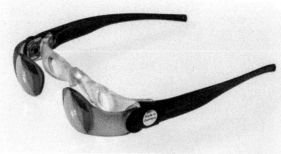

D

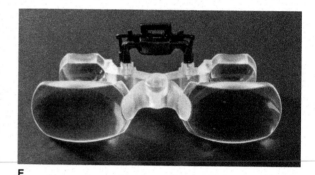

E

▲ Figure 24–5. Telescopes. **A:** Hand-held monocular. **B:** Spectacle-mounted for close tasks. **C:** Spectacle-mounted for distance viewing, including focusable (right). **D:** Spectacle-mounted for distance viewing with independent focusing for each eye. **E:** Clip-on for middle-distance viewing.

illumination, but the amount of magnification is limited, and there may be problems with distortion and light reflection.

Hand magnifiers (Figure 24–4F–L) that can have colored illumination are convenient for shopping, reading dials and labels, identifying money, etc. They are often used by older people in conjunction with their reading glasses to enlarge print. The advantage is a greater working space between the eye and lens, but holding a lens may be a disadvantage for a trembling hand or stiff joints. Hand magnifiers are available from 4 to 68 diopters. Stand magnifiers (Figure 24–4M) are convex lenses mounted on a rigid base whose height is related to the power of the lens, for example, a 10-diopter lens is just under 10 cm from the page, writing on the material being read being possible with the lower magnification devices. Because the lens mounting may block light, a battery-powered light may be helpful. For both hand and stand magnifiers, an LED light source improves illumination and battery life and reduces glare.

TELESCOPES (FIGURE 24–5)

Telescopes are the only devices that can be focused from infinity to near. All telescopes share the disadvantage of a small field diameter and shallow depth of field. The simplest device is the hand-held monocular telescope (Figure 24–5A) used for short-term viewing, particularly of signs. The practical limit of power for hand-held units is 2–8×. For close tasks and vocational or hobby interests, telescopes mounted in (Figure 24–5B–D) or clipped on (Figure 24–5E) a spectacle frame are practical but difficult to use above 6×.

NONOPTICAL DEVICES (ADAPTIVE AIDS) (FIGURE 24–6)

Many practical items can augment or replace visual aids. They are traditionally called "nonoptical devices," although "adaptive aids" is probably a better term. In daily life,

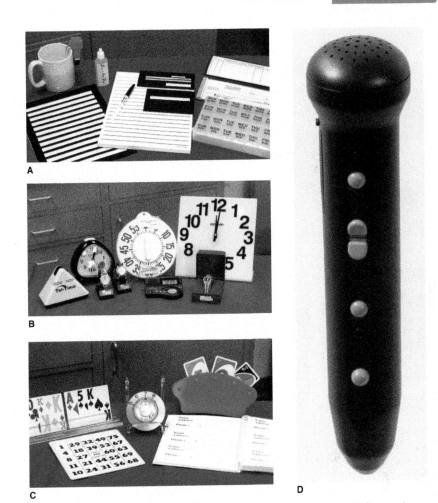

▲ **Figure 24–6.** Nonoptical devices. **A:** Reading and writing guides, marking devices, pill organizer, and liquid level indicator. **B:** Large numeral and talking clocks, watches, and timers. **C:** Large print address book, bingo card, playing cards, and thermostat. **D:** Audio labeler.

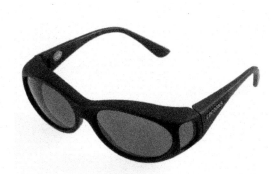

▲ **Figure 24–7.** Amber-tinted wraparound glasses.

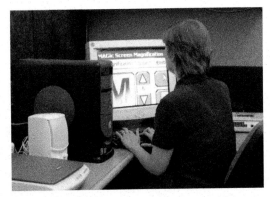

▲ **Figure 24–8.** Computer reading system with image scanner and magnification software.

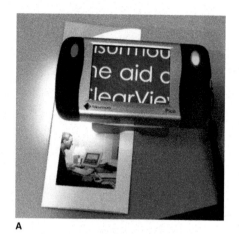

A

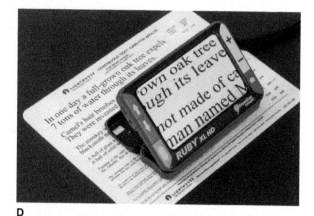

D

B

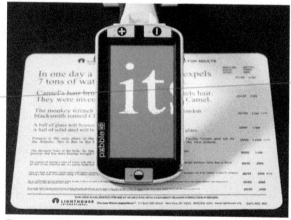

E

C

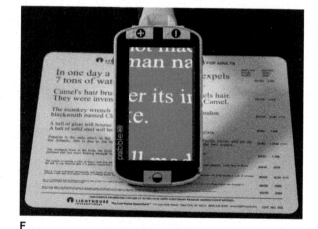

F

▲ Figure 24–9. **A–H:** Portable video magnifiers.

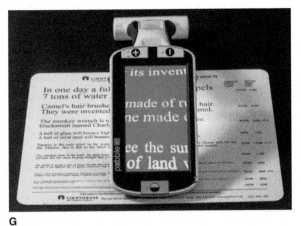

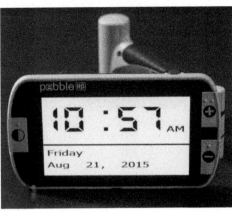

G H

▲ **Figure 24–9.** (*Continued*)

difficulty in reading is not the only frustrating experience for the low-vision person. Cooking, setting thermostats and stove dials, measuring, reading a scale, putting on makeup, selecting the correct illumination, identifying banknotes, and playing cards are only a few things that sighted people take for granted. Many devices are available for the visually impaired to assist in performing these tasks. The field is expanding rapidly, and it is important to keep up to date with available aids and resources.

TINTS, COATINGS, AND ILLUMINATION

Many low-vision patients complain of poor contrast and glare, which particularly hinders traveling around on their own. Light or medium gray lenses are prescribed to reduce light intensity, and amber or yellow lenses improve contrast and reduce the effect of short-wave light rays (Figure 24–7). Devices designed specifically for low-vision patients offer nonchangeable filters and photochromic (variable intensity tint) lenses. An additional antireflective coating should be considered for glare-sensitive patients. Trial lenses are advisable because each patient responds differently to the various available tints and to the degree of light transmission that the lens provides.

Adequate task and ambient lighting is essential for persons who depend principally on the macula for vision, enhancing contrast, reducing glare, and simulating natural lighting. Light that is too bright may cause strain, glare, and photophobia, which may be relieved by introducing amber to yellow filters that block ultraviolet and visible blue light below 527 nm. Patients with early cataracts, macular changes, and corneal dystrophies may have difficulty reading with their current lighting. Older patients also notice difficulties with near tasks after changing to energy-saving light sources known as compact fluorescent light (CFL). Before

changing the incandescent bulb to a CFL, it is important to select the proper CFL bulb, one designated as "warm or soft light." Full-spectrum bulbs can improve lighting, eliminating glare and improving efficiency. Light that does not scatter and is aimed directly on the print or task is preferred.

ELECTRONIC AND PORTABLE VIDEO MAGNIFIERS AND READING SYSTEMS (FIGURES 24–8 AND 24–9)

A closed-circuit television reading machine (CCTV) consists of a high-resolution monitor with a built-in camera with a zoom lens, if necessary an illumination system, and in the desktop models, an X-Y reading platform. Magnification from 1.5× to 45× is possible with adjustable font sizes, and the background can be reversed from white to dark gray. Image scanning and software programs enhance flexibility (Figure 24–8). Such systems encourage a natural reading posture and are a good choice for school children to help them see their class work and view graphs, diagrams, or photos.

Portable video magnifiers (Figure 24–9) allow the visually impaired to read medication labels, mail, price tags, and menus, or view videos. The devices have built-in illumination and allow for contrast enhancement, color display, and variable magnification. Many are small enough to fit in a pocket or purse. Some have a built-in distance camera to allow viewing of signs, arrival and departure boards at airports, and classroom lectures. Electronic portable reading devices can download printed material such as books and newspapers, which can be read or listened to using text to speech options. Other functions include audible clock and calendar. Some cellular phones can perform some of these tasks.

The rapid development of devices for the general population has benefited visually impaired patients by increasing choice and reducing cost, allowing them to regain their independence more easily.

THE EFFECT OF THE EYE DISORDER

Treatment plans should take into account the effect of the eye disorder on both visual acuity and visual field. The type and strength of visual aid are influenced by the type and extent of the deficit.

Diseases resulting in low vision can be classified into three categories (Figure 24–10): (1) blurred or hazy vision throughout the visual field, characteristic of cloudy media; (2) central scotomas, characteristic of macular disorders and optic nerve disease; and (3) peripheral scotomas, such as the generalized constriction typical of retinitis pigmentosa and other peripheral retinal disorders, and advanced glaucoma, or homonymous hemianopia due to central nervous system disorders such as stroke.

BLURRED, HAZY VISION (FIGURE 24–10B)

Any corneal disease, cataract, capsular opacification, or vitreous opacity interferes with refraction of light rays entering the eye. Such random refraction causes reduced acuity, glare, and decreased contrast. Pupillary miosis further restricts the

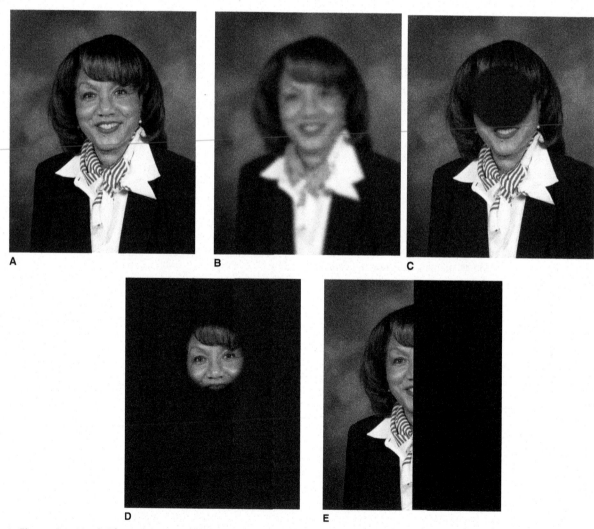

▲ Figure 24–10. **A:** Normal image. **B:** Blurred image. **C:** Central scotoma. **D:** Peripheral scotoma of peripheral retinal disorders or advanced glaucoma. **E:** Right homonymous hemianopia due to left cerebral hemisphere stroke.

quantity of light reaching the retina. Patients have difficulty seeing stairs and steps and other low-contrast objects. Acuity varies with ambient light.

Useful parameters of visual function include visual acuity, glare, and contrast sensitivity. A potential acuity meter (PAM) used in conjunction with a glare test helps to differentiate retinal from media pathology.

▶ Management

Refraction should always be carefully done, including multiple pinholes, stenopeic slit, and keratometry. Modification of illumination and attention to details of room and task lighting are most important. Antireflective lens coatings and neutral gray lenses reduce light intensity (and therefore glare). Yellow and amber lenses enhance contrast. Ultraviolet filters should be used particularly for pseudophakic patients. Large bold print provides the higher contrast the patient needs.

Magnification may or may not be effective depending on the patient's level of contrast sensitivity. A magnified image itself has low contrast. The glare from an illuminated stand magnifier may actually reduce reading acuity. Large bold print may be a better choice than a magnifier—or in case of surface glare from paper, a reading slit of matte black plastic to reduce glare and outline the text. Contact lenses, keratoplasty, corneal laser refractive surgery, posterior capsulotomy, and cataract surgery may also be indicated.

If cataract seems to be interfering with optimal function, a combination of contrast sensitivity and glare tests may indicate the best time for surgery. The intraocular lens should contain an ultraviolet blocking agent. The surgeon may wish to discuss overcorrecting the power of the implant by a few diopters. The resulting myopia will provide clear intermediate distance vision without correction, which is more important for a visually impaired person than clear far-distance vision.

CENTRAL SCOTOMAS (FIGURE 24–10C)

Central retinal (macular) function, predominantly utilizing cone photoreceptors, is essential for detailed, color, and daylight (photopic) vision. The two most common causes of macular disease are atrophic (dry) and neovascular (exudative, wet) age-related macular degeneration, both of which are increasingly prevalent in today's aging society. Other causes are macular holes, myopic macular degeneration, and congenital macular disorders. Optic nerve disease also predominantly affects central vision.

In the early stages of atrophic age-related macular degeneration, patients most often report blurred or distorted central vision. Peripheral vision is unaffected unless there is cataract. The loss of central vision interferes with reading and seeing details, including facial features. Dense scotomas are not present in atrophic macular degeneration and usually not in exudative disease unless there is retinal fibrosis

following choroidal or subretinal hemorrhage. Contrast sensitivity decreases as the disease extends beyond the fovea. Macular degeneration generally does not hinder safe travel because the preserved peripheral vision is effective for orientation purposes. Effective treatment of exudative age-related macular degeneration has increased the number of patients with macular degeneration who can benefit from low-vision rehabilitation.

▶ Management

Patients with moderately advanced macular disease often spontaneously adopt an eccentric head tilt or eye turn to move images from nonseeing retina to a viable parafoveal area, known as a preferred retinal locus (PRL), of which there may be more than one in each eye. The ability to move the scotoma may be demonstrated to a patient during the Amsler grid test. Some patients respond to bilateral prisms in spectacles to relocate the image. Other patients may benefit from training to utilize a PRL, or to utilize another area of parafoveal retina, a trained retinal locus (TRL), that is more advantageous. Such training can be undertaken by occupational therapists or certified low-vision therapists and can be facilitated with a scanning laser ophthalmoscope (SLO).

Magnifying lenses enlarge the retinal image, allowing use of eccentric fixation by compensating for lower retinal sensitivity in the parafoveal area. The power of the lens is related to the contrast sensitivity, as well as location and density of the scotoma. Patients may use different types of devices for various tasks: spectacles for reading, hand magnifier for shopping, or CCTV for writing and typing. Most people learn to use low-vision aids successfully, particularly after instruction sessions to reinforce correct usage. Older people may require more time and repetition.

PERIPHERAL SCOTOMA (FIGURE 24–10D AND E)

Scotomas in the peripheral field are characteristic of end-stage glaucoma, retinitis pigmentosa, other peripheral retinal disorders including proliferative diabetic retinopathy treated with panretinal photocoagulation, and central nervous system disorders such as tumor, stroke, or trauma. The peripheral field is essential for orienting oneself in space, detecting motion, and awareness of potential hazards in the environment. The predominantly rod vision is most sensitive in twilight and at night. A person with a constricted field may be able to read small print yet need a cane or guide dog to get around.

▶ Management

If the central field diameter is less than 7°, magnification may not be advantageous. Telescopes and spectacle magnifiers may enlarge the image beyond the useful field. Hand magnifiers and closed-circuit television or computers may be the equipment of choice because the size of the image can be adjusted to match the size of the field.

Mainly for patients with homonymous hemianopia, various training techniques, such as vision restoration therapy and explorative saccade training, have been advocated and are being evaluated.

REFERENCES

Agarwal A et al: Prognosis and treatment of visual field defects. Semin Neurol 2015;35:549. [PMID: 26444400]

Altpeter EK et al: Requirements for low vision magnification aids in age-related macular degeneration: Data from the Tübingen low vision clinic (comparison of 2007-2011 with 1999-2005). Ophthalmologe 2015;112:923. (German) [PMID: 26040791]

American Academy of Ophthalmology Preferred Practice Pattern Committee: Vision Rehabilitation Preferred Practice Pattern Guidelines. American Academy of Ophthalmology, 2012. Available at www.aao.org/ppp.

Burggraaff MC et al: Randomized controlled trial on the effects of training in the use of closed-circuit television on reading performance. Invest Ophthalmol Vis Sci 2012;53:2142. [PMID: 22427558]

Chavda S et al: Low-vision rehabilitation methods in children: A systematic review. Can J Ophthalmol 2014;49:e71. [PMID: 24862788]

Das A et al: New approaches to visual rehabilitation for cortical blindness: Outcomes and putative mechanisms. Neuroscientist 2010;16:374. [PMID: 20103505]

Decarlo DK et al: Use of prescribed optical devices in age-related macular degeneration. Optom Vis Sci 2012;89:1336. [PMID: 22902420]

Dilks DD et al: Reorganization of visual processing in age-related macular degeneration depends on foveal loss. Optom Vis Sci 2014;91:e199. [PMID: 24978868]

Do AT et al: Effectiveness of low vision services in improving patient quality of life at Aravind Eye Hospital. Indian J Ophthalmol 2014;62:1125. [PMID: 25579355]

Downes K et al: SKread predicts handwriting performance in patients with low vision. Can J Ophthalmol 2015;50:225. [PMID: 26040223]

Dundon NM et al: Visual rehabilitation: Visual scanning, multisensory stimulation and vision restoration trainings. Front Behav Neurosci 2015;9:192. [PMID: 26283935]

Faye EE (editor): *Clinical Low Vision*, 2nd ed. Little, Brown, 1984.

Faye EE: Low vision aids. In: *Clinical Ophthalmology, Vol 1: Refraction.* Duane TD (editor). Harper & Row, 1990.

Faye EE: Pathology and visual function. In: *Functional Assessment of Low Vision.* Rosenthal BP, Cole RG (editors). Mosby, 1996.

Faye EE et al: *The Aging Eye and Low Vision: A Study Guide.* The Lighthouse, 1995.

Forooghian F et al: Visual acuity outcomes after cataract surgery in patients with age-related macular degeneration: Age-Related Eye Disease Study Report No. 27. Ophthalmology 2009;116:2093. [PMID: 19700198]

Goldstein JE et al: Clinically meaningful rehabilitation outcomes of low vision patients served by outpatient clinical centers. JAMA Ophthalmol 2015;133:762. [PMID: 25856370]

Goodwin D: Homonymous hemianopia: Challenges and solutions. Clin Ophthalmol 2014;8:1919. [PMID: 25284978]

Gordon K et al: Comprehensive vision rehabilitation. Can J Ophthalmol 2015;50:85. [PMID: 25677290]

Gothwal VK et al: Assessing the effectiveness of low vision rehabilitation in children: An observational study. Invest Ophthalmol Vis Sci 2015;56:3355. [PMID: 25829416]

Gothwal VK et al: Outcomes of multidisciplinary low vision rehabilitation in adults. Invest Ophthalmol Vis Sci 2015;56:7451. [PMID: 26595605]

Hamade N et al: The effects of low-vision rehabilitation on reading speed and depression in age related macular degeneration: A meta-analysis. PLoS One 2016;11:e0159254. [PMID: 27414030]

Ho AC et al: Long-term results from an epiretinal prosthesis to restore sight to the blind. Ophthalmology 2015;122:1547. [PMID: 26162233]

Jobke S et al: Vision restoration through extratriate stimulation in patients with visual field defects: A double-blind and randomized experimental study. Neurorehabil Neural Repair 2009;23:246. [PMID: 19240199]

Lam N et al: Low-vision service provision by optometrists: A Canadian nationwide survey. Optom Vis Sci 2015;92:365. [PMID: 25599339]

Leat SJ: A proposed model for integrated low-vision rehabilitation services in Canada. Optom Vis Sci 2016;93:77. [PMID: 26583792]

Lighthouse Continuing Education: Annual catalog of courses, seminars and symposia. http://www.lighthouse.org/about/education/programs.htm, Fax: 212-821-9707; e-mail: education@lighthouse.org.

Lighthouse Information and Resource Service: Information and pamphlets about eye conditions, visual impairment, and blindness. http://www.lighthouse.org/services/rehab.htm, Tel: 800-829-0500.

MacKeben M et al: Random word recognition chart helps scotoma assessment in low vision. Optom Vis Sci 2015;92:421. [PMID: 25946100]

Markowitz SN: State-of-the-art: low vision rehabilitation. Can J Ophthalmol 2016;51:59. [PMID: 27085259]

Markowitz SN et al: The relationship between scotoma displacement and preferred retinal loci in low-vision patients with age-related macular degeneration. Can J Ophthalmol 2010;45:58. [PMID: 20130712]

Mohler AJ et al: Factors affecting readiness for low vision interventions in older adults. Am J Occup Ther 2015;69:6904270020p1. [PMID: 26114465]

Monteiro MM et al: Optical and nonoptical aids for reading and writing in individuals with acquired low vision. Arq Bras Oftalmol 2014;7:91. [PMID: 25076472]

Moshtael H et al: High tech aids low vision: A review of image processing for the visually impaired. Transl Vis Sci Technol 2015;4:6. [PMID: 26290777]

Natarajan S. Low vision aids: A boon. Indian J Ophthalmol 2013;61:191. [PMID: 23760451]

Nollett CL et al: Depression in Visual Impairment Trial (DEPVIT): A randomized clinical trial of depression treatments in people with low vision. Invest Ophthalmol Vis Sci 2016;57:4247. [PMID: 27548898]

Pascolini D et al: Global estimates of visual impairment: 2010. Br J Ophthalmol 2012;96:614. [PMID: 22133988]

Rainey L et al: Comprehending the impact of low vision on the lives of children and adolescents: A qualitative approach. Qual Life Res 2016;25:2633. [PMID: 27076189]

Renieri G et al: Changes in quality of life in visually impaired patients after low-vision rehabilitation. Int J Rehabil Res 2013;36:48. [PMID: 22890293]

Robinson JL et al: Usage of accessibility options for the iPhone and iPad in a visually impaired population. Semin Ophthalmol 2017;32:163-171. [PMID: 26154395]

Roth T et al: Comparing explorative saccade and flicker training in hemianopia: A randomized controlled study. Neurology 2009;72:324. [PMID: 19171828]

Ryan B et al: Effectiveness of the community-based Low Vision Service Wales: A long-term outcome study. Br J Ophthalmol 2013;97:487. [PMID: 23410732]

Shima N et al: Concept of a functional retinal locus in age-related macular degeneration. Can J Ophthalmol 2010;45:62. [PMID: 20130713]

Stelmack JA et al: The effectiveness of low-vision rehabilitation in 2 cohorts derived from the Veterans Affairs Low-Vision Intervention Trial. Arch Ophthalmol 2012;130:1162. [PMID: 22965592]

Thayaparan K et al: Clinical assessment of two new contrast sensitivity charts. Br J Ophthalmol 2007;91:749. [PMID: 17166891]

van Rheede JJ et al: Improving mobility performance in low vision with a distance-based representation of the visual scene. Invest Ophthalmol Vis Sci 2015;56:4802. [PMID: 26218908]

Wittich W et al: Usability of assistive listening devices by older adults with low vision. Disabil Rehabil Assist Technol 2016;11:564. [PMID: 25945610]

Internet Resources

www.afb.org/seniorsitehome.asp

www.cdc.gov/visionhealth/

www.cdc.gov/visionhealth/pdf/improving_nations_vision_health.pdf

www.independentliving.com/products.asp?dept=30&deptname=Portable-Systems

www.lighthouse.org/

www.nei.nih.gov/nehep/programs/lowvision/index.asp

www.nei.nih.gov/nehep/newsletter/index.asp

http://one.aao.org/CE/EducationalContent/Smartsight.aspx http://www.spedex.com/napvi/

http://www.preventblindness.org/vpus/

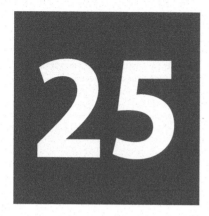

Vision Rehabilitation

August Colenbrander, MD

Vision is the most important source of information about our environment. Loss of vision reduces the ability to perform activities of daily living, and affects safety and quality of life. Most of this book deals with reducing the *causes* of vision loss. Vision rehabilitation deals with reducing its *consequences*.

In developed countries, and increasingly in developing countries, the majority of irreversible vision loss occurs in the elderly and will represent an ever increasing part of ophthalmic practice (see Chapter 20). Unfortunately, many patients and caregivers still consider vision loss as an inevitable result of aging and often do not seek the help that is available. It is the task of the ophthalmologist to tell them that even if *"nothing more can be done"* about their reduction of vision, *"much can be done"* to deal with the consequences of vision loss for the person.

STAGES OF VISUAL PROCESSING

When dealing with the consequences of vision loss, it is important to recognize that vision is a complex, multistage process. Dysfunction at the different stages of visual processing causes different problems that require different solutions. The first is the *optical* stage, which puts an image of the outside world on the retina. The second is the *receptor* stage, which translates the optical image into neural impulses. The third stage is *neural processing*, which starts in the inner retina and proceeds via the visual cortex to higher cortical centers, where it eventually gives rise to visually guided behavior.

The *optical* stage can be disrupted by refractive errors and media opacities. Letter chart acuity is a good tool to evaluate this stage, and magnification devices (see Chapter 24) are the natural choice to counteract this type of vision loss.

The *receptor* stage can be disrupted by retinal disease. If foveal function is reduced, visual acuity is reduced. If foveal function is absent, causing a central scotoma, a pseudo-fovea or preferred retinal locus (PRL) must take over fixation. This

eccentric area will have a reduced receptor density, which causes further reduction of visual acuity.

For retinal disorders, letter chart acuity is important but tells only part of the story, since it describes only the function at the point of fixation and tells us nothing about the condition of the surrounding retina (even a 20/200 letter covers less than a 1° area). Normal vision involves constant eye movements, which may move the object of attention in and out of the best-functioning area. This *scotoma interference*, which may be apparent as hesitation during testing, is not quantified by visual acuity and cannot be remedied with magnification devices. Patients need *training and practice* to improve their fixation stability. This may be provided by occupational therapists or vision rehabilitation specialists, but it is up to ophthalmologists to recognize the need for this training and to make the appropriate referral.

Neural processing comprises the third and most complex stage. Awareness of vision problems related to the processing of visual information is increasing. It includes the perceptual consequences of traumatic brain injury (TBI) in adults, cerebrovascular accidents (CVAs) in the elderly, and cerebral (cortical) visual impairment (CVI) in children. In this area, the ophthalmologist may need to cooperate and communicate with social workers and educators.

Some cerebral defects produce obvious impairments of visual acuity and visual field (visual impairment). More subtle defects (visual dysfunction) may exist in the presence of normal performance on standard clinical testing. A patient with optical or retinal problems may stumble over a curb because of lack of contrast, whereas a patient with a cerebral injury may be able to detect the change in contrast but may be unable to decide whether this is a line on the ground or the edge of a step. In this case, *vision enhancement* (better illumination, contrast) will not help, and *vision substitution* (use of senses other than vision such as a cane to tactically determine the step) may be more appropriate. Full assessment of impaired cerebral processing may involve other professionals and neuropsychological testing, but preliminary assessment by ophthalmologists can often be the starting point.

ASPECTS OF VISION LOSS

A convenient framework to discuss the various impacts of vision loss considers four aspects of visual functioning: *organ structure, organ function, individual abilities, and societal consequences* (Figure 25–1).

Macroscopic and microscopic examination of tissues may reveal *structural changes*, such as scarring, degeneration, and atrophy. This is the domain of the ocular pathologist. But these changes do not necessarily indicate how well the organ functions. To assess this, we need tests, such as visual acuity, visual field, and contrast sensitivity, which determine *organ function*. This is the domain of the ophthalmologist. However, *"how well the eyes function"* does not yet assess *"how well the person functions"* in performing various activities of daily living (ADL) and various *visual abilities*, such as reading, getting around, or recognizing faces. This is the domain of occupational therapists and other rehabilitation professionals, who need to work with patients and teach them how to use their residual vision most effectively. Finally, there is a need to assess how these changes affect the person's role and *participation in society*, since this is the ultimate goal of all interventions at whichever level. From this short summary, it should be clear that comprehensive vision care cannot be the work of one person; it requires team work, and the patient needs to be a part of this team.

Traditional textbooks describe these four aspects from left to right in the sequence from causes to consequences. For patients, however, the starting point is on the right, since they experience primarily the societal consequences. The patient may come with a complaint: *"Doctor, I cannot read"*; the doctor translates this to a statement about the eyes: *"She has lost three lines."* The doctor is primarily interested in the *"how the eyes function"* and wants to find and treat the underlying causes; the patient is primarily interested in

"how the person functions" and wants to alleviate the consequences. It is the task of rehabilitation to bridge this gap.

Recognizing how doctors and patients approach medical conditions from different points of view is essential for effective communication. Seemingly similar tests may have to be done in somewhat different ways. Clinicians, who are interested in how each eye functions, will measure visual acuity for *each eye separately*. However, to determine how the person functions, whether for employment, for a driver's license, for education, or simply for quality of life, we must measure visual acuity with *both eyes open*, since that is how people live their lives. Although we have two eyes, those eyes are part of a single visual system that generates a single visual perception. This shift in emphasis was explicitly recognized by the World Health Organization in a 2003 consultation, which acknowledged the fact that health statistics are not only a tool to detect eye disease, but also to describe the burden of vision loss in a population. At the individual level, this is also important. Refractive surgeons are becoming increasingly aware of the need to individualize treatment to the patient's needs. A comprehensive reading assessment should not only determine the smallest print size read, but also reading speed, reading endurance, reading enjoyment, and reading comprehension.

COMPREHENSIVE VISION REHABILITATION

Considering all of these aspects, it should be clear that comprehensive vision rehabilitation extends beyond the provision of low-vision aids, although that is still vitally important (see Chapter 24). Since any rehabilitation requires teamwork involving different professionals to deal with the various components and since vision loss is the common denominator, the ophthalmologist should coordinate the team.

▶ History and Goal Setting

Before considering a rehabilitation plan, the patient's goals and needs must be clarified. For the general ophthalmologist,

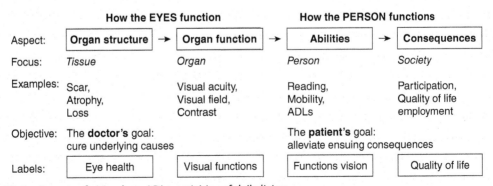

▲ **Figure 25–1.** Aspects of vision loss. ADLs, activities of daily living.

this may involve only a general question, such as, *"How does your vision loss bother you most?"* or *"Can you still read the newspaper?"* If the answer reveals a problem, clinicians should do the same as they do for retinal, glaucoma, or other problems and tell the patient, *"I understand your problem and I will refer you to someone who can help you."*

When future deterioration is a possibility, it is not necessary to wait until there is severe vision loss before recommending action. Early adaptations to minor loss can facilitate later adaptations to major loss. The possibility of deterioration of vision is best made known from the beginning but must be accompanied with advice about the availability of skilled professionals and resources. Unfortunately, many practitioners are poorly trained in conveying bad news, a skill that should be taught and practiced in medical school. All ophthalmologists should master this skill, which includes informing the patient about options and knowing the appropriate referral sources.

The American Academy of Ophthalmology (AAO) recognizes several levels of competence in vision rehabilitation. Some ophthalmology practices may employ professionals who can provide basic services in-house. For more complex cases, referral to specialized vision rehabilitation services is appropriate.

To determine the range of services that are appropriate, the AAO recommends the following checklist:

- **Reading**—For many patients, this is their foremost concern.
- **Activities of daily living (ADLs)**—Even though reading may be the most prominent complaint, most people spend the larger part of their day performing a variety of other activities.
- **Safety**—Are people at risk for falls? How do they cross the street?
- **Community participation**—Can they still participate in community events or at church?
- **Physical, cognitive, and psychosocial well-being**—Since many patients with vision loss are elderly, this is an important aspect that should not be overlooked. If problems exist, they may affect the recommendations to be made.

Not all areas may have problems, but the simple 5-point checklist is important so that priorities can be set and specific rehabilitation goals formulated that reflect the patient's needs and desires, not just the practitioner's expectations.

Examination

The standard ophthalmic examination, including identification of any conditions amenable to specific treatment, needs to be adapted as discussed in Chapter 24.

Observation of visual performance is important in young children, where regular testing may not be possible. Reports from parents and teachers are often as informative as direct observation in the office. Even for adults, observation of the

performance of daily living tasks can be helpful. It provides a baseline against which future progress can be measured. It can also give insight in the patient's problem-solving skills and motivation.

Questionnaires can assess the subjective difficulty of tasks, including those that cannot be assessed in the office. A disadvantage is that the responses are subjective, with some patients exaggerating their difficulties and others understating them.

Assessment of mobility, including identification of peripheral visual field loss, is very important since impaired mobility should trigger referral for assessment by an orientation and mobility (O+M) instructor. Mobility training may be crucial to reestablishing independence. Patients also need to be made aware of the importance of appropriate signaling of their visual impairment. Many feel that carrying a long cane or similar aid publicizes their vulnerability to individuals who might take advantage of it, but well-meaning individuals need to be made aware of the patient's visual impairment, so that they can provide assistance where needed.

Comprehensive Rehabilitation Plans

A comprehensive vision rehabilitation plan requires attention to more than just how the eyes function. Figure 25–2 provides a summary of the possible interventions. It is useful to use this as a checklist, although not all parts will be needed in every case.

Vision Enhancement (See Chapter 24)

- **Vision substitution** refers to the use of senses other than vision. Common examples include talking books and voice-output devices (see Chapter 24), Braille, and long canes. Vision enhancement and vision substitution are not mutually exclusive but complementary. A patient may use a magnifier to read price tags and talking books for recreational reading. A patient with retinitis pigmentosa, who has normal mobility in the daytime, may need a cane at night. Audio cassettes may have Braille labels.
- **Assistance** is a form of vision substitution using the eyes of others. Family members, caregivers, and office personnel should be familiar with sighted-guide techniques to effectively assist visually impaired patients with minimal embarrassment. Guide dogs are another possibility. They require training of the dog as well as of the patient, who needs to be physically active and able to manage the dog.
- **Coping skills:** Vision loss often causes reactive depression, which renders the patient less receptive to rehabilitative suggestions. Conversely successful rehabilitation can be therapeutic and motivate the patient to pursue further improvements. Dealing with severe depression may involve other professionals, but the authority of the ophthalmologist can play a major role in convincing patients that they can do far more than they may believe after the initial shock of vision loss.

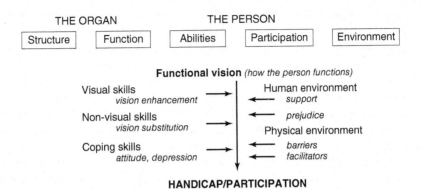

Figure 25–2. Comprehensive rehabilitation.

- **Human environment:** As patients go through the stages of adaptation to vision loss, a supportive home environment is essential, and it is important to include spouses, children, and significant others in the counseling process. The clinician should make sure that the significant others understand the underlying condition, what can be expected, and how to support the patient. Answering their questions directly, by having them attend the examination, is often better than leaving this to the patient, who initially may not have absorbed everything that was said. An overprotective environment that deprives patients of opportunities to do things themselves can be as detrimental as an overdemanding one that puts too much emphasis on the patient's shortcomings. The same applies to work, school, and social groups. Initially, patients often feel isolated and believe that they are the only ones experiencing these problems. This is where *peer support groups* can be helpful; in these groups, they can experience how others are dealing with similar problems.

- **Physical environment:** An uncluttered environment, where things have a defined, fixed place is helpful because it eliminates the need for searching. Good general illumination and task lighting often help, because at higher illumination levels retinal cells that are damaged but not dead can still contribute. Good contrast is important; for instance, milk should not be served in a white Styrofoam cup and edges of steps and stairs should be marked.

CONCLUSION

The patient's life does not end with the diagnosis of visual impairment. Similarly, the responsibility of the ophthalmologist does not end with the treatment of eye disease, but extends to counseling the patient and initiating rehabilitation, based on knowledge of the available resources and referral pathways.

RESOURCES

Searching business telephone directories (yellow pages) and the Internet under visual impairment, low vision, blindness, and rehabilitation can provide useful information on local rehabilitation resources.

General Information

The SmartSight initiative of the American Academy of Ophthalmology (www.AAO.org, search SmartSight) contains handouts for patients as well as for practitioners (including an extensive list of resources).

The American Foundation for the Blind (www.AFB.org/) contains many resources for various age groups and conditions.

The MDsupport website (www.MDsupport.org) specializes in support for age-related macular degeneration.

The Lighthouse International in New York (www.lighthouse.org) offers extensive resources for all forms of vision loss.

These websites contain links to many more websites with additional information and often can provide information about local resources.

Personnel

Occupational Therapists (OT) (www.aota.org). This profession evolved in the health care field. They have broad rehabilitation training, but traditionally learned little about vision. This is changing as the demand for vision rehabilitation grows.

Another group includes Certified Low Vision Therapists (CLVT), Certified Orientation and Mobility Specialists (COMS), and Certified Vision Rehabilitation Therapists (CVRT). These professions evolved from the education field. Their training is vision-specific, but traditionally focused on students and younger age groups. They are certified by the

Academy for Certification of Vision Rehabilitation & Education Professionals (www.acvrep.org).

For both groups, their state chapters may provide information about available manpower.

Devices, Technology

Low-tech devices, such as magnifiers and telescopes, are available from many suppliers, who have their own websites. They are relatively low cost and can serve a large number of patients. High-tech devices, such as video-magnifiers, cost more and evolve more rapidly. For these, it is important to get up-to-date information from a specialist (see Chapter 24).

The Library of Congress provides an extensive library of free talking books.

Financial Support, Social Services

Financial support and social service programs may vary from state to state. All states have vocational rehabilitation programs. Special services are available for veterans through the Veterans Affairs Blind Rehabilitation Centers. Local agencies are often the best source of information.

REFERENCE

Consultation on Development of Standards for Characterization of Vision Loss and Visual Functioning. WHO, Geneva, 2003. Available at http://apps.who.int/iris/bitstream/10665/68601/1/WHO_PBL_03.91.pdf.

APPENDIX
Functional Vision Score
August Colenbrander, MD

HISTORY

Vision loss is a complex phenomenon that cannot be fully understood unless many different aspects are considered (see Chapter 25). Yet, for certain applications, it may be desirable to reduce this complex reality to a single number. Administrators prefer the oversimplification of the single number approach when they have to decide on eligibility for benefits or for worker's compensation cases, where the outcome also is a single number: the amount of compensation.

Formulas to calculate what was then called "Visual Economics" were first proposed in Germany in the late 1800s. In 1925, Snell proposed to the American Medical Association (AMA) a simpler formula for "Visual Efficiency." This formula, reflecting an 80% loss of employability for a visual acuity loss to 20/200, served until 2000. In its fifth (2001) and sixth (2008) editions the AMA *Guides to the Evaluation of Permanent Impairment* adopted the "Functional Vision Score" (FVS), which reflects an estimate of the ability to perform activities of daily living (ADL).

On the new scale, 20/200 acuity is rated as an estimated 50% loss of ADL ability, rather than as an 80% loss of employability. Other changes include no longer considering the two eyes as separate organs, vision with both eyes open being the normal condition. The new scale has been shown to correlate well with other measures of ability.[1]

CALCULATING THE FUNCTIONAL VISION SCORE

Figure A–1 represents the steps in calculating the functional vision score and its use in calculating an AMA impairment rating.

Functional Acuity Score

The first step is measuring the visual acuity. Use of an ETDRS-type chart with a logarithmic progression of letter sizes and five letters on each line is preferred. The best corrected acuity is measured for each eye and with both eyes open.

According to the Weber-Fechner law, visual *ability* is proportional to the logarithm of the visual *acuity* value. This is reflected in the **visual acuity score (VAS)** (Table A–1). On an ETDRS-type chart, the VAS increases by 1 point for every letter read correctly; the scale is anchored at 20/20 = 100.

Next, the three VAS values—both eyes (OU), right eye (OD), left eye (OS)—are combined to provide a single **functional acuity score (FAS)**, with 60% weighting being given to the acuity with both eyes open and 20% to each of the monocular values.

Functional Field Score

In a similar way, a **visual field score (VFS)** and **functional field score (FFS)** are calculated. The VFS is determined with a grid (Figure A–2) that allocates 50 points to the central 10° (radius) area and 50 points to the remainder of the visual field reflecting the representation of the central 10° of visual field over about 50% of the primary visual cortex. It also divides the score evenly between the central area, which is important for reading and detailed vision, and the outer area, which is important for orientation and mobility.

The points are allocated along two meridians in each of the upper quadrants and three meridians in each of the lower quadrants. On each meridian, 5 points (2° apart) are assigned to the central area and 5 points (10° apart) to the outer area, with their distribution being approximately logarithmic. The lower visual field is weighted 50% more than the upper visual field because of its greater importance in functional vision. The primary meridians are not used, to avoid the need for special rules for hemianopias.

The VFS is determined by counting the number of points seen within the visual field delineated by the Goldmann III4e (or equivalent, eg, Humphrey 10 dB) isopter. The FFS is calculated from the three VFS values using the same weighted formula for calculating the FAS from the three VAS values (60% OU + 20% OD + 20% OS).

Finally, the FAS and FFS are combined into a single **functional vision score (FVS)**. Thus far, the calculation follows strict mathematical rules. If there are other vision

---

[1]Fuhr PSW et al. The AMA Guides Functional Vision Score is a better predictor of vision-targeted quality of life than traditional measures of visual acuity or visual field extent. *Vis Impairment Res* 2003;5:137.

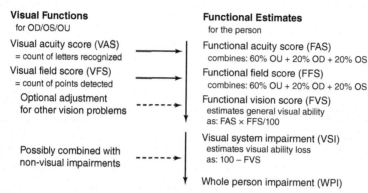

Visual Functions
for OD/OS/OU

Visual acuity score (VAS)
= count of letters recognized

Visual field score (VFS)
= count of points detected

Optional adjustment
for other vision problems

Possibly combined with
non-visual impairments

Functional Estimates
for the person

Functional acuity score (FAS)
combines: 60% OU + 20% OD + 20% OS

Functional field score (FFS)
combines: 60% OU + 20% OD + 20% OS

Functional vision score (FVS)
estimates general visual ability
as: FAS × FFS/100

Visual system impairment (VSI)
estimates visual ability loss
as: 100 − FVS

Whole person impairment (WPI)

Using the WPI calculation and other factors to determine monetary compensation is a separate,
administrative decision, beyond the scope of the AMA guides.

▲ **Figure A–1.** Steps in calculating the Functional Vision Score (FVS) and the AMA impairment ratings.

problems that are not reflected in a visual acuity or visual field loss, the examiner may apply an adjustment of maximally 15 points. Such an adjustment must be properly argued and documented.

CALCULATING THE AMA IMPAIRMENT RATING

The FVS reflects visual function (20/20 = 100), whereas the AMA impairment rating reflects loss (20/20 = no loss = 0). Therefore, the AMA impairment rating is calculated by subtracting the FVS from 100.

Table A–1. Visual Acuities (VA), ETDRS Letters (ETDRS), and Visual Acuity Scores (VAS)

VA	ETDRS	VAS	VA	ETDRS	VAS
20/10	100	115	20/200	35	50
20/12.5	95	110	20/250	30	45
20/16	90	105	20/320	25	40
20/20	85	100	20/400	20	35
20/25	80	95	20/500	15	30
20/32	75	90	20/640	10	25
20/40	70	85	20/800	5	20
20/50	65	80	20/1000	0	15
20/63	60	75	20/1250	0	10
20/80	55	70	20/1600	0	5
20/100	50	65	20/2000	0	0
20/125	45	60	CF < 2 ft	0	0
20/160	40	55	HM < 10 ft	0	0

Note that the VA column lists a geometric (logarithmic) sequence of visual *acuity* values, whereas the ETDRS letters column lists a linear sequence of visual *acuity* values. The VAS column provides the corresponding linear sequence of visual *ability* estimates.
Also note that the VAS scale is not capped at 20/20, although American Medical Association impairment ratings only reflect the loss relative to the 20/20 level. Similarly the ETDRS letters scale is referenced to 20/10 rather than 20/20, and thus, there is a constant difference between ETDRS letters and VAS. CF, counting fingers; HM, hand motion.

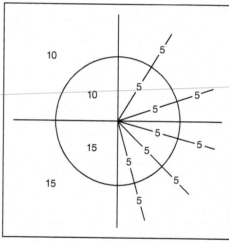

▲ **Figure A–2.** Visual field score grid, showing the total number of points in each region (left half) and how the points are allocated along the five meridians (right half). The radius of the circle is 10°.

Furthermore, a distinction is made between **visual system impairment (VSI)** and **whole person impairment (WPI)**. One hundred percent VSI (total blindness) does not equal 100% WPI (death). Therefore, a gradual correction is made from VSI = 50% to VSI = 100%, so that 100% VSI = 85% WPI. This adjustment is justified by the increasing use of visual substitution skills (see Chapter 25) at lower visual acuity levels.

If there are impairments in other organ systems, these may be combined (through special tables) with the visual WPI percentage.

For a more detailed discussion with examples, the reader is referred to the AMA publication: Rondinelli RD (ed). *Guides to the Evaluation of Permanent Impairment*, 6th edition. American Medical Association, 2008.

Glossary

Accommodation: The adjustment of the eye for seeing near objects, accomplished by increasing the power of the crystalline lens by changing its shape through the action of the ciliary muscle.

Acquired: Contracted after birth.

Agnosia: Inability to recognize common objects despite an intact visual apparatus.

Albinism: A hereditary deficiency of melanin pigment in the retinal pigment epithelium, iris, and choroid.

Alternate cover test: Determination of the full extent of strabismus (heterotropia and heterophoria) by alternately covering one eye and then the other with an opaque object, thus eliminating fusion.

Amaurosis fugax: Transient loss of vision. Usually reserved for transient loss of vision due to retinal embolus.

Amblyopia: Reduced visual acuity in the absence of sufficient eye or visual pathway disease to explain the level of vision.

Ametropia: See Refractive error.

Amsler grid: A grid of vertical and horizontal lines to test the central 20° square of visual field.

Angiography: Imaging of the vascular system. The ocular circulation can be highlighted by intravenous injection of either fluorescein, which particularly demonstrates the retinal circulation, or indocyanine green, to demonstrate the choroidal circulation.

Aniridia: Congenital absence of the iris.

Aniseikonia: Image seen by one eye differs in size from that seen by the other.

Anisocoria: Unequal pupillary size.

Anisometropia: Difference in refractive power of the two eyes.

Anophthalmos: Absence of the globe.

Anterior chamber: Space bounded anteriorly by the cornea and posteriorly by the iris that is filled with aqueous.

Aphakia: Absence of the crystalline lens.

Aqueous: Clear, watery fluid that fills the anterior and posterior chambers.

Asthenopia: Eye fatigue from muscular, environmental, or psychological causes.

Astigmatism: Different power of refraction in various meridians.

Axis: The meridian specifying the orientation of a cylindrical lens.

Binocular vision: Ability of both eyes to focus on an object and fuse the two images into one.

Biomicroscope: See Slitlamp.

Blepharitis: Inflammation of the lids.

Blepharoptosis (ptosis): Drooping of the upper lid.

Blepharospasm: Involuntary spasm of the lids.

Blind spot: "Blank" area in the visual field corresponding to the position of the optic nerve.

Blindness: In the United States, the usual definition of blindness is corrected visual acuity of 20/200 or less in the better eye, or a visual field of no more than 20° diameter in the better eye.

Botulinum toxin: Neurotoxin A of the bacterium *Clostridium botulinum* injected into extraocular or facial muscles to produce temporary paralysis.

Buphthalmos: Enlarged globe in infantile glaucoma.

Canal of Schlemm: A circular modified venous structure in the anterior chamber angle that drains aqueous to the aqueous veins.

Canaliculus: Small tear drainage tube in inner aspect of upper and lower lids leading from the punctum to the common canaliculus and then to the tear sac.

Canthotomy: Usually implies lateral canthotomy—cutting of the lateral canthal tendon for the purpose of widening the palpebral aperture.

Canthus: The outer (lateral) or inner (medial) angle at either end of the lid aperture.

Cataract: Opacity of the crystalline lens.

Chalazion: Granulomatous inflammation of a meibomian gland.

Chemosis: Conjunctival edema.

Choroid: The vascular middle coat between the retina and sclera.

Ciliary body: Portion of the uveal tract between the iris and the choroid. It consists of ciliary processes and the ciliary muscle.

Coloboma: Congenital cleft due to incomplete development of some portion of the eye or ocular adnexa.

Color blindness (deficiency): Diminished ability to perceive differences in color.

Concave lens: Lens having the power to diverge rays of light; also known as diverging, reducing, negative, or minus lens; denoted by the sign (–); and used to correct myopia.

Cones and rods: Two kinds of retinal photoreceptor cells. Cones are primarily involved in fine visual discrimination (optimal visual acuity) and color vision; rods in peripheral vision and vision in decreased illumination.

Congenital: Existing at or before birth but not necessarily inherited (hereditary).

Conjunctiva: Mucous membrane that lines the posterior aspect of the lids and covers the anterior sclera.

Contact lenses: Lenses that fit directly on the globe, usually on the cornea but sometimes on the sclera.

Convergence: The process of inward rotation of both eyes to direct their visual axes to a near point.

Convex lens: Lens having power to converge rays of light and to bring them to a focus; also known as converging, magnifying, or plus lens; denoted by the sign (+); and used to correct hyperopia and presbyopia.

Cornea: Transparent portion of the outer coat of the globe forming the anterior wall of the anterior chamber.

Corneal graft (keratoplasty): Replacement of a portion of the cornea, either involving the full thickness (penetrating keratoplasty), only a superficial layer (lamellar keratoplasty), or only the endothelium (endothelial keratoplasty), with donor cornea from the same human (autograft), or another human (homograft).

Cover test: Determination of the presence and degree of manifest strabismus (heterotropia) by covering one eye with an opaque object and examining for any movement of the uncovered eye to fixate a target.

Cross cylinder: A specialized spherocylindrical lens to measure astigmatism.

Crystalline lens: Transparent biconvex structure suspended behind the iris between the aqueous and the vitreous. Its function is to focus the visual image on the retina. Accommodation is achieved by changing its shape to increase its power. (Usually called simply the lens.)

Cyclodestructive procedures: Destruction of portions of the ciliary body to reduce aqueous production in the treatment of intractable glaucoma, using cryotherapy (cyclocryotherapy), laser (cyclophotocoagulation), or diathermy.

Cycloplegic: Drug that relaxes the ciliary muscle, paralyzing accommodation.

Cylindrical lens: Segment of a cylinder, the refractive power of which varies in different meridians, used to correct astigmatism.

Dacryocystitis: Infection of the lacrimal sac.

Dacryocystorhinostomy: Formation of an opening between the nasolacrimal duct and the nasal cavity to relieve an obstruction in the nasolacrimal duct, or sac.

Dark adaptation: The ability to adjust vision to decreased illumination.

Diopter: Unit of measurement of refractive power of lenses.

Diplopia (double vision): Seeing one object as two. It is usually binocular, being overcome by covering one eye, due to misalignment of the eyes. Monocular diplopia is usually due to focusing abnormality.

"E" test: A system of testing visual acuity in illiterates, particularly preschool children.

Ectropion: Turning out of the lid.

Emmetropia: Absence of refractive error.

Endolaser: Application of laser from a probe inserted into the globe.

Endophthalmitis: Extensive intraocular infection.

Enophthalmos: Abnormal retrodisplacement of the eyeball.

Entropion: Turning inward of the lid.

Enucleation: Complete removal of the globe.

Epicanthus: Congenital skin fold that overlies the inner canthus.

Epi-LASIK: Corneal excimer laser ablation under an epithelial flap created by a mechanical keratome to treat refractive error.

Epiphora: Excessive tearing.

Esophoria: Tendency of the eyes to converge (latent convergent strabismus).

Esotropia: Manifest inward deviation of one eye (manifest convergent strabismus).

Evisceration: Removal of the contents of the globe.

Exenteration: Removal of the contents of the orbit, including the globe and part or all of the lids.

Exophoria: Tendency of the eyes to diverge.

Exophthalmos: Abnormal protrusion of the globe.

Exotropia: Manifest outward deviation of one eye.

Familial: Pertaining to traits, either hereditary or acquired, occurring in families.

Far point: The point at which the eye is focused when accommodation is completely relaxed.

Farsightedness: See Hyperopia.

Field of vision: The entire area that can be seen without shifting gaze.

Floaters: Moving images in the visual field due to vitreous opacities.

Focus: A point to which rays of light are brought together to form an image; focal distance is the distance between a lens and its focal point.

Fornix: Junction of the palpebral and bulbar conjunctiva.

Fovea: 1.5-mm-diameter zone of the central retina, characterized histologically by thinning of the outer nuclear layer.

Foveola: 0.3-mm-diameter thinnest (0.25 mm) area of the central retina, clinically apparent as a depression, in which there are only cone photoreceptors and which provides optimal visual acuity. It corresponds to the retinal avascular zone on fluorescein angiography.

Fundus: The posterior portion of the eye visible through the pupil.

Fusion: Combining the images received by the two eyes into one image.

Glaucoma: Disease characterized by optic disk cupping and reduction of visual field, usually associated with raised intraocular pressure.

Gonioscopy: Examination of the anterior chamber angle that requires a special corneal contact lens.

Hemianopia: Reduction of one side of the field of vision of one or both eyes.

Heterophoria (phoria): See Strabismus.

Heterotropia (tropia): See Strabismus.

Hippus: Exaggerated spontaneous rhythmic movements of the iris.

Hordeolum, external (sty): Infection of gland of Moll or Zeis.

Hordeolum, internal: Infection of meibomian gland.

Hyperopia, hypermetropia (farsightedness): Refractive error in which light rays from a distant object are focused behind the retina.

Hyperphoria: Latent vertical strabismus.

Hypertropia: Manifest vertical strabismus.

Hyphema: Blood in the anterior chamber.

Hypopyon: Pus in the anterior chamber.

Hypotony: Abnormally low intraocular pressure (5 mm Hg or less).

Inherited (hereditary): Transmitted from parents to offspring.

Injection: Congestion of blood vessels.

Iridectomy: Excision of a sector of iris to form a direct communication between the anterior and posterior chambers.

Iridoplasty, peripheral (laser) iridoplasty: Procedure to contract the iris stroma by application of usually argon laser burns to the peripheral iris.

Iridotomy, peripheral (laser): Formation of a hole in the iris to form a direct communication between the anterior and posterior chambers, usually performed with the neodymium:YAG laser.

Iris: Colored, annular membrane, suspended behind the cornea and immediately in front of the lens.

Ishihara color plates: Test for color vision using pseudoisochromatic multicolored charts.

Isopter: Boundary of the visual field to a particular target. Isopters to targets of different colors and sizes allow differentiation of relative from absolute visual field defects.

Jaeger test: Near vision test using various sizes of type.

Keratic precipitate (KP): Accumulation of inflammatory cells on the posterior cornea in uveitis.

Keratitis: Inflammation of the cornea.

Keratoconus: Cone-shaped deformity of the cornea.

Keratomalacia: Corneal softening, usually due to vitamin A deficiency.

Keratometer: Instrument to measure the curvature of the cornea, used to diagnose and monitor corneal disease, fit contact lenses, and determine intraocular lens power prior to cataract surgery.

Keratopathy, bullous: Edema of the cornea with painful epithelial blisters (bullae).

Keratoplasty: See Corneal graft.

Keratoprosthesis: Implant surgically placed in an opaque cornea to achieve optical clarity.

Kerato-refractive surgery (refractive keratoplasty): Corneal surgery to correct refractive error.

Keratotomy: Incision in the cornea. In arcuate keratotomy, circumferential incisions are made to correct astigmatism.

Koeppe nodule: Accumulation of inflammatory cells on the iris in uveitis.

Lacrimal sac: Dilated area at the junction of the nasolacrimal duct and canaliculi.

Laser epithelial keratomileusis (LASEK): Corneal excimer laser ablation under an epithelial flap to treat refractive error.

Laser in situ keratomileusis (LASIK): Corneal excimer laser ablation under a stromal flap to treat refractive error.

Lens: A refractive medium having one or both surfaces curved. (See also Crystalline lens.)

Lensometer: Instrument for measuring the power of optical lenses.

Limbus: Junction of the cornea and sclera.

Macula: 5.5- to 6-mm-diameter area of central retina bounded by the temporal retinal vascular arcades. It is known to anatomists as the area centralis, to differentiate it from the macula lutea, and is defined as the part of the retina in which the ganglion cell layer is more than one cell thick.

Macula lutea: 3-mm-diameter area of the central retina defined anatomically by the presence of yellow xanthophyll pigment.

Maddox rod: Lens composed of parallel strong cylinders through which a point of light is seen as a line—used to quantify heterophoria.

Magnification: Ratio of the size of an image to the size of its object.

Megalocornea: Abnormally large cornea (> 13 mm diameter).

Metamorphopsia: Wavy distortion of vision.

Microphthalmos: Abnormally small globe with abnormal function (see Nanophthalmos).

Miotic: Drug causing pupillary constriction.

Mydriatic: Drug causing pupillary dilation.

Myopia (nearsightedness): Refractive error in which light rays from a distant object are focused anterior to the retina.

Nanophthalmos: Abnormally small globe with normal function (see Microphthalmos).

Near point: The point at which the eye is focused when accommodation is fully active.

Nearsightedness: See Myopia.

Nystagmus: Involuntary rhythmic oscillation of the globe that may be horizontal, vertical, torsional, or mixed.

Ophthalmia neonatorum: Conjunctivitis in the newborn.

Ophthalmoscope: Instrument with special illumination system for viewing the inner eye, particularly the retina and associated structures.

Optic atrophy: Optic nerve degeneration, manifesting clinically as pallor of the optic disk.

Optic disk: Ophthalmoscopically visible portion of the optic nerve.

Optic nerve: The nerve that carries visual impulses from the retina to the brain.

Orbital cellulitis: Inflammation of the orbital tissues surrounding the globe.

Orthoptics: Study and treatment of defects of binocular visual function or of the muscles controlling movement of the eyes.

Oscillopsia: Subjective illusion of movement of objects caused by ocular instability such as nystagmus.

Palpebral: Pertaining to the lid.

Pannus: Infiltration of the cornea with blood vessels.

Panophthalmitis: Inflammation of the globe and orbital tissues.

Papilledema: Swelling of the optic disk due to raised intracranial pressure.

Papillitis: Inflammatory swelling of the optic nerve head.

Partially seeing child: For educational purposes, a partially seeing child is one who has a corrected visual acuity of 20/70 or less in the better eye.

Perimeter: Instrument for quantifying the field of vision.

Peripheral vision: Ability to perceive the presence and movement of objects outside the direct line of vision.

Phacoemulsification and phacofragmentation: Techniques of extracapsular cataract surgery in which the nucleus of the lens is disrupted into small fragments by ultrasound, thus allowing its aspiration through a small wound.

Phakomatoses: Group of hereditary diseases characterized by the presence of spots, cysts, and tumors in various parts of the body—for example, neurofibromatosis, Von Hippel-Lindau disease, and tuberous sclerosis.

Phlyctenule: Localized lymphocytic infiltration of the conjunctiva.

Phoria: See Strabismus.

Photochemical damage: Tissue damage due to creation of oxygen free radicals by excessive exposure to visible or near ultraviolet light that can be used for corneal disease (crosslinking) or retinal disease (photodynamic therapy).

Photodecomposition: Tissue damage by direct separation of chemical bonds by absorption of very-short-wavelength ultraviolet light (eg, from excimer lasers).

Photodynamic therapy (PDT): Retinal laser augmented by intravenous injection of a dye (verteporfin).

Photomechanical damage (photodisruption/plasma-mediated ablation): Tissue damage produced by the breakdown of "plasma," which is a state of ionization created by spot focusing a high-energy laser source (eg, neodymium:YAG).

Photophobia: Abnormal sensitivity to light.

Photopsia: Visual sparks or flashes due to abnormal retinal stimulation.

Photorefractive keratectomy (PRK): Surface corneal excimer laser ablation to treat refractive error.

Phototherapeutic keratectomy (PTK): Surface corneal excimer ablation to treat anterior corneal disorders such as recurrent corneal erosion.

Photothermal damage: Thermal damage to tissues due to absorption of high levels of light (including laser) energy, resulting in small rise (10–20°C) in temperature (photocoagulation) or large rise in temperature (reaching 100°C) (photovaporization).

Phthisis bulbi: Atrophy of the globe with blindness and decreased intraocular pressure, due to end-stage intraocular disease.

Placido disk: Disk with concentric rings used to determine the regularity of the cornea by observing the ring's reflection on the corneal surface.

Poliosis: Depigmentation of the eyelashes.

Posterior chamber: Space filled with aqueous anterior to the lens and posterior to the iris.

Presbyopia ("old sight"): Physiologically blurred near vision, commonly evident soon after age 40, due to reduction of power of accommodation.

Prism: Wedge of transparent material that deviates light rays without changing their focus.

Prism cover test: Extension of the alternate cover test using different strength prisms to quantify the total magnitude of strabismus.

Prism diopter: Unit of prism power.

Pseudoisochromatic charts: Charts with colored dots of various hues and shades forming numbers, letters, or patterns, used for testing color discrimination (see Ishihara color plates).

Pseudophakia: Presence of artificial intraocular lens implant following cataract extraction.

Pterygium: Triangular growth of tissue that extends from the conjunctiva over the cornea.

Ptosis: Drooping of the upper lid.

Puncta: External orifices of the upper and lower canaliculi.

Pupil: Round hole in the center of the iris that corresponds to the aperture of a camera.

Refraction: (1) Deviation in the course of rays of light in passing from one transparent medium into another of different density. (2) Determination of refractive error of the eye and its correction by lenses.

Refractive error (ametropia): Optical defect that prevents light rays from being brought to a single focus on the retina.

Refractive index: Ratio of the speed of light in a vacuum to the speed of light in a given material.

Refractive media: The transparent parts of the eye having refractive power, of which the cornea is most powerful but the (crystalline) lens is under voluntary control (see Accommodation).

Retina: Innermost coat of the eye, consisting of the sensory retina, which is composed of light-sensitive neural elements connecting to other neural cells, and the retinal pigment epithelium.

Retinal detachment: Separation of the neurosensory retina from the retinal pigment epithelium and choroid.

Retinitis pigmentosa: Hereditary degeneration of the retina.

Retinoscope: Instrument for objective determination of refractive error.

Rods: See Cones and rods.

Sclera: The white part of the eye—a tough covering that, with the cornea, forms the external protective coat of the eye.

Scleral spur: Normal protrusion of sclera into the anterior chamber angle.

Scotoma: Blind or partially blind area of the visual field.

Slitlamp biomicroscope: A combination light and microscope for examination of the eye, particularly allowing stereoscopic imaging.

Small incision lenticule extraction (SMILE): Excision of a portion of corneal stroma with a femtosecond laser to treat refractive error.

Snellen chart: Test of visual acuity consisting of lines of letters or numbers, graded in size according to the distance at which they can be discriminated by a normal eye.

Sphincterotomy: Incision of the iris sphincter muscle.

Staphyloma: Thinned part of the wall of the globe, resulting in protrusion of intraocular structures.

Strabismus: Misalignment of the eyes (ocular deviation) that may be present under binocular viewing conditions (manifest strabismus, manifest ocular deviation, heterotropia) or only when binocular vision has been interrupted by occlusion of one eye (latent strabismus, latent ocular deviation, heterophoria).

Sty: See Hordeolum, external.

Symblepharon: Adhesions between bulbar and palpebral conjunctiva.

Sympathetic ophthalmia: Intraocular inflammation (uveitis) in both eyes following trauma.

Synechia: Adhesion of the iris to the cornea (anterior synechia) or lens (posterior synechia).

Syneresis: Degenerative process within a gel; specifically applied to the vitreous.

Tarsorrhaphy: Surgical procedure to join the upper and lower lid margins such as to protect the cornea.

Tonometer: Instrument to measure intraocular pressure.

Trabeculectomy: Surgical procedure to create an additional aqueous drainage channel in the treatment of glaucoma.

Trabeculoplasty: Laser photocoagulation of the trabecular meshwork in the treatment of open-angle glaucoma.

Transpupillary thermotherapy: Diffuse treatment of fundal lesions with low-energy diode laser.

Trichiasis: Rubbing of the eyelashes against the globe.

Tropia: See Strabismus.

Uncover test: Extension of the cover test to determine the presence of heterophoria by detection of corrective movement of the covered eye as it is uncovered.

Uvea (uveal tract): Iris, ciliary body, and choroid.

Uveitis: Inflammation of one or all portions of the uveal tract.

Visual acuity: Measure of the spatial resolution of the eye.

Visual axis: Imaginary line connecting a point in space (point of fixation) with the foveola.

Vitiligo: Localized patchy decrease or absence of skin pigment.

Vitrectomy: Surgical removal of the vitreous to clear vitreous hemorrhage, allow treatment of retinal detachment or retinal vascular disease, or treat intraocular infection or inflammation.

Vitreous: Transparent, colorless, gel filling the globe behind the crystalline lens.

Xerosis: Drying of tissues of surface of the globe.

Zonule: One of numerous fibrils that arise from the surface of the ciliary body and insert into the equator of the crystalline lens to hold the crystalline lens in place.

INDEX

NOTE: Page numbers followed by *f* and *t* denote figures and tables, respectively.